ASSESSMENT AND PREDICTION OF SUICIDE

ASSESSMENT AND PREDICTION OF SUICIDE

Edited by

Ronald W. Maris, Ph.D.
CENTER FOR THE STUDY OF SUICIDE
UNIVERSITY OF SOUTH CAROLINA

Alan L. Berman, Ph.D.
WASHINGTON PSYCHOLOGICAL CENTER
NATIONAL CENTER FOR THE STUDY AND PREVENTION OF SUICIDE

John T. Maltsberger, M.D.
HARVARD MEDICAL SCHOOL
McLEAN HOSPITAL
BOSTON PSYCHOANALYTIC SOCIETY AND INSTITUTE

Robert I. Yufit, Ph.D.
SUICIDE ASSESSMENT PROGRAM
NORTHWESTERN UNIVERSITY MEDICAL SCHOOL

*An Official Publication
of the American Association of Suicidology*

THE GUILFORD PRESS
New York   London

© 1992 The Guilford Press
A Division of Guilford Publications, Inc.
72 Spring Street, New York, NY 10012

Printed in the United States of America

This book is printed on acid-free paper.

Last digit is print number: 9 8 7 6 5 4 3 2 1

Library of Congress Cataloging-in-Publication Data

Assessment and prediction of suicide / edited by Ronald W. Maris . . .
[et al.].
    p. cm.
    "An official publication of the American Association of
Suicidology."
    Includes bibliographical references and indexes.
    ISBN 0-89862-791-5
    1. Suicide—Risk factors. 2. Suicide—Prevention.   I. Maris,
Ronald, W.   II. American Association of Suicidology.
    [DNLM: 1. Suicide—prevention & control.   HV 6545 A846]
RC569.A77 1992
616.85′8445075—dc20
DNLM/DLC
for Library of Congress   91-35408
                                                                    CIP

Contributors

Angela M. Adan is a Ph.D. candidate of Psychology at the University of Illinois at Urbana/Champaign.

Cheryl L. Addy, Ph.D., is Assistant Professor of Biostatistics at the University of South Carolina, Columbia, and Statistical Editor of *Suicide and Life-Threatening Behavior*. She is doing biostatistical research and categorical data analysis in a longitudinal study of adolescent depression and suicidality. She coauthored, with Carol Z. Garrison, "A Longitudinal Study of Suicide Ideation in Young Adolescents" in *The Journal of the American Academy of Child and Adolescent Psychiatry*.

Aaron T. Beck, M.D., is Professor of Psychiatry at the University of Pennsylvania, Philadelphia. He has been elected Fellow of the Royal College of Psychiatrists and has received an honorary doctor of medical science degree from Brown University. His current work in progress is a longitudinal (prospective) study of prediction of suicide, cognitive therapy of panic, drug abuse, and depression. His most recent publication is *Cognitive Therapy of Personality Disorders*.

Alan L. Berman, Ph.D., is in private practice at the Washington Psychological Center, Washington, D.C., Director of the National Center for the Study and Prevention of Suicide at the Washington School of Psychiatry, Washington, D.C. and Case Consultation Editor of *Suicide and Life-Threatening Behavior*. The bulk of his research focuses on suicidal multiple sclerosis patients. He coauthored *Adolescent Suicide: Assessment and Intervention* with D. A. Jones.

Bruce Bongar, Ph.D., is Associate Professor in the Clinical Psychology Program at the Pacific Graduate School of Psychology, Palo Alto, Calif.; Adjunct Associate Professor of Psychiatry at the University of Massachusetts Medical School, Worcester; Chair of the American Association of Suicidology Training Committee; and Consulting Editor of *Suicide and Life-Threatening Behavior*. He has conducted extensive research on the chronically suicidal patient and is an authority on suicide, malpractice, and standards of care. He most recently authored *The Suicidal Patient: Clinical and Legal Standards of Care* and edited *The Assessment and Management of Suicide in Clinical Practice.*

Ronald L. Bonner, Psy.D., is Chief Psychologist at the Federal Correctional Institution at Shuylkill, Minersville, Penn.; is in private practice in Harrisburg and Selinsgrove, Penn.; and is Consulting Editor for *Suicide and Life-Threatening Behavior.* His research interests include clinical models of depression and suicidal behavior, and his most recent publication is "Suicide Prevention in Correctional Facilities," in *Innovations in Clinical Practice.*

Gerald L. Brown, M.D., is Clinical Section Chief of the Laboratory of Clinical Studies, Division of Intramural Clinical and Biological Research, at the National Institute of Alcohol Abuse and Alcoholism, Bethesda, Md. His current research is on aggressive suicidal behavior and its relationship to behavior disturbance and alcohol abuse. He is the coauthor of the paper *Probability and Pedigree Studies Review a Lack of Association between the Botanine and D_2 Receptor and Genan Alcoholism.*

David C. Clark, Ph.D., is Associate Professor of Psychiatry and Psychology at Rush Medical College; Director of the Center for Suicide Research at Rush-Presbyterian-St. Luke's Medical Center, Chicago, Ill; and Associate Editor of *Suicide and Life-Threatening Behavior.* He is currently comparing community-based samples of adolescents who died by suicide and by car accident, and is studying a community-based sample of older adults who died by suicide. His most recent publication is on the relationship between physically reckless behavior and suicidal tendencies in adolescents.

Denys de Catanzaro, Ph.D., is Associate Professor of Psychology at McMaster University, Hamilton, Ontario, Can., and Consulting Editor of *Suicide and Life-Threatening Behavior.* He also holds a University Research Fellowship from the Natural Sciences and Engineering Research Council of Canada. His most recent publication, "Evolutionary Limits to Self-Preservation" in *Ethology and Sociobiology,* modifies the theory of senescence to account for the evolution of conditional self-destructive genetic expression. He is also researching hormonal mediation of psychogenic pregnancy blocks and other reproductive failures in laboratory animals.

James R. Eyman, Ph.D., is a staff psychologist and Director of the Suicide Research Project of The Menninger Clinic, Topeka, Kans. He is also a faculty member in the Department of Psychology at the Karl Menninger School of Psychiatry and Mental Health Sciences, Topeka, Kans. His current research in progress centers on the assessment of suicide potential and the subsequent treatment of suicidal individuals. His latest publication is "Countertransference When Counseling Suicidal School-Aged Youth" in *Suicide Prevention in Schools.*

Susanne Kohn Eyman, Ph.D., is in private practice at Mental Health Associates, Manhattan, Kan. Her current research involves the assessment of suicide potential. She coauthored, with James R. Eyman, "Suicide Risk and Assessment Instruments" in *Issues, Assessment and Intervention* (P. Cimbolic and D. Jobes, eds.).

Robert D. Felner, Ph.D., is Director of the Center for Prevention, Research and Development, and Professor of Public Policy, Psychology, Education, and Social Welfare at the University of Illinois at Urbana/Champaign; and is Consulting Editor of *Suicide and Life-Threatening Behavior.*

Prudence Fisher, M.S., is with the New York State Psychiatric Institute, New York.

Carol Z. Garrison, Ph.D., is Associate Professor and Chair of Epidemiology at the University of South Carolina, Columbia, and Consulting Editor of *Suicide and Life-Threatening Behavior.* She is the principal investigator of an epidemiologic study of depression and suicidal behaviors in young adolescents and the coinvestigator of a study of interventions to reduce posttraumatic stress in adolescents. She is coauthor with Cheryl L. Addy of "A Longitudinal Study of Depressive Symptomatology in Young Adolescents" in the *Journal of the American Academy of Child and Adolescent Psychiatry.*

Carol Geer-Williams, Ph.D., is a Clinical Psychologist with the Psychology Service of the National Rehabilitation Hospital, Washington, D.C. She is currently studying the management of difficult patients in medical facilities. Her most recent publication is "Union Personality Types as a Predictor of Attendance at the Black College Day March" in *Psychological Reports.*

Fredrick K. Goodwin, M.D., is Chief Administrator for the Alcohol, Drug Abuse, and Mental Health Administration, Rockville, Md. His research has focused on manic-depressive illness, aggression, and suicide. He recently published *Manic-Depressive Illness* and "Comorbidity of Mental Disorders with Alcohol and Other Drug Abuse . . ." in the *Journal of the American Medical Association.*

Madelyn S. Gould, Ph.D., M.P.H., is Associate Professor of Psychiatry and of Public Health at the College of Physicians and Surgeons of Columbia University, New York, N.Y., and is a Research Scientist at the New York

State Psychiatric Institute, New York. Her current work in progress includes the identification of risk factors for teenage suicide, as well as a number of studies examining the role of suicide contagion among adolescents. She is a coauthor of "Time-Space Clustering of Teenage Suicide" in the *American Journal of Epidemiology*.

Sara L. Horton-Deutsch, M.S., R.N., is a Research Associate at the Center for Suicide Research at Rush-Presbyterian-St. Luke's Medical Center, Chicago, Ill., and is a Ph.D. candidate in the Department of Psychiatric Nursing there. She has collaborated with David C. Clark in a study on psychological autopsies of elderly suicides and a study of the relationship between respiratory distress and suicidal acts among the elderly.

Marjorie Kleinman, M.S., is with the New York State Psychiatric Institute, New York.

Antoon A. Leenaars, Ph.D., C.Psych., is in private practice in Windsor, Ontario, Can.; is President of the Canadian Association for Suicide Prevention; and is Special Issue Editor of *Suicide and Life-Threatening Behavior*. His current work in progress focuses on suicide and the older adult. He is Editor of *Life Span Perspectives of Suicide*.

David Lester, Ph.D., is Professor of Psychology at Stockton State College, Pomona, N.J.; is at the Center for the Study of Suicide, Blackwood, N.J.; and is Consulting Editor of *Suicide and Life-Threatening Behavior*. His research in progress is an exploration of predictors of suicide in Terman's sample of gifted children. His book *Understanding and Preventing Suicide* explores the application of criminological theory to suicide in order to generate new theories and new approaches for preventing suicide.

Katherine Lesyna, M.A., is a graduate student of Sociology at the University of California at San Diego. She is interested in studying deviant behavior, the sociology of gender, and mass media.

Markku I. Linnoila, M.D., Ph.D., is a Research Scientist at the Laboratory of Clinical Studies, Division of Intramural and Biological Research, National Institute on Alcohol Abuse and Alcoholism, Bethesda, Md.

Robert E. Litman, M.D., is Clinical Professor of Psychiatry at the University of California at Los Angeles; Attending Psychiatrist at Cedars-Sinai Hospital, Los Angeles; and Consulting Editor of *Suicide and Life-Threatening Behavior*. He is working on a book reviewing his 30 years of experience in suicidology, and his most recent publication is "Long-Term Treatment of Chronically Suicidal Patients" in *Bulletin of the Menninger Clinic*.

John T. Maltsberger, M.D., is Associate Psychiatrist at Harvard Medical School; Senior Consultant in the Psychosocial Program at McLean Hospital, Belmont, Mass.; a member of the Boston Psychoanalytic Society and Institute; and Consulting Editor of *Suicide and Life-Threatening Behavior.* His current work in progress is an examination of disturbances of the body image in relation to suicide. His is the author of the book *Suicide Risk: The Formulation of Clinical Judgment.*

Ronald W. Maris, Ph.D., is the Director of the Center for the Study of Suicide and Professor of Preventive Medicine at the University of South Carolina, Columbia. His current research centers on suicide in midlife and forensic investigation of death. He is Editor-in-Chief of *Suicide and Life-Threatening Behavior.* His most recent publications are "Suicide" in the *Encyclopedia of Human Biology* and "Forensic Suicidology" in *The Assessment and Management of Suicide in Clinical Practice* (Bruce Bongar, ed.).

David J. Mayo, Ph.D., is Professor of Philosophy at the University of Minnesota, Duluth, and Consulting Editor of *Suicide and Life-Threatening Behavior.* His recent work is in medical and other areas of applied ethics. His most recent major publication was *AIDS, Testing and Privacy,* coauthored by M. Gunderson and F. Rhame. His work in progress includes an examination of ethical dilemmas associated with the testing of an HIV vaccine; an analysis of the role of slippery-slope arguments in public policy debates on subjects such as euthanasia; and the ethics of "outing."

John L. McIntosh, Ph.D., is Associate Professor of Psychology at Indiana University at South Bend, and Consulting Editor of *Suicide and Life-Threatening Behavior.* His current work centers on survivors of elderly and young suicides and the reactions of and attitudes toward survivors of suicide. His most recent publication is "Trends in Racial Differences in U.S. Suicide Statistics" in *Death Studies.*

Alyssa Morishima, M.S., is with the New York State Psychiatric Institute, New York.

Jerome A. Motto, M.D., is Professor of Psychiatry at the University of California at San Francisco, School of Medicine, and Consulting Editor of *Suicide and Life-Threatening Behavior.* His work in progress is an analysis of data to clarify the role of time in the estimation of suicide risk. His most recent publication is "Empirical Indicators of Near-Term Suicide Risk" in *Crisis,* coauthored with A. Bostrom.

Daniel Paight, M.A., is a graduate student of Sociology at the University of California at San Diego. He is interested in studying deviant behavior, mass media, the sociology of science, and the sociology of culture.

David P. Phillips, Ph.D., is Professor of Sociology at the University of California at San Diego. His current research is an examination of the misclassification of cause of death and age—factors affecting the difference in life expectancy of males and females, and the diffusion of scientific information. His most recent publication is "Postponement of Death Until Symbolically Meaningful Occasion" in the *Journal of the American Medical Association.*

Alex D. Pokorny, M.D., is Emeritus Professor of Psychiatry at Baylor College of Medicine, Houston, Texas. Although he is retired, he participates in the Psychiatry Residency Program at Baylor College of Medicine; is a consultant to the drug abuse treatment program at the Houston Veterans Administration Medical Center; and has conducted numerous research projects. His most recent publication is "Can Death Be Postponed? The Death-Dip Phenomenon in Psychiatric Patients" in *Omega,* coauthored by T. Greiner.

Joseph M. Rothberg, Ph.D., is Research Mathematician with the Department of Military Psychiatry, Walter Reed Army Institute of Research, Washington, D.C., and Adjunct Associate Professor in the Department of Psychiatry of the F. Edward Hébert School of Medicine, Uniformed Services University of the Health Sciences, Bethesda, Md. He is currently studying health in the Army. His most recent publication is "Life and Death in the U.S. Army" in the *Journal of the American Medical Association.*

Alex Roy, M.D., is Director of the Affective Disorders Program at Hillside Hospital, Glen Oaks, N.Y. He is currently working on the set up of a suicide research center. His most recent publication is "Suicide in Twins" in *Archives General Psychiatry.*

David Shaffer, M.D., F.R.C.Psych., is Professor of Psychiatry at Columbia University, New York, N.Y. and at the New York State Psychiatric Institute, New York. He has made a major contribution to research on adolescent suicide, especially in the area of suicide prevention in schools. His most recent publication is in the *Journal of the American Medical Association.*

Robert E. Sherman, Ph.D., is with the Hennepin County Office of Planning and Development, Minneapolis, Minn. He is a coauthor of "Use of Case Vignettes in Suicide Risk Assessment" in *Suicide and Life-Threatening Behavior.*

Edwin S. Shneidman, Ph.D., is Professor of Thanatology Emeritus at the University of California at Los Angeles, and Editor Emeritus of *Suicide and Life-Threatening Behavior.* He is currently working on a long-term project with Gordon Strauss, M.D., of U.C.L.A. on selected men from the Terman Study, who Shneidman intensively studied as septuagenarians in the 1980s.

His most recent publication is "A Life in Death" in *The History of Clinical Psychology in Autobiography* (C. Eugene Walker, ed.). He is the founder of the American Association of Suicidology.

Morton M. Silverman, M.D., is Director of the Student Counseling and Resource Service at the University of Chicago, Chicago, Ill., Special Issue Coeditor of *Suicide and Life-Threatening Behavior.*

Steven Stack, Ph.D., is Professor of Sociology and Director of the Criminal Justice Program at Wayne State University, and Consulting Editor of *Suicide and Life-Threatening Behavior.* He is working on the statistical analysis of suicide and homicide rates in Eastern and Western Europe. His most recent publication is "The Effect of Divorce on Suicide in Denmark, 1950–1980" in *Sociological Quarterly.*

Zigfrids T. Stelmachers, Ph.D., is Clinical Professor of Psychology at University of Minnesota, Minn.; Director of the Crisis Intervention Center, Minneapolis, Minn.; and the Chief Clinical Psychologist of the Hennepin County Medical Center, Minneapolis, Minn. His research focuses on the exploration of the use of chaos theory in suicide prediction. His most recent publication is "Use of Case Vignettes in Suicide Risk Assessment" (with Robert E. Sherman) in *Suicide and Life-Threatening Behavior.*

Bryan L. Tanney, M.D., F.R.C.P.(C.), is Associate Professor of Psychiatry at the University of Calgary, and Canadian Editor of *Suicide and Life-Threatening Behavior.* Currently he is working on the large-scale dissemination of a preventive intervention program for caregivers working with persons at risk of suicide. His most recent publication is "Comprehensive School Suicide Prevention Programs" in *Death Studies*, with coauthors Tierney, Ramseay, and Lang.

Ira M. Wasserman, Ph.D., is Professor of Sociology at Eastern Michigan University, Ypsilanti, and Consulting Editor of *Suicide and Life-Threatening Behavior.* He is currently working on a number of projects: First, he has reformulated Durkheim's thesis regarding the impact of war and political crises on suicide, and is testing this reformulated model using the United States between 1910 and 1920, and 1933 and 1977. Second, he is testing models statistically regarding the causes of lynching behavior in the American South. Third, he is examining the relationship between the woman suffrage movement and the prohibition movement. Fourth, he is examining changing suicide patterns in Quebec Province in Canada. His most recent publication is "The Effects of War and Alcohol Consumption Patterns on Suicide: United States, 1910–1933" in *Social Forces.*

Marjorie E. Weishaar, Ph.D., is Clinical Assistant Professor of Psychiatry and Human Behavior at Brown University. She is a consultant on grants for in-patient treatment of depression. Her most recent publication is "Hopelessness and Suicide" in the *International Review of Psychiatry.*

Robert I. Yufit, Ph.D., is Associate Professor of Clinical Psychology at Northwestern University Medical School, Chicago, Ill., and Consulting Editor of *Suicide and Life-Threatening Behavior.* He is currently involved in the development of assessment techniques to identify suicide potential and evaluate degree of lethality. His most recent publication is "Assessment of Suicide Potential" in *Clinical and Diagnostic Interviewing* (R. J. Craig, ed.).

Foreword

This excellent volume brings the reader up to date on the assessment and prediction of who is at risk for suicide. It will prove of considerable interest to both clinicians and researchers.

The book has 32 chapters, and the reader will appreciate the variety of approaches and ideas, with some chapters more meaningful or informative than others. In other words, there is something here for both the clinician and the scientist. The overall structure of the book highlights the importance of utilizing clinical judgment, intuition, and insight in order to derive empirically an aggregate of hypothetical predictors of suicide. A section of the book dealing with the evaluation and testing of a variety of rating instruments illustrates how the clinician and the scientist struggle in an effort to address a clinical problem by a scientific experiment. The clinician tries to decide who is at risk for suicide within the next few hours or days. The scientist tries to predict who is at risk for suicide over the next few months or years. Future research will attempt a greater convergence of these aims.

A unique aspect of the book is the use of the five case studies, which each author has examined and discusses. One can see how both clinician and scientist attempt to analyze these cases. The last chapter reveals the true outcome of these cases and permits the reader to test his or her own clinical judgment against that of the experts. The book does not, however, attempt to provide a specific answer to the question, Who is going to commit suicide and who is not? For no one has the gift of prophecy.

In the Old Testament prophets were denounced as false when their prophecies of favorable events turned out to be incorrect. At the same time, the prediction of an adverse event that did not then occur was not equated with false prophecy because of the possibility of divine mercy and intervention. Applying this model to the prediction of suicide as an adverse event, one of the chapter authors, Dr. Pokorny, was able to predict 55% of the actual suicides in his follow-up study. In this pivotal study 45% of the suicides were not predicted. Thus, his instruments suggested that 45% of the suicides were going to survive, but they did not. As clinicians and scientists we are able to do a reasonable job of predicting suicide, but our failures prove that we do not meet the Old Testament's criteria for prophets. This has long been recognized by clinicians and underscores the need for a comprehensive review of the success rate in suicide risk assessment in terms of research and clinical practice.

Thirty-three thousand Americans die by suicide each year. More Americans die by suicide in 2 years than died in the entire Vietnam war. This cause of death, which is largely associated with psychiatric illness, represents a major challenge to our health care system. Clinicians should endeavor to improve their level of expertise in detecting these patients, and this book will help them in that goal.

Investigators in the field of suicidology will also find this volume a valuable statement of the extent of our knowledge in this field at the present time. This book has set our current standard, and it identifies where we should go next. The widespread mortality and morbidity that result from suicide and attempted suicide present the health care professionals with an enormous challenge. We must commit our best resources to meet this challenge at the clinical level by the recognition and treatment of high-risk patients, and at the research level by improving our tools for the recognition of those who are at risk.

J. John Mann, M.D.
Professor of Psychiatry
Western Psychiatric Institute
Pittsburgh

Preface

It goes without saying that suicide is a major public and mental health problem. Suicide is usually a premature, tragic loss that causes anguish in survivors and represents at least some threat to the social order. In recent years there have been about 31,000–33,000 completed suicides annually in the United States. Suicide is the eighth leading cause of death (ahead of cirrhosis and liver disease and just behind diabetes mellitus) and has been moving up that list in this century.

Of course, completed suicides are only the tip of the self-destructive iceberg, so to speak. It is also estimated that there are 250,000–600,000 nonfatal suicide attempts each year, and that each suicide on average leaves behind six survivor victims. While suicide may solve problems for the suicide, it certainly creates problems for those left behind. And we must add to this list the thousands of walking wounded who live with chronic partial self-destruction—the alcoholics, the depressives, the deliberate self-harmers, the excessive risk takers, whose lives are shortened and crippled in part from their own inability to live better. If we take into account all completed suicides, nonfatal suicide attempts, survivor victims, and premature natural deaths related to self-abusive lifestyles, roughly half a million people in the United States are affected by self-destructive behaviors each year.

To all those who suffer and feel they might be better off dead (and to those clinicians who work daily with such people), this volume attempts to provide some alternatives. But before we can be of any help to suicidal people, we must first be able to identify and understand them. This book arose out of our work face-to-face with suicidal individuals. For example, in Maris and Berman's forensic suicide practices we asked, Should these unfortunate deaths have been foreseeable? Maltsberger's long-time psychoanalytic therapy with suicidal clients was recently crystallized in his book, *Suicide Risk: The Formulation of Clinical Judgment* (1986). And Yufit devoted the

---

Much of what appears in a traditional preface (viz., an overview of the book, theory and concepts, a listing of key issues to be addressed, and a review, in the case of this particular text, of the specific single predictors of suicide) is to be found in the Introduction (Chapter 1). There is also a helpful synopsis of all chapters in the Appendix.

major theme of the annual American Association of Suicidology conference in New Orleans (1990) during his presidency (and presently) to the assessment of suicide potential in clinical practice.

Although the book before you grew out of our clinical practice, it also attempts to bridge the gap between clinical work and basic science, as Dr. Mann notes in his Foreword. It should be clear that we believe suicide and its assessment and prediction are multidisciplinary problems. With this in mind we have attempted to present a vehicle for "cross-cultural" communication among diverse professional perspectives. Clinicians tend to get caught up in the practical exigencies of nonrandom samples of diverse self-destructive populations, and few of them have either the time or the inclination to do basic research or to write. Still, one cannot be fully effective without empirically based understanding. Accordingly, we have intentionally kept the scope of this volume broad. For example, we have included chapters from basic scientists (Beck, Brown, de Catanzaro, Felner, Goodwin, Linnoila, Roy, Shaffer, et al.), biostatisticians (Addy), and philosophers (Mayo).

However, another unique feature of this book is the inclusion of five clinical cases on which all contributors, including the basic scientists, have been asked to comment, predict the suicidal outcome, and discuss etiology from their subdisciplinary perspectives. Throughout the book these cases provide a state-of-the-art litmus test, giving a measure of accountability for individual hypotheses and predictions. Thus, our treatment of suicide assessment and prediction shifts back and forth from broad categorical group traits and abstract scientific generalizations to specific individual patient traits and clinical insight. For those who want to try their own hand at assessment and prediction, the actual suicide outcome of our five cases is revealed in the last chapter.

Given the length and scope of this book, there is some unavoidable overlap or redundancy, but we enlisted the very best suicidological specialists available and gave them relatively free rein in writing their chapters. Some chapter authors were selected because of their expertise with specific suicide predictors, others because of their special knowledge of statistics, genetics, pharmacology, and so on. Still others were asked to synthesize specific predictors, as well as to integrate the particular findings of chapter authors.

Can suicide be predicted? In a sense Dr. Mann (in his Foreword) is right, of course. Individual suicides are very difficult to predict; especially *when* the suicide will occur, as opposed to *if* it will. Given the current state of the science and art of suicide assessment and prediction we generate far too many false positives. But for groups we can certainly predict suicide risk over periods of 1 to 5 years, and we can then determine which types of patients/clients to give special attention to. In fact we do this every day in psychiatric hospitals when we put depressed, or agitated, or psychotic patients on suicide precautions. Perhaps using the collective knowledge and skills represented in this volume, in the future we will improve our prediction of individual suicide within relatively short time frames. Only research like that of Dr. Pokorny (Chapter 6) and longitudinal work like that of Drs. Weishaar and Beck (Chapter 22) will tell.

One final note. This book is not primarily about suicide prevention and treatment. As important as those subjects are, one cannot cover all aspects in a single volume. Although we make a somewhat modest attempt to relate prediction and assessment to treatment in Chapter 32 and sporadically throughout the book, treatment is not considered thoroughly here. Yet we invite the reader to consider assessment and prediction as fundamental to treatment—in establishing an effective treatment plan, in evaluating the success of treatment efforts, and so on—in short, to think of assessment and prediction as essential steps in the process of treatment of suicidal individuals and suicide prevention.

Ronald W. Maris, Ph.D.
Alan L. Berman, Ph.D.
John T. Maltsberger, M.D.
Robert I. Yufit, Ph.D.

Acknowledgments

This multidisciplinary volume on suicide assessment and prediction was truly a cooperative effort. The book was conceived in December 1989 by the senior editor, Ronald Maris. Maris was joined in the spring of 1990 by coeditors Berman, Maltsberger, and Yufit and 44 individual chapter authors. Two years in the making, this volume got started in earnest at a workshop by the same name at the 1990 annual meeting of the American Association of Suicidology (AAS) in New Orleans. The editors gratefully acknowledge the financial support of the AAS for that workshop and for making this volume an official publication of the AAS. Twenty-five percent of all royalties generated by this book will be returned to the American Association of Suicidology to further its work in suicide prevention and suicidology.

Although all of the editors worked hard and responsibly in producing this book, special thanks is due to coeditor Dr. Alan Berman, who produced the cases, carefully read the entire manuscript, and critically reviewed it. At Guilford special thanks to Editor-in-Chief Seymour Weingarten who alternately gave us votes of confidence and chastized our occasional poor judgments, and to Production Editor Anna Brackett, who showed incredible diligence and patience in getting the manuscript in order and keeping after chapter authors to stay on schedule. In South Carolina the day-to-day mailings, phone calls, record keeping, permissions requests, letter writing, etc., were all ably performed by Dr. Maris's research assistants, Miriam Lee Suen and Cimberlie Chambers.

Contents

PART VI
SYNTHESIS AND CONCLUSIONS

P A R T   I

Introduction

Overview of the Study of Suicide Assessment and Prediction

Ronald W. Maris, Ph.D.
University of South Carolina

After the fact of a suicide, it is tempting to become righteously indignant. Surely someone should have realized when a person was acutely suicidal? There often seem to be plenty of clues to suicide. The person may have even stated the intention of killing himself or herself. Of course, suicidal hindsight is 20/20. But *before* the fact of suicide, everything is usually not so obvious. Indeed, many situations in which individuals appear suicidal do not result in completed suicides. Psychiatrist Alex Pokorny has even argued that suicide cannot be predicted using widely acknowledged "high-risk group" factors without identifying unworkably large numbers of false positives (Pokorny, 1983; see Chapter 6 of this book). One might cynically conclude that only suicide "predicts" suicide.

A single, comprehensive, up-to-date reference book on the assessment and prediction of suicide is sorely needed. As far as can be determined, the last comprehensive book on the topic was Beck, Resnik, and Lettieri's *The Prediction of Suicide* in 1974. This significant book was a valuable reference in its time, but was rather small (14 chapters), omitted some important topics, and is now badly out of date. Of course, there have been significant scientific articles on the subject of suicide assessment and prediction in the last 15 to 20 years, but these references are fragmented and scattered.

ISSUES

Suicide Assessment versus Suicide Prediction

If we are to have any hope of producing a more comprehensive and up-to-date reference book on the assessment and prediction of suicide, several important issues and definitions have to be considered. An initial issue suggested by the title of the present book is this: How are suicide assessment and suicide prediction different? "To predict" literally means "to make known beforehand" or "to foretell." Suicide prediction has a kind of zero-sum quality to it: One either "gets it right" or not. As we shall see, unfortunately suicides are mispredicted more often than not. Given the current state of the art, suicide prediction is not very precise or useful. This is one reason why many suicidologists may prefer to speak of assessment. "Assessment" originally meant a determination of the amount of taxes to be paid. More generally, it means to set an estimated value on something. For example, in the present context we might wish to assess suicide potential or suicide intent, or to identify those at risk of suicide. In most cases the concept of suicide assessment implies less precision than that of suicide prediction. "Assessment" also tends to be a more clinical term that "prediction."

Definitions and Types of Suicide

A second issue is: What exactly do we wish to predict or assess? Often we naively assume that suicide is a unidimensional concept or behavior (see my discussion in Chapter 4, and Mayo's in Chapter 5). It most clearly is not. To cite Shneidman's (1985) definition (see also Chapter 3), "suicide is a conscious act of self-induced annihilation, best understood as a *multidimensional* malaise in a needful individual who defines an issue for which the suicide is perceived as the best solution" (p. 203; emphasis added). One common mistake is to equate completed suicides with nonfatal suicide attempts. This is absurd on the face of it, since in the first case people die and in the second they do not. It is amazing how many clinical researchers study nonfatal suicide attempts and then claim to understand completed suicides. The truth is that 85–90% of suicide attempters never go on to complete suicide.

The suicidal continuum includes completions, nonfatal attempts, gestures, partial self-destruction, indirect suicide, and ideation (Farberow, 1980; Menninger, 1938). These self-destructive acts and thoughts (and there are others) are sufficiently different from one another to require somewhat different explanations or independent predictor variables. There are probably at least as many explanations of suicide as there are types of suicide (see Chapter 4). Although types of self-destruction may overlap (Blumenthal & Kupfer, 1990), they are also each in a way unique. One only need remind oneself of the differences among a mutilating adolescent prisoner, an older alcoholic male on skid row, a teenage girl who obsesses about death and dying but never actually makes a suicide attempt, the middle-aged professional who is grossly overworked and overstressed, the teenage male who drives too fast and abuses drugs, the diabetic who refuses to take insulin, or an overweight black female who chain-smokes cigarettes.

In addition to the continuum from completed suicide to partial self-destruction to "simple" ideation, there is also variation *within* each of these categories. Most suicidologists believe that within the category of completed suicide there are at least 4 to 12 fundamental types. Durkheim (1897/1951) claimed that there are "egoistic," "anomic," "altruistic," and "fatalistic" suicides, with seven subtypes and two mixed types. Baechler (1975/1979) argued that all suicides are "escapist," "aggressive," "oblative" (self-sacrificing), or "ludic" (risk-taking), or one of 11 subtypes. Menninger (1938) spoke of sucides dominated by either revenge (a "wish to kill"), depression (a "wish to die"), guilt (a "wish to be killed"), or some combination of the three elements. Similar within-category differentiations can be made for nonfatal suicide attempts, gestures, partial self-destruction, and ideation.

The picture that emerges is complex. If our predictions and assessments of suicidal behaviors are ever to be accurate, then at the very least we must specify our dependent variable in sufficient detail to encompass the basic types of suicidal behaviors (and their major subsets—see Chapter 4, this volume). Since suicide is a rare behavior, we need to be careful as well not to make too many subtle distinctions. This is a methodological as well as a practical consideration. In specifying the full range of our dependent variable, we could end up with too few cases to do meaningful analyses or statistical differences that really do not make much of a practical difference.

Scales and Tests

A third issue to be considered in this book is whether there are scales or tests that predict suicide with any degree of reliability, validity, sensitivity, and specificity. Of course, it would be useful if an individual could fill out a brief questionnaire or take a projective test that would allow us to know the probability of his or her committing suicide within a specific (preferably short) time frame. Such tests may be general, such as the Minnesota Multiphasic Personality Inventory (Hathaway & McKinley, 1943), the Rorschach (Klopfer, 1954–1970), the Diagnostic Interview Schedule (Robins, Helzer, Croughan, Williams, & Spitzer, 1981), the Schedule for Affective Disorders and Schizophrenia (Spitzer & Endicott, 1978), the Family History—Research Diagnostic Criteria (Endicott, Andreasen, & Spitzer, 1978), or the Symptom Checklist 90 (Derogatis, Lipman, & Covi, 1973). They may be specific for depressive illness, such as the Hamilton Depression Rating Scale (Hamilton, 1960), the Beck Depression Inventory (Beck, 1967), or the Zung Self-Rating Scale for Depression (Zung, 1965). Or they may be specific for suicide, such as the Scale for Assessing Suicide Risk (Tuckman & Youngman, 1968), the Los Angeles Suicide Prevention Center (LASPC) Scale (Beck et al., 1974), the Index of Potential Suicide (Zung, 1974), the Scale for Suicide Ideation (Beck, Kovacs, & Weissman, 1979), the Suicide Probability

Scale (Cull & Gill, 1982), or the Clinical Instrument to Estimate Suicide
Risk (Motto, Heilbron, & Juster, 1985).

All of these psychological tests and others are critically reviewed elsewhere in this book (see Eyman & Eyman, Chapter 9, and Rothberg & Geer-
Williams, Chapter 10). At this point I wish simply to call attention to four
aspects of such scales or tests: their reliability, validity, sensitivity, and
specificity. Since most readers are already familiar with the general concepts
of reliability and validity, little needs to be added here. If an instrument or
prodedure is "reliable," then it produces consistent results (Maris, 1988,
p. 87). For example, suppose a psychologist administers the LASPC Scale to
a patient and the patient scores a 3. To make sure of this finding, the
psychologist repeats the test, but this time the patient scores a 9. Such a test
would be unreliable. "Validity," on the other hand, means that a test
actually measures what it is intended to measure. For example, many suicide
prediction tests measure depressive illness instead of suicide potential. Note,
too, that scales can be reliable but not valid, and that there are several
subtypes of reliability and validity.

Most readers are probably less familiar with the concepts of "sensitivity" and "specificity." Thus, it may be helpful to define them and then give
a specific numerical example. There are four possible outcomes for any
prediction of suicide:

1. True positives (predict suicide, get suicide)
2. False positives (predict suicide, get nonsuicide)
3. True negatives (predict nonsuicide, get nonsuicide)
4. False negatives (predict nonsuicide, get suicide)

"Sensitivity" is the proportion of correctly identified positive cases (i.e., the
true positives; Andreasen, Rice, Endicott, Reich, & Coryell, 1986). Sensitivity can be calculated as follows:

$$\text{Sensitivity} = \frac{\text{TP}}{\text{TP} + \text{FN}} \times 100$$

"Specificity" is the proportion of correctly identified negative cases (i.e., the
true negatives). It can be calculated as follows:

$$\text{Specificity} = \frac{\text{TN}}{\text{FP} + \text{TN}} \times 100$$

An ideal predictive test would produce high sensitivity and specificity
scores, and low false-positive and false-negative scores. Actual suicide prediction tests, as we shall see throughout this book, unfortunately produce
large numbers of false positives. In fact, they usually produce so many that

the false positives cannot be distinguished from the true positives. In Chapter 6 of this book, Pokorny describes a study in which 4,800 psychiatric patients were followed for 5 years. From this original group, there were 67 suicides over the 5 years. Using the best available predictive tests, Pokorny achieved the following results:

True positives   =   35 (of 63)   = 55% (sensitivity)
False positives   = 1,206 (of 4,641) = 30%
True negatives   = 3,435 (of 4,641) = 74% (specificity)
False negatives =   28 (of 63)   = 44%

    Total n = 4,704

Note the high number of false positives in Pokorny's study. Out of 1,241 cases predicted as suicides, only 35 were in fact suicides. How would any clinician determine which of the 1,241 patients to be concerned about, give special treatments to, and so forth? Such data cause Pokorny to conclude that suicide cannot be predicted, since our current tests or scales do not have high enough sensitivity and specificity scores, and since suicide has such a low base rate. Suicides typically occur at the rate of 1 to 3 cases for every 10,000 people in the general population. Ironically, if we predicted no suicide in every case, our results would be highly accurate. But we would also identify no suicides before they died.

The predictive value of a scale or test is given as follows:

$$\frac{TP}{TP + FP} \times 100$$

With the Pokorny data, the predictive value of the tests utilized (the proportion of true suicides out of all positive predictions) was only 2.8%, hardly an impressive result! In fact, with rare behaviors like suicide, we would have to have sensitivity and specificity scores approaching 99% each to reach predictive values of roughly 80%.

The Role of Clinical Judgment

Given studies like that of Pokorny, many suicidologists (especially clinicians) remain highly skeptical of the usefulness of *any* empirical approach to the prediction and assessment of suicide. This raises a fourth important issue: What is the role of clinical judgment of suicide potential, and how do such judgments relate to more quantitative techniques of assessment and prediction? An argument can be made that suicide prediction scales, psychological tests, statistics (e.g., analysis of variance), suicide checklists, and other quantitative procedures only take us so far. Such procedures are usually not flexible, individualized, specific, or thorough enough. For example, no suicide prediction scale ever considers all relevant factors or changing weights of factors in changing circumstances. The argument goes that the skilled clinician can read between the lines or numbers, as the case may be. What does a clinician do when a test indicates that a patient is at no or low suicide risk and the clinician simply does not believe it?

Clinical judgment tends to emphasize "soft" indicators (e.g., "How does the patient make me feel? Am I worried about his or her imminent suicide?"). One important factor can overwhelm all others (e.g., a sudden, profound loss of support or relationships) and yet may not reveal high suicide risk, since most scales assign limited weight to any single variable. It should be noted in passing that the concept of "high suicide risk" is usually a misnomer. Even when the risk of suicide goes from about 1 in 10,000 (the rate in the general population) to 1 in 10 (the lifetime rate of prior suicide attempters), it still is not a "high" risk. How much would you be tempted to wager on an outcome that had a 10% probability of happening (and suicide predictions with even a 10% probability in a short time frame are very seldom obtained)?

For further explorations of the role of clinical judgment in suicide assessment and prediction, the reader is referred to the chapters by Maltsberger (2), Shneidman (3), Litman (21), Weishaar and Beck (22), and Motto (31). The concepts introduced in these chapters are strikingly different from those in the formal suicide scales. For example, Maltsberger talks about profound aloneness, the inability to tolerate solitude, self-hatred, murderous rage, and abrupt loss of external resources. There are also many detailed accounts of individual suicide cases, as opposed to group data and suicide rates. Clinicians tend to deal with very small numbers of patients, rather than large, random samples.

Of course, clinical judgment can be combined with empirically sound methods. One good contemporary example of this approach is the work of Smith (1985) on ego vulnerabilities. Smith still sounds like Maltsberger or Menninger (1938) when he identifies such suicide-predicting variables as high self expectations, an ambivalent attitude toward death, a suppressive stance toward painful feelings, an inability to mourn overly narcissistic or romantic gratifications, and rigidity in perception. The difference is that Smith tends to derive his concepts from systematic research and not from insight alone.

This is important, because clinical judgment has a tendency to be somewhat mystical and private. An example of this can be seen in Shneidman (1971). Shneidman studied 30 cases taken from the Terman prospective study of high-IQ whites male Stanford students (1921–1960 in this instance). Five of these 30 cases were completed suicides. All explicit references to mode of death were edited out, and then the files of the suicide completers were mixed in with those of the others (who either had died natural deaths or were still living). Using clinical judgment, Shneidman pored over the files and ranked the cases from 1 (definite suicide) to 30 (definite non-suicide). He got the first four right; they were all suicides. His fifth-ranked case was not a suicide, but his sixth-ranked one was. Shneidman stated that the probability of correctly predicting the first four out of five as suicide was roughly .001. Impressive as all this was and is, when it came to saying how he did it Shneidman waffled a little. He vaguely mentioned the role of the significant other and "burning out"—hardly concepts that would allow *others* to make such accurate predictions. We may well wonder why the clinical judgment of suicide risk by skilled clinicians like Shneidman, Maltsberger, Litman, Motto, and others cannot be routinized and packaged for the general public. Can we not explicate or "unpack" what skilled clinicians do in assessing or predicting suicide, and then (say) write a computer program for ordinary mortals that would help them manage their own suicidal clients?

Specific Predictors of Suicide

Regardless of whether we utilize clinical judgment or more quantifiable empirical procedures (such as suicide prediction scales), a critical fifth issue is this: What items ought to be attended to? Obviously, we cannot pay attention to all potential attitudinal, situational, and other clues to suicide. Table 1.1 attempts to list 15 single-variable predictors (ignoring for a moment the crucial problem of comorbidity or interaction effects) that almost everyone agrees are present in most suicides. In fact, our detailed examina-

TABLE 1.1. Common Single Predictors of Sucide

1. Depressive illness, mental disorder (2, 7, 14, 21, 22, 29)
2. Alcoholism, drug abuse (15, 18, 28)
3. Suicide ideation, talk, preparation; religious ideas (9, 16, 22, 26)
4. Prior suicide attempts (17)
5. Lethal methods (18)
6. Isolation, living alone, loss of support (2, 19)
7. Hopelessness, cognitive rigidity (22)
8. Being an older white male (23)
9. Modeling, suicide in the family, genetics (24, 28)
10. Work problems, economics, occupation (25)
11. Marital problems, family pathology (26)
12. Stress, life events (27)
13. Anger, aggression, irritability, 5-HIAA (29)
14. Physical illness (28, 30)
15. Repetition and comorbidity of factors 1–14; suicidal careers

Note. Relevant book chapters from this volume are noted in parentheses after each predictor. 5-HIAA, 5-hydroxyindoleacetic acid.

tion of these predictors constitutes the majority of the present volume (see especially Part V, Chapters 14–30). Accordingly, book chapters that consider each predictor most explicitly are listed in parentheses next to each item in Table 1.1. Item 15 reminds us that in all actual suicide cases or circumstances, single suicide predictors are variously weighted; they mix and meld (comorbidity) in different complex "suicidal careers" or conditions over time (see Brent, Kupfer, Bromet, & Dew, 1988; Maris, 1981; see also Shneidman, Chapter 3, and Addy, Chapter 11, this volume).

I now provide a brief overview of specific suicide predictors. This is clearly in no way a substitute for the detailed chapters that follow. However, the chapters themselves do not refer extensively to one another; thus, it is important for the reader to have some sense of an integrated set of suicide predictors. The issue of how single-variable predictors are interrelated is taken up again in Part VI of the book (chapters 31 and 32). None of the single predictors occurs in a vacuum in real life. Thus, interaction effects or models cannot be specified with any detail or precision, nor do I claim to present an exhaustive list of single predictors.

Mental Disorder

Almost all individuals who commit suicide have a diagnosable mental disorder, usually one of the affective disorders, although suicide risk is also high among individuals with schizophrenia and some personality disorders. It has been estimated that about 15% of depressives eventually commit suicide and that about two-thirds of suicides have a primary depressive illness (Black & Winokur, 1986). Suicide is particularly likely when a depressive illness starts to lift and a patient now has sufficient energy to carry out a suicide plan. The tension reduction of the decision to resolve his or her life problems by committing suicide often makes the patient seem dramatically improved. Depression is more suicidogenic if a patient is living alone and has had persistent insomnia (especially terminal insomnia). Psychotic depression can cause the risk of suicide to soar (however, see Fawcett et al., 1990). In general, the relationship of psychosis to suicide is complex and multifaceted (Buie & Maltsberger, 1989, p. 65). A pattern of repeated depressive illnesses can lead to hopelessness, which Weishaar and Beck argue is more highly related to a suicidal outcome (see Chapter 22).

Alcoholism and Drug Abuse

Alcoholism is another major predictor of completed suicide. In a large series of studies of alcoholics, Roy and Linnoila (1986) found that on average 18% of all alcoholics eventually commit suicide. In Robins's (1981) St. Louis research, 72% of completed suicides were either depressed (47%) or alcoholic (25%). No other single predictor was present in more than 5% of the suicides.

Alcoholism has a complex relationship to suicide. Often in the short run alcoholism seems to protect against suicide (perhaps by transiently raising low brain serotonin levels; Roy & Linnoila, 1986), but in the long run (on average, about 25 years) it is related to higher rates of suicide. A major factor in alcoholic suicide is increased disruption of interpersonal relations and social supports. Although the data on nonalcoholic drug abuse are more equivocal, such abuse is also related to completed suicide, especially among younger drug abusers (see Lester, Chapter 15). One should not forget that patients can and often do use their antidepressant medications to overdose.

Ideas, Talk, Preparation

Ideas about suicide, talk of suicide, and preparation for suicide occur in most cases, especially if one pays careful attention to what a person is saying or doing. It has been estimated that as many as 75 to 80% of all suicides given presuicidal clues of their suicidal intentions (Shneidman & Farberow, 1957). Although the relation of ideation to action is not isomorphic, sometimes the best predictor of suicide is simply to *ask* people whether they are thinking about killing themselves. It is also useful to ask, "If you were going to commit suicide, how would you do it [what methods, specific plans, when, etc.]?" The literature suggests paying attention to new wills, new or altered life insurance policies, giving away valued possessions, death or suicide talk, and the like. Partially self-destructive behaviors may indicate ideas about suicide. For example, is the individual drinking heavily, abusing drugs, acting out sexually, having numerous accidents, or missing work or school uncharacteristically? Religious ideas and behaviors can be relevant, too. Does the individual believe in an afterlife? What does he or she think happens after death (is there a hell, does one get punished for suicide, does one join deceased loved ones in heaven, is death more attractive than life, etc.)? Behaviorally, has the individual stopped attending church or synagogue or participating in religious rituals?

Prior Suicide Attempts

Of course, before one can kill oneself, one must make a suicide attempt. Any individual with a history of one or more prior nonfatal suicide attempts is at much greater risk for suicide than most of those who have never made a suicide attempt. About 15% of nonfatal suicide attempters will die by suicide (Maris, 1981). In the general population, the suicide rate is only 12 per 100,000, or .0001. Thus, prior suicide attempts raise the risk of suicide dramatically. However, among older whites males (the typical suicide) who attempt suicide, almost 90% die the first time they attempt it (mainly because they shoot themselves in the head). When someone makes only one fatal suicide attempt, the suicide attempt obviously cannot be used as a signal that the person is about to commit suicide and it is time to intervene. Nonfatal suicide attempts are more likely among younger persons, especially females. Suicide attempts within this group are a useful predictor of completed suicide. With most older males, however, we need to specify precursors of suicide attempts.

Lethality of Method

This brings us to the method used to attempt suicide and its lethality. It seems obvious that men are more likely to die when they attempt suicide, since they usually employ more lethal methods than females do. "Lethality" refers to the probability of a fatal outcome (Smith, Conroy, & Ehler, 1984). "Acute lethality" indicates the probability of suicidal death in a short time frame (e.g., tonight, this weekend, in a few weeks, if treatment is not initiated, etc.). "Chronic lethality" is the long-term probability of suicidal death. Both types of lethality have ranges from low to high on specific scales. The more lethal the method used, the more likely it is that a suicide will be completed.

Since 1980, both men and women have preferred firearms as the method of choice for suicide. In that year, 63% of male completers and 39% of female completers used guns. The second most common method of suicide for males in 1980 was hanging (15%) and for females was poisoning (27%) (Centers for Disease Control, 1985). (Percentages for 1987 were about the same; see Garrison, Chapter 23.) Overall, men choose relatively few, highly lethal methods to commit suicide; women use a much greater variety of methods, many of which are of relatively low lethality. Thus, it is no surprise that men on average have a suicide rate three or four times higher than that of women. Of course, we still have not determined *why* women are more likely to utilize less lethal methods to attempt suicide. It should be noted in passing that suicide prevention is often gun control. If one can remove the gun or limit access to guns, the risk of suicide plummets. It simply is not true that a determined individual will just find another way to commit suicide if the preferred method is controlled. For example, it is well known that in Great Britain, when toxic gas in the home was detoxified, the suicide rate dropped significantly (Kreitman, 1976).

Social Isolation

As long as social interaction is not negative (e.g., driving a person to suicide), social involvement of all sorts reduces suicide potential, and social isolation or living alone increases the risk of suicide. For example, in one study of suicidal depressives versus nonsuicidal depressives, 42% of the suicides lived alone as opposed to only 7% of the nonsuicidal depressives (Maris, 1981).

In my Chicago research (Maris, 1981), 50% of the completed suicides had no close friends, compared to 20% of the nonfatal suicide attempters. As Harvard psychiatrist Avery Weisman used to say, we all need at least one significant "udder." Weisman and Worden's (1974) "risk–rescue ratio" calculates not only suicide risk, but also the probability of rescue or intervention. Clearly, when one is alone or isolated, the possibility of rescue is diminished.

Finally, the relevance of isolation to jail and hospital suicides should be noted (see Bonner, Chapter 19, and Litman, Chapter 21). Suicide is the leading cause of death in jails and hospitals, and it often occurs in large part because an inmate or patient is isolated from other people in the institution. In a suicide crisis, it is common to have someone within arm's reach of the potential suicide for 24 hours a day. It only takes 3 or 4 minutes for someone to die of asphyxiation. In a real suicide crisis, 15-minute logged checks (the norm in most hospitals and jails) are totally insufficient.

Hopelessness

Beck and colleagues' studies (see Weishaar & Beck, Chapter 22) reveal that hopelessness is a better predictor of suicide, suicidal ideation, or the wish to die than is depressive illness. Suicidal hopelessness often involves no perceived alternatives to suicide, rigid thinking, or "tunnel vision." In fact, Shneidman (1985) has claimed that the "four-letter word" in suicidology is "only" (as in "Suicide was the only thing I could do"). Sometimes a small gain, minute change, or just-noticeable difference can give a suicidal individual hope, and thus (at least in the short run) can prevent suicide. Included here would be a slight reduction in physical pain or a supportive relationship.

Age, Race, Sex

Demographically or epidemiologically speaking, one striking trait of suicide completers is that about 70% of them are white males (see Garrison, Chapter 23). The celebrated rise of the suicide rates of U.S. adolescents in the late 1960s and early 1970s took place almost exclusively among males. Even with these changes in adolescent rates, completed suicide rates are still highest among older males. The most recent data (1987 rates) indicate significant increases in the suicide rates of older white males (McIntosh, 1992). Only 22% of all suicides are white females, and very few nonwhites are suicidal (with the exception of some inner-city blacks and Native American adolescents). Some have even claimed that maleness (in the biological, genetic, or chromosomal sense) is related to premature death and to suicide in particular. For example, even the *in utero* death rate of males is higher than that of females.

Genetic and Modeling Influences

Suicides and depressive illnesses tend to run in families. In my Chicago research (Maris, 1981), 11% of suicides had at least one other suicide among their first-degree relatives, but none of the natural death sample did. This may indicate either genetic (see Roy, Chapter 28) or modeling (Phillips, Lesyna, & Paight, Chapter 24) influences. One study of suicide and affective disorder among the Amish (Egeland & Sussex, 1985) found that both outcomes were gene-related (specifically, related to a narrow portion of chromosome 11). However, a study by Phillips and Carstensen (1986) suggests modeling or imitation as a predictor of suicide. Adolescent suicide rates rose 6.9% above the expected rates 7 to 10 days after New York City suicide stories were broadcast on television. Adult suicide rates showed only a 0.5% rise in the same circumstances. (These findings are not without their critics; e.g., see Phillips, Lesyna, & Paight, Chapter 24.) Still another possibility is that of sociobiological factors, such as having dependent children or being beyond the years of reproductive fitness (see de Catanzaro, Chapter 30).

Work Problems

Although suicide occurs in all census occupational categories (see Wasserman, Chapter 25) and in all social classes (i.e., it is very "democratic"), it does seem to be the case that work or productive life activities protect one against suicide and that work problems are related to suicidal outcomes. In my own studies (Maris, 1981), about one-third of all suicides were unemployed at the time of their death. Suicides typically have erratic work or job histories.

Marital Status and Family Factors

Marriage and having a family (other things being equal) are usually associated with lower rates of suicide (see Stack, Chapter 26). Conversely, suicide rates are almost always highest among the divorced and widowed. Suicide completers are also more likely to have never been married than are individuals who die natural deaths. Studies of family development have suggested that certain kinds of family pathology (e.g., early object loss; early separation from one's mother for long periods of time; physical and emotional abuse by one's father or mother, including incest; frequent moving; etc.) are all related to subsequent suicide as an adult. One study by Shneidman (1971) claims that men's disrupted, hostile, competitive, nonsupportive relations as adults with their wives or lovers are especially predictive of suicide.

Stress and Life Events

Suicide is sometimes triggered by undesirable life events or stress (see Yufit & Bongar, Chapter 27) over fairly long periods of time ("suicidal careers").

These events can include blows to self-esteem, shame, guilt, fear, legal problems, interpersonal discord, loss of important relationships, threat of jail or imprisonment, loss of status, just being repeatedly overworked, and so forth. Most stress is chronic and accumulates slowly. There can be a few intense, acute, "triggering" events preceding a suicide, but without a history of stress most of us can tolerate time-limited, single, dramatic episodes of stress without resorting to suicide. Triggering events are usually not substantially different from the chronic stressors in one's life. Thus, when the suicide threshold is crossed, friends and relatives of the suicide may not notice anything special going on and often express surprise that the death occurred when it did.

Aggression and Anger

Because suicide is a violent act, it usually requires some minimal aggressive energy (see Brown, Linnoila, & Goodwin, Chapter 29). In addition to being depressed and hopeless, most suicides are also angry, irritated, or dissatisfied. Freud argued that suicides are disguised murders of introjected objects. As Menninger (1938) put it, suicide is "murder in the 180th degree." Murderous revenge is particularly likely among younger suicides, for whom interpersonal factors are more salient. Among older suicides, anger and dissatisfaction are more likely to be directed at life itself than at specific individuals. One significant biological finding (see Brown et al., Chapter 29) is that impulsive, violent suicides are likely to have lower cerebrospinal fluid levels of 5-hydroxyindoleacetic acid (5-HIAA). The aggressive component in suicide may also help account for the excess of male suicides, in terms of both socialization to be violent and hormonal concentrations of testosterone.

Physical Illness

Finally, we know that about 35–40% of all suicides have some significant physical illness (see Roy, Chapter 28, and de Catanzaro, Chapter 30). Diseases that have been found to be related to suicide include epilepsy, malignant neoplasms, gastrointestinal problems, and musculoskeletal disorders (e.g., arthritis or lower back pain). As with any other single predictor of suicide, physical illness in and of itself is usually insufficient to cause a suicide. In passing, it should be commented that aging is related both to physical illness and to suicide.

Comorbidity and Interaction of Factors

Item 15 in Table 1.1 reminds us that most people bear up under initial insults to their adaptive repertoire. Suicidal coping breaks down gradually after about 40–50 years of certain kinds of lives. These patterns leading up to suicide can be thought of as "suicidal careers." As I have said at the very beginning of these comments on single suicide predictors, comorbidity and interaction are crucial considerations in predicting suicide. There are different predictive or causal models for different types of suicides. The following examples suggest only a few of the possible variety of predictor combinations: (1) an old white male with no family, who is an alcoholic, is living in the street, and is physically ill; (2) a black adolescent female in the rural South who lives with a physically and sexually abusive stepfather and is doing poorly in school; (3) a white teenage athlete who is sociopathic, is out of work, has just had his fifth arrest for driving while intoxicated, and is in jail; or (4) an elite soldier captured by the enemy as a spy who is about to be tortured. Obviously, this list could be extended almost indefinitely.

Different Levels of Assessment and Prediction

There are three other important assessment and prediction issues, although space precludes developing them here as completely as the first five issues have been discussed. The sixth issue is: Are there different levels of suicide assessment and prediction? The second issue (see above) focuses on individuals and different types of individual suicide. In fact, by consciously highlighting five cases in this book (see "Plan of the Book," below), we are accentuating assessment and prediction of individual suicide. But clearly there is also what we might call "social suicide." As a case in point, federal, state, and local governments need to have some idea about trends in suicide rates to budget health care dollars, to fund community mental health centers, to manage epidemics (one thinks of AIDS, but there was about 250% increase in teen suicides from 1950 to 1977 and elderly suicide rates have increased recently), and so forth.

A related question is that of why certain nations, cultures, ethnic groups, economics eras, and so on have high or low suicide rates (see Hendin, 1982; Easterlin, 1980). One especially striking contrast is that between predominantly Catholic countries (which usually have low rates) and predominantly Protestant countries (which usually have high suicide rates). Other possible examples of social suicide factors include nuclear war, industrial pollution, inner-city blight, housing and business decay in capitalist economies, or mass suicides (e.g., the People's Temple suicide in Jonestown, Guyana). An important corollary of this sixth issue is that disciplinary levels of explanation also vary. Regardless of whether we are considering suicide on an individual or a social level, assessment and prediction need to be multidisciplinary. There are, at a minimum, social, psychological, psychiatric, biological, cultural, and economic dimensions to suicide—all of which make distinctive contributions to the assessment and prediction of suicide. Disciplinary specialties furnish overlapping contributions (as in a Venn diagram) to our understanding and explanation of suicide (Blumenthal & Kupfer, 1990).

Different Settings or Contexts for Suicide

Not only are there individual and social levels of suicide assessment and prediction; there are different settings or contexts of suicide as well. A seventh issue is: What are these different settings or contexts in which suicide needs to be assessed or predicted, and how are needs specific to a setting? Suicides occur in a wide variety of settings or contexts, each of which has unique problems of assessment and prediction. A partial list of these contexts might include the following:

1. Outpatient therapy
2. Jails, prisons, correctional facilities
3. Hospitals
4. Public buildings, skyscrapers, bridges
5. Homes
6. Workplaces or jobs
7. Schools
8. Life insurance companies
9. Drug companies
10. The law
11. Public health, government
12. Survivors

Contextual differences may be illustrated with a few examples. A person who works for a life insurance company needs to know on average over a specified period of time (usually annually) how many policy holders can be expected to commit suicide. (Most life insurance companies, of course, do know this and adjust all policy holders' premiums accordingly, in addition to having a 2-year suicide exclusion clause.) A survivor, by contrast, may feel a compelling need to know whether the family member's death was preventable or whether the children in the family now have an increased risk of suicide. A civil engineer or architect needs to know the probability that an interior hotel design or bridge is suicide-proof. (Some hotels with high inside courtyards almost seem to invite jumping deaths.) Drug companies are concerned about product liabilities for their antidepressants, narcotics, benzodiazepines, and other products (e.g., consider the current Prozac litigation; *New York Times*, August 16, 1990). One important factor is the ratio of a drug's therapeutic dose to its effective dose. Several recent drug cases have focused on benzodiazepines such as Halcion and their relationship to paradoxical rage reactions, anterograde amnesia, depression, and suicide (American Psychiatric Association, 1990). Clearly, all of these contexts raise somewhat different ad hoc assessment and prediction issues.

Statistics, Designs, and Methods

Eighth, and finally, there are statistical, design, and methods issues (see Addy, Chapter 11, and Section III in general). I have only skirted these issues in discussing the third and fourth issues, above. To predict suicide, explicit causal models of suicide outcome are needed in which predictors (the independent variables) are temporally ordered and then tested statistically (see Blumenthal & Kupfer, 1990). Since suicide is a dichotomous, nominal scale outcome (one either commits suicide or does not), only certain statistics for predicting suicide are appropriate (viz., logistic regression, the probit model, discriminant-function analysis, or log-linear models especially; see Chapter 11). Logistic regression, which utilizes the likelihood ratio test of statistical inference, is the optimum statistical method for most suicide prediction problems.

The preferred prediction research design is probably a case–control method (Schlesselman, 1982). Here the cases are various samples of suicide completers (not just suicide attempters). An important question is what kind of controls suicide completers should be compared with (individuals who died natural deaths; living normal matched for age, sex, and race; persons who died by homicide or accident; psychiatric patients; etc). To determine appropriate sample sizes, power equations need to be calculated. To do this, one needs to specify the relative risk of suicide to be detected; to determine the exposure rates among the control group(s); to set significance and power levels; and to estimate the proportion of cases in various strata. The appropriate sample size can then be derived. Usually one calculates several different equations and gets a range of sample sizes. Suicide prediction designs can be retrospective or prospective. Truly predictive studies probably need to be prospective, but prospective studies of infrequent events like suicide are difficult to do and are rare. Some suicidologists argue that constructing causal models with merely probable outcomes is really not very useful, and that instead one needs to actually intervene in a hypothesized causal chain and to observe the outcome (see Felner, Silverman, & Adan, Chapter 20).

PLAN OF THE BOOK

These, then, are the major issues the present volume attempts to address and resolve. In order to accomplish this, I and my coeditors have divided the book into six major sections: I, "Introduction," II, "Concepts and Theories," III, "Methods and Quantification," IV, "The Cases," V, "Specific Predictors," and VI, "Synthesis and Conclusions." These sections and their contents are indicated by the chapter titles they subsume and are fairly straightforward.

We start off in Section II with generic definitions and broad concepts. The focus is on Shneidman's (1985) definition of suicide as a "multidimensional malaise in a needful individual who defines an issue for which suicide is perceived as the best solution." Chapters 3, 4, and 5 examine our dependent variable, suicidal outcomes. They ask: How are suicides alike and different? What do we mean by "suicide"? How many fundamental or basic types of suicide are there? What is it exactly that we are trying to assess or predict? Do the predictors (and the causal models) that explain suicide vary with each different suicidal outcome? What about life-threatening outcomes short of completed suicide? And what are the major theories and specific hypotheses about the etiology of suicide? Maltsberger (Chapter 2) and Shneidman (Chapter 3) also begin to sketch the major psychological independent variables that are thought to predict suicide (lack of self-regulation, profound aloneness, murderous rage, crucial loss, self-contempt, intolerable psychological pain, frustrated psychological needs, hopelessness–helplessness, ambivalence, constriction of thought, egression, and cessation of consciousness, among others). Coeditor John T. Maltsberger is primarily responsible for developing Section II.

Section III, "Methods and Quantification," is the generic empirical counterpart to Section II (see the discussion of the eighth issue, above). Concepts are crucial in the assessment and prediction of suicide, but eventually one must examine some data. This section of the book asks whether suicide can be predicted at all (Pokorny, Chapter 6), and, if so, what empirical and statistical procedures are most appropriate (Addy, Chapter 11). Special attention is given to logistic regression, discriminant-function analysis, log-linear methods, and the probit model. The case–control design and related sampling issues are also considered (Gould, Shaffer, Fisher, Kleinman, & Morishima, Chapter 7). In addition, the problems that arise from utilizing after-the-fact data (as in the "psychological autopsy") are considered (Clark & Horton-Deutsch, Chapter 8). Finally, scales or psychological tests that claim to predict or assess suicide are examined (Eyman & Eyman, Chapter 9; Rothberg & Geer-Williams, Chapter 10). Section III generally examines questions of sampling, statistics, research design, probable outcomes, relative risks, odds ratios, control groups, reliability and validity, sensitivity and specificity, false positives and false negatives, and other broad methodological issues. This section is coedited by Robert I. Yufit.

Section IV, "The Cases," is coedited by Alan L. Berman. Often one is interested in whether or not a specific individual will commit suicide, or one wants to assess an individual's suicide potential. (Of course, one could want to predict suicide rates in groups, or another nonindividual outcome; see the discussion of the sixth issue, above). Accordingly, we have selected five individual cases, which are described in detail in Chapter 12 and referred to in most of the other chapters. The five cases are (1) "Heather B," a 13-year-old white female; (2) "Ralph F," a 16-year-old white male; (3) "John Z," a 39-year-old white male; (4) "Faye C," a 49-year-old white female; and (5) "José G," a 64-year-old Hispanic male. Of course, one could quibble with this case selection; for example, there are no black cases. However, the age and sex spans are fairly well covered. The chapter authors were all asked to relate their topics to one or more of these five cases. Chapter authors were not told the actual suicide outcome of any of the cases (i.e., whether or not the individuals killed themselves; see Berman, Chapter 12). In Chapter 13, Stelmachers and Sherman introduce the "case vignette" method of suicide assessment.

The content of Section V, "Specific Predictors," which I have edited, has been described extensively above in the discussion of the fifth issue and need not be reviewed further here. Finally, Section VI, "Synthesis and Conclusions," lives up to its title. In Chapter 31, psychiatrist Jerome Motto (after reviewing Chapters 1-30 and utilizing his own data as well) attempts to create an integrated approach to predicting suicide. In the concluding chapter, Chapter 32, I and my coeditors summarize the major results and/or conclusions of the respective book sections. We make a collective effort to describe the current state of the art of suicide assessment and prediction.

We have labored to produce a comprehensive, systematic, readable, and up-to-date reference book on suicide assessment and prediction. In an effort to avoid platitudes and superficiality, we have turned to the experts. Indeed, we have had little choice, since suicide is far too complex and multifaceted a subject for any one or two authors to master. The results are great detail and some highly technical chapters. Editorially, we have tried to compensate for this by making every effort to integrate, blend, and coordinate the products of our multidisciplinary team of specialist authors. Finally, we have tried to maintain an applied, clinical focus and to keep in mind that we tend to save or lose lives one at a time. We hope you are pleased with the results.

REFERENCES

American Psychiatric Association. (1990). *Benzodiazepine dependence, toxicity, and abuse.* Washington, DC: Author.

Andreasen, N. C., Rice, J., Endicott, J., Reich, T., & Coryell, W. (1986). The family history approach to diagnosis. *Archives of General Psychiatry, 43,* 421-429.

Baechler, J. (1979). *Suicides* (B. Cooper, Trans.). New York: Basic Books. (Original work published 1975)

Beck, A. T. (1967). *Depression: Clinical, experimental, and theoretical aspects.* New York: Harper & Row.

Beck, A. T., Kovacs, M., & Weissman, A. (1979). Assessment of suicidal intent: The Scale for Suicide Ideation. *Journal of Consulting and Clinical Psychology, 47*, 343-352.

Beck, A. T., Resnik, H. L. P., & Lettieri, D. J. (Eds.). (1974). *The prediction of suicide.* Bowie, MD: Charles Press.

Black, D. W., & Winokur, G. (1986). Prospective studies of suicide and mortality in psychiatric patients. *Annals of New York Academy of Science, 487*, 106-113.

Blumenthal, S. J., & Kupfer, D. J. (Eds.). (1990). *Suicide over the life cycle: Risk factors, assessment, and treatment of suicidal patients.* Washington, DC: American Psychiatric Press.

Brent, D. A., Kupfer, D. J., Bromet, E. J., & Dew, M. A. (1988). The assessment and treatment of patients at risk for suicide. In A. J. Frances & R. E. Hales (Eds.), *Review of psychiatry* (Vol. 7, pp. 353-385). Washington, DC: American Psychiatric Press.

Buie, D. H., Jr., & Maltsberger, J. T. (1989). The psychological vulnerability to suicide. In D. J. Jacobs and H. N. Brown (Eds.), *Suicide: Understanding and responding—Harvard Medical School perspectives* (pp. 59-72). Madison, CT: International Universities Press.

Centers for Disease Control. (1985). *Suicide surveillance, 1970-1980.* Atlanta, GA: Author.

Cull, J. G., & Gill, W. S. (1982). *Suicide Probability Scale manual.* Los Angeles: Western Psychological Services.

Derogatis, L. R., Lipman, R. S., & Covi, L. (1973). SCL-90: An outpatient psychiatric rating scale—preliminary report. *Psychopharmacology Bulletin, 9*, 13-28.

Durkheim, E. (1951). *Suicide: A study in sociology* (J. A. Spaulding & G. Simpson, Trans.). Glencoe, IL: Free Press. (Original work published 1897)

Easterlin, R. A. (1980). *Birth and fortune: The impact of numbers on personal welfare.* London: Grant McIntyre.

Endicott, J., Andreasen, N., & Spitzer, R. L. (1978). *Family History—Research Diagnostic Criteria.* New York: New York State Psychiatric Institute.

Egeland, J., & Sussex, J. (1985). Suicide and family loading for affective disorders. *Journal of the American Medical Association, 254*, 915-918.

Farberow, N. L. (Ed.). (1980). *The many faces of suicide: Indirect self-destructive behavior.* New York: McGraw-Hill.

Fawcett, J., Scheftner, W. A., Fogg, L., Clark, D. C., Young, M. A., Hedeker, D., & Gibbons, R. (1990). Time-related predictors of suicide in major affective disorder. *American Journal of Psychiatry, 147*, 1189-1194.

Hamilton, M. (1960). A rating scale for depression. *Journal of Neurology, Neurosurgery and Psychiatry, 23*, 56-62.

Hathaway, S. R., & McKinley, M. D. (1943). *Minnesota Multiphasic Personality Inventory.* New York: Psychological Corporation.

Hendin, H. (1982). *Suicide in America.* New York: Norton.

Klopfer, B. (Ed.). (1954-1970). *Developments in the Rorschach technique.* New York: World.

Kreitman, N. (1976). The coal gas story: United Kingdom suicide rates 1960-71. *British Journal of Preventive and Social Medicine, 30*, 86-93.

Maris, R. W. (1981). *Pathways to suicide: A survey of self-destructive behaviors.* Baltimore: Johns Hopkins University Press.

Maris, R. W. (1988). *Social problems.* Belmont, CA: Wadsworth.

McIntosh, J. L. (1992). Older adults: The next suicide epidemic? *Suicide and Life-Threatening Behavior, 22*(3).

Menninger, K. (1938). *Man against himself.* New York: Harcourt, Brace & World.

Motto, J. A., Heilbron, D. C., & Juster, R. P. (1985). Development of a clinical instrument to estimate suicide risk. *American Journal of Psychiatry, 142,* 680–686.

New York Times. (1990, August 16). Eli Lilly facing million-dollar suits on its antidepressant drug Prozac, p. B13.

Phillips, D. P., & Carstensen, L. L. (1986). Clustering of teenage suicides after television new stories about suicide. *New England Journal of Medicine, 315,* 685–689.

Pokorny, A. D. (1983). Prediction of suicide in psychiatric patients: Report of a retrospective study. *Archives of General Psychiatry, 40,* 249–257.

Robins, E. (1981). *The final months.* New York: Oxford University Press.

Robins, L. N., Helzer, J. E., Croughan, J., Williams, J. B. W., & Spitzer, R. L. (1981). *NIMH Diagnostic Interview Schedule.* Washington, DC: National Institute of Mental Health.

Roy, A., & Linnoila, M. (1986). Alcoholism and suicide. In R. W. Maris (Ed.), *Biology of suicide* (pp. 162–191). New York: Guilford Press.

Schlesselman, J. J. (1982). *Case-control studies: Design, conduct, and analysis.* New York: Oxford University Press.

Shneidman, E. S. (1971). Perturbation and lethality as precursors of suicide in a gifted group. *Suicide and Life-threatening behavior, 1,* 23–45.

Shneidman, E. S. (1985). *Definition of suicide.* New York: Wiley.

Shneidman, E. S., & Farberow, N. L. (1957). *Clues to suicide.* New York: McGraw-Hill.

Smith, K. (1985). Suicide assessment: An ego-vulnerabilities approach. *Bulletin of the Menninger Clinic, 49*(5), 489–499.

Smith, K., Conroy, R. W., & Ehler, R. (1984). Lethality of Suicide Attempt Rating Scale. *Suicide and Life-Threatening Behavior, 14,* 215–242.

Spitzer, R. L., & Endicott, J. (1978). *Schedule of Affective Disorders and Schizophrenia.* New York: New York State Psychiatric Institute.

Tuckman, J., & Youngman, W. F. (1968). Assessment of suicide risk in attempted suicides. In H. L. P. Resnik (Ed.), *Suicidal behaviors: Diagnosis and management* (pp. 190–197). Boston: Little, Brown.

Weisman, A., & Worden, W. J. (1974). Risk–rescue rating in suicide assessment. In A. T. Beck, H. L. P. Resnik, & D. J. Lettieri (Eds.), *The prediction of suicide* (pp. 193–213). Bowie, MD: Charles Press.

Zung, W. W. K. (1965). A self-rating depression scale. *Archives of General Psychiatry, 12,* 63–70.

Zung, W. W. K. (1974). Index of Potential Suicide. In A. T. Beck, H. L. P. Resnik, & D. J. Lettieri (Eds.), *The prediction of suicide* (pp. 221–249). Bowie, MD: Charles Press.

PART II
Concepts and Theories

CHAPTER 2

The Psychodynamic Formulation: An Aid in Assessing Suicide Risk

John T. Maltsberger, M.D.
Harvard Medical School, Department of Psychiatry
McLean Hospital, Belmont, Massachusetts
Boston Psychoanalytic Society and Institute

THE VARIETY OF SUICIDE TYPES

What do people who commit suicide have in common, beyond the fact that they deliberately bring about their own deaths? Students of suicide sift through the lives of such unfortunates and scrutinize the circumstances in which they lived; they winnow out patterns, classes, and types, hoping to arrive at some understanding, aspiring also to devise means for prediction and even prevention. Establishing classes implies the discovery of common characteristics according to which groupings can be derived. Here inquirers into suicide meet their first obstacle: The variety they encounter in looking through the records of history, the clinic, the public health statistics, and the other sources beggars imagination. The casual inquirer, surveying the complex suicide panorama, might conclude that the only thing suicides have in common is the way they die.

How is a Japanese kamakaze pilot of World War II akin to Sylvia Plath, the poet who asphyxiated herself in 1963? What have these cousins in death in common with the Greek philosopher Zeno, who, his life lived out (he was 98), disgusted with the painful toe he had dislocated in a stumble, went home and hanged himself? With an American high school student who joins the rest of his "gang" in their "cluster," commiting another of the group's serial suicides? With the 16th-century sea captain Sir Richard Grenville and his crew, who blew up their vessel, the *Revenge*, rather than fall into the grip of the Spanish Armada? With a derelict who throws himself in front of a subway train? All these, and other suicides as well, do indeed have characteristics in common. Edwin Shneidman (1985) describes 10, which he calls the "commonalities of suicide"; however, the phenomenon they embrace is multiplex, so his commonalities are general in scope.

Many scholars have classified suicide. Durkheim (1897/1951) is always remembered first; Baechler (1975/1979) has recently entered the lists. Scholars of the classifying sort typically strive to include all possible different kinds of suicide types, many of which are unusual. Durkheim, for instance, included in his list "fatalistic suicides"—those who take their lives because the social milieu in which they are trapped leaves them with no other acceptable choice. Slaves or prisoners whose futures are hopelessly bleak might commit fatalistic suicide, for example.

Those of us chiefly concerned with the clinical assessment of suicide risk hardly ever come on cases of the rare types. Who among us has encountered a suicidal virgin choosing death before dishonor? Or an "exhibitionistic" suicide, such as that of the disgruntled 19th-century eccentric who tied himself to a rocket and, lighting the fuse, projected himself defiantly into the sky (Fedden, 1938)? For the most part, we only read of such persons.

This want of experience in arcane reaches of suicide impoverishes us ordinary clinicians; we must be content to dig in the ordinary field among the ordinary cases. But the constriction simplifies our task. Most of the cases we meet seem comparatively familiar; we have some notion about how to proceed with them. Hardly ever, for instance, does a suicidal patient come to our attention who is not suffering from a diagnosable mental illness (most commonly a major depressive episode or schizophrenia, often superimposed on a personality disorder, and frequently aggravated by alcoholism). There are exceptions, of course. Rarely, a suicidal patient appears who seems to suffer from no more than a "narcissistic personality disorder." We may then indeed wonder just what manner of person confronts us; such an appellation does no more than put a vague name to an immediate clinical puzzle.

The difficulties of classification do not much daunt us in the clinic. Even though the want of accurate classification may disappoint and occasionally confuse us, our patients must be cared for. We make the best of what we have, usually the standard diagnostic nomenclature. "A clinical suicidologist is interested in that which is useful and makes sense, not in what has specious accuracy" (Shneidman, 1986, p. 3).

THE ASPIRATION TO PREDICT, THE NEED TO ASSESS

One psychiatric resident in an eminent teaching hospital recently told another that since suicide prediction is impossible, the best one can do in caring for patients who threaten to take their own lives is to flip a coin and go forward. The startled trainee who was given this grim advice declined to take it, but it did make him think.

It is not impossible to predict the weather, after all, but it cannot be predicted very accurately. We accept the auguries of the weather bureau and plan our lives accordingly. Sometimes, in the short run, weather prediction can be very good indeed, but applied meteorology often fails us. In our chagrin, we may indeed say that we should have tossed a coin.

In later sections of this compendium, the difficulties in accurate suicide prediction will receive a thorough discussion. By way of overture, I mention a few here.

We do not know how much force each of the known morbid factors exerts in impelling a patient down the final common path to suicide and out of this life. We do not know how the force of each is augmented or diminished according to the presence or absence of other suicide-inviting factors in the clinical mix. We do not even know what all the suicide-inviting factors are, and we know less yet about the preservative factors that protect against suicide. Rosen (1954) has pointed out that because suicide is a comparatively rare event, an unacceptably large number of "false positives" will be identified by any but the most exquisitely discriminating tests. Exquisite discrimination is something we do not have.

Nevertheless, a clinical plateau remains where we can stand between the unattainable pinnacle of sure prediction and the slough of predictive despond into which that coin-tossing psychiatric resident fell. Clinical assessment should, of course, come as close to correct prediction as possible. Just as the passionate wish for some scientifically unassailable prediction tool tempts some to dismiss the whole task of clinical assessment as contemptibly crude, the very cloudiness of the problem invites others to impose their favorite theories on it. These sometimes claim more for their schemes than even clinical practice and experience will support.

Practical clinical assessment is different from scientific suicide prediction research in method, scope, and goal. The usual predictive studies (as the reader will see) concern themselves with forecasting over a lifetime, or over some stipulated future term (rarely less than a year). Clinical assessment concerns itself with estimating suicide risk over short periods—hours, days, or weeks. Pokorny (1983; see Chapter 6, this volume) has emphasized this point, going so far as to suggest that the clinical problem is not suicide prediction, but the identification of a suicide crisis that is already developing.

Fawcett and his colleagues have separated which factors predispose individuals to suicide over a shorter time period as opposed to a longer one (Fawcett et al., 1987, 1990). They have shown that six clinical features are associated with suicides occurring within the first year of posthospital follow-up: panic attacks, severe psychic anxiety, diminished concentration, global insomnia, moderate alcohol abuse, and severe loss of interest or capacity for pleasure. Clark (in press) suggests that suicides occurring immediately following hospital treatment (in the first 6–12 months after discharge) have a distinct character all their own, and observes that when short-term and long-term suicides are lumped together in a single large group in order to derive a suicide risk profile, the qualitatively short- and long-term factors are likely to confound one another in the course of statistical analysis.

Clinicians in the pursuit of their task have many more observational opportunities than most researchers attempting to predict suicide. The researchers concern themselves with groups of patients, not individuals. They limit themselves to the information they can glean from a questionnaire or test administered once or twice over a long period of time. By contrast, clinicians return weekly or even hourly, not to a group, but to one patient. The researchers do not study one patient with a microscope over a long period on the clinical plateau. They watch, as it were, from afar, from a mountain, by telescope, and concern themselves with the behavior of observationally remote groups.

What the clinicians can glean helps the researchers to lay out their plans of investigation, to develop hypotheses, and to test them by group observation over an extended period. What scientific answers come down from the pinnacle can guide the clinicians in their day-to-day close study of the individual patient. So it is that clinical work and scientific investigation go hand in hand, supporting and helping each other.

SUICIDE ASSESSMENT: THE PERSPECTIVE FROM THE CLINICAL PLATEAU

Close to the patients, where copious information is readily obtainable and frequent observation possible, how do clinicians organize their thinking in the day-to-day task of assessing suicide risk? They assume, probably correctly, that the patients whom they identify as suicidal and choose to study over an extended period are in fact at high risk to destroy themselves, and are not among Rosen's (1954) "false positives." Clinicians concern themselves for the most part with high-risk cases. Patients admitted to a psychiatric hospital after lethal suicide attempts occurring in the context of significant mental illness are very likely to go on to die by their own hands in a subsequent try. One group of such patients showed a suicide mortality of 22%. Furthermore, most such suicides occur within the first year of follow-up (Moss & Hamilton, 1956; Motto, 1965).

Clinicians must assume that their work with high-risk patients is therapeutically effective. They trust that their efforts (especially if continued after hospital discharge over many months or years) prevent suicide, and that these efforts improve the quality of their patients' lives.

If our therapeutic effectiveness has not been refuted by empirical demonstration, it has not been thoroughly established either. The view from the pinnacle via sociological telescope makes it plain that suicide rates in the population at large have not declined since the introduction of antidepressant drugs, for instance. Viewed from afar, the clinical workers seem to toil on a murky plain.

Maris (1969) has asserted that suicide is not being prevented in this country. Litman, Farberow, Wold, and Brown (1986) have averred that nobody knows to what extent the clinical labors put forth in hospitals and clinics are effective, or whether psychotherapy, electroconvulsive treatment, psychotropic drugs, community mental health centers, or emergency telephone services are really effective in preventing suicide. Strictly speaking, they are correct: We clinicians do not know for sure that our work does any good except for one patient at a time. Certainly we do not know how much good we do for the entire population of suicidal patients who come our way. In the clinic workers press on, trusting that they do good, not falling into skeptical paralysis. We have evidence that some of these doubts are ill founded. There is reason to believe that treatment for properly selected patients does protect against suicide (Huston & Locher, 1948a, 1948b; Tsuang, Dempsey, & Fleming, 1979). It is true that our therapeutic bustle has not reduced the suicide rate in the population at large, but it may have reduced the rate in the subgroup that comes to clinical attention and receives intelligent treatment.

There is a definitive experiment that would show whether or to what extent clinical efforts are truly helpful, but it should never be carried out. It would require the identification of a large sample of patients who are at serious risk for suicide (say, several hundred with major depressive illness and an immediate past history of a serious attempt). This sample would then have to be randomly divided: Half the sample would be assigned to receive treatment, whereas the other half would be denied it. A follow-up analysis 5 years later would answer the question.

THE RAW INFORMATION AT HAND
FOR CLINICAL ASSESSMENT

The reader will have noticed that the task of clinical assessment can proceed only after much circumscriptive exclusion. I have set aside three desiderata that are of great interest and importance for the larger work of suicide study: precise, inclusive classification; scientifically established risk prediction of high accuracy and precision; and scientific demonstration of the results of therapeutic and prophylactic intervention. Clinicians have to clear away the underbrush in order to make a tillable field. At present, perhaps, they have no other choice; they cannot work effectively in a forest. No harm will follow if they do not forget that their vision is limited. They must not imagine that the perspective from their plateau is as broad as the perspective from the pinnacle.

A clinician is trained to address each new patient by taking a "history" and by carrying out a "mental state examination." A history is a systematic inquiry into the patient's biography. The clinician looks into as many areas as possible, so that nothing pertinent to the clinical assessment of his patient will be neglected. Obviously, history taking has to be inclusive, but it also has to be selective. Every area of the patient's past is investigated, from family history, prenatal course, infancy, and childhood, on through every aspect and vicissitude of development. Yet some areas will be studied in greater detail according to the clinical purpose at hand. If a clinician were primarily interested in coming to grips with a digestive disturbance, the history taking would delve into infant feeding, food tolerances, behavior at the supper-table, the details of defecation, belly aches, and groceries. Suicide assessment requires attention to other areas, but the clinician systematically inquires into the same *general* sectors of the patient's life, whatever the disturbance: the history of the present illness, the developmental history from conception, family history, the character of parent and siblings, preschool history, school history, sexual history, work history, military history, the history of medical and surgical illness, and marital history.

A complete discussion of how to proceed in examining suicide cases is available elsewhere (Maltsberger, 1986). For present purposes, suffice it to say that we try to gather enough information to answer certain specific questions about the patient and his environment. Next, the clinician attempts to construct some overall picture of the patient's personality—its strengths, vulnerabilities, and patterns of reaction. The clinician studies in particular how the patient responds in times of stress and at moments of narcissistic injury. In taking the history, however, because we are especially concerned with suicide assessment, we will take care not to omit systematic inquiry into certain areas that are known to be particularly pertinent to the special task at hand.

Personal Factors

Let us concern ourselves first with a list of special personal details that are relative to the matter of suicide risk:

Age
Sex
Race
Marital status
Living arrangements
Employment status
Physical health

Mental condition (including alcohol and/or drug abuse)
Medical care within 6 months
Previous suicide attempt or threat
Recent loss
Childhood losses
Separations
Family history of mental illness
History of physical, sexual, emotional abuse

The association between suicide and the first 10 items in this list has been statistically demonstrated (Tuckman & Youngman, 1968). Suicide is commoner among the elderly, among males, among whites, and among single people; moreover, living alone is more suicide-inviting than living with others (Sainsbury, 1986). In addition, 85–90% of patients who commit suicide suffer from diagnosable psychiatric illnesses. About 70% have significant depressive illnesses or alcoholism, or both. Another 5% satisfy the criteria for schizophrenia, and a further 10% meet the criteria for some other illness, including borderline personality disorder (Barraclough, Bunch, Nelson, & Sainsbury, 1974; Dorpat & Ripley, 1960; Robins, Murphy, Wilkinson, Gassner, & Kayes, 1959; Stone, 1990).

More than half the patients who commit suicide have consulted a physician within a month or less of their deaths (Robins et al., 1959), and a high proportion of them, especially if they are older, suffer not only from psychiatric illness but from physical ailments as well. Fifteen studies of the prevalence of physical illness in suicide have been reviewed by Whitlock (1986). About a third of these patients are physically sick. Patients with brain diseases, perhaps because so many of them fall into depression, are startlingly high in risk for committing suicide. The rate in epilepsy is said to be much greater than the general prevalence rate; the risk is also elevated in cases of brain damage following head injury, multiple sclerosis, stroke, Huntington's chorea, and progressive organic deteriorative dementia (Barraclough & Hughes, 1987). In cancer the suicide rate is certainly elevated, but how much it is elevated remains unclear. Sainsbury (1955) found a rate 20 times greater than the expectable one; Dorpat and Ripley (1960) found a rate 15 times greater. Later studies restricted to a review of suicide deaths in patients included in a tumor registry, however, suggest that the increased risk is much less, not even rising to a factor of 2 (Fox, Stanek, Boyd, & Flannery, 1982; Louhivuori & Hakama, 1979). The rate of suicide in patients receiving dialysis after renal transplant may be 100 times greater than that in the general population (Lowry, 1979; Haenel, Brunner & Gattegay, 1980; Abrams, Moore, & Westervelt, 1971).

Finally, patients who have made threats and previous attempts are well known to be at increased risk for suicide. Dorpat and Ripley (1967) have shown that between 10% and 20% of all suicide attempters go on to completed suicide; whether a more lethal suicide attempt portends a greater likelihood of future suicide death remains uncertain (Motto, 1965; Cohen, Motto, & Seiden, 1966).

Clinicians are likely to look for still other details, though their close association with suicide may remain unproven. In two kinds of cases, the suicide-promoting influence of loss has in fact been empirically demonstrated: in alcoholics (Robins, 1981) and in patients with borderline personality disorder (Kullgren, 1988; Kullgren, Renberg, & Jacobsson, 1986). Every patient's loss history is of interest, not only because of the developmental impact that losses are likely to have in themselves, but also because a clinician wants to know whether the patient has been able to sustain a loss, at whatever time in life, without resultant reactive illness and subsequent scarring.

Fairly recent loss of a parent through bereavement seems to be significantly associated with suicide, although early parental bereavement may or may not be (Bunch, Barraclough, Nelson, & Sainsbury, 1971). The patient's reactions to separations of all sorts in childhood and afterward are also of interest because suicide-prone people are separation-intolerant (Cross & Hirschfeld, 1986; Crook & Raskin, 1975). The clinician estimates the patient's capacity to make and keep emotionally deep attachments to others, and studies the nature of the attachments he forms, whether narcissistic or mature in form. The history of major mental illness in the family—suicide and suicide attempts in particular—is also ascertained. Suicide and depression are probably partly genetically determined; they are assuredly familial (Barraclough & Hughes, 1987; Kety, 1986; Bunch & Barraclough, 1971). Finally, the clinician determines the presence of any abuse history in the patient's biography—sexual, physical, or psychological (Goodwin, 1982; Goodwin, Cheeves, & Connell, 1988; Yates, 1987; Beres, Eissler, Freud, & Glover, 1951; Jaffe, Wolfe, Wilson, & Zak, 1986; Straus, Gelles, & Steinmetz, 1980).

Exterior Factors

In collecting the history, the clinician will to some extent take into consideration a wide variety of exterior, environmental phenomena that are impersonal. Other environmental details impinge more personally on the individual patient. The exterior phenomena are important not only as influences on the patients in the immediate present, whether toward or away from suicide; they matter also as important influences in character formation. Some of these exterior factors are listed below.

Broad social and cultural influences
    Ratio of old to young in the general population

Suicide characteristics of the patient's age cohort
War and peace
Economic conditions
Availability of means, especially guns
Country of origin
State in which patient resides
Social influences
Socioeconomic class
Greater peer group
Immediate peer group
Attitudes of close friends
Cohesion of social group
Suggestion; media influences
Family influences
Tradition, patterns, and attitudes
Family style of dealing with conflict
Scapegoating
Family dynamics

The broad social influences known by epidemiologists to favor suicide are, for the most part, so remote from the individual case that they are clinically disregarded. In the first place, we do not understand how the broad factors affect the suicide rate in the general population. It is beyond clinical skill to discern which patients are going to be touched in particular by these larger forces which are in some way at work on everyone. It *is* known that the suicide proclivity of each age cohort, taken by decade, differs from that in other cohorts, and that when the population of large groups has a high proportion of young people the rate rises. Suicide rates decrease in wartime and increase during economic depressions. Natives of some countries are at greater risk of committing suicide than those of others; Icelanders, for instance, are at greater risk than Italians. Similarly, those living in Nevada are at greater risk than the citizens of Massachusetts. Considerations such as these rarely enter the minds of clinicians in their daily work of suicide assessment.

The availability of firearms, toxic medicines, or rope for hanging is much more likely to be taken into account. When most clinicians ask about means, they are trying to assess how thoughtfully and completely the patient has worked out a suicide plan. They are weighing not so much the availability of lethal devices as a general suicide promoting factor. Once it is plain that a suicide is in the offing, inquiries about available means follow quickly because it becomes important to get them out of the way. After all, a piece of hefty rope can be had at the nearest hardware store, and (in the United States at least), buying a handgun is not much more complicated.

The clinician will take morbid social influences into account according to his sense of the patient's sensitivity to them. An adolescent boy saturated in the "pop culture," devoted to death-preoccupied music groups, and sharing his peers' scorn for the federal government's hesitant attitude toward environmental protection and conservation is much more likely to feel socially alienated than a Republican businessman active in the Kiwanis or Lions Club who has never smoked marijuana or picked up a copy of *Rolling Stone* magazine. A sensitive clinician will take more time asking about the social milieu of the adolescent than about that of the middle-aged businessman, once satisfied that the businessman is well integrated into his milieu.

A clinician will pay more attention to exterior factors as the factors become more immediate in the patient's life. The discovery that an adolescent boy spends several hours every day listening to a rock group whose music extols suicide and sadomasochism would be worrisome. It would be more worrisome still to learn that the patient's friends idealize the rock group and that some have attempted suicide. Questions in the mind of the assessing clinician would be these: How suggestible is this patient? To what extent does his immediate social milieu suggest and support suicide? To what extent does it discourage it?

Clinicians do not doubt that suggestion can trigger suicide when patients are suicide-ready. Experience in psychiatric hospitals suggests that this is true; the controversial work of Phillips (1974) argues to the same end (see also Phillips, Lesyna, & Paight, Chapter 24, this volume). Although the sociologists do not agree as to the extent and means whereby suggestion and imitation operate in bringing about suicide, clinicians treat it as significant (Maris, 1989).

If clinicians pay little attention to broad societal influences as they go about the work of assessing suicide risk, they conversely pay great attention to family attitudes. Family influences are of great importance as they play out their part in propelling patients toward or holding them back from the suicidal brink. They are also critical in their formative effect on patients' personalities and may reinforce any congenital suicidal proclivity.

To what extent does a patient's family, explicitly or implicitly, foster the idea that suicide is an acceptable way to deal with the problems of living? In some families there is a legacy of suicide that may go back over several generations (Roy, 1983). Children who commit suicide have had contact with a friend or relative who has threatened or attempted it five times more often than those in a matched group of controls (Shafii, Carrigan, Whittinghill, & Derrick, 1985). Pfeffer (1986) has emphasized the importance of suicidal behavior in families of children, and clinicians know that family scapegoating can be suicide-promoting (Sabbath, 1969; Richman, 1986). So important are family and other relationships in suicidal cases that a clinician routinely searches the scene for anyone who might wish the patient dead.

Mental State Phenomena

We may now turn to the third sector of raw information included in clinical suicide assessment—the data from the mental state examination. As in history taking, one does not restrict oneself only to observations that pertain to suicide risk. The entire mental state of the patient is weighed, but the clinician bears in mind the special findings that bear on suicide. Some of these mental state details are listed below:

Mental content
    Suicidal preoccupation, especially planning
    Fantasies about death
Cognition
    Capacity for reality testing
    Capacity for self–object differentiation
    Delusions
    Hallucinations
    Formal thought disorder
    Constriction
Affect
    Presence and intensity of suicide-inviting affects (self-hate, aloneness [terror], murderous hate)
    Fatigue
    Despair (hopelessness)
    Depersonalization
Intellectual functioning: disorientation and delirium
Attitude toward the examiner (health-accepting vs. help-rejecting)

Obviously, the clinician will need to know to what extent the patient is preoccupied with committing suicide. The patient to whom the idea occurs occasionally as a passing fantasy is obviously different from the one who broods about it for hours at a time. Has the patient elaborated a suicide plan? If so, the clinician will wish to know the details: How lethal is the scheme the patient has in mind (Weisman & Worden, 1986)? In some suicide scenarios the clinician may detect unconsciously built-in provisions for rescue, or may discern no coherent plan at all. Other plans will be clearly thought out, devised to prevent interference from others, and frighteningly likely to succeed.

Systematic inquiry into the patient's beliefs and daydreams about death is routine. Quite often patients imagine they can be reunited with others who have died before them, or that they will be transported through dying into a better world without sorrow and suffering. Others believe it is a way to come into the loving embrace of God, who will wipe away the tears from their eyes. Some daydream about suicide as a means to punish others. Others contemplate suicide as a means to escape from persecutors, real or imaginary (Maltsberger, 1986; Maltsberger & Buie, 1980; Friedlander, 1940). How emotionally valuable to the patient is his fantasy about death, the clinician will ask, and how much does he believe that suicide can really bring it about?

These last questions bring us to an examination of the patient's cognition. Emotionally healthy people have their favorite daydreams, of course, but at the same time they maintain a good capacity to tell the difference between fact and fiction. In psychosis this is not true; some patients develop extraordinary ideas and remain convinced they are correct, in spite of overwhelming evidence to the contrary. Delusional people such as these may be more likely to commit suicide when depressed than ordinary depressives are, though reports in the literature are conflicting (Roose, Glassman, Walsh, Woodring, & Vital-Herne, 1983; Wolfersdorf, Keller, Steiner, & Hole, 1987; Black, Winokur, & Nasrallah, 1988).

The examiner should take care not to fall into the mistaken belief that reality testing is impaired only in the presence of fixed delusions. All of us, when sufficiently distressed, are likely to suffer from transient disturbances in reality testing, and suicidal people are very distressed indeed. Under such circumstances, a daydream ordinarily recognizable as sweet but unrealistic can grow into a precious last hope worth the final gamble of a serious suicide attempt.

Not only patients with frank psychosis, but those who suffer from borderline personality disorder as well, may have difficulty in discerning where their own bodies leave off and those of others begin. Many primitive patients are confused about who owns their bodies, and carry out self-attacks in the belief that in doing so they injure somebody else's most precious possession (Zilboorg, 1936; McGlashan, 1983; Maltsberger, 1986). Learning about uncertain self–object differentiation may not always be so straightforward as clinicians might wish; questioning in the course of history taking may not bring it to light, and on the initial mental status examination there may be no clues. Such disturbances are likely to emerge as a course of psychotherapy progresses and the transference unfolds.

The importance of "command hallucinations" in suicide assessment is controversial, but a clinician should nevertheless look for them. Although some intrepid students claim that patients who hear hallucinated commands to kill or harm themselves are not more likely to do so than those who are hallucination-free, most clinicians treat orders from unseen voices to jump off high buildings as danger signals (Hellerstein, Frosch, & Koenigsberg, 1987).

Not all patients disclose their inner experiences to us, especially if they are psychotic. There is, after all, the matter of trust: Many patients, though convinced of the reality of their hallucinatory experiences or beliefs, know very well that psychiatrists and psychologists are skeptics. Therefore they sometimes conceal such information. In the course of an examination, the clinician must remain on the alert for any manifestation of formal thought disorder (e.g., loose or "klang" associations, concretisms, neologisms) that may betray the presence of a not otherwise obvious psychosis.

Shneidman (1985, 1989; see also Chapter 3, this volume) points to cognitive constriction as the perceptual state common to all suicides. (By "perceptual" he means not only sensory perception, but self-perception also. He implies in his use of the word "constriction" a disturbance in the patient's insight and grasp.) When patients fall into an acutely suicidal state, sometimes they can think of nothing but finishing their deadly task. They can be single-minded in the extreme. Their thinking, under great affective press, runs along one channel only. In great urgency they prepare to die, brushing all alternatives for other solutions aside, if they think of them at all.

The driving force behind almost every suicide, clinically speaking, is mental pain. The novelist William Styron (1990), a sufferer from depression, calls such pain a "howling tempest in the brain" and counts off a variety of components in that unholy wind: Self-loathing, anxiety, confusion, loss of concentration and memory, stupor, vague dread, "dank joylessness," and continuous horror. The three basic suicide-inviting affects are self-hate, aloneness, and murderous hate. They usually appear in some combination clinically, and they are frequently combined with other painful affects (such as depersonalization) that are probably not suicide-inviting when they occur alone.

Self-hate impels the victim of melancholia over the suicidal brink in most cases. It is an experience of relentless, burning scorn from within that over time can assume the quality of an interior persecution: One part of the self sets itself over against the rest. It is often compounded by a sense of unbearable inner terror from which the patient can find no relief. The second suicide-inviting affect, that of aloneness, is timeless. It is a state that seems always to have been and that will never end. It is an experience of utter isolation, often accompanied by some sense of unreality; it has the quality of emptiness, horror, devastation, and impending disintegration (Adler & Buie, 1979).

Some patients struggle endlessly with homicidal fury. They sometimes do away with themselves in order to protect others, or they put themselves down in the way one might put down a rabid dog (Maltsberger, 1986).

The clinician studies the affective experience of the patient, watching for indications of the three lethal emotions. If any such indications are present, the clinician attempts to determine what (if anything) the patient does or has done to obtain relief from them, as well as what makes them worse.

The experience of suicidal affects over long periods of time is emotionally exhausting; the clinician must notice how close the patient has come to wearing out and surrendering. One young woman compared her struggle against melancholia to competing in a long-distance run. In such races, she had often heard the footfall and the heavy breathing of a competitor coming up from behind her. She described her efforts to outrun her inner enemy as similar: She said that she was almost worn out, that she could hear it and feel it gaining on her. Exhaustion, moreover, is closely related to despair. The clinician must ask whether the patient has given up on himself; hopelessness is known to be much more highly associated with suicide than the severity of depression is (Minkoff, Bergman, Beck, & Beck, 1973; Yufit & Benzies, 1973).

The integrity of the patient's intellectual functioning (orientation, memory, level of consciousness) also concerns the examiner, inasmuch as many who commit suicide in general hospitals and nursing homes are confused and delirious. The final item on the mental status list is the attitude of the patient toward the examiner. The patient who repudiates help, refuses to cooperate, and wants nothing to do with those who are prepared to help keep him alive is worrisome; such a patient is at special risk to commit suicide (Litman et al., 1986).

THE INTEGRATION OF INFORMATION BEARING ON SUICIDE RISK

We have now surveyed three kinds of information that a clinician assembles in trying to decide whether a patient will commit suicide in the near future. When the clinician finishes collecting the large mass of data from the clinical history and mental state examination, he must try to integrate it. Because no one knows how to do this precisely and with empirical certainty, the clinician is forced to rely on clinical experience and on inductive reasoning. He does not know how important each datum may be in comparison to the others that have been collected. It is true, generally speaking, that the patient who appears to be profoundly hopeless may be, on the basis of that observation alone, more in danger of committing suicide than the patient who has recently developed epilepsy. (We know that both these findings invite suicide to some degree.) The difficulty, however, is in considering multiple variables and their relation to one another. For instance, I believe that epilepsy predisposes a patient to suicide because of its effect on the patient's level of depression and impulsivity, but this would be very difficult to verify. Similarly, it is almost impossible to tell which of two hypothetical combinations would be more dangerous: a diagnosis of carcinoma for a patient with a formal thought disorder, or the death of a parent for a patient who has recently lost his job. Too many other factors must weigh heavily in each case.

We cannot tell how the occurrence of one factor in combination with another augments or diminishes the suicidal force with which the original factor operates. The collective pattern of augmentation or diminution of risk when a large number of factors are present together is not measurable at present. Very roughly speaking, however, if we group the raw data discussed above as I have grouped them—that is, into personal factors (p), exterior factors (e), and mental state factors (ms)—then the risk of suicide (R) will be a rough function of the sum of all of these:

$$R = f(p + e + ms)$$

This state of affairs is obviously very unsatisfactory, because we do not know how to weight most of the variables at hand, and also because many of the variables depend on each other. For instance, the weight assigned one of the p variables (say, a history of a previous suicide attempt) may be radically increased when one of the ms variables (perhaps terror) is included in the assessing. Add to this darkening picture one of the e variables (e.g., a close relative wants the patient dead), and the risk would probably increase more. Yet we cannot say how much more.

Is the assessing clinician at this juncture able to do no more than to think over the assembled data and arrive at a decision about suicidal danger on the basis of intuition? Motto (1989; see also Chapter 31, this volume) perceives it that way. This is the argument: Because it is impossible to quantify certain forces in the patient's life, whether helpful or morbid, and because the clinician can do no more than estimate their importance, the matter is reduced to intuitive judgment, no matter what dynamic considerations are taken into account. "Intuition" means "immediate understanding and grasp, knowing something *without having recourse to inference or reasoning*" (Gove, 1969, p. 1187; my italics).

Inductive arguments cannot be justified as satisfying deductive standards of correctness, but they are nevertheless rational, not intuitive. They infer generalities from factual particulars. According to logic, induction is the process of discovering principles by the observation and combination of particular instances. Strictly speaking, the formulation of suicide risk is not formal induction, because it does not seek to establish general principles about all suicide cases. It does, however, assist the clinician in choosing between two immediate hypotheses at a specific clinical moment: that the patient at hand either will or will not soon attempt to commit suicide. The choice of hypothesis is governed by inference from clinical facts at hand; it is therefore a reasoned, inductive, nonintuitive choice (Sturt, 1910). It is *not* simple intuition.

Between the pinnacle of scientific certainty and the slough of intuitive guesswork lies the considerable territory of inductive clinical reasoning. The principal work that takes place on the inductive plateau is the integration of the information gathered into the context of what is known about the character of a given patient, after which certain inferences that stop short of certainty may be drawn. Researchers whose primary work is the construction and testing of suicide rating scales typically leave character variables in the background. Character traits are difficult to quantify. A variable such as "capacity to bear depression" or "impulsivity" is hard to rate. This is not to say that character-related items do not appear in the checklists; assuredly, they do. But in good clinical assessment, *all* the data gathered are examined through the lens of character. In clinical work, character phenomena are brought into the foreground, not left in the background.

Shneidman's (1985) "cubic" model of suicide is a way of integrating clinical information, and in it considerations of character are prominent. He separates three vectors that can drive a patient to suicide: press, pain, and perturbation. Under the rubric "press," he subsumes a number of events and factors—personal and external, interior and exterior—that push patients in the direction of suicide (losses, rejections, illness, and poverty are among the things he mentions as exterior factors). Press also includes the patient's reaction to such vicissitudes: "But what we are talking about mostly is the press that comes as the mind mediates (or exaggerates or even imagines) the negative press that it perceives or misperceives" (Shneidman, 1989, p. 23).

"Pain" arises from the frustration of certain basic psychological needs (for instance, needs for achievement, succorance, and avoidance of shame and humiliation) as set forth by the late Henry Murray (1938). In discussing pain in this way, Shneidman addresses the important matter of narcissistic equilibrium and reminds us of some of the ways in which it may be disturbed. Finally, he deals with "perturbation," which has two components: constriction of the cognitive and perceptual ranges, and an increased penchant for action. When the three vectors act together and reach critical intensity, suicide takes place, as Shneidman views the matter.

PSYCHODYNAMIC FORMULATION

Implicit in each of Shneidman's three vectors are matters that bear on the character of the patient under consideration. Press refers not only to the vicissitudes of the patient's journey through life—losses, humiliations, physical ills—but also specifically to the way in which he perceives or misperceives them. Psychoanalytically speaking, press must therefore depend in part on the patient's patterns of ego defense. Pain, the suffering arising from frustrated needs, plainly refers to the integrity of the patient's narcissism. Nobody can maintain an intact self in the face of unlimited emotional frustration; the capacity to tolerate emotional injury is greater or lesser, according to the patient's capacity to bear psychic pain. Perturbation, referring as it does to constriction and the patient's penchant for action, raises again the matter of defense and adaptation.

Psychodynamic formulation is an attempt to assist and stabilize the work of clinical inference. Through it, the patient's potential reaction to present stress can be put into perspective from the vantage of character. Assessing the patient's character reveals his narcissistic strengths and vulnerabilities. It arms us with an understanding of the patient's disposition to react adaptively or maladaptively (perhaps suicidally) to emotional injury, because the clinician has been at pains to see how the patient has reacted over the course of his life to a variety of injuries (Maltsberger, 1986).

When a patient is narcissistically vulnerable, the assembled stresses as described above (i.e., the p, e, and ms factors) may be expected to bring him low, possibly into the zone of suicidal danger. When a patient is narcissistically sturdy, he will be more resistant. Our risk formula may be revised to take the factor of character into account. I suggest that suicide risk is directly proportional to the sum of the p, e, and ms forces, and inversely proportional to character strength, $f(c)$.

$$R = \frac{f(e + p + ms)}{f(c)}$$

"Character strength" is very much an inferential matter; at present, its scientific quantification is beyond us. Furthermore, character is the consequence of exterior (notably familial) influences operating on the constitutionally given (biological) matrix of a developing person over a period of time. Let us begin the discussion of character by listing certain items in the now-familiar form.

Pattern of reaction to loss and separation
Vulnerability to suicide-inviting affects
Capacity to bear anxiety and depression: impulsivity
Strength of self-sustaining narcissistic capacities
   Autonomous self-esteem regulation
   Autonomous anxiety regulation
   Autonomous capacity to feel real
Reliance on exterior sustaining resources
Patterns of ego defense
Stability of reality testing
Reliability of capacity for self–object differentiation
Strength of object attachment
Reliance on fantasy, especially death fantasy

Maturation inevitably progresses across separations and losses; each person must come to terms in some way with the distancing experiences that life imposes. These begin with weaning and continue through the discovery that one's mother will not inevitably appear when called, through going to school, the surrender of parents in adolescence, and finally the losses of adulthood and old age. Sometimes, more serious and less ordinary losses are visited on a child before maturity: The mother may die; the parents may divorce. The clinician forms an estimate of how well or how ill a patient responds to loss by noticing how he has done so over the course of his life.

The case of young Ralph F (see Berman, Chapter 12, this volume), admitted to the hospital because of depression, drinking, and suicidal concerns, illustrates the point. Ralph had begun to drink at the age of 12 when his parents separated. His drinking worsened with the suicide of his aunt. The parents had separated at least eight times previously. His emotionally troubled mother was admitted to a psychiatric hospital for 2 weeks when Ralph was 5 years old. The information available is scant—we would like more—but it suggests that Ralph never developed much capacity to stand alone and hold himself together autonomously.

Psychological survival in adulthood is impossible without a modicum of self-regard and freedom from panic. It is almost impossible unless one can "feel real" (believe in one's existence) most of the time. In the ordinary course of events, adults develop sufficient capacity for autonomous regulation of self-esteem, anxiety, and the sense of personal reality to enable them to manage reasonably well when stressed (as when afflicted by loss). Their autonomous *self-sustaining capacities* are adequate. They have enough interior narcissistic reserve to hold themselves together without overreliance on exterior resources. (The term "narcissistic" can be defined as applying to inner resources, psychic structures, functions, relationships, and exterior resources that are used to preserve the integration and integrity of the self; see Stolorow, 1975.) Buie, to whom we are indebted for this theoretical development, is describing the self-sustaining resources in more detail in a forthcoming paper (Buie, 1991).

For present purposes, it is sufficient to point out that when one cannot maintain reasonable self-esteem in a neutral or even moderately unfriendly environment, and when one cannot soothe oneself sufficiently under stress, crises of self-contempt, panic, or rage may be expected. As we have seen, these may be intense enough to invite suicide. Every adult under stress grows anxious to some degree; depression is another universal experience. Commonly, anxiety and depression occur together. In assessing a patient's character, a clinician tries to learn how he may have fared in anxious or depressing past times. The clinician wants to know as much as possible about the patient's capacity to bear emotional pain without being overwhelmed. When anxiety and depression become unendurable, patients may act impulsively, fall into psychosis, or attempt suicide. What, we ask, is the characteristic reaction pattern of this particular patient (Zetzel, 1949/1970, 1965/1970)?

To the extent that the patient cannot hold together with whatever inner narcissistic resources he can command, he must look for exterior sustaining supplies to avoid getting into a narcissistic crisis (Kohut, 1971, 1977). Most of the time, narcissistically crippled patients lean on other people. In formulating a patient's psychodynamic character, a clinician will often notice that the patient has been able to hold together as long as there was somebody else available. The clinician tries to learn whether the patient must have one special person only for a buttress, or whether one *type* of person is acceptable (i.e., can the patient tolerate substitutions?). The clinician then tries to define just what functions that person (or persons) performs for the patient.

Faye C, the 49-year-old spinster who developed a psychotic depression (see Chapter 12 for more details), may have been such an externally dependent person. The illness into which she fell took place as her parents aged and their deaths neared. The patient was acutely aware that she could not hold on to them forever; we are told of no other important people in her life. There is no suggestion that the patient had ever been able to substitute anyone else for her parents. She was vulnerable to flooding with both self-loathing and terror when threatened with losing them, and she could not "feel real."

Some patients rely less on other people and more on work (or the admiration and praise that work brings) for narcissistic support. They feel good about themselves and reasonably calm as long as they can perform their self-bolstering task. José G, the 64-year-old railroad foreman (see Chapter 12), developed a depression after he hurt his hand and could no longer work. "The railroad is in my blood. I've worked and slept railroads all my life!" he said. How much he relied on his wife or children to sustain him is not clear from the record, but the vital importance of his work as a stabilizing bulwark stands out.

Murderous fury may follow the loss of vitally needed exterior sustaining resources. José was enraged at the railroad for which he had worked because it no longer appeared to esteem him. Indeed, he felt that the railroad investigator blamed him for causing his hand injury, and that the company officials dismissed his many years of loyalty as meaningless. Kohut (1972) has discussed this kind of fury, calling it "narcissistic rage"; he relates it to fantasies and schemes for revenge. José had a narcissistically vulnerable character; he depended significantly on the constancy of his work as an exterior sustaining resource. Deprived of this resource, he fell into a state of narcissistic rage that conceivably could develop into killing intensity. Suicide could follow its turning around against himself.

An important consideration that the clinicians must bear in mind when formulating the immediate risk of suicide is the degree of narcissistic shock from which the patient suffers. A vulnerable person suddenly and devastatingly deprived of supports may be so thrown out of emotional balance that suicide-forcing affect floods him. If the patient's view of possible options becomes constricted, he may commit suicide. Only a few days may suffice for recovery if the patient can remain alive long enough without being swept away by the pain. Sometimes supportive others can regroup around him, or skillful intervention can help reduce the pain enough so that narcissistic reintegration can occur.

At this juncture we may turn to the next item on the list of character aspects—patterns of ego defense. To the extent that any depressed person is self-hating, we may infer that anger is being turned against the self. More primitive patients are likely to turn to denial, distortion, and projection at times of crisis in order to assign the blame for what to them is an intolerable situation to somebody or something else. José chose the inspector and the officers of the railroad. Distortion is obvious here. The inspector, alert that some employees wanting to "go on disability" deliberately hurt themselves, asked pointed questions; he may have been suspicious: José convinced himself that the inspector was accusing him and distorted the difference. The protocol in Chapter 12 does not suggest that denial played a major part in José's thinking (he did not, for instance, convince himself that his injury was trifling and that he could return to work in a week or two). There is, however, evidence for projection. José attributed much of his anger to the railroad officials. He convinced himself that they bore him serious animus, when in reality they were guilty of no more than ordinary insensitive bureaucratic indifference.

The patient in a narcissistic rage with a tendency to distort, deny, and project will have difficulty separating fact from fiction. With fragile reality-testing capacity, such a person is likely to develop delusions, whether transient or fixed. If the capacity to distinguish where the self leaves off and another person begins is disturbed, the patient may develop the idea that he (1) can read the minds of others (or that others can read his mind); (2) can discern secret motives in the minds of others; or (3) can tell that others want him dead. A past history of psychosis, however brief, alerts us to the possibility that the patient may become fantasy-driven when under stress. The patient Faye was obviously such a person; she described a wide variety of omnipotent delusions. She asserted that the intake interviewer was a malignant magician, for instance. Fantasy-driven patients can become suicidal when an emotionally powerful daydream of rejoining a lost person through death preoccupies them.

A patient who can make and maintain attachments to others will rely less on fantasy for comfort than on real relationships. Good capacity for relatedness protects against suicide; constricted attachments to others invite it. Unfortunately, when depressive illness is sufficiently intense, the patient may abandon belief in the love and constancy of others, or may develop a conviction that they would be better off without him. Affiliative characters are less likely to commit suicide than solitary ones, unless the affiliative persons depend excessively on their relationships with others for exterior sustaining support. Narcissistic affiliations protect against suicide also, but the loss of a critical relationship of that kind can precipitate a crisis.

Only some of the considerations that a clinician takes into account in constructing a psychodynamic formulation lend themselves to numerical quantification. A skillful clinician can readily say, however, whether any given factor is present or absent. We can systematically look over the data of the clinical history and mental status examination to estimate (if not to measure) a variety of phenomena. The clinician can say, for instance, that factor *x* is absent, minimally at work, moderately at work, or strongly at work. This is quantification of a sort, although it is subjective and inexact.

Clinical inductive work differs from simple intuition in a number of respects. First of all, it searches out which exterior stressors are present or absent in the patient's current life. Then it takes note of the patient's specific narcissistic vulnerabilities. These are identified by an examination of the patient's lifetime reaction patterns to emotional stress and injuries, especially losses and separations. Furthermore, it surveys what exterior sustaining resources the patient has required in the past to avoid emotional crises, or to extricate himself from them when they occur. Formulation also takes into account whether the exterior sustaining resources the patient needs are available or not available in the present difficulty; whether they are likely to be lost; or, if they are lost, whether they are likely to be restored. Finally, it gauges the severity of the patient's present suffering and ventures to predict whether it is likely to worsen or improve, with special reference to the presence of fatigue and hopelessness.

REFERENCES

Abrams, H. S., Moore, G. L., & Westervelt, F. B. (1971). Suicidal behavior in chronic dialysis patients. *American Journal of Psychiatry, 127,* 1199–1204.

Adler, G., & Buie, D. H. (1979). Aloneness and borderline psychopathology: The possible relevance of child developmental issues. *International Journal of Psycho-Analysis, 60,* 83–96.

Baechler, J. (1979). *Suicides* (B. Cooper, Trans.). New York: Basic Books. (Original work published 1975)

Barraclough, B., Bunch, J., Nelson, B., & Sainsbury, P. (1974). A hundred cases of suicide: Clinical aspects. *British Journal of Psychiatry, 125,* 355–373.

Barraclough, B. M., & Hughes, J. (1987). *Suicide: Clinical and epidemiological studies.* London: Croom Helm.

Beres, D., Eissler, R., Freud, A., & Glover, E. (1951). Vicissitudes of superego function and superego precursors in childhood. *Psychoanalytic Study of the Child, 13,* 324–351.

Black, D. W., Winokur, G., & Nasrallah, A. (1988). Effect of psychosis on suicide risk in 1593 patients with unipolar and bipolar affective disorders. *American Journal of Psychiatry, 145,* 849–852.

Buie, D. H. (1991). *Essential self-sustaining functions*. Manuscript in preparation.

Bunch, J., & Barraclough, B. M. (1971). The influence of parental death anniversaries upon suicide dates. *British Journal of Psychiatry, 118*, 621-626.

Bunch, J., Barraclough, B. M., Nelson, B., & Sainsbury, P. (1971). Suicide following bereavement of parents. *Social Psychiatry, 6*, 193-199.

Clark, D. C. (in press). Suicide risk assessment and prediction in the 1990s. *Crisis*.

Cohen, E., Motto, J., & Seiden, R. (1966). An instrument for evaluating suicide potential: A preliminary study. *American Journal of Psychiatry, 122*, 886-891.

Crook, T., & Raskin, A. (1975). Association of childhood parental loss with attempted suicide and depression. *Journal of Consulting and Clinical Psychology, 43*, 277.

Cross, C. K., & Hirschfeld, R. M. A. (1986). Psychosocial factors and suicidal behavior: Life events, early loss, and personality. *Annals of the New York Academy of Sciences, 487*, 77-89.

Dorpat, T. L., & Ripley, H. S. (1960). A study of suicide in the Seattle area. *Comprehensive Psychiatry, 1*, 349-359.

Dorpat, T. L., & Ripley, H. S. (1967). The relationship between attempted suicide and committed suicide. *Comprehensive Psychiatry, 8*, 74-79.

Durkheim, E. (1951). *Suicide: A study in sociology* (J. A. Spaulding & G. Simpson, Trans.). Glencoe, IL: Free Press. (Original work published 1897)

Fawcett, J., Scheftner, W. A., Clark, D. C., Hedeker, D., Gibbons, R., & Coryell, W. (1987). Clinical predictors of suicide in patients with major affective disorders: A controlled prospective study. *American Journal of Psychiatry, 144*, 35-40.

Fawcett, J., Scheftner, W. A., Fogg, L., Clark, D. C., Young, M. A., Hedeker, D., & Gibbons, R. (1990). Time related predictors of suicide in major affective disorder. *American Journal of Psychiatry, 147*, 1189-1194.

Fedden, H. R. (1938). *Suicide: A social and historical study*. London: Peter Davies.

Fox, B. H., Stanek, E. J., Boyd, S. C., & Flannery, J. T. (1982). Suicide rates among cancer patients in Connecticut. *Journal of Chronic Disease, 35*, 89-100.

Friedlander, K. (1940). On the longing to die. *International Journal of Psycho-Analysis, 21*, 416-426.

Goodwin, J. (1982). *Sexual abuse: Incest victims and their families*. Littleton, MA: PSG.

Goodwin, J., Cheeves, K., & Connell, V. (1988). Defining a syndrome of severe symptoms in survivors of extreme incestuous abuse. *Dissociation, 1*, 11-16.

Gove, P. B. (Ed.). (1969). *Webster's third new international dictionary of the English language unabridged*. Springfield, MA: G. & C. Merriam.

Haenel, T., Brunner, F., & Gattegay, R. (1980). Renal dialysis and suicide: Occurrence in Switzerland and in Europe. *Comprehensive Psychiatry, 21*, 140-145.

Hellerstein, D., Frosch, W., & Koenigsberg, H. W. (1987). The clinical significance of command hallucinations. *American Journal of Psychiatry, 144*, 219-221.

Huston, P. E., & Locher, L. M. (1948a). Involutional psychosis—course when untreated and when treated with electric shock. *Archives of Neurology and Psychiatry, 59*, 385-394.

Huston, P. E., & Locher, L. M. (1948b). Manic depressive psychosis—course when treated and untreated with electric shock. *Archives of Neurology and Psychiatry, 60*, 37-48.

Jaffe, P., Wolfe, D., Wilson, S. K., & Zak, L. (1986). Family violence and child adjustment: A comparative analysis of girls' and boys' behavioral symptoms. *American Journal of Psychiatry, 143,* 74-77.

Kety, S. (1986). Genetic factors in suicide. In A. Roy (Ed.), *Suicide* (pp. 41-45). Baltimore: Williams & Wilkins.

Kohut, H. (1971). *The analysis of the self.* New York: International Universities Press.

Kohut, H. (1972). Thoughts on narcissism and narcissistic rage. *Psychoanalytic Study of the Child, 27,* 360-400.

Kohut, H. (1977). *The restoration of the self.* New York: International Universities Press.

Kullgren, H. (1988). Factors associated with completed suicide in borderline personality disorder. *Journal of Nervous and Mental Disease, 176,* 40-44.

Kullgren, G., Renberg, E., & Jacobsson, L. (1986). An empirical study of borderline personality disorder and psychiatric suicides. *Journal of Nervous and Mental Disease, 174,* 328-331.

Litman, R. E., Farberow, N. L., Wold, C. I., & Brown, T. R. (1986). Prediction models of suicidal behaviors. In A. T. Beck, H. L. P. Resnik, & D. J. Lettieri (Eds.), *The prediction of suicide* (2nd ed., pp. 141-162). Philadelphia: Charles Press.

Louhivuori, K. A., & Hakama, M. (1979). Risk of suicide among cancer patients. *American Journal of Epidemiology, 109,* 59-65.

Lowry, M. R. (1979). Frequency of depressive disorder in patients entering home dialysis. *Journal of Nervous and Mental Disease, 167,* 199-204.

Maltsberger, J. T. (1986). *Suicide risk: The formulation of clinical judgment.* New York: New York University Press.

Maltsberger, J. T., & Buie, D. H. (1980). The devices of suicide: Revenge, riddance and rebirth. *International Review of Psychoanalysis, 7,* 61-72.

Maris, R. W. (1969). *Social forces in urban suicide.* Homewood, IL: Dorsey Press.

Maris, R. W. (1989). The social relations of suicide. In D. Jacobs, & H. N. Brown (Eds.), *Suicide: Understanding and responding* (pp. 87-125). Madison, CT: International Universities Press.

McGlashan, T. H. (1983). The "we-self" in borderline patients: Manifestations of the symbiotic self-object in psychotherapy. *Psychiatry, 46,* 351-361.

Minkoff, K., Bergman, E., Beck A. T., & Beck, R. (1973). Hopelessness, depression and attempted suicide. *American Journal of Psychiatry, 130,* 455-459.

Moss, L., & Hamilton, D. (1956). The psychotherapy of the suicidal patient. *American Journal of Psychiatry, 112,* 814.

Motto, J. A. (1965). Suicide attempts: A longitudinal view. *Archives of General Psychiatry, 13,* 516-520.

Motto, J. A. (1989). Problems in suicide risk assessment. In D. Jacobs & H. N. Brown (Eds.), *Suicide: Understanding and responding* (pp. 129-142). Madison, CT: International Universities Press.

Murray, H. A. (1938). *Explorations in personality.* New York: Oxford University Press.

Pfeffer, C. R. (1986). *The suicidal child.* New York: Guilford Press.

Phillips, D. P. (1974). The influence of suggestion on suicide. *American Sociological Review, 39,* 340-354.

Pokorny, A. D. (1983). Prediction of suicide in psychiatric patients: Report of a prospective study. *Archives of General Psychiatry, 40,* 249-257.

Richman, J. (1986). *Family therapy for suicidal people.* New York: Springer.

Robins, E. (1981). *The final months.* New York: Oxford University Press.

Robins, E., Murphy, G. E., Wilkinson, R. H., Jr., Gassner, S., & Kayes, J. (1959). Some clinical considerations in the prevention of suicide based on a study of 134 successful suicides. *American Journal of Public Health, 49,* 888-899.

Roose, S. P., Glassman, A. H., Walsh, B. T., Woodring, S., & Vital-Herne, J. (1983). Depression, delusions, and suicide. *American Journal of Psychiatry, 140,* 1159-1162.

Rosen, A. (1954). Detection of suicidal patients: An example of some limitations in the prediction of infrequent events. *Journal of Consulting Psychology, 18,* 397-407.

Roy, A. (1983). Family history of suicide. *Archives of General Psychiatry, 40,* 971-974.

Sabbath, J. C. (1969). The suicidal adolescent—the expendable child. *Journal of the American Academy of Child Psychiatry, 8,* 272-289.

Sainsbury, P. (1955). *Suicide in London: An ecological study.* London: Chapman & Hall.

Sainsbury, P. (1986). The epidemiology of suicide. In A. Roy (Ed.), *Suicide* (pp. 17-40). Baltimore: Williams & Wilkins.

Shafii, M., Carrigan, S., Whittinghill, J., & Derrick, A. (1985). Psychological autopsy of completed suicide in children and adolescents. *American Journal of Psychiatry, 142,* 1061-1064.

Shneidman, E. S. (1985). *Definition of suicide.* New York: Wiley.

Shneidman, E. S. (1986). Some essentials of suicide and some implications for response. In A. Roy (Ed.), *Suicide* (pp. 1-16). Baltimore: Williams & Wilkins.

Shneidman, E. S. (1989). Overview: A multidimensional approach to suicide. In D. Jacobs & H. N. Brown (Eds.), *Suicide: Understanding and responding* (pp. 1-30). Madison, CT: International Universities Press.

Stolorow, R. D. (1975). Toward a functional definition of narcissism. *International Journal of Psycho-Analysis, 56,* 179-185.

Stone, M. H. (1990). *The fate of borderline patients.* New York: Guilford Press.

Straus, M. A., Gelles, R. J., & Steinmetz, S. K. (1980). *Behind closed doors: Violence in the American family.* Garden City, NY: Doubleday/Anchor.

Styron, W. (1990). *Darkness visible: A memoir of madness.* New York: Random House.

Sturt, H. (1910). Induction. In H. Chisholm (Ed.), *Encyclopaedia Britannica* (11th ed., Vol. 14, p. 503). Cambridge, England: Cambridge University Press.

Tsuang, M. T., Dempsey, G. M., & Fleming, J. A. (1979). Can ECT prevent premature death and suicide in schizoaffective patients? *Journal of Affective Disorders, 1,* 167-171.

Tuckman, J., & Youngman, W. F. (1968). A scale for assessing suicidal risk in attempted suicide. *Journal of Clinical Psychology, 24,* 17-19.

Weisman, A., & Worden, J. W. (1986). Risk-rescue rating in suicide assessment. In A. T. Beck, H. L. P. Resnik, & D. J. Lettieri (Eds.), *The prediction of suicide* (2nd ed., pp. 193-213). Philadelphia: Charles Press.

Whitlock, F. A. (1986). Suicide and physical illness. In A. Roy (Ed.), *Suicide* (pp. 151–170). Baltimore: Williams & Wilkins.

Wolfersdorf, M., Keller, F., Steiner, B., & Hole, G. (1987). Delusional depression and suicide. *Acta Psychiatrica Scandinavica, 76,* 359–363.

Yates, A. (1987). Psychological damage associated with extreme eroticism in young children. *Psychiatric Annals, 17,* 257–261.

Yufit, R., & Benzies, B. (1973). Assessing suicide potential by time perspective. *Suicide and Life-Threatening Behavior, 3,* 270–282.

Zetzel, E. R. (1970). Anxiety and the capacity to bear it. In E. R. Zetzel, *The capacity for emotional growth* (pp. 33–52). London: Hogarth Press. (Original work published 1949)

Zetzel, E. (1970). On the incapacity to bear depression. In E. R. Zetzel, *The capacity for emotional growth* (pp. 82–114). London: Hogarth Press. (Original work published 1965)

Zilboorg, G. (1936). Differential diagnostic types of suicide. *Archives of Neurology and Psychiatry, 35,* 270–291.

CHAPTER 3

A Conspectus
of the Suicidal Scenario

Edwin S. Shneidman, Ph.D.
University of California at Los Angeles

THE EXPERIENCE OF SUICIDE:
ACCOUNTS OF THREE CASES

Let us consider some verbatim excerpts from the case transcripts of three "failed suicides"—each of whom performed an act that is ordinarily fatal, and fortuitously, against all realistic odds, survived to tell us something about the inside view of the suicidal scenario. What are the common threads of psychological gold and silver in the ore and slag of these heated reports? Both as a preview to all of the following text and as a guide to the proactive reading of the three excerpts, let us keep in mind these half-dozen key words (to be defined and discussed in this chapter): "pain," "needs," "frustration" (of needs), "constriction," "ambivalence," and "cessation" (of pain).

> *Immolator:* I remember sitting in the car, and it was sort of like a blank in my mind. I felt very calm. I felt a kind of hush over my body. That everything was going to be OK. And I remember then pouring the gasoline first over the front seat, and of course over myself to a great extent. Even then, no thoughts went through my head at all of the pain that it was going to entail, the misery, hurt, any of that. I guess I didn't think that burns would really hurt, but none of that went through my head. It just felt good. It was the first time, in fact, that I had felt at peace, that I wasn't hurting inside. And for once it seemed like I had taken care of my problems and that my pain would just go away. It was not going to exist any more, especially my mental pain. And I remember very slowly striking the match and at that moment the fumes ignited, just a tremendous explosion.

Portions of this chapter have previously appeared in other publications (Shneidman, 1973, 1980, 1984, 1986, 1987, 1989, 1990).

Jumper: I was so desperate, I felt, My God, I can't face this thing. Everything was like a terrible whirlpool of confusion. And I thought to myself, There's only one thing to do: I just have to lose consciousness. That's the only way to get away from it. The only way to lose consciousness, I thought, was to jump off something good and high. I just figured I had to get outside. I just slipped out. No one saw me. And I got to the other building by walking across that catwalk thing, sure that someone would see me, you know, out of all those windows. The whole building is made of glass. And I just walked around until I found this open staircase. And as soon as I saw it, I just made a beeline right up to it. And then I got to the fifth floor and everything got very dark all of a sudden, and all I could see was this balcony. Everything around it just blacked out. It was just like a circle. That was all I could see, just the balcony. I climbed over it and I just let go. I was so desperate.

Shooter: There was no peace to be found. I had done all I could and was still sinking. I sat many hours seeking answers and all, but there was a silent wind and no answers. The answer was in my head. It was all clear now: Die. The next day a friend of mine offered to sell me a shotgun. I bought it. My first thought was What a mess this is going to make. The next day I began to say goodbye to people. Not actually saying it, but expressing it silently. I didn't sleep. The dreams were reality and reality dreams. One by one I turned off my outside channels to the world. My mind became locked on my target. My thoughts were Soon it will all be over. I can obtain the peace I have sought so long for. The will to survive and succeed had been crushed and defeated. I was like a general alone on a battlefield being encroached upon by my enemy and its hordes: fear, hate, self-depreciation, desolation. I felt I had to have the upper hand, to control my environment, so I sought to die rather than surrender. Destiny and reality began to merge. Those around me were as shadows, apparitions, but I was not actually conscious of them, only aware of myself and my plight. Death swallowed me long before I pulled the trigger. I was locked within myself. The world through my eyes seemed to die with me. It was like I was to push the final button to end this world. I committed myself to the arms of Death. There comes a time when all things cease to shine, when the rays of hope are lost. As I look back on that day it is as if this was another person's life. I was ending. I placed the gun under my chin. Then I remember a tremendous explosion of lights like fireworks consumed within a brilliant radiance. Thus did the pain become glorious, becoming an army rallied to the side of death to help destroy my life which I could feel leaving my body with each rushing surge of blood. I was engulfed in total darkness.

It is possible to conceptualize the commonalities of these (and all other) suicides in terms of the basic and omnipresent elements of the suicidal scenario—a "conspectus" of suicide, as it were. These fundamentals are as follows:

1. A sense of unbearable psychological *pain,* which is directly related to thwarted psychological *needs.*

2. Traumatizing *self-denigration*—a self-image that will not include tolerating intense psychological pain.
3. A marked *constriction* of the mind and an unrealistic narrowing of life's actions.
4. A sense of *isolation*—a feeling of desertion and the loss of support of significant others.
5. An overwhelmingly desperate feeling of *hopelessness*—a sense that nothing effective can be done.
6. A conscious decision that *egression*—leaving, exiting, or stopping life—is the *only* (or at least the best possible) solution to the problem of unbearable pain.

All these elements combine to result in suicide.

THE 10 COMMONALITIES OF SUICIDE

In previous publications (Shneidman, 1985, 1986, 1987, 1989, 1990b), I have referred to "the 10 commonalities of suicide"—specifically, the common psychological features in human self-destruction. They are reproduced in Table 3.1 and are discussed briefly below. But first, a few preliminary remarks.

Suicidal phenomena can be understood in various ways. (I discuss these different approaches at the end of the chapter.) Clearly, one of the principal ways is the psychological approach, and the key to the psychological understanding of suicide is *pain*—psychological pain, the pain that the suicidal individual feels in *that* situation in his or her life. In this sense, suicide is a

TABLE 3.1. The 10 Commonalities of Suicide

I. The common purpose of suicide is to seek a solution.	VI. The common cognitive state in suicide is ambivalence.
II. The common goal of suicide is cessation of consciousness.	VII. The common perceptual state in suicide is constriction.
III. The common stimulus in suicide is intolerable psychological pain.	VIII. The common action in suicide is egression.
IV. The common stressor in suicide is frustrated psychological needs.	IX. The common interpersonal act in suicide is communication of intention.
V. The common emotion in suicide is hopelessness–helplessness.	X. The common consistency in suicide is with lifelong coping patterns.

Note. From *Definition of Suicide* (pp. 121–149) by E. S. Shneidman, 1985, New York: Wiley. Copyright 1985 by Edwin S. Shneidman.

practical act intended to stop to unbearable flow (in consciousness) of intolerable pain. As Murray (1938) says in his great book, *Explorations in Personality*, suicide is clearly not adaptive, but it is just as clearly uniquely adjustive. Similarly, Baechler (1975/1979), in his intensive book-length essay on suicide, tells us that in order to understand a specific case of suicide we must know what problem it was intended to solve. And Kelly (1961), in a way that is both philosophical and psychological, views suicide by proposing that each individual has his or her own private (unique, idiosyncratic) epistemology—his or her personal construct of the world—and that a suicide is to be understood as that individual's efforts to validate this personal construct.

Let us now consider the 10 psychological commonalities of suicide (see Table 3.1), together with some illustrative quotations from the three suicidal vignettes presented above:

I. The common purpose of suicide is to seek a solution. First of all, suicide is not a random, pointless, or purposeless act. To the sufferer, it seems to be the only available answer to a real puzzler: "How am I to get out of this? What am I to do?" Its purpose is to seek a solution to a perceived crisis—the problem of overwhelming pain—that is generating intense suffering. To understand what a suicide is about, one must know the psychological problems it was intended to resolve. The general question one must put to the suicidal person is this: "What is going on?"

Excerpts: "And for once it seemed like I had taken care of my problems."

"And I thought to myself, 'There's only one thing to do . . .'"

"The answer was in my head."

II: The common goal of suicide is cessation of consciousness. Suicide is both a moving toward and a moving away. The common practical goal of suicide is the stopping of the painful flow of consciousness. Suicide is best understood not so much as a movement toward a reified Death as it is in terms of "cessation"—the complete (and irreversible) stopping of one's consciousness of unendurable pain. Suicide, as R. E. Litman (personal communication, 1990) points out, involves not only pain, but the individual's unwillingness to tolerate that pain, the decision not to endure it, and the active will to stop it. This means that in psychotherapy one needs to focus on the amelioration of the pain, as well as the "character" that has chosen not to tolerate it.

Excerpts: "It [the mental pain] was not going to exist any more."

"I felt, 'My God, I can't face this thing. . . . I just have to lose consciousness.'"

"'Die. . . . Soon it will all be over.'"

III. The common stimulus in suicide is unendurable psychological pain. In any close analysis, suicide is best understood as a combined movement toward cessation *and* a movement away from intolerable, unendurable, unacceptable anguish. It is psychological pain of which I am speaking: "metapain," the pain of feeling pain. From a traditional psychodynamic view, hostility, shame, guilt, fear, protest, longing to join a deceased loved one, and the like have singly and in combination been identified as the root factor(s) in suicide. It is none of these; rather, it is the pain involved in any or all of them, together with the unwillingness to endure that idiosyncratically defined pain. Psychological pain is the center of suicide and constitutes the chief hurdle that must be lowered before any kind of therapy can be effectively life-saving. The basic clinical rule is this: If the level of suffering is reduced (often just a little bit), the individual can choose to live.

Excerpts: "It was the first time . . . that I wasn't hurting inside. And for once it seemed . . . the [mental] pain would just go away."

"I was so desperate."

"'I can obtain the peace I have sought so long for.'"

IV. The common stressor in suicide is frustrated psychological needs. The psychological pain that is central to suicide is driven, created by, and sustained by frustrated, blocked, or thwarted psychological needs. Suicide is best understood not so much as an unreasonable act—every suicide seems logical to the person who commits it (given that person's major premises, styles of syllogizing, and constricted focus)—as it is a reaction to unfulfilled psychological needs.

In order to understand suicide in this kind of context, we need to ask a much broader question, which I believe is the key: What purposes do most human acts (including suicide) intend to accomplish? The best nondetailed answer to that question is that, in general, human acts are intended to satisfy a variety of human needs. There is no compelling *a priori* reason why a typology (or classification or taxonomy) of suicidal acts might not parallel a general classification of human needs. Such a classification of psychological needs can be found in Murray's *Explorations in Personality* (1938). Murray's discussion of human needs is a ready-made, viable taxonomy of the essential underpinnings of suicidal behaviors. Table 3.2 presents a partial listing of Murray's explication of psychological needs.

Most suicides represent combinations of various needs, so that a particular case of suicide may properly be understood in terms of two or more different need categories. There are many pointless deaths, but never a needless suicide. If the frustrated needs are addressed, the pain they cause will be lessened, and the suicide will not occur. The therapist's function is to decrease the patient's acute discomfort and to increase the patient's comfort.

One way to operationalize this task is to focus on the thwarted needs. Questions such as "Where do you hurt?" can be useful in clarifying the suicidal picture.

The assessment of needs related to suicide may be a more complicated epistemological task than the identification of the other commonalities of suicide. Psychological needs are more conceptual and abstract, and there is more inference necessary to name them. One requires access to a detailed anamnestic record or case history for the raw data from which inferences can reasonably be made. In the case of the shooter whose words are quoted above, I have concluded that the half-dozen most important needs (see Table 3.2) related to his suicidal state were the needs for dominance, autonomy, counteraction, succorance, affiliation, and order. These constitute a quite different constellation of vital psychological needs from the frustrated needs that ignited the immolator or those that pushed the jumper. I should note also that the use of the language of psychological needs immediately and radically changes the way in which one then conceptualizes that individual's suicidal behavior and in which one can think of ways to help the suicidal person.

> *Excerpts:* "I was like a general . . . being encroached upon by my enemy and its hordes: fear, hate, self-depreciation, desolation."

V. The common emotion in suicide is helplessness-hopelessness. In the suicidal state, there is a pervasive feeling of helplessness-hopelessness: "There is nothing I can do [except to commit suicide] and there is no one who can help me [with the pain that I am suffering]." Underlying all of the emotions—hostility, guilt, shame—is the emotion of impotent ennui, the feeling of helplessness-hopelessness. The most effective way to reduce the elevated lethality is to reduce the elevated perturbation of which the feelings of helplessness-hopelessness are an integral part.

> *Excerpts:* "There comes a time when all things cease to shine, when the rays of hope are lost."

VI. The common cognitive state in suicide is ambivalence. The (non-Aristotelian) accommodation to the psychological realities of mental life—simultaneous contradictory feelings (such as love and hate toward the same person)—is called "ambivalence." It is the common internal attitude toward suicide: to feel that one has to do it, and at the same time to yearn (even to plan) for rescue and intervention. The therapist uses this ambivalence, and plays for time so that the affect rather than the bullet can be discharged.

> *Excerpts:* "[I was] sure that someone would see me [and rescue me] . . . The whole building is made of glass."

TABLE 3.2. A Partial Listing of the Murray Psychological Needs

Abasement. To submit passively to external force. To accept injury, blame, criticism, punishment. To surrender. To become resigned to fate. To admit inferiority, error, wrongdoing, or defeat. To confess and atone. To blame, belittle, or mutilate the self. To seek and enjoy pain, punishment, illness, and misfortune.

Achievement. To accomplish something difficult. To master, manipulate, or organize physical objects, human beings, or ideas. To do this as rapidly and independently as possible. To overcome obstacles and attain a high standard. To excel oneself. To rival and surpass others. To increase self-regard by the successful exercise of talent.

Affiliation. To draw near and enjoyably cooperate or reciprocate with an allied other (who resembles the subject or who likes the subject). To please and win affection of a respected person. To adhere and remain loyal to a friend.

Aggression. To overcome opposition forcefully. To fight. To attack or injure another. To oppose forcefully or punish another.

Autonomy. To get free, shake off restraint, break out of social confinement. To resist coercion and restriction. To avoid or quit activities prescribed by domineering authorities. To be independent and free to act according to desires. To defy convention.

Counteraction. To master or make up for a failure by restriving. To obliterate a humiliation by resumed action. To overcome weakness; to repress fear. To efface a dishonor by action. To seek for obstacles and difficulties to overcome. To maintain self-respect and pride on a high level.

Defendance. To defend the self against assault, criticism, or blame. To conceal or justify a misdeed, failure, or humiliation. To vindicate the ego.

Deference. To admire and support a superior. To praise, honor, or eulogize. To yield eagerly to the influence of an allied other. To emulate an exemplar. To conform to custom.

Dominance. To control one's human environment. To influence or direct the behavior of others by suggestion, seduction, persuasion, or command. To dissuade, restrain, or prohibit.

Exhibition. To make an impression. To be seen and heard. To excite, amaze, fascinate, entertain, shock, intrigue, amuse, or entice others.

Harmavoidance. To avoid pain, physical injury, illness, and death. To escape from a dangerous situation. To take precautionary measures.

Infavoidance. To avoid humiliation. To quit embarrassing situations. To avoid conditions that lead to scorn, derision, or indifference of others. To refrain from action because of fear of failure.

Inviolacy. To protect the self. To remain separate. To resist attempts of others to intrude upon or invade one's own psychological space. To maintain a psychological distance. To be isolated, reticent, concealed, immune from criticism.

Nurturance. To give sympathy and gratify the needs of another person, especially an infant or someone who is weak, disabled, tired, inexperienced, infirm, defeated, humiliated, lonely, rejected, sick, or mentally confused. To feed, help, support, console, protect, comfort, nurse, heal; to nurture.

Order. To put things or ideas in order. To achieve arrangement, organization, balance, tidiness, and precision among things in the outer world or ideas in the inner world.

Play. To act for "fun" without further purpose. To like to laugh and make jokes. To enjoy relaxation of stress. To participate in pleasurable activities for their own sake.

TABLE 3.2. (*continued*)

Rejection. To separate oneself from a negatively viewed person. To exclude, abandon, expel, or remain indifferent to an inferior person. To snub or jilt another.

Sentience. To seek and enjoy sensuous experience. To give an important place to creature comforts of taste, touch, and the other senses.

Succorance. To have one's needs gratified by the sympathetic aid of another person. To be nursed, supported, sustained, protected, loved, advised, guided, indulged, forgiven, consoled, taken care of. To remain close to a devoted protector. To have a supporter.

Understanding. To ask and answer questions. To be interested in theory. To speculate, formulate, analyze, and generalize. To want to know the answers to general questions.

Note. Adapted from *Explorations in Personality* (pp. 142–242) by H. A. Murray, 1938, New York: Oxford University Press. Copyright 1938 by Oxford University Press. Adapted by permission.

VII. The common perceptual state in suicide is constriction. Suicide is not best understood as a psychosis, a neurosis, or a character disorder (100% of suicides are highly perturbed). It is more accurately seen as a more or less transient psychological constriction of affect and intellect. A synonym for "constriction" would be a "tunneling" or "focusing" or "narrowing" of the range of options usually available to that individual's consciousness when the mind is not panicked into dichotomous thinking: either some specific (almost magical) good solution or cessation; *Caesar aut nihil*; all or nothing. The range of life choices has narrowed to two—not very much of a range. The usual life-sustaining images of loved ones are not even within the mind. The fact that suicide is committed by individuals who are in a special constricted condition suggests that no one should ever commit suicide while disturbed. It takes a mind capable of scanning a range of options greater than two to make a decision as important as taking one's life. At the outset, it is vital to counter the suicidal person's constriction of thought by widening the mental blinders and increasing the number of options beyond only two dichotomous options of either achieving a magical resolution or being dead. The dangerous word that the therapist must be alert for is the word "only."

> *Excerpts:* "[It] was sort of like a blank in my mind. . . . I didn't think that burns would really hurt . . ."
>
> "'There's only one thing to do . . . That's the only way . . .' The only way to lose consciousness, I thought, was to jump off something good and high. . . . [E]verything got dark all of a sudden . . . Everything around it just blacked out. It was just like a circle. That was all I could see . . ."
>
> "My mind became locked on my target. . . . I sought to die rather than surrender."

VIII. The common action in suicide is egression. "Egression" or escape is a person's intended departure from a region of distress. Suicide is the ultimate egression, besides which all others (running away from home, quitting a job, deserting an army, leaving a spouse) pale. The therapist needs to give the person other exits, other ways of doing something. (The therapist and those close to the patient also need to close a possible lethal exit by, for example, removing a gun.) This notion is very much related to expanding the patient's constriction.

Excerpts: "It [I] was not going to exist any more . . ."
"'I just have to lose consciousness.'"
"I committed myself to the arms of Death."

IX. The common interpersonal act in suicide is communication of intention. Perhaps the most interesting finding from large numbers of psychological autopsies of suicidal deaths is that in most cases (80%) there were clear verbal or behavioral clues to the impending lethal event. Individuals who are intent on committing suicide (albeit ambivalent about it) consciously or unconsciously emit signals of distress, whimpers of helplessness, or pleas for response; or they provide opportunities for rescue in the usually dyadic interplay that is an integral part of the suicidal drama. The common interpersonal act of suicide is paradoxical communication of intention with the usual verbal and behavioral clues.

Excerpt: "The next day I began to say goodbye to people."

X. The common consistency in suicide is with lifelong coping patterns. In suicide, one may be initially thrown off the scent because suicide is an act that, by definition, that individual has never committed before; thus, there seems to be no precedent. And yet there are some deep consistencies with lifelong coping patterns. The therapist must look at previous episodes of deep perturbation, distress, duress, and threat, and at the person's capacity to endure psychological pain, for patterns of egression in that person's life.

Excerpt: "I felt I had to have the upper hand, to control my environment, so I sought to die rather than surrender."

A THEORETICAL MODEL OF SUICIDE

It is now possible to combine these 10 items into a more succinct theoretical model. Let us imagine a cube (see Figure 3.1) made up of 125 cubelets, with

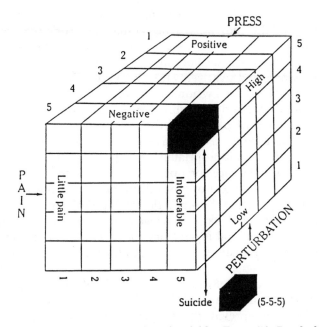

FIGURE 3.1. A theoretical cubic model of suicide. From "A Psychological Approach to Suicide" by E. S. Shneidman, 1987, in G. R. VandenBos and B. K. Bryant (Eds.), *Cataclysms, Crises and Catastrophes: Psychology in Action*. Washington, DC: American Psychological Association. Copyright 1987 by the American Psychological Association. Reprinted by permission.

25 squares on a plane, and 5 cubelets in each row and each column. I call these three faces of the cube (and the three corresponding components of this theoretical model) "pain," "perturbation," and "press," which are defined as follows:

1. *Pain.* "Pain," represented on the front of the cube, refers to the psychological pain resulting from thwarted psychological needs. The leftmost column of cubelets represents little or no pain, the next column some bearable pain, and so on until the rightmost column, which represents intolerable psychological pain.

2. *Perturbation.* "Perturbation," assigned to the side plane of the large cube, is a general term meaning the state of being upset or perturbed. Ranked here on a 5-point rating scale, perturbation includes everything in the *Diagnostic and Statistical Manual of Mental Disorders*, third edition, revised (DSM-III-R; American Psychiatric Association, 1987). In relation to suicide, perturbation includes (a) perceptual constriction, and (b) a pen-

chant for precipitous self-harm or inimical action. "Constriction" refers to the reduction of the individual's perceptual and cognitive range. At its worst, the individual reduces the viable options to two, and then to one. On this plane in the cube, the bottom row reflects open-mindedness, wide mentational scope, and relatively clear thinking. The top row reflects constriction of thought, tunnel vision, and a narrowing of focus to few options, with cessation, death, and egression as one (and ultimately the only) solution to the problem of pain and frustrated needs. "Penchant for action" refers to something akin to impulsiveness—a tendency to get things over with; to bring them inappropriately to a quick resolution; to have little patience and low tolerance for open and stressful situations; to jump to conclusions; and to jump at opportunities for more immediate resolution. The column of cubelets at the rear reflects a high tolerance for ambiguity, a capacity for patience and waiting. As we move forward (toward us) on this plane, we come closer to this tendency for precipitous and consummatory action, this lethal impulsivity. That is what the foremost column on the side plane represents.

3. *Press.* Murray (1938) may have had the word "pressure" in mind when he decided to use the word "press" ("press" is both the singular and the plural form) to represent those aspects of the inner and outer world or environment that impinge on, move, touch, or affect the individual and make a difference. The term refers to the things done *to* the individual (and the way they are incorporated and interpreted), to which he or she reacts. There is positive press (good genes and happy fortune), and there is negative press (conditions or events that perturb, threaten, stress, or harm the individual). It is the latter that are relevant to suicide. Press includes both actual and imagined events, in the sense that everything is mediated by the mind. In this cubic model, press ranges from positive (in the back row of the top plane) to negative (in the front row of the top plane).

In this theoretical cube of 125 cubelets, there is only one cubelet that is numbered 5-5-5. Not every individual who is in a 5-5-5 cubelet commits suicide—he or she may commit homicide, or go crazy, or become amnesic, or destroy a career—but in this conceptual model no one commits suicide *except* those in the 5-5-5 cubelet (maximum pain, maximum perturbation, maximum negative press). The implications for therapy and life-saving redress would seem to be obvious: Reduce any of these three dimensions from a 5 to a 4 (or less); preferably, reduce all three. Individuals can lead long, unhappy lives as 4's and 3's, but the specific goal in suicide prevention is to remove the individual from the 5-5-5 cubelet—to save his or her life. All else (demographic variables, family history, previous suicidal history) is peripheral, except as those and other factors bear on the presently felt pain, perturbation, and negative press.

TABLE 3.3. Various Contemporary Approaches to the Study
of Suicidal Phenomena

Sector	Key references	Principal assertion: That suicide is best understood primarily—
Life history	Allport (1937) Murray (1967) Runyon (1982)	As an episode in a long life history; precursors of the suicidal death can be seen in previous patterns of response to comparable life situations.
Personal documents	Allport (1942) Shneidman & Farberow (1957) Leenaars (1988)	Through the analysis of such personal documents as letters, diaries, autobiographies, and especially suicide notes.
Demographic; epidemiological	Graunt (1662) Sussmilch (1741) Dublin (1963) Hollinger & Offer (1986)	In terms of "census" data (the statistics for sex, age, race, religious affiliation, marital status, socioeconomic status, etc.).
Systems theoretical	Blaker (1972) Miller (1978) Tyler (1984)	As an act within a living system; both the individual and the individual-within-the-society are considered as living systems.
Philosophical; theological	Pepper (1942) Fowles (1964) Choron (1972) Battin (1982)	In terms of answers to questions such as these: What is the purpose of life? Are there forces beyond ourselves? What is our relation to the universe? Is there life after death?
Sociocultural	Hendin (1964) Lifton, Kato, & Reich (1979) Iga (1986)	In terms of sociocultural data (e.g., knowledge of various countries and cultures such as Sweden, Japan, etc.).
Sociological	Durkheim (1897/1951) Douglas (1967) Maris (1981)	In terms of an individual's relationship to his or her society (estrangement from it, ties to it).
Dyadic and family	Pfeffer (1986) Richman (1987)	In terms of the stressful interaction between two people or within a family nexus.
Psychiatric	Kraepelin (1883/1915) American Psychiatric Association (1987)	In terms of mental illnesses (e.g., depression, schizophrenia, alcoholism).
Psychodynamic	Freud (1910/1967) Zilboorg (1937) Menninger (1938) Litman (1967)	In terms of unconscious conflicts, especially unconscious hostility toward the father; suicide is seen as unconscious murder.

(continued)

TABLE 3.3. (*continued*)

Sector	Key references	Principal assertion: That suicide is best understood primarily—
Psychological	Murray (1938) Shneidman (1985)	In terms of psychological pain, produced by the frustration of psychological needs.
Constitutional	Roy (1986) Kety (1986)	As an expression of inborn (constitutional or genetic) factors.
Biological; biochemical	Bunney & Fawcett (1965) Asberg, Nordstrom, & Traskman-Bendz (1986)	As a result of biochemical imbalances in the body fluids (blood) or organs (brain).

CONCLUSION: FIELDS CONTRIBUTING TO SUICIDOLOGY

Now, finally, to put this presentation of the psychological approach to suicide in a wider perspective, I can speak of a variety of fields of knowledge that have a legitimate interest in suicidology (see Table 3.3). Each of these approaches can contribute to our knowledge of suicidal phenomena. In this same sense, any one of them errs when it claims that *its* sector represents the whole circle of etiology—that it is clearly the only way to achieve a real understanding of suicide. Furthermore, proponents of all the approaches need to be vigilant that they do not confuse concomitance (events [in the brain, in the blood, in society, in interpersonal relations, within the psyche] that happen at the same time as heightened suicidality) with causality (events that necessarily must precede the onset of a suicidal state). It is the causally related events that present us with reasonable avenues to effective prevention).

REFERENCES

Allport, G. (1937). *Personality: A psychological interpretation.* New York: Holt, Rinehardt & Winston.

Allport, G. (1942). *The use of personal documents as psychological science.* New York: Social Science Research Council.

American Psychiatric Association. (1987). *Diagnostic and statistical manual of mental disorders* (3rd ed., rev.). Washington, DC: Author.

Asberg, M., Nordstrom, P., & Traskman-Bendz, L. (1986). Biological factors in suicide. In A. Roy (Ed.), *Suicide.* Baltimore: Williams & Wilkins.

Baechler, J. (1979). *Suicides* (B. Cooper, Trans.). New York: Basic Books. (Original work published 1975)

Battin, M. P. (1982). *Ethical issues in suicide.* Englewood Cliffs, NJ: Prentice-Hall.

Blaker, K. P. (1972). Systems theory and self-destructive behavior. *Perspectives in Psychiatric Care, 10,* 168-172.

Bunney, W. E., & Fawcett, J. A. (1965). Possibility of a biochemical test for suicide potential. *Archives of General Psychiatry, 13,* 232-239.

Choron, J. (1972). *Suicide.* New York: Scribner's.

Douglas, J. D. (1967). *The social meaning of suicide.* Princeton, NJ: Princeton University Press.

Durkheim, E. (1951). *Suicide: A study in sociology* (J. A. Spaulding & G. Simpson, Trans.). Glencoe, IL: Free Press. (Original work published 1897)

Dublin, L. I. (1963). *Suicide: A sociological and statistical study.* New York: Ronald Press.

Fowles, J. (1964). *The aristos.* Boston: Little, Brown.

Freud, S. (1967). Comments on suicide. In P. Friedman (Ed.), *On suicide* (E. Fitzgerald, Trans.). New York: International Universities Press. (Original work published 1910)

Graunt, J. (1662). *Natural and political annotations . . . upon the bills of mortality.* London.

Hendin, H. (1964). *Suicide in Scandinavia.* New York: Grune & Stratton.

Hollinger, P. C., & Offer, D. (1986). *Sociodemographic, epidemiologic and individual attributes of youth suicides.* Bethesda, MD: Department of Health and Human Services.

Iga, M. (1986). *The thorn in the chrysanthemum: Suicide and economic success in modern Japan.* Berkeley: University of California Press.

Kelly, G. A. (1961). Suicide: The personal construct point of view. In N. Farberow & E. S Shneidman (Eds.), *The cry for help.* New York: McGraw-Hill.

Kety, S. (1986). Genetic factors in suicide. In A. Roy (Ed.), *Suicide.* Baltimore: Williams & Wilkins.

Kraepelin, E. (1915). *Textbook of psychiatry.* (Original work published 1883)

Leenaars, A. A. (1988). *Suicide notes.* New York: Human Sciences Press.

Lifton, R. J., Kato, S., & Reich, M. R. (1979). *Six lives/six deaths.* New Haven, CT: Yale University Press.

Litman, R. E. (1967). Sigmund Freud on suicide. In E. S. Shneidman (Ed.), *Essays in self-destruction.* New York: Science House.

Maris, R. (1981). *Pathways to suicide: A survey of self-destructive behaviors.* Baltimore: Johns Hopkins University Press.

Menninger, K. A. (1938). *Man against himself.* New York: Harcourt, Brace & World.

Miller, J. G. (1978). *Living systems.* New York: McGraw-Hill.

Murray, H. A. (1938). *Explorations in personality.* New York: Oxford University Press.

Murray, H. A. (1967). Dead to the world: The passions of Herman Melville. In E. S. Shneidman (Ed.), *Essays in self-destruction.* New York: Science House.

Pepper, S. (1942). *World hypotheses.* Berkeley: University of California Press.

Pfeffer, C. (1986). *The suicidal child.* New York: Guilford Press.

Richman, J. (1986). *Family therapy for suicidal individuals.* New York: Springer.

Roy, A. (Ed.). (1986). *Suicide.* Baltimore: Williams & Wilkins.

Runyon, W. M. (1982). *Life histories and psychobiography: Explorations in theory and method.* New York: Oxford University Press.

Shneidman, E. S. (1973). Suicide. In *Encyclopaedia Britannica* (14th ed., Vol. 21). Chicago: William Benton.

Shneidman, E. S. (1980). *Voices of death.* New York: Harper & Row.

Shneidman, E. S. (1984). Aphorisms of suicide and some implications for psychotherapy. *American Journal of Psychotherapy, 38,* 319–328.

Shneidman, E. S. (1985). *Definition of suicide.* New York: Wiley.

Shneidman, E. S. (1986). Some essentials of suicide and some implications for response. In A. Roy (Ed.), *Suicide.* Baltimore: Williams & Wilkins.

Shneidman, E. S. (1987). A psychological approach to suicide. In G. R. VandenBos & B. K. Bryant (Eds.), *Cataclysms, crises and catastrophes: Psychology in action.* Washington, DC: American Psychological Association.

Shneidman, E. S. (1989). A multidisciplinary approach to suicide. In D. Jacobs & H. Brown (Eds.), *Suicide: Understanding and responding: Harvard Medical School perspectives.* Madison, CT: International Universities Press.

Shneidman, E. S. (1990). A life in death: Notes of a committed suicidologist. In C. E. Walker (Ed.), *A history of clinical psychology in autobiography.* Pacific Grove, CA: Brooks/Cole.

Shneidman, E. S., & Farberow, N. (Eds.). (1957). *Clues to suicide.* New York: McGraw-Hill.

Sussmilch, J. (1741). *Die Göttliche Ordnung in den Veränderungen des Menschlichen Geschlechts, aus der Gerburt, dem Tode, und der Fortsflanzug desselben erwiesen.* Berlin: J. C. Spenser.

Tyler, L. (1984). *Thinking creatively.* San Francisco: Jossey-Bass.

Zilboorg, G. (1937). Considerations in suicide with particular reference to that of the young. *American Journal of Orthopsychiatry, 7,* 15–31.

CHAPTER 4

How Are Suicides Different?

Ronald W. Maris, Ph.D.
University of South Carolina

In spite of the fact that suicides tend to share common traits, obviously not all suicides are alike. Some are younger, others are older. Most suicides are males, but there are, of course, female suicides. A substantial majority of suicides have a recognizable mental disorder, but by no means all do. Most suicides use highly lethal methods (e.g., guns), but some other suicides employ methods of relatively low lethality (e.g., reversible poisons). In short, the variability in suicidal outcomes is immense.

The complexity, variability, or multidimensionality of suicide has some very pragmatic consequences. In order to be able to predict suicide or assess suicidality accurately, we must specify the type of suicide as exactly as possible. One reason for this is that the predictor variables of suicide and their weights vary with the type of suicide. For example, Lettieri and Nehemkis (1974), in a book chapter on suicidal death prediction scales, distinguished four basic types of individuals committing suicide: younger males, older males, younger females, and older females. The number, varieties, and weights of predictor variables varied considerably among these four basic types. Among older males, there were seven primary predictors (relative importance was derived empirically by means of discriminant-function analysis; this is the short list):

1. Divorce status
2. Depression (vegetative symptoms)
3. Irritation, rage, violence
4. Refusal of help now
5. Divorce in last 6 months
6. Repetition of suicide attempts
7. Role failure

The variable with the highest single weight was recent divorce. Among younger females, by contrast, there were only three predictor variables (short list):

1. Friends in the vicinity
2. Dependent versus independent (high = independent)
3. Inability to maintain warm, interdependent relationships

Not only were there fewer significant predictor variables for the younger females, but these were very different from those for the older males. The variable with the highest single weight for younger females was being independent. Obviously, it is very important to be able to specify types of suicides.

The crucial question asked in this chapter is this: "Is suicide one thing or many?" Given this choice, it seems clear that the answer is "many." But how many? In the extreme case, a few clinicians might argue that every individual suicide is unique—that no two suicides are the same. If this is true, then prediction of suicide is virtually impossible. Logically, if all suicidal careers were unique, we could only understand what caused a suicide after it happened, and then it would obviously be too late to predict that suicide. Furthermore, given the assumed uniqueness of suicides, any one case of completed suicide would have little bearing on the dynamics of any other future suicide. Fortunately, almost no one believes that all suicides are absolutely unique.

What is more plausible to most suicidologists is that suicides share some traits but not others. Figure 4.1 depicts three hypothetical suicides and some of their presumed attributes. Note that each of the suicides in this example was unique in some aspects (and any prediction or assessment would have to take this into consideration): Suicide 1 was epileptic, suicide 2 was black, and suicide 3 was female. All of the suicides were clinically depressed and used a gun to kill themselves. Suicides 1 and 2 were both alcoholic and male; suicides 1 and 3 were both divorced and unemployed at the time of their deaths; and suicides 2 and 3 both had prior nonfatal suicide attempts.

Of course, if there are too many different types of overlaping suicides, then the prediction and assessment problem becomes extremely complex. For example, in the revised third edition of the *Diagnostic and Statistical Manual of Mental Disorders* (DSM-III-R; American Psychiatric Association, 1987), there are 18 major types of mental disorders, about 300 subtypes, and a multiaxial system of classification. As the reader is well aware, the unreliability and invalidity of specific psychiatric diagnoses are notorious (Kendall, 1975). Most suicidologists define three or four basic types of completed suicides and two to three subtypes for each basic type. There are good reasons for limiting types of suicides. Empirically, when a suicide researcher

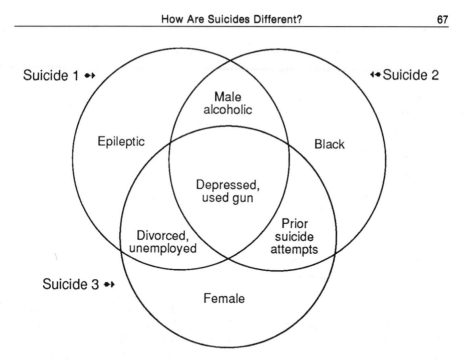

FIGURE 4.1. Overlap of traits of three hypothetical suicide cases.

goes beyond 4 to 12 suicide types, he or she runs the risk of having too small a sample to analyze meaningfully. It must be remembered that completed suicide is a rare behavior (viz., 1 to 3 per 10,000 in the general population). Theoretically, we could specify a virtually unlimited number of suicide types, but to do so is at some point to create differences that do not really make a difference (i.e., specious differences).

TYPES OF SUICIDES

In this section, I review briefly the classical suicide typologies of Durkheim, Freud, Menninger, Baechler, and Shneidman. (Of course, there are many others.) All of these typologies tend to be biased according to the disciplines of their creators. For example, Durkheim focused on social types, whereas the others have taken a psychological or psychiatric approach. At this point, we should be careful to distinguish "types of suicides" from "types of suicidologists." Quite understandably, we all tend to see suicide through our disciplinary glasses. Suicidology has its own "Rashomon effect," so to speak. That is, our perspectives on types of suicides reflect our professional training and biases. Some of the different types of suicidologists, each with their own disciplinary approach or emphasis (and there are subtypes within each of these disciplines), are as follows:

- Psychiatrists, physicians
- Psychologists
- Sociologists
- Biologists, geneticists, neurobiochemists
- Nurses
- Social workers
- Epidemiologists, demographers, biostatisticians
- Philosophers, ethicists
- Lawyers
- Theologians
- Politicians
- Educators, counselors

Most of the typologies of sucide reflect the disciplinary biases of sociologists, psychiatrists, or psychologists. Clearly, there can be typologies based on any of the other disciplinary perspectives. For example, there are biological, biochemical, genetic, endocrinological, neurotransmitter-based, and other such typologies of suicide (see Maris, 1986, 1991). The reader should be reminded that some suicidologists believe that *any* attempt at classification or taxonomy of suicide is specious (see Shneidman, 1985, pp. 30–40).

Durkheim's Typology

The French sociologist Emile Durkheim was one of the founders of the scientific study of suicide. Durkheim (1897/1951) argued that there are four basic types of completed suicides (with seven subtypes and six mixed types; see Tables 4.1 and 4.2). The four basic (pure or ideal) types of suicide are (1) "egoistic," (2) "altruistic," (3) "anomic," and (4) "fatalistic." Egoistic and altruistic suicides are polar types, as are anomic and fatalistic. It should be noted that Durkheim was interested in the broad social conditions of sucide, not in the attributes of individual suicides, and that his pure types of suicides are in fact mixed in real-life situations.

Durkheim hypothesized that suicide rates vary inversely with the degree of social integration of the groups of which the individual formed a part. For example, egoistic suicide results from excessive individuation or lack of social integration. Other things being equal, Protestants (who, in the tradition of Martin Luther, tend to advocate a "priesthood of all believers") should have higher suicide rates than Catholics or Jews (who are more socially and ritually homogeneous—bound by traditions, catechisms, the Torah, etc.; see Stack, Chapter 26, this volume). On an individual level, male

TABLE 4.1. Durkheim's Typology of Suicide (Pure Types)

Basic types	Characteristics	Paradigms	Secondary types
A. Egoistic	Excessive individuation. Apathy. Results from man no longer finding a basis for existence in life.	Within religions, family (domestic society), and politics (wars and revolutions). Protestants vis-à-vis Jews. Skid row pariahs.	A1. Melancholic languor Depressed and inactive. Reflection is egoistic. A2. Epicurean Skeptical, disillusioned matter-of-factness.
B. Altruistic	Insufficient individuation. Energy of passion or will. Activity. Basis for existence appears situated beyond life. Eastern-like asceticism; try to achieve *moksha* or *nirvana*. "Heroic" suicide.	Lower societies, soldiers, religious martyrs, etc. Hara-kiri, suttee, the kamikaze.	B1. Obligatory Duty. This is clearest type of altruistic suicide; e.g., North American Indians, Polynesians. B2. Optional Mystical enthusiasm. B3. Acute Renunciation itself is praiseworthy; e.g., India. NB.: B2 and B3 derive from B1.
C. Anomic	Literally "deregulation," lack of normative restraint. Irritation, disgust. Anger and weariness. Often violence (nonegoistic) and murder (nonaltruistic). Unregulated emotions. Always accompanied by a morbid desire for the infinite. Lack of power controlling individuals gives rise to anomic suicide. Abrupt social change. Poverty restrains it.	Economic crises, sudden social changes, widowhood, divorce, liberal occupations.	C1. General Violent recriminations against life in general. C2. Particular Violent recriminations against life in particular; e.g., against one specific person (homicide–suicide).
D. Fatalistic	Excessive regulation.	Very young husbands. Childless married women. Slaves and prisoners.	

Note. From *Social Forces in Urban Suicide* (p. 39) by R. W. Maris, 1969, Homewood, IL: Dorsey Press. Copyright 1969 by Wadsworth Publishing Co. Reprinted by permission.

TABLE 4.2. Durkheim's Typology of Suicide (Mixed Types)

Mixed types	Characteristics	Paradigms
AB. Ego-altruistic	Melancholy tempered with moral fortitude.	Stoic.
AC. Ego-anomic	Mixture of agitation and apathy, of action and reverie.	Upswing of depressive reactions.
AD. Ego-fatalistic	Hyperregulation and apathy.	Prisoners, slaves.
BC. Anomic-altruistic	Exasperated effervescence.	Bankrupt family man.
BD. Altruistic-fatalistic	Forced obligation.	Elite soldiers.
CD. Anomic-fatalistic	Mixture of normative deregulation and hyperregulation.	Juvenile delinquents.

Note. From Social Forces in Urban Suicide (p. 40) by R. W. Maris, 1969, Homewood, IL: Dorsey Press. Copyright 1969 by Wadsworth Publishing Co. Reprinted by permission.

"skidrow" outcasts would be close to the egoistic suicide type. Apathy is thought to characterize egoistic suicides.

Altruistic suicide, on the other hand, results from insufficient individuation and is characterized by energy or activity, rather than by apathy. The altruistic suicide type typically finds the basis for existence beyond earthly life. Examples would include religious martyrs; soldiers who die for their country, (e.g., Japanese kamikaze pilots in World War II); or Indian widows, who until fairly recently were expected to sacrifice themselves on their husbands' funeral pyres (the custom of suttee).

If egoistic and altruistic suicides are defined by the degree of social participation or involvement anomic and fatalistic suicides have to do with social deregulation or hyperregulation. In a sense, then, egoistic and altruistic suicides operate on the level of horizontal or social restraint, whereas anomic and fatalistic suicides result from a temporary but abrupt disruption of normative (vertical) restraint. "Anomie" literally means "without norms," and anomic suicide results from a temporary but abrupt disruption of normative restraint. Suicides following stock market crashes or high rates of divorce could be considered anomic.

Fatalistic suicide (which Durkheim [1897/1951] only considered in a footnote) is suicide generated by excessive regulation. Examples would be jail or prison suicides or suicides of very young married couples. Most real-world suicides have both anomic and egoistic traits (see Table 4.2). It should be noted, too, that suicide only varies negatively with soical integration, if the society's or group's norms prohibit suicide. As a case in point, in the mass suicide of People's Temple members in Jonestown, Guyana (and, perhaps, in Iraq in 1991) and social integration were positively (not in versely) related. Finally, Durkheim maintained that "pure" altruistic and fatalistic suicidal types are relatively rare.

Freud's and Menninger's Typologies

Psychiatric and psychological types of suicide were developed early on by the celebrated Viennese physician Sigmund Freud (1917/1957), and later by the American psychiatrist Karl Menninger (1938), among others. As Menninger (and, to a lesser extent, Freud) saw it, all suicides have three fundamental dimensions: hate, depression (or melancholia), and guilt. It follows that all suicides are of three interrelated types (cf. Shneidman & Farberow, 1957, p. 41 ff.): (1) revenge (a "wish to kill"), (2) depression/hopelessness (a "wish to die"), and (3) guilt (a "wish to be killed"). The loss of an important love object (such as the death of one's father, as in the case of the American poet Sylvia Plath), who has been internalized as part of one's own ego ("introjection"), often results in adult melancholia or depression. Freud believed that all suicides involve hostility or a death wish originally directed at an external object (father, mother, lover, spouse, etc.). Accordingly, one type of suicide is based on anger, rage, hatred, revenge, or a wish to kill (see Maltsberger, Chapter 2, this volume). Thus, Menninger called suicide "murder in the 180th degree" (retroflexed anger).

Psychologically, trying to kill an introjected object results in ego splitting and regression (Litman, 1967). The person also feels guilty for harboring murderous wishes toward loved ones. Thus, suicides involve not only a "wish to kill," but also a "wish to be killed" or punished. Finally, suicides are depressed, hopeless, and cognitively constricted. As one's ego is destroyed by self-hatred and guilt, a "wish to die" arises. Freud also thought that the processes of civilization require collective repression of sexuality and aggression, which in turn are channeled into a punitive group superego, fragmenting and otherwise diminishing healthy egos. In a sense, as Freud saw it, higher suicide rates are one cost of civilization.

Baechler's Typology

In a more recent interdisciplinary synthesis, French social philosopher Jean Baechler (1975/1979) contends that there are 11 types of suicides (see Table 4.3; he includes nonfatal suicide attempts as well), fitting into four broad categories: (1) "escapist," (2) "aggressive," (3) "oblative," and (4) "ludic." In all escapist suicides, the central intention is to take leave. There are three subtypes: flight (to avoid an intolerable situation), grief (to deal with a loss), and punishment (to atone for a fault). In my own research (Maris, 1981), I have found that about 75% of completed suicides are of the escapist variety. Usually, suicides are trying to escape pain, loss, shame, physical illness,

TABLE 4.3. Baechler's Typology of Suicide

1. Escapist
   1.1 Flight
   1.2 Grief
   1.3 Punishment
2. Aggressive
   2.1 Vengeance
   2.2 Crime
   2.3 Blackmail
   2.4 Appeal
3. Oblative
   3.1 Sacrifice
   3.2 Transfiguration
4. Ludic
   4.1 Ordeal
   4.2 Game

Note. From *Suicides* (p. 63) by J. Baechler, 1979 (B. Cooper, Trans.), New York: Basic Books (original work published 1975). Copyright 1979 by Basic Books, Inc. Reprinted by permission.

aging, failure, fatigue, or the like. As such, suicide is problem-solving behavior. Such people often believe that the only real, lasting solution to their life problems is to die. In a sense they are right, since death resolves many problems that are sometimes otherwise insoluble. Hopelessness and repeated depressive illness figure prominently in escapist suicides.

Aggressive suicides are directed against another person or persons, and consist of four subtypes: vengeance (to achieve revenge—to provoke a response or to inflict community opprobrium), crime (to kill another person as well as oneself—i.e., murder–suicides), blackmail (to put pressure on another person), and appeal (to cry for help or sound an alarm). In my judgment, roughly 20% of all suicides are primarily aggressive suicides. Such suicides have strong interpersonal components and include motivations of anger, retribution, manipulation, and so forth. Aggressive suicides tend to be more common among younger persons.

Baechler's oblative suicides are reminiscent of Durkheim's altrusitic suicide. There are two subtypes: sacrificial (to gain a greater value than one's own life) or transfigurational (to obtain a heightened state, such as religious martyrdom). Finally, ludic suicides are either of the ordeal type (to prove something or to solicit the judgment of others) or the game type (to play with or to risk one's life). Baechler is probably most innovative in designating ludic suicides. Many people are willing to risk death in order to intensify or enhance the quality of their lives, without explicitly intending or wanting to die. With ludic suicides, the individuals usually wish to live life to its fullest, even if it kills them or reduces their normal life expectancy.

Farberow (1980) has called such behavior "indirect self-destructive behavior." Some suicidologists are doubtful that risk taking should be called "suicide" at all, since the conscious intention to die is often missing or unmeasurable.

Shneidman's Evolving Typologies

One of the founding fathers of American suicidology, Edwin Shneidman, originally (Shneidman, 1968) argued that all completed suicides were either (1) "egotic," (2) "dyadic," or (3) "ageneratic." Egotic suicides result from an intrapsychic debate characterized by a sharply narrowed focus of attention (cf. Neuringer's [1964] "rigid thinking" or Breed's [1972] "tunnel vision"); self-denigrating depression; and a focus on the utter misery of oneself to the exclusion of considerations of the welfare of loved ones, children, or significant others (Shneidman, 1985). Egotic suicides thus are essentially "psychological," not sociological. The external environment, one's job, one's physical health, and the like all become secondary. I think of Herman Melville's "Bartleby the Scrivener" as a classic example of egotic suicide.

Shneidman's dyadic and ageneratic suicide types are both primarily social phenomena. The dyadic suicide's death results from unfilled needs or wishes related to his or her most important interpersonal partner; the "dyad" is that of the suicide and the significant other. Although the specific affects or the interpersonal problems in dyadic suicides vary immensely, the key to the suicide is always found in the formulaic statement, "If only he [or she] would _____." One is reminded of Ernest Becker's (1973, Ch. 7) discussion of the impossible burden put on heroes and lovers—the "transference" problems caused by depending upon presumably unconflicted, larger-than-life others to resolve one's own life needs. Ageneratic suicides not only fall out with crucial individual significant others, but also become alienated from human history itself—from their ancestors, from generations, from the whole human race. Such suicides are truly alone and isolated. There are clear ties between ageneratic suicides and de Catanzaro's argument (Chapter 30, this volume) that suicides tend to occur when individuals have lost their ability to reproduce or need to nurture their offspring.

Having posited these three suicidal types in his earlier work, Shneidman has more recently eschewed the very attempt at taxonomy (Shneidman, 1985). He now claims that classifications and typologies of suicide are "not useful." One of his reasons for this assertion is that taxonomies tend to be biological in the sense of Linnaeus or Darwin. Thus, typologies tend to force a biological overlay on an essentially psychological event. Shneidman believes that we should focus on egotic suicide, since suicide is ultimately existential and concerns primarily "personology." That is, regardless of suicides' differences, types, classes, and so on, each and every suicide occurs in the mind of a unique individual human being (Shneidman, 1985, p. 202). Each suicide is also multifaceted, with various mixtures of biological, cultural, social, psychological, and other factors.

Thus, Shneidman concludes that "suicide is a conscious act of self-induced annihilation, best understood as a multidimensional malaise in a needful individual who defines an issue for which suicide is perceived as the best solution" (1985, p. 203). Shneidman's points are well taken, but suicidologists cannot avoid the need to specify different types of suicides. One is forced to reply to Shneidman: Which dimension? What need? Which issue? That is, what *exactly* are we talking about in a particular instance or case of suicide? To fail to specify types is to lapse into mysticism and dogmatism, not the scientific study of suicide. "Precision" need not be a dirty word, and "personological" reduction (or any other) is not a great deal better than biological reductionism.

Not only are completed suicides different; there are also other different types of self-destructive behaviors. To oversimplify matters considerably, self-destruction constitutes a continuum (actually, probably interrelated, multidimensional continua) that begins with completed suicide and includes at least nonfatal suicide attempts, partial self-destruction, indirect self-destructive behaviors, self-destructive gestures (suicidal behaviors short of an explicit attempt), and suicidal ideas and thoughts (Beck et al., 1973; Pokorny, 1974; McIntosh, 1985; Jobes, Berman, & Josselson, 1987; Weishaar & Beck, 1990). Related concepts include parasuicide, acute and chronic lethality, seriousness of intent to die, accident-proneness, pseudocide (apparently suicidal behavior that is in fact nonsuicidal), risk taking, self-mutilation, deliberate self-harm, and many others (Kreitman, 1977; Farberow, 1980; Favazza, 1989).

TYPES OF NONFATAL SUICIDE ATTEMPTS

One absolutely fundamental basis for differentiation of self-destructive behaviors is that of whether a person dies or not. Predicting and assessing completed suicides is very different from predicting and assessing nonfatal suicide attempts, even though there is some overlap between the two outcomes. Since these issues are considered elsewhere in this book (e.g., see Chapter 17), they are not reviewed in any great detail here. From 85% to 90% of those who make nonfatal suicide attempts never die by suicide (Maris, 1981, Ch. 10). Although prior nonfatal suicide attempts greatly increase the lifetime probability of a completed suicide (crudely, from 12 per 100,000 [.0001] to 10 per 100 [.10]), they are of limited value as predictors. The reasons for this are as follows: (1) Most suicide attempters die natural deaths; (2) the .10 probability of completed suicide among nonfatal suicide attempters is a *lifetime* probability (i.e., it is usually spread over 30–40 years); and (3) other factors (third variables) are crucial in determining which nonfatal suicide attempters will actually complete suicide.

I should note in passing that there are at least as many different types of suicide attempters as there are types of suicide completers (i.e., at least four to six basic types and two or three subtypes for each main type). For example (after controlling for age, sex, and race, and keeping it simple by considering only dichotomies), one can think of the following distinctions: psychotic versus nonpsychotic, organic versus nonorganic, interpersonal versus noninterpersonal, self-harm versus harm to others, hopeless versus change-motivated, altruistic versus "narcissistic," risk taking versus a genuine wish to die, single versus multiple attempts, and so on. Most of these differences in suicide attempts and combinations of the differences would need to be specified in any reasonable effort at assessment or prediction of nonfatal suicide attempts.

Beck et al. (1973) have recommended that both completed suicides and attempted suicides be differentiated by factors of certainty, lethality, intent, mitigating circumstances, and methods (scales for all variables except methods are zero, low, medium, and high). "Certainty" refers to the rater's confidence that the particular behavior is suicidal. "Lethality" means danger to life in a medical or biological sense, and is often differentiated into "acute" (short-term) and "chronic" (long-term) lethality (e.g., see Smith, Conroy, & Ehler, 1984). "Intent" means the seriousness of the subject's action in ending his or her life. "Mitigating circumstances" refers to such factors as degree of alcoholic toxicity, age, intelligence, and the like. "Method" is simply the method used to attempt or complete suicide. Sometimes it is extremely difficult to specify intention (especially after death). Thus, Kreitman (1977) focuses on behavioral factors (not on intention, which is more subjective and hidden), and speaks of "parasuicide" (i.e., "the nonfatal act of deliberate self-injury," regardless of the intention to die). It is not clear, though, whether "deliberate" is much of an improvement over "intentional."

TYPES OF INDIRECT SELF-DESTRUCTIVE BEHAVIORS, IDEAS, AND OTHER DEATHS

Perhaps the largest group of self-destructive behaviors are what Farberow (1980) has called "indirect self-destructive behaviors." Included here are self-mutilation, deliberate self-harm, mismanagement of some physical illnesses, participation in risky sports, car accidents, gambling, alcoholism, drug abuse, cigarette smoking, obesity and overeating, anorexia nervosa and bulimia nervosa, overwork and excessive self-imposed stress, sexual promiscuity, and much more. Of course, to call such diverse behaviors "suicidal" is vague at best and results in a whole host of operational and measurement problems. Some behaviors can be partially self-destructive and partially self-preservative, and we cannot always tell the difference (Menninger, 1938). Given the complex measurement problems involved with indirect self-destructive behavior, many suicidologists prefer to focus only on explicit suicide completions or attempts.

Suicidal thoughts or ideas need at least to be mentioned. It has been estimated that about 20% of the general population has considered committing or attempting suicide at some point (Linehan & Laffaw, 1982). If this is true, obviously many people think about suicide who never attempt or complete suicide. Included here are individuals who plan, obsess, save their pills, consider special circumstances for suicide (e.g., irreversible terminal illness), make living wills, ruminate, talk about suicide, threaten, fantasize, communicate ideas about suicide, and so forth. Although it is important, suicidal talk is clearly different from suicidal behavior, and probably more difficult to measure and assess.

One final differentiation is that of self-destructive deaths versus all other deaths. Forensically or pathologically, suicides are often defined by elimination; that is, a suicide is *not* a natural death, an accident, or a homicide. Most death certificates employ the so-called "NASH" classification system of death (Shneidman, 1980; Jobes, Berman, & Josselson, 1987). After an autopsy and/or death investigation, the pathologist must check a box on most death certificates indicating the manner of death as "natural," "accidental," "suicidal," or "homicidal." In some instances, such a neat classification is impossible. There may need to be a fifth residual category or box labeled "undetermined" or "decision deferred" or "pending."

Of course, how one decides in which "NASH" pigeonhole to put a particular death is a complex problem with a long history (see Litman, Curphey, Shneidman, Farberow, & Tabachnick, 1963; Murphy, 1974; Pokorny, 1974; Jobes et al., 1987; Pescosolido & Mendelsohn, 1986). Theoretically, suicides are intentional, natural deaths are nonintentional, accidents are unintentional or subintentional, and homicides are contraintentional. Furthermore, the degree of intention to die could be specified (say, as high, medium, low, or zero; see Shneidman, 1980, Beck et al., 1973). But there are problems with this: Measuring intention (especially after death) is very difficult. In real life, modes or manners of death are often "equivocal" (Litman et al., 1963); that is, we are unsure just what the manner of death actually is. To complicate matters further, manners of death commonly overlap. For example, we may only be able to classify a death as "suicide-accident–undetermined," "probable suicide," or the like (Shneidman, 1980).

Medical examiners and behavioral scientists now tend to employ a forensic tool that has come to be known as a "psychological autopsy" (a retrospective investigation of the psychosocial factors and relevant life history of the decedent), in an effort to help resolve the mode of equivocal deaths (Jobes, Berman, & Josselman, 1986; Brent, Perper, Kolko, & Zelenak, 1988; Clark & Horton-Deutsch, Chapter 8, this volume). However, the psychological autopsy is not yet standardized; in fact, the term refers vaguely to many diverse procedures that mask inherent confusion in the definition and operationalization of what we mean by "suicide." One result is that the reliability and validity of suicide reports in death certificates and vital statistics remain highly suspect, although these sources may furnish the best data we have at present (Pescosolido & Mendelsohn, 1986).

CLASSIFICATION OF SUICIDAL BEHAVIOR AND IDEAS

Given all the variation in self-destructive behaviors and ideas, the scientific study of suicide ("suicidology") would be advanced immensely by the creation of a single, standardized classification system, similar to the DSM-III-R, the forthcoming DSM-IV, or the ninth edition of the *International Classification of Diseases* (ICD-9; U.S. Department of Health and Human Services, 1980). Since suicide is not a mental disorder, it appears nowhere in the DSM-III-R. Suicide ideation is cross-referenced as a symptom of major depressive episode (code 296.xx) and borderline personality disorder (301.83). Self-destructive behaviors are also implied by scores of 1 to 20 on the DSM-III-R Axis V Global Assessment of Functioning Scale. The ICD-9 references suicide in association with codes 300.9 (neurotic disorder) and 959.9 (Trauma, not an exclusive category). Usually, psychiatric classification schemes view suicide as a possible complication, symptom, or consequence of mood disorders.

Theoretically, there is no reason why a diagnostic and statistical manual of suicidal behaviors (and perhaps ideas) could not be developed. One could easily imagine 12 to 18 basic types of suicidal behaviors, each with 6 to 12 subtypes, and even a multiaxial system of classification like that of the DSM. Of course, to develop such a standardized classification of suicide outcomes would be a prodigious and costly undertaking. For example, the American Psychiatric Association (1987) lists some 431 individuals (many names are repeated on different committees) and 31 committees as having helped to produce the DSM-III-R.

The Beck Committee's Classification Scheme

In effect, the National Institute of Mental Health, Center for the Studies of Suicide Prevention, did just this in 1972–1973. Sixty-two medical and behavioral suicidologists met in Phoenix, Arizona, to consider various aspects of suicide prevention. One of the six committees (chaired by Aaron T. Beck) developed a classification and nomenclature scheme for suicidal behaviors (see Table 4.4); Beck still regards the scheme as basically appropriate even

TABLE 4.4. The Beck Committee's Classification of Suicidal Behaviors

I. Completed suicide (CS)
  A. Certainty of rater (0–100%)
  B. Lethality (medical danger to life)
    (zero, low, medium, high)
  C. Intent (to die)
    (zero, low, medium, high)
  D. Mitigating circumstances (confusion, intoxication, etc.)
    (zero, low, medium, high)
  E. Method
II. Suicide attempt (SA)
  A. Certainty (0–100%)
  B. Lethality (medical danger to life)
    (zero, low, medium, high)
  C. Intent (to die)
    (zero, low, medium, high)
    Includes consideration of subject's statements, the likelihood of rescue, past history, and other evidence; requires inference and judgment on part of the rater.
  D. Mitigating circumstances
    (zero, low, medium, high)
  E. Method
III. Suicidal ideas (SI)
    Includes all overt suicidal behavior and communications except for overt acts classifiable under suicide attempt or completed suicide. Includes suicide threats, suicide preoccupation, expressions of wish to die, and indirect indicators of suicide planning, etc.
  A. Certainty (0–100%)
  B. Lethality (medical danger to life)
    (undetermined, low, medium, high)
    Refers to the consequences if life-threatening plan is carried out.
  C. Intent (to die)
    (zero, low, medium, high)
    Includes consideration of subject's current statements, reports of his previous statements and his actions by others, past history and other evidence; requires inference and judgment on part of the rater.
  D. Mitigating circumstances
    (confusion, intoxication, and other transient modifying factors in operation at time of suicide ideas)
  E. Method
    (Name the method. Multiple methods may be listed. In some cases method may be unknown. Not an ordinal scale.)

Note. From "Classification and Nomenclature" (p. 8) by A. T. Beck, J. H. Davis, C. J. Frederick, S. Perlin, A. D. Pokorny, R. E. Schulman, R. H. Seiden, & B. J. Wittlin, 1973, in H. L. P. Resnik and B. C. Hathorne (Eds.), *Suicide Prevention in the Seventies* (pp. 7–12). Washington, DC: U.S. Government Printing Office.

today (personal communication, 1990). This suicide classification scheme has been discussed above and need not be elaborated at much greater length here. Essentially, suicidal phenomena are considered either as completions, as nonfatal suicide attempts, or as suicidal ideas. Each of these three types is further specified by (A) certainty of the rater (0–100%), (B) lethality (zero, low, medium, or high), (C) intent to die (zero, low, medium, or high) (D) mitigating circumstances (zero, low, medium, or high), and (E) method (list actual method used).

Although the Beck et al. scheme has the advantage of parsimony, it does not approach the sophistication of such mental disorder classification schemes as the DSM-III-R. Most obviously, all suicides, nonfatal attempts, and ideation are considered in the same way; intention is usually not obvious and is difficult to measure; basic demographic differences are not recorded; and indirect self-destructive behaviors are left out entirely.

The Jobes and Ellis Classification Systems

Jobes et al. (1987)—plus a committee of scholars from the American Academy of Forensic Sciences, the American Association of Suicidology, the Association for Vital Statistics and Health Sciences, the Centers for Disease Control, the National Association of Medical Examiners, the National Center for Health Statistics, and other organizations—elaborated upon the Beck et al. classification system, but focused only on completed suicide (see Table 4.5). They argued that all suicides must be self-inflicted and that the deceased must intend to die. One advance of the Jobes et al. classification is that it allows for *indirect* evidence of intent to die (11 criteria for intent are specified). However, only completed suicide is classified; also, as in the Beck et al. (1973) scheme, no subtypes are delineated.

Ellis (1988) has explored what he calls the "dimensions" of self-destructive behavior (see Table 4.6). The Ellis classification does encompass all major types of self-destruction (including ideation and parasuicide), as well as other descriptive, situational, psychological/behavioral, and teleological concomitants. However, Ellis comes close to confusing predictors with outcomes or causes with classes. Many of his dimensions are not so much types of self-destruction as they are hypothesized *causes* of self-destruction. Definitions should not be explanations. There are other small problems with the Ellis dimensions; for example, it is not clear how "parasuicide" and "self-destructive behavior without conscious ideation" are different. A possible advantage of the Ellis schema is that different dimensions of basic self-destructive types are separated from one another. To illustrate, "escapist suicide" has descriptive, situational, psychological/ behavioral, and teleological components or dimensions that perhaps should be differentiated.

TABLE 4.5. Operational Criteria for Classification of Suicide

I. *Self-inflicted*: There is evidence that death was self-inflicted. This may be determined by pathological (autopsy), toxicological, investigatory, and psychological evidence, and statements of the decedent or witnesses.

II. *Intent*: There is evidence (explicit, implicit, or both) that at the time of injury the decedent intended to kill himself or herself or wished to die, and that the decedent understood the probable consequences of his or her actions.

A. Explicit verbal or nonverbal expression of intent to kill self.

B. Implicit or indirect evidence of intent to die, such as the following:

- Preparations for death inappropriate to or unexpected in the context of the decedent's life.
- Expression of farewell or the desire to die or an acknowledgment of impending death.
- Expression of hopelessness.
- Expression of great emotional or physical pain or distress.
- Effort to procure or learn about means of death or to rehearse fatal behavior.
- Precautions to avoid rescue.
- Evidence that decedent recognized high potential lethality of means of death.
- Previous suicide attempt.
- Previous suicide threat.
- Stressful events or significant losses (actual or threatened).
- Serious depression or mental disorder.

Note. From "Improving the Validity and Reliability of Medical–Legal Certifications of Suicide" (p. 323) by D. A. Jobes, A. L. Berman, and A. R. Josselson, 1987, *Suicide and Life-Threatening Behavior, 17*(4), 310–325. Copyright 1987 by the American Association of Suicidology. Reprinted by permission.

The Maris Classification Scheme

Although it is far from a finished product and has its own obvious shortcomings, I offer Table 4.7 as a further classification step in the right direction. First, on Axis I, the rater has to decide whether a suicidal outcome (the focus is on just one outcome at a particular time) is a completion (code I), a nonfatal attempt (code II), an idea (code III), or a mixed or uncertain outcome (code IV). Second, I have assumed from the prior review of the suicide literature that suicidal phenomena are fundamentally either (A) escape, (B) revenge, (C) altruistic, (D) risk-taking, or (E) mixed. Each type is elaborated to be as broad as possible and still relatively homogeneous, and yet to be reasonably exclusive with other basic types of suicidal behaviors. For example, "escape suicides" (IA) include Shneidman's egotic suicide, Maltsberger's concept of aloneness (see Chapter 2, this volume), Durkheim's egoistic suicide, Menninger's depressed/hopeless suicide, and so on. "Revenge suicides" (IB) include a saliency of interpersonal traits: hatred, aggression, manipulation, Shneidman's dyadic suicide, appeal, blackmail, guilt, and so forth. "Altruistic suicides" (IC) include self-sacri-

TABLE 4.6. Dimensions of Self-Destructive Behavior

I. Descriptive
    A. Suicidal behavior
        1. Suicide
        2. Parasuicide
        3. Ideation only
        4. Self-destructive behavior without conscious ideation
    B. Method
    C. Lethality
    D. Communication (direct or indirect)
    E. Other victim
    F. Prior attempts/threats/ideation
II. Situational
    A. Loss
        1. Interpersonal
        2. Achievement
        3. Health
        4. Material
    B. Interpersonal conflict
    C. Stimulus characteristics
    D. Reinforcement contingencies
    E. Lack of clear precipitant
III. Psychological/behavioral
    A. Mood disorder
    B. Substance abuse
    C. Psychosis
    D. Organic brain dysfunction
    E. Cognitive distortions
        1. Hopelessness
        2. Dysfunctional attitudes/beliefs
    F. Skill deficit
        1. Interpersonal
        2. Coping/problem solving
        3. Emotion regulation
IV. Teleological
    A. Instrumental
        1. Elimination of pain
            a. Physical
            b. Emotional
        2. Interpersonal change
        3. Self-punishment
        4. Other punishment
        5. Cry for help
    B. Cessation
        1. Lack of reason to live
        2. Philosophical
    C. Unknown/impulse attempt

Note. From "Classification of Suicidal Behavior: A Review and Step toward Integration" (p. 366) by T. E. Ellis, 1988, *Suicide and Life-Threatening Behavior, 18*(4), 359–371. Copyright 1988 by the American Association of Suicidology. Reprinted by permission.

TABLE 4.7. Multiaxial Classification of Suicidal Behaviors and Ideation

Suicidal behaviors/ideas	1. Check (√)	1. Primary type	2. Certainty	3. Lethal-ity	4. Intent	5. Circum-stances	6. Method	7. Sex	8. Age	9. Race	10. Marital status	11. Occupa-tion
I. Completed suicides												
A. Escape, egotic, alone, no hope												
B. Revenge, hate, aggressive												
C. Altruistic, self-sacrificing, transfiguration												
D. Risk-taking, ordeal, game												
E. Mixed												
II. Nonfatal suicide attempts												
A. Escape, catharsis, tension reduction												
B. Interpersonal, manipula-tion, revenge												
C. Altruistic												
D. Risk-taking												
E. Mixed												
F. Single vs. multiple												
G. Parasuicide												
III. Suicidal ideation												
A. Escape, etc.												
B. Revenge, interpersonal, etc.												
C. Altruistic, etc.												
D. Risk-taking, etc.												
E. Mixed												
IV. Mixed or uncertain mode												
A. Homicide–suicide												
B. Accident–suicide												
C. Natural–suicide												
D. Undetermined, pending												
E. Other mixed												
V. Indirect self-destructive be-havior (not an exclusive category)												
A. Alcoholism												
B. Other drug abuse												
C. Tobacco abuse												
D. Self-mutilation												
E. Anorexia–Bulimia												
F. Over- or underweight												
G. Sexual promiscuity												
H. Health management prob-lem, medications												
I. Risky sports												
J. Stress												
K. Accident-proneness												
L. Other (specify)												

Note. Certainty: Rate 0–100%.
Lethality (medical danger to life): Rate zero, low, medium, high (0, L. M. H).
Intent: Rate zero, low, medium, high.
Mitigating circumstances (psychotic, impulsive, intoxicated, confused): Rate zero, low, medium, high.
Method: firearm (F); poison (solid and liquid) (P); Poison (gas) (PG); hanging (H); cutting or piercing (C); jumping (J); drowning (D); crushing (CR); other (O); none (N).
Sex: Male (M) or female (F).
Age: Record actual age at event.
Race: White (W), black (B), Asian (A), other (O).
Marital status: Married (M), single (S), divorced (D), widowed (W), other (O).
Occupation: Manager, executive, administration (M); professional (P); technical workers (T); sales workers (S); clerical worker (C); worker in precision production (mechanic, repairer, construction worker) (PP); service worker (SW); operator, laborer (OL); worker in farming, forestry, fishing (F); other (O); none (N).

fice, duty, obligation, Baechler's oblative suicide, transfiguration or self-change, dying for a higher good or cause, and the like. "Risk-taking suicides" (ID) include suicidal ordeals, games, Baechler's ludic suicide, being willing to lose one's life without having death in mind as the primary goal (e.g., the wish to have a stimulating existence or to enhance the quality rather than the length of life), and the like. Finally, suicides can be of the "mixed" type (IE). For example, a case can have strong escape and revenge components virtually equally present. Mixed types should be specified (e.g., as A and B). If one type is clearly predominant or primary, it is best not to code the case as mixed. The primary type of suicidal behavior should be checked in column 1.

Like Beck's committee, I recommend that the rater record the certainty of the type (0–100%—column 2), the lethality or medical danger to life (column 3), the degree of intent to die (column 4), and the mitigating circumstances (column 5). In addition, the method, sex, age, race, marital status, and census occupational category should be coded for each case (columns 6 to 11; see footnotes to Table 4.7); these variables are *not* part of the definition, however. Category V records all known indirect self-destructive behaviors (the rater should check all copresent traits in row V, column 1). Category V can be completed for all cases (if the relevant traits are present) and is not an exclusive code; categories I to IV are mutually exclusive, however. The rater should note that homicide–suicide, uncertain modes of death, and other mixed modes get category IV codes.

In effect, suicidal behaviors are being coded in Table 4.7 on three axes: Axis I (primary type), Axis II (secondary characteristics), and Axis III (indirect self-destructive behaviors). For example, the code "IA/75,H,H,M,F,M, 55,W,D,P/A,C,H" would indicate an escape suicide with a 75% certainty, high lethality and intent, medium mitigating circumstances, and death by a firearm; the individual in this case was male, 55 years old, white, divorced, and a professional. The category V codes (A, C, H) indicate that this man had indirect factors of alcoholism, tobacco abuse, and health management problems. Table 4.7 is admittedly incomplete, in that it does not rate social or many biological types explicitly. The chapter now concludes with an attempt to classify five clinical cases by means of the Table 4.7 scheme.

Application of the Maris Scheme to the Five Cases

Table 4.8 attempts to classify the five clinical cases discussed in this book (Heather B., Ralph F., John Z., Faye C., and José G.; see Chapter 12 for full descriptions). We are at a disadvantage, since we do not know (yet) which (if any) of the five cases actually completed suicide. It is *predicted* here that all cases except Heather were in fact completed suicides. Furthermore, classifying suicidal outcomes differs considerably from assessing or predicting suicide. As a predictive tool, Table 4.7 has many insufficiencies. Most

TABLE 4.8. Application of Table 4.7's Classification Scheme to the Five Clinical Cases

	Case				
Factor	1 Heather B	2 Ralph F	3 John Z	4 Faye C	5 José G
1. Completed suicide[a]	N	Y	Y	Y	Y
2. Suicide attempt	Y?	N	Y	N	N
3. Suicide ideation	Y	Y	Y	Y	Y
4. Sex	F	M	M	F	M
5. Age	13	16	39	49	64
6. Race	W	W	W	W	O (Hispanic)
7. Marital status	S	S	M	S	M
8. Occupation	N[b]	N[b]	N[c]	P?	N[c]
9. Table 4.7 type	IIB	IA	IA	IA	IA
10. Certainty (0–100%)	100%	75%	75%	60%	90%
11. Lethality	L	H	H	L?	H?
12. Intent	M	H	M	M?	H?
13. Circumstances	M	H	H	H	H
14. Method	N?	J?	O?	N?	F?
Category V items					
A. Alcoholism	N	Y	N?	N	Y
B. Other drug abuse	N?	N?	N	N	N
C. Tobacco abuse	?	Y	N	N	Y
D. Self-mutilation	Y	N	N	N	N
E. Anorexia–bulimia	N	N	Y	?	N
F. Over- or underweight	N	N	Y	?	N?
G. Sexual problem, promiscuity	Y	Y	N	Y	N
H. Health problem	N	Y	N	N	Y
I. Risk taking	Y	Y	N	N	Y?
J. Stress	Y	Y	Y	Y	Y
K. Accident-proneness	N	N	N	N	Y?
L. Other (specify)	School problems	Suicide in family, depression	Considerable depression, work problem	Schizophrenia	Anger, hopelessness

[a]Predicted only.
[b]Student.
[c]Out of work.
[d]? indicates uncertainty or missing information.

notably, several standard predictors of suicide are missing (e.g., mental disorders such as depressive disorders or schizophrenia; degree of social isolation; treatment history; etc.). We also do not know for sure which method was used to commit suicide (if any). In fact, in several categories the information is simply missing or uncertain information (often indicated in Table 4.8 by question marks).

However, this attempt to apply the classification scheme to five actual cases of suicidal behaviors makes some deficiencies in the scheme readily apparent. First, instead of merely checking the primary types in column 1, it would be better to check the primary type but also to rate ("yes" or "no") other relevant categories, too. For example, Ralph is predicted to have committed suicide, made no nonfatal attempts, and had suicidal ideation. Heather is not predicted to have completed suicide, but probably attempted suicide (self-mutilation) and definitely had ideas about suicide. Second, the major types probably need to be elaborated into more subtypes. In Table 4.8, all the (predicted) completed suicides are classified as primarily escape suicides (viz., as "IA"), in spite of the fact that they have some obvious differences. In effect, four of five cases are classified as having had the same outcome, when the four cases have very different profiles. Probably these different profiles ought to be reflected in at least some different subtype classifications of suicides.

Third, it might be useful for the classification scheme to include a subjective factor, such as the rater's "gut feeling" or "clinical judgment" about the case's suicidality. For example, I find myself feeling that José and Ralph were highly suicidal, but their factor profiles really did not indicate why I feel this way. This suggests that an important class or factor may be missing from the Table 4.7 scheme in any given individual case, or that one or two factors may be more heavily weighted than others. Finally, many classes or codes in Table 4.7 remain vague or uncertain. In some cases this is because of missing information; in others it is because Table 4.7 needs better, more explicit operational definitions of its classes.

REFERENCES

American Psychiatric Association. (1987). *Diagnostic and statistical manual of mental disorders* (3rd ed., rev.). Washington, DC: Author.

Baechler, J. (1979). *Suicides* (B. Cooper, Trans.). New York: Basic Books. (Original work published 1975)

Beck, A. T., Davis, J. H., Frederick, C. J., Perlin, S., Pokorny, A. D., Schulman, R. E., Seiden, R. H., & Wittlin, B. J. (1973). Classification and nomenclature. In H. L. P. Resnik & B. C. Hathorne (Eds.), *Suicide prevention in the seventies* (pp. 7-12). Washington, DC: U.S. Government Printing Office.

Becker, E. (1973). *The denial of death.* New York: Macmillan.

Breed, W. (1972). Five components of a basic suicide syndrome. *Suicide and Life-Threatening Behavior, 2,* 3-18.

Brent, D. A., Perper, J. A., Kolko, D. J., & Zelenak, J. P. (1988). The psychological autopsy: Methodological considerations for the study of adolescent suicide. *Journal of the American Academy of Child and Adolescent Psychiatry, 27*(3), 362-366.

Durkheim, E. (1951). *Suicide: A study in sociology* (J. A. Spaulding & G. Simpson, Trans.). Glencoe, IL: Free Press. (Original work published 1897)

Ellis, T. E. (1988). Classification of suicidal behavior: A review and step toward integration. *Suicide and Life-Threatening Behavior, 18*(4), 358-371.

Farberow, N. L. (1980). *The many faces of suicide: Indirect self-destructive behavior.* New York: McGraw-Hill.

Favazza, A. R. (1989). Why patients mutilate themselves. *Hospital and Community Psychiatry, 40*(2), 137-145.

Freud, S. (1957). Mourning and melancholia. In J. Strachey (Ed. and Trans.), *The standard edition of the complete psychological works of Sigmund Freud* (Vol. 4, pp. 237-260). London: Hogarth Press. (Original work published 1917).

Jobes, D. A., Berman, A. L., & Josselson, A. R. (1986). The impact of psychological autopsies on medical examiners' determination of manner of death. *Journal of Forensic Sciences, 31*, 177-189.

Jobes, D. A., Berman, A. L., & Josselson, A. R. (1987). Improving the validity and reliability of medical–legal certifications of suicide. *Suicide and Life-Threatening Behavior, 17*(4), 310-325.

Kendall, R. E. (1975). *The role of diagnosis in psychiatry.* Oxford: Blackwell Scientific.

Kreitman, N. (1979). *Parasuicide.* New York: Wiley.

Lettieri, D. J., & Nehemkis, A. M. (1974). A socio-clinical scale for certifying mode of death. In A. T. Beck, H. L. P. Resnik, & D. J. Lettieri (Eds.), *The prediction of suicide* (pp. 119-140). Bowie, MD: Charles Press.

Linehan, M. M., & Laffaw, J. A. (1982). Suicidal behaviors among clients of an outpatient psychology clinic versus the general population. *Suicide and Life-Threatening Behavior, 12*, 234-239.

Litman, R. E. (1967). Sigmund Freud on suicide. In E. S. Shneidman (Ed.), *Essays in self-destruction* (pp. 324-344). New York: Science House.

Litman, R. E., Curphey, T., Shneidman, E. S., Farberow, N. L., & Tabachnick, N. (1963). Investigations of equivocal suicides. *Journal of the American Medical Association, 184*, 924-929.

Maris, R. W. (1969). *Social forces in urban suicide.* Homewood, IL: Dorsey Press.

Maris, R. W. (1981). *Pathways to suicide: A survey of self-destructive behaviors.* Baltimore: Johns Hopkins University Press.

Maris, R. W. (Ed.). (1986). *Biology of suicide.* New York: Guilford Press.

Maris, R. W. (1991). Suicide. In R. Dulbecco (Ed.), *Encyclopedia of human biology* (pp. 327-335). San Diego, CA: Academic Press.

McIntosh, J. L. (1985). Definitions and varieties of self-destructive behavior. In J. McIntosh, *Research on suicide* (pp. 18-32). Westport, CT: Greenwood Press.

Menninger, K. (1938). *Man against himself.* New York: Harcourt, Brace & World.

Murphy, G. E. (1974). The clinical identification of suicidal risk. In A. T. Beck, H. L. P. Resnik, & D. J. Lettieri (Eds.), *The prediction of suicide* (pp. 119-140). Bowie, MD: Charles Press.

Neuringer, C. (1964). Rigid thinking in suicidal individuals. *Journal of Consulting Psychology, 28*, 54-58.

Pescosolido, B. A., & Mendelsohn, R. (1986). The social organization of suicide rates. *American Sociological Review, 51*, 80-100.

Pokorny, A. D. (1974). A scheme for classifying suicidal behaviors. In A. T. Beck, H. L. P. Resnik, & D. J. Lettieri (Eds.), *The prediction of suicide* (pp. 29–44). Bowie, MD: Charles Press.

Shneidman, E. S. (1968). Classifications of suicidal phenomena. *Bulletin of Suicidology, 1*, 1–9.

Shneidman, E. S. (1980). *Voices of death.* New York: Harper & Row.

Shneidman, E. S. (1985). *Definition of suicide.* New York: Wiley-Interscience.

Shneidman, E. S., & Farberow, N. L. (1957). Suicide and age. In E. S. Shneidman & N. L. Farberow (Eds.), *Clues to suicide* (pp. 41–49). New York: McGraw-Hill.

Smith, K., Conroy, R. W., & Ehler, R. (1984). Lethality of Suicide Attempt Rating Scale. *Suicide and Life-Threatening Behavior, 14*, 215–242.

U.S. Department of Health and Human Services. (1980). *International classification of diseases* (9th ed., 2nd rev.). Washington, DC: U.S. Government Printing Office.

Weishaar, M. E., & Beck, A. T. (1990). Cognitive approaches to understanding and treating suicidal behavior. In S. J. Blumenthal & D. J. Kupfer (Eds.), *Suicide over the life-cycle* (pp. 469–498). Washington, DC: American Psychiatric Press.

C H A P T E R   5

What Is Being Predicted?: The Definition of "Suicide"

David J. Mayo, Ph.D.
University of Minnesota, Duluth

"What is suicide?" A straightforward answer to this question is that to commit suicide is to end one's own life intentionally. This strikes me as the correct definition of "suicide," and one I explicate and defend in this chapter.

On first glance, this definition seems uncontroversial and hardly in need of either explication or defense. If John Z had died when his depression drove him to put a plastic bag over his head, or if Ralph F had actually jumped from a high bridge to his death (see Chapter 12 for details on both these cases), surely these would have counted as suicides. However, all cases are not so clear. What if Heather B (see Chapter 12) had been brought to the emergency room after being found unconscious on her mother's bed next to an empty bottle of sleeping pills? Suicidal behaviors such as Heather's may or may not mean that the person really intended to die (a question quite distinct from the question of whether or not he or she really *did* die!). And what of deaths that are self-willed in some straightforward sense, but with which we are generally more sympathetic? What of Socrates, who willingly cooperated in carrying out his own death sentence by drinking the hemlock the state provided him with, rather than escaping, as the state was rather hoping and his friends were urging? Or Samson, who brought down the temple on himself and his enemies? What of modern-day martyrs—aviators who stay with falling planes to pilot them into open areas, rather than bail out and risk letting the planes crash into populated areas; or soldiers who leap on grenades to protect their fellow-soldiers from the blasts; or people who starve or immolate themselves, for political causes? Or what of persons who refuse medical treatment—cancer patients, or even patients whose lives could be prolonged indefinitely by treatments such as renal dialysis, because they would rather die than continue to suffer or to impose burdens on others? What of terminally ill persons who request and are given lethal injections (as in The Netherlands), or (in the United States) doses of morphine so massive that everyone realizes they will slow respiration and kill the patient, even though everyone insists that the intention is simply to kill the pain?

How one answers these questions will depend on how one understands the concept of suicide, and there exists a considerable literature which debates how this should be done. In my defense of the definition of suicide as the intentional ending of one's own life, I look at the themes raised by these problem cases. First, however, let me offer some general remarks about the nature of definitions.

THE NATURE OF DEFINITIONS

A definition articulates the meaning of a term. If a term has a precise meaning, a correspondingly precise definition is possible. A "square", for instance, can be defined as an equilateral rectangle. A precise definition will represent an equivalence proposition: The *definiens*, or statement of meaning, can replace the *definiendum*, or term being defined, in all but intentional contexts, without changing the original meaning or the truth value of the utterance. Many terms, however, lack precise meaning and are vague in some way. In that case, it is no more possible to give a precise definition of the term than it is to give the exact dimensions of an inexact object such as a cloud, or to say *exactly* when a mood began.

The meaning of terms can be imprecise in any of a number of ways, only two of which need concern us here. The first of these occurs when a word that appears in the definition of some other term is vague. A "father" for instance, can be defined as "a male parent." But does "parent" here necessarily mean "biological parent"; does it refer to anyone in the social role of parent; or is it a legal notion? To take another example, a "living person" can be defined as "a person who is not dead." But the pressing need for organs has prompted some debate over the definition of "death," and we now find confusing newspaper accounts of people who are "brain-dead," about which we may not know *what* to think. Are these people alive, and if not, why do they receive all that expensive medical attention in the intensive care unit? I refer to this kind of vagueness as "inherited vagueness," because the term derives or inherits its vagueness from a vague term in the *definiens*.

The second kind of vagueness relevant for our purposes occurs when the applicability of a term depends on some matter of degree. "Old" means "having been around a long time," but how long? "Rich" means "having a lot of money," but how much? Similarly, "wisely," "lazy," "ambitious," "colorfully," "healthy," "sunny," "messy," "entertaining," "indecent," and many other adjectives and adverbs are vague in this way. So is the word "vague" itself.

Sometimes these two kinds of vagueness combine: One term will inherit vagueness from a term in the *definiens* that is vague by virtue of involving some matter of degree. Specifically, I wish to argue that this is true of "intention," "intentional," and "intentionally"—a cluster of notions that figure prominently in the definition of suicide. The term "intentionally" is vague for several reasons. The first involves matters of degree: Someone may do something more or less intentionally, or with more or less clear intentions about it. I may act with clear intention when I reluctantly drive downtown, head straight for the post office, and pick up the package I have been waiting for that the mail carrier tried to deliver when I was not home. At the other extreme, I may be a person who loves crowds, loves to shop, and has noticed a number of tempting ads in the paper, including one for a shirt I really cannot afford. I may be troubled by my debts and wracked with ambivalence about my spending habits. I head downtown "just to window-shop," but while there I buy the coveted shirt. Did I go downtown intending to buy the shirt?

The second reason for the vagueness of "intention" is that people can have multiple intentions, all of which point in the same direction. I explore this source of vagueness in what follows.

The second vague term in the definition of suicide is the term "end." "To end" is "to bring something to a close," or, more precisely, "to behave in such a way as to bring something to a close." But there is some vagueness about the range of behavior that will count if I am to be regarded as the agent in bringing something to a close. How, and how directly, must one's behavior be linked to an event before one can be said to end it? If, at a dinner, people leave after I conspicuously fold my napkin, place it on the table during a lull in the conversation, say quite loudly "Well, this has been lovely," and start to push my chair from the table, I will have ended the dinner. But what if I try to slip off quietly, but the other guests notice me discreetly thanking the hostess, and get up and leave as well? What if people leave a party I am hosting shortly after I "do nothing," but simply quit offering the guests more food or drink, and perhaps fall silent? Certainly people often *do* things by inaction. (I could insult another guest by not speaking to him or her all evening.) I argue here that persons may commit suicide by inaction, when they refrain from some action with the intention of bringing about their own deaths.

These remarks notwithstanding, I believe that when we look closely at the definition of suicide, we find it surprisingly precise. One way in which the definition of the term "suicide" is *not* vague is that it does *not* contain any normative component. Words such as "courage," "cowardice," "duty," or "immoral" carry value judgments *as part of their very meaning*. This being so, the statements "It is wrong to do something immoral" and "Cowardice is bad" do not tell us anything about life; they are simply tautologies that are true strictly by virtue of the meaning of the words they contain, like the tautologies that "Terrible wine is bad wine," or "A square has four sides." By contrast, any value judgments that attach to suicide *do not attach to it as part of its meaning.* The claims that "Suicide is wrong" or "Suicide is not praiseworthy," or "Suicide is irrational," if they are true at all, are *not* so by virtue of the definition of suicide, but for other reasons, which must be made out independently.

I mention this because much of the controversy in the literature about euthanasia and suicide (and about the definitions thereof) is obfuscated by the suspicious premise that anything that can properly be labeled "suicide" is to be condemned, discouraged, pitied, or treated. Thus, for instance, some advocates of euthanasia, which can be defined as intentionally ending one's life before the ravages of disease do so more slowly and painfully, feel it necessary to insist as part of their defense that euthanasia is not suicide; in turn, some critics of euthanasia feel that they need do no more to condemn it than to insist that it is a form of suicide. (This dialogue played itself out, for instance, in the case of Elizabeth Bouvia, a woman who decided she would rather die than continue to live with cerebral palsy that left her almost totally immobile, and tried to refuse food to that end.) None of this, however, genuinely advances the debate about either the morality of euthanasia or the morality or rationality of suicide. Instead, such discussions simply trade on the general presumption that anything that is suicide ought never to be encouraged.

This presumption is far from obvious, however. A number of suicides are referred to in the Bible with no hint of condemnation, and even so prominent a suicidologist as Edwin Shneidman (1985) grants that Socrates' death was a suicide, without for a minute suggesting that it was anything but praiseworthy. Frey (1980) and Martin (1980) also argue that noble self-sacrifices ought to be classified as suicides, and that these show that suicide can sometimes be admirable.

Indisputably, most suicides are tragedies. However, this fact must not eclipse thoughtful debate over the question of whether intentionally ending one's life can *ever* be rational or praiseworthy. This question will obviously become ever more important as new medical technology makes possible progressively longer life, much of it of progressively lower quality, and almost certainly at progressively greater expense. If this debate is to proceed in a clear-headed way, it is important to be clear on what is meant by "suicide," and to define the term in a way that is neutral on the normative issue, so that this issue can be debated independently. To do otherwise would be as unhelpful for the debate as it would be unhelpful for the abortion debate to define "abortion" at the outset as the "killing of a tiny baby."

THE DEFINITION OF "SUICIDE"

With these preliminaries out of the way, we may now turn to the definition of "suicide" proper. There are four elements to the definition I am proposing (namely, that to commit suicide is to end one's own life intentionally): (1) the fatality of suicide, (2) the reflexivity of suicide, (3) the fact that the agency of suicide can be either active or passive, and (4) the issue of intentionality. I consider each of these in turn.

The Fatality of Suicide

The first feature outlined above stipulates that a suicide has taken place only if death occurs. Someone may attempt to end his or her life, and fail. Such a person has *attempted* suicide, or made a suicide attempt; however, an attempt is not a suicide unless it is successful—that is, unless the attempt ends in death. This requirement is not unique to suicide, but is absolutely general and applies to anything one can be said to attempt. Someone who attempts to become a parent or a movie star or to graduate from college, but fails, is not a parent or a movie star or a college graduate. Obviously, some people who attempt suicide do not succeed.

This, of course, is not to deny that the study of suicidal behavior (specifically, the study of suicide prediction and prevention) will be equally concerned with both those who successfully commit suicide and those who make nonfatal attempts; the psychosocial dynamics of the case will be nearly identical in either case. Moreover, the field of study will also extend to persons who do not intend to kill themselves, but engage in *suicidal gestures*—that is, who stage insincere suicide attempts—with the intention not of dying, but of drawing attention to their need for help. In practice, of course, the intentions of a person who engages in suicidal behavior may be so ambivalent and murky (even to that person) that there will never be a clear answer as to whether he or she intended suicide, or merely intended a suicidal gesture. This is another reason why the psychosocial dynamics may be similar. I return to the distinction between suicide attempts and suicidal gestures shortly.

The Reflexivity of Suicide

For a death to be a suicide, it must be one's own doing, in some straightforward sense. A death that is suicide must be a death that was intended by, and then effected by, the person who died.

This does not mean, however, that a person must act alone in committing suicide. Both ordinary language and the law speak of "assisted suicide." (Again, the point is completely general; many of the things we do intentionally we do with the assistance of others.) The most straightforward kind of assisted suicide involves a person who has decided to end his or her life but lacks the means to do it alone (e.g., because of physical disability or lack of access to the means), and who successfully elicits the assistance of another person by openly sharing his or her intentions. In this case the person assisting becomes the agent of the suicidal person, in the sense that he or she acts at that person's behest. This is the sort of assistance that is proscribed by law, even in states in which committing or attempting suicide is not proscribed. Moreover, a case can be described as an assisted suicide, regardless of whether the assistance consists only of providing someone with the means or of taking a more aggressive role. Assisting someone with any act clearly admits of degrees: One can provide more or less assistance. And even in states where assisting suicide is proscribed by law, there is no univocal and straightforward legal standard specifying how much assistance is proscribed. (Issues of free speech come into play, for instance, if the alleged assistance consists only of providing general information, or of providing it in a public format or forum.)

Significantly, we can also assist people in carrying out their intentions (suicidal or otherwise) without being aware of those intentions. By loaning a friend my hunting rifle, or driving him or her to a scenic overlook, I may assist that friend's suicide, even though I am totally unaware of his or her intentions and hence not acting as the friend's agent. In this case, of course, my action, though regrettable, remains morally (and legally) innocent. I mention this case only as a preliminary to a cluster of more interesting cases, in which a suicidal person dares or manipulates another person into murdering him or her. According to one study (Kobler, 1980), as many as 25% of all homicides are provoked by their victims.

In some of these cases, one person may actually intend to die, and manipulate the other into murdering simply by provoking him or her without sharing the suicidal intent. In others, one party may dare the other to kill, for a range of intentions: The provoker may want the other to kill him or her, so the killer will feel shame or be hurt. At the other extreme, the provoker may dare simply as an act of bravado, not intending to die but willing to risk it. (Games of Russian roulette are similar in this respect.) Whether such cases of homicide also constitute suicide will depend upon whether the provoker intends to die or is merely willing to risk it to achieve some end that does not require his or her death. (I return to intention shortly.) When the intention is to die, the death meets our definition of suicide. Intuitively, it strikes me as correct to describe such deaths as suicides; again, there are many ends I may be able to achieve by daring or taunting others into doing what I want them to do.

Legally, since deaths are classified in only one of several categories, a death classified as a homicide cannot also be classified as a suicide. This, however, strikes me as a defect in the law. I suggest that the most straightforward view is that such a case is both a suicide and a homicide. It is a suicide because the deceased has ended his or her own life intentionally (by provoking the other to kill), and it is a homicide because one party has killed another. One can hardly argue that it is not a suicide by virtue of involving the participation of a second party, for that is also true of the sort of assisted suicide mentioned in proscriptions against assisted suicide in the criminal code. The same consideration undercuts any claim that the person has not ended *his or her own* life, since someone else has done so. Here, as elsewhere, the law recognizes that two people can both be responsible for a (two-person) deed. (See Frey, 1981, for further defense of the view that suicide can also be homicide.) If the provoker intends suicide, (i.e., intends to provoke the other person to homicide), but the murderer is not aware of the suicidal intentions of the victim/provoker, the crime of which the murderer is guilty is not assisting suicide, but some other form of homicide. He or she is as innocent of the *crime* of assisting suicide as I would be if I were naively to drive my suicidal friend to the scenic overlook.

The Action-Inaction Distinction

Must suicide involve a physical *action* of some sort, or can a person commit suicide by opting for appropriate *inaction* that leads to death? I wish to defend the latter view.

Undeniably, committing suicide usually involves suicidal *acts*. Nevertheless, there are cases of persons' intending and realizing their own deaths through appropriate types of *inaction*, which seem to meet the definition, and which I see no reason to deny are suicides. One classic (though undoubtedly rare) case is that of persons who lie down on the railroad tracks and wait for the train to kill them. Others involve refusals of life-sustaining or life-prolonging medical treatment by people intent on ending their lives.

One might object that although the former individuals are suicides, they are not inactive, since they act by lying down on the tracks. I suggest, however, that what is essential here is not how they get onto the tracks, but that they intend their own deaths and remain inactive (i.e., lie on the tracks) in order to realize that intention. If, say, a person who is depressed and weary of life, and intends suicide but is unable to decide upon the method, awakes to *find himself or herself* on the track for some reason and opts to stay there, the case is not fundamentally different.

More typical cases of suicide by inaction involve failure to take (or refusal to permit) life-sustaining treatments. Some renal dialysis patients find their quality of life so greatly diminished by renal failure that they eventually elect to forgo the treatment needed to sustain their lives. I have noted earlier that when Elizabeth Bouvia expressed her intention to die by starvation, there was criticism of what she was proposing *on the grounds that it amounted to suicide.*

It seems that what is often driving the impulse to deny (or insist) that certain "passive" self-willed deaths are suicides is the desire to show that they are not (or are) morally blameworthy. Again, in the euthanasia debate, critics are often quick to claim that voluntary euthanasia amounts to suicide, whereas advocates of euthanasia are often equally quick to claim (lamely, in my view) that it is nothing of the kind. But, *unless one assumes at the outset* that suicide is immoral, none of this is germane either to the definition of suicide or to the morality of these proposed deaths. What is germane to the question of whether or not a death of this type constitutes a suicide is the intention behind the action or inaction. Sometimes people can achieve their ends through overt physical action, but sometimes what is needed is inaction (and perhaps patience). Moreover, we may be held morally or legally culpable for certain kinds of inaction just as clearly as for action. In May 1990, for example, Peggy Barsness was convicted of homicide by a Minneapolis jury for leaving her infant daughter alone and unattended for 2 weeks while she flew to California for a few weeks to visit her boyfriend. Surely persons can commit suicide by either allowing, refraining from getting out of, or suffering situations that will lead to their deaths, and doing so because they intend to die. Again, the point is completely general: People can achieve (and can be responsible for achieving) all sorts of intended objectives in this way. It is a mistake to focus too much attention on whether or not a person acts physically, when what is really at issue is what the person's intentions are in behaving as he or she does.

The Intentionality of Suicide

Intentionality is by far the most subtle feature of the definition I wish to defend. Committing suicide involves *intentionally* ending one's life. Minimally and uncontroversially, this feature serves to distinguish suicide from accidental self-inflicted death. A person who accidentally shoots himself or herself while cleaning a shotgun, who drives into a post at high speed while trying to adjust the controls on the car radio, or who dies as a result of an overdose of tranquilizers taken to help sleep off a night of heavy drinking is clearly not a suicide, but an accidental death.

Although medical examiners recognize this distinction, it is often difficult to distinguish in practice between an accidental death and a suicide. There are two quite different kinds of reasons for this. The first is that by the time the death has occurred, the relevant distinguishing elements—namely, the intentions of the deceased, which after all are states of mind—no longer exist and are at best only indirectly knowable. The second is that even if they are or were totally accessible, those states of mind may be inherently murky and ambivalent.

The first problem can manifest itself in several ways. A person committing suicide may disguise the deed as an accident. Alternatively, even if the person completing suicide does not try to conceal his or her intentions, he or she may still leave no clear evidence one way or the other about whether the death is accidental or intentional. Finally, the person may intentionally undertake what I call a suicidal "gesture" (e.g., Heather's hypothetical overdose of sleeping pills, mentioned above), in which the intent is *not* to die, but rather to express despair or helplessness, or to utter a "cry for help" in an effort to improve the person's life. Although death is self-caused in lethal cases involving suicidal gestures, such persons do not *intend* to die. Suicidal gestures and suicide attempts are conceptually quite distinct, because they are defined in terms of intentions that are quite distinct. (What could be more different than the intention to risk everything in an attempt to improve one's life, and the intention to end it?) For that reason, it seems to me that the common practice of lumping suicidal gestures that accidentally prove fatal with suicides is a common but serious mistake. For instance, Alvarez (1980) discusses Sylvia Plath's death as if it were a suicide, then notes parenthetically that her death resulted accidentally when an improbable set of circumstances frustrated her careful plans for the discovery of her suicidal gesture. The actual outcome in cases such as Plath's is neither intended nor desired. They are accidents; death is *not* the desired outcome. These are surely accidental deaths. That is not altered by the fact that such accidents occur in the context of an attempt to imitate or even to create the illusion of a sincere suicide attempt, nor by the fact that many of the psychosocial dynamics may be the same in the two cases.

I emphasize that there is a clear conceptual distinction between suicide gestures and sincere suicide attempts, even though I acknowledge that distinguishing them in practice can be extraordinarily difficult. The difficulty of distinguishing them when they end in death has been addressed above. But even when they do not, the issue remains murky, precisely because the intentions of very depressed individuals are murky—rendered so by depression, tunnel vision, and above all ambivalence. Shneidman (1985) goes so far as to say that "the prototypical suicidal state is one in which an individual cuts his throat and cries for help at the same time, and is genuine in both of these acts" (p. 135). It is probably even fair to say that ambivalence of this sort is the norm for most suicidal individuals, so that for the purposes of learning to assess and prevent persons from killing themselves, the distinction is not central. That should not obscure the important conceptual point, however, that by anyone's definition suicide involves intentionally ending one's life. By even the loosest reading of "intention," suicidal gestures by individuals who want to remain alive do *not* involve the intention to end their lives, but rather are desperate attempt to improve them.

Unfortunately, the distinction between genuine suicide attempts and mere suicidal gestures does not spell the end of either the conceptual or the empirical troubles associated with intentionality. A three-way distinction— tricky to articulate and even more difficult to interpret in practice—remains to be drawn among cases in which death is (1) intended as an end in itself;

(2) intended as a means to an end; and (3) not intended at all, but foreseen as a consequence of what is intended. We must try to tease apart these three different sorts of cases.

Some persons may simply decide that they are weary of life and kill themselves because they long for death. They are not suffering; their thinking is not structured around what they will escape by death. Rather, they simply and genuinely wish to be and look forward to being dead. (Looking forward to being dead is not, I would argue, an incoherent notion. As I nervously await surgery, I can genuinely *look forward* to being put under, without any illusions about being conscious to savor it once it happens.) Such a case, rare as it may be, would be a case in which a person intends his or her own death as an end in itself.

Much more common are cases in which persons end their lives, not because they find death attractive, but as a means to an end. Most often, persons who commit suicide do so because they find life highly unattractive. Most people who genuinely attempt suicide do so to escape the pain (Shneidman, 1985). In these cases, suicide is a means to an end—the end being, in this case, to put an end to suffering that has become unbearable.

Although this may be the most typical end suicide serves, it is not the only possible one. People may kill themselves as a means of impressing or hurting or getting even with others (perhaps, but not necessarily, deluding themselves that they will somehow survive their own deaths and be able to savor the effect of their suicides on others). Again, people may kill themselves for loftier or much more altruistic ends: to spare their families further problems or expense, to save face or maintain honor, or to further or express support for a cause (Wood, 1980). Soldiers or spies provided with a quick means of ending their lives, for instance, may use them to kill themselves as a means of avoiding torture and/or revealing secrets to the enemy. In each of these cases death is intended, but as a means to some further end.

The use of the distinction I am introducing here has been criticized, and I wish to address two such criticisms. The first, a conceptual claim made by Joseph Margolis (1973), is that only cases in which death is willed as an end in itself qualify as suicides. This claim strikes me (and other commentators) as implausible, first because it is completely at odds with ordinary usage, and second because it would make suicide very rare indeed. Indisputably, most of the people who actually attempt suicide are "troubled" and do so in order to escape pain. Moreover it may often be difficult to distinguish these cases in practice from cases in which people end their lives not because their lives pain them, but because life simply no longer interests them and they want death as an end in itself.

This brings me to the second claim I wish to dispute, which is an empirical one—namely, the claim that people never kill themselves simply because they find death attractive as an end. In this view, anyone who commits suicide must *ipso facto* be troubled, deranged, or suffering from some other mental condition that is diagnosable (or would be, if only the diagnosticians were clever enough and had enough data). In response, let me stress my acknowledgment that most actual suicides are committed by such persons. However, this is obviously not true of all suicides. Not even the most rabid opponents of rational suicide insist upon this interpretation for most altruistic suicides, for instance. (Instead, they usually try to deny on an ad hoc basis that praiseworthy altruistic deaths are suicides.) All I am claiming is that these appear to be cases in which persons who are not troubled in any obvious way may simply decide they have "had enough" and no longer value living, and the reasons for assimilating such cases to those of tormented individuals who commit suicide to escape the pain seem uncompelling. Moreover, these reasons seem to me to be driven by value-laden dogma rather than good empirical science. The dogma is the one I have spoken of earlier—namely, that suicide is always "a mistake," and one that can be undertaken only by a person who is troubled or confused in some way, irrational, and/or suffering from some diagnosable mental condition.

In addition to self-willed deaths that are intended (either as means or ends), there is the third category of self-willed deaths: those that are not intended at all, but merely foreseen consequences of the pursuit of ends that people value even more than they value their own lives. People often risk their lives in dramatic ways to save the lives of others (e.g., firefighters, or the Armenian woman buried with her baby in the rubble of the 1989 earthquake for several days who decided to use a sharp bit of glass to cut her own finger, so she could save her dehydrated baby by offering her own blood for it to drink). People even pursue life-threatening goals (altruistic or otherwise) when the loss of their own lives is not merely a risk, but a virtual certainty. A few persons may climb out of an overcrowded lifeboat into a freezing ocean fully expecting to die, in order to save others in the boat. Although such persons intentionally embark on courses of action that will lead to their deaths, their deaths are not a direct part of their "plan," but only unwanted but unavoidable side effects.

These are *not* suicides. Although these persons act intentionally, and even kill themselves knowingly by acting intentionally as they do, it would be misleading to say that they intentionally kill themselves, and certainly wrong to say that their intentions are to kill themselves. These cases are not rare, and they are problematic because the phrase "He intentionally killed himself" is so crucially ambiguous. Lifeboat martyrs do, after all, kill themselves while acting intentionally. This makes it tempting to concede that they are intentionally ending their own lives. However, this would be a mistake if it is taken to imply that they act *with the intention* of ending their lives—in other words, that they are committing suicide. The temptation and the confusion are only compounded by the fact that from the point of view of an external observer, the martyrs' action is indistinguishable from that of persons who *are* committing suicide: In both cases, the persons climb out of the boat into the water, fully expecting to freeze to death.

Let us consider now some of the puzzling cases posed at the outset of this chapter, in light of this distinction. Socrates drank the hemlock in order to respect the laws of Athens, and killing himself was the preferred means to that end. So Socrates drank the hemlock *intending to end his life* as a means of respecting the laws of Athens. The death of Socrates was a suicide (see Frey, 1980). By contrast, Samson's intention was not to end his own life, but to bring the temple down on his enemies *in spite of the fact that it meant his death* as well as theirs. Unfortunately, the only means available to him also rendered his own death a near-certainty. But unlike Socrates, Samson did not include his own death as an integral part of his plan: His dying was neither a means nor an end, but simply a foreseen (though unfortunate) consequence of achieving his ends. The distinction can be brought home as follows: Socrates' death was essential to his course of action's coming to fruition, whereas the case was otherwise with Samson. Samson's survival of the collapse of the temple would not have constituted a failure of his plan of action.

Some of the modern cases of martyrdom fall each way. Aviators who stay with their falling planes do not do so *in order that* they will die, and, like Samson, can survive crashes without having their intentions thwarted. Similarly, soldiers who leap on grenades and survive the experience (either because the grenades fail to go off, or because they survive the blast) suffer no frustration of their goals and hence are not committing suicide (unless, of course, their intention is to die in the line of duty—a suicidal desire). By contrast, the deaths of spies who try to kill themselves in order to avoid capture or torture or revealing secrets to the enemy are *integral components* of their plans, and if they do not die, their plans go unrealized. Thus they do commit suicide. Whether or not martyrs who starve or immolate themselves for a cause are suicides depends upon whether they intend to die for the cause, or whether they are merely risking their lives in the hopes of achieving social change. (Again, the critical question is this: Do their deaths represent integral features of their plans, or merely unavoidable risks? To put it differently, will their plans be thwarted if they do not die?)

Similarly, some of the medical cases involve suicide, and others do not. Dialysis patients who decide to forgo treatment, because they believe that death is preferable to the quality of life that is possible given their renal failure, have committed suicide. On the other hand, patients who refuse some invasive or mutilating surgery even if the refusal costs them their lives may not necessarily *want* to die, but may be willing to die in order to avoid the surgery. Even some cancer cases fall each way. Some commit suicide by forgoing treatment so that they can die and bring an end to the suffering caused by the cancer; others, who would still like to live, nevertheless decide

to forgo chemotherapy or other treatments because they are too high a price
to pay for the short period of extended life they might purchase.

Even granted the clarity of the conceptual distinction between intended
and foreseen self-willed deaths, there will of course still be problems with its
application. The problem here is similar to that involved in distinguishing
accidental (unintended) death from suicide (intended death), only here it
involves the possibility of multiple intentions. According to the present
analysis, a martyr who leaves a lifeboat (only) in order to save the lives of the
others is not a suicide. But what if this person is tired of life and was
plotting suicide when the plane crashed and they were all whisked aboard
the lifeboat? If this person sees the situation as a golden opportunity to end
his or her life and at the same time save family members from embarrassment—if, that is, the person's *primary* intention is to end his or her life, and
the overcrowding of the boat merely provides a convenient opportunity—
the death *is* a suicide. But what is one to say if both intentions are present? I
believe the correct answer is that the death is a suicide, *since* the person is
ending his or her life intentionally. It is true to say that he or she intends to
die. The person is not merely *risking* his or her life, but trying to end it, and
some sort of miraculous survival would thwart part of the plan. Part of the
person's plan is to commit suicide.

Analogously, if the *real intentions* of both a doctor and a terminal,
suffering patient are merely to kill the patient's pain with a lethal dose of
morphine, then the death is not an assisted suicide. However *if*, as one
suspects, the patient's real intention here is simply to "get it over with,"
then it is simply a dishonest charade to deny that suicide, euthanasia, or
intentional killing is involved.

To those versed in medical ethics, all of this may sound suspiciously
like the principle of double effect. The distinction between intended and
foreseen consequences is at the center of that principle for the moral evaluation of certain actions. However, I want to stress that while I am invoking
the same distinction, its import is completely different here. In medical
ethics, it is used to draw a distinction between morally permissible and
morally impermissible actions. Here, on the contrary, I have tried to stress
the folly of using "suicide" as an evaluative term. Even if the person
climbing over the side of the lifeboat, or the person begging for the dose of
morphine that everyone realizes will prove lethal, intends to die, no moral
judgment follows from that fact alone. Rather, I submit that attaching such
moral approbrium to the notion of intentionally ending one's own life both
begs important moral questions at the theoretical level about the possibility
of praiseworthy suicide, and also invites dishonesty and self-deception about
one's true intentions in practical situations (such as the one involving the
cancer patient begging for more morphine, in which it is difficult enough
for well-intentioned moral agents to figure out how they ought to conduct
themselves). Surely in these situations we must, at the very least, do every-

thing we possibly can to encourage clear and honest assessment of the situation, and not invite misrepresentions of everyone's true intentions by proclaiming that it is perfectly all right to administer a lethal dose of morphine, just as long as the people who must make such a difficult decision can convince themselves that its lethality is not integral to their intentions.

REFERENCES

Alvarez, A. (1980). The background. In M. P. Battin & D. J. Mayo (Eds.), *Suicide: The philosophical issues* (pp. 7-32). New York: St. Martin's Press.

Frey, R. G. (1980). Did Socrates commit suicide? In M. P. Battin & D. J. Mayo (Eds.), *Suicide: The philosophical issues* (pp. 35-38). New York: St. Martin's Press.

Frey, R. G. (1981). Suicide and self-inflicted death. *Philosophy, 56*, 193-202.

Kobler, A. (1980). Suicide: Right and reason. *Bioethical Quarterly, 2*, 46-55.

Margolis, J. (1973). Suicide. In J. Margolis (Ed.), *Negativities: The limits of life* (pp. 23-36). Columbus: Charles Merrill.

Martin, R. M. (1980). Suicide and self-sacrifice. In M. P. Battin & D. J. Mayo (Eds.), *Suicide: The philosophical issues* (pp. 48-68). New York: St. Martin's Press.

Shneidman, E. S. (1985). *Definition of suicide*. New York: Wiley.

Wood, D. (1980). Suicide as instrument and expression. In M. P. Battin & D. J. Mayo (Eds.), *Suicide: The philosophical issues* (pp. 151-160). New York: St. Martin's Press.

PART III

Methods
and Quantification

CHAPTER 6

Prediction of Suicide in Psychiatric Patients: Report of a Prospective Study

Alex D. Pokorny, M.D.
Baylor College of Medicine

This chapter is based on two assumptions: (1) Suicide is an undesirable event; (2) suicide in patients should be prevented if possible. Although each of these points is arguable, these are the positions from which physicians in the medical system generally work.

METHODS OF SUICIDE PREVENTION

There are three basic approaches to preventing suicide in patients. The first is to physically prevent the act (by locking patients up, watching or restraining them, removing harmful objects, etc.). This has been the traditional approach with patients on suicidal precautions. However, these precautions are all somewhat demeaning and infantilizing, and they pit the treatment staff against the patients to see who can outwit the other. There are also practical limits to the number of persons who can be kept under such precautions and to the duration of enforcement.

The second approach is to remove the distress or dysphoria that is feeding the suicidal urge. This goal might be achieved by social changes, medication, psychotherapy, or other treatment or rehabilitative measures. Such an approach has the advantage of placing the treating team and the patient more nearly on the same side, both fighting the "disease," distress, or discomfort. Unfortunately, not all distress, dysphoria, or misery can be removed.

This chapter originally appeared in *Archives of General Psychiatry*, 1983, *40*, 249-257. Copyright 1983 by the American Medical Association. Reprinted by permission.

The third possibility is to instill some ethical or moral barriers to the act of suicide, making such behavior less "available" to the patient. It is questionable whether this can be done in adulthood, after suicidal behavior or preoccupation has already appeared. It may work only if taught or instilled during childhood.

Each of these three approaches requires considerable time and individual attention. It is not feasible to apply them to whole populations or even sizable subsets of whole populations. We need to apply them to those persons who will almost certainly commit suicide unless prevented. Hence, there is a pressing need for "prediction" of suicide (i.e., identification of the persons who will commit suicide unless stopped).

EARLIER STUDIES

The relationship of various characteristics to suicide or suicide attempts has been the subject of hundreds of published studies. Most of them have been correlational in nature and have identified "significant" relationships. Many have claimed to be "predictive of suicide," which has almost always meant that a subgroup was identified that had a suicide rate significantly greater than the base rate or the rate of a comparison group.

The research findings on suicide between 1882 and 1969 were summarized in a 1972 book by Lester. Although that book concludes that research into suicide tends to be repetitive, uninspired, and sterile, it provides a good summary of the demographic, sociological, psychopathological, and other characteristics related to suicide.

Another useful review, focusing on prediction of suicide, is a 1974 book edited by Beck, Resnik, and Lettieri. In it, a chapter by Diggory notes the limitations of prior prediction efforts and strongly recommends the use of multiple-regression methods. The book includes a review of the suicide prediction "scales" in use at the time (Litman, Farberow, Wold, & Brown, 1974).

Another excellent review of the topic was published in 1972 by Brown and Sheran. It summarized information on predictive signs based on a person's attributes, behavior, and surroundings. Brown and Sheran concluded that results of such research are equivocal and that it is not possible to predict suicide at *useful levels* from single signs, psychological tests, specially devised tests, clinical judgments, or special scales. They urged researchers to put more stress on subgroupings, interactions, and duration of indicators.

Murphy reviewed these same issues in 1972 and illustrated the impracticality of available suicide predictors, using hypothesized data and data from previously published reports. He then sidestepped the issue to a degree by arguing that if the treatment offered was relatively innocuous and appropriate in its own right, the issue of false-positive predictions is not a serious one. He acknowledged, however, that if the required "treatment" was long-term hospitalization, too many false positives would be impractical.

MacKinnon and Farberow (1975) stressed the difficulties in identifying specific cases, because of low base rates and the error rate of our prediction "instruments." They presented a simulated exercise in prediction of suicide with a hospital population, using an imaginary instrument having idealistically low false-positive and false-negative rates of 1%. Even under these circumstances, only 20% of the predictions of suicide would be valid (true positives). Because any currently conceivable prediction instrument or shceme would perform more poorly (with more inherent error), the actual results would be far worse.

PREVIOUS WORK BY AUTHOR

The present study was based in part on my earlier studies of suicidal behavior, which were carried out at the Houston Veterans Administration Medical Center (VAMC) (Pokorny, 1960, 1964, 1966, 1967). One study (Pokorny, 1964) derived suicide rates for diagnostic groupings, all strikingly higher than the current U.S. suicide rate of 10 per 100,000 per year and the calculated expected rate of 22.7 per 100,000 per year for the male war veterans in Texas.

Another study followed up 618 patients who had initially been seen in psychiatric consultation for suicide attempts or threats, preoccupation, or ideation (Pokorny, 1966). Of that group, 615 were successfully traced for a period averaging 4.6 years, and 21 (3.4%), all male, had committed suicide. By computing man-years of risk for each case and summing these results by categories, the following suicide rates were derived: all 615 subjects, 740 per 100,000 per year; male suicidal patients, 786 per 100,000 per year; suicide attempters, 805 per 100,000 per year; suicide threateners, 710 per 100,000 per year; and patients with suicidal ideas, 704 per 100,000 per year. The period of greatest risk was the first 2 years after the initial suicidal behavior; during the first 3 months, the incidence of suicide was almost 1% of the entire group. It was concluded that suicide attempts, threats, and ideas were strong indicators of future completed suicide, stronger than the psychiatric diagnostic grouping. Male patients who had shown suicidal behavior had about 35 times the expected suicide rate.

Another study investigated the matter of suicide rates in veterans generally (Pokorny, 1967), to see whether war veterans were significantly more suicidal than the general population. My colleagues and I examined the absolute and relative suicide rates in three groups: Texas males, Texas male veterans, and male former psychiatric inpatients of the Houston VAMC. Suicide rates in veterans did not differ from those in the general population for persons of the same age and sex, but suicides in veterans tended to occur at an earlier age.

RATIONALE FOR CURRENT PROJECT

The study reported herein was designed as a definitive test of whether, in a high-risk population, the particular persons who would later commit suicide could be identified at a practical or feasible level (i.e., without too many false positives). The population consisted of all patients admitted to an inpatient psychiatric service, a group already shown to have a suicide rate nine times that in the general population of the same age and sex (Pokorny, 1967). The project was designed to include, in each patient's admission workup, inquiries regarding most of the previously reported "predictors" of suicide.

There are several general problems in research on completed suicide: (1) Suicide is a rare event, so there are few positive cases; (2) subjects are not available for direct study after committing suicide; (3) retrospective data are likely to be distorted; and (4) when observers encounter a strong indicator (such as the statement "I am going to kill myself today"), they immediately attempt to prevent a suicidal outcome, which, from a research standpoint, weakens the relationship of predictors to outcome.

My colleagues and I attempted to avoid some of these problems, as follows. By enrolling a very large number of subjects, we ensured that even such a rare event as suicide would occur in a reasonably large number of cases. To further increase the probability of having cases of suicide within the population, the study used a sample of subjects known to have a high suicide rate—namely, psychiatric inpatients. The study was prospective. This meant that the subjects were alive and available for study at the time of intake, and also that the distortion found in retrospective data could be avoided. We had no solution for the fourth problem.

Our "solutions" introduced three new problems. First, to follow up so many cases is a formidable task, although with a VA sample this was facilitated through use of the elaborate and comprehensive VA records system. Second, the need to include a large number of subjects meant that multiple raters had to be used, which very probably introduced greater variability and more error into the ratings. Third, the need to process so many cases necessarily limited the time that could be spent with any individual subject. This required the streamlining, abbreviation, and selection of items from the large number of available rating instruments and scales.

SUBJECTS AND METHODS

We assembled and developed a set of rating instruments, using items from established rating scales and incorporating most of the items that have been shown to predict higher rates of suicide. These were applied to 4,800 patients consecutively admitted to the psychiatry inpatient service of the Houston VAMC. Informed consent was obtained from each subject after the nature of the procedures had been explained. All 4,800 subjects were followed up for the duration of the study, to identify subsequent instances of (1) actual suicide, (2) suicide attempts or suicidal ideation leading to rehospitalization, (3) behavior or events that might have served as "alternatives to suicide" (including accidental death, death from cirrhosis, death as homicide victim, hospitalization for psychosis, and rehospitalization for alcoholism, or drug abuse), and (4) death from any cause. This chapter reports only subsequent suicides and suicide attempts. The data collected were analyzed through item-by-item analysis in terms of prediction of completed suicide, and also by grouped or summary scores for the various rating instruments. The good predictor items were then combined into predictor scales by various techniques, including discriminant-function analysis.

Sample

The sample included all consecutive "first admissions" (defined as the first admission to occur after the start of the project) to the nine psychiatry inpatient wards of the Houston VAMC. The service included two alcoholism wards and one drug abuse ward, so these two disorders were well represented.

A "high-risk" subsample, about 15% of the total sample, was also selected for study, according to a formula using conventional indicators of increased suicide risk, such as history of attempted suicide, presence of depression, or being widowed or divorced. The 21 items making up this formula were selected on the basis of previous reports, many based on studies of the general population. It was recognized that "conventional" indicators of high suicide risk for the population at large might not apply in the same manner to a population of psychiatric patients.

The subsample subjects were given additional interviews and ratings, as a second screening, to see whether this additional information might help identify future suicides. These additional ratings were too time-consuming to be used with the entire sample of 4,800 patients. However, they were also administered to a randomly selected subgroup of 668 subjects, to permit comparisons with the high-risk subgroup on these additional items.

Rating Instruments

The selection of items and scales was based on the following considerations:

1. Those items that had proved to be good predictors in previous VAMC studies (Pokorny, 1960, 1964, 1966, 1967) were assembled into structured interview and rating forms, to be completed by the physician examining the patient immediately after admission and by a research clerk who reviewed and abstracted all prior hospital and claims records.

2. Ratings reported in the literature (Lester, 1972; Diggory, 1974; Brown & Sheran, 1972) as predictive of suicide were also performed; these included standard demographic items, items from the scales of Tuckman and Youngman (1968) and Cohen, Motto, and Seiden (1966), and ratings of depression.

3. The Brief Psychiatric Rating Scale (BPRS; Overall & Gorham, 1962), with 24 items added for greater breadth of coverage, was administered as a general assessment of psychopathological condition.

4. The Nurses' Observation Scale for Inpatient Evaluation (NOSIE-30) (Honigfeld & Klett, 1965) was used to assess behavior and symptoms observed by nursing personnel.

In addition, the "high-risk" subsample, about 15% of the entire group, answered a 94-item questionnaire containing the Zung Self-Rating Depression Scale (Zung, 1965), the Rosenberg Self-Derogation Scale (Kaplan & Pokorny, 1969; Kaplan, 1975), the Brief Michigan Alcoholism Screening Test (MAST; Pokorny, Miller, & Kaplan, 1972), a drug abuse identification scale, and portions of scales intended to rate anxiety, somatization, general state of health, subjective life expectancy, and attitudes toward death. Additionally, a research social worker interviewed each patient and completed several ratings. For suicide attempters and ideators, the appropriate Beck intentionality scales were completed, along with the Beck hopelessness and depression scales (Beck, Schuyler, & Herman, 1974; Beck, Weissman, Lester, & Trexler, 1974). These same additional ratings were given to a randomly selected group of 668 subjects.

Raters

The research social worker did all of the additional ratings in the high-risk group. The regular ward physician performed the examination and completed the BPRS. The NOSIE-30 was completed by the ward nursing staff. The records review was done by a research clerk. Each of the raters was given initial training in completion of the rating forms, followed by continual supervision by the investigators.

Follow-Up

All 4,800 patients were followed up for a period of 4 to 6 years (mean, 5 years), using several sources of data. Instances of completed suicide and death from any cause were identified by (1) word of mouth, (2) local newspaper stories and obituary columns, (3) information from VA officials, (4) monthly report of death certificates for veterans in Texas, and (5) a yearly search of the VA national record system. These sources are listed in order of increasing completeness, but decreasing immediacy. We used all of these systems to be able to follow up completed suicide instances as soon after the event as possible. We also studied records of admission to any VA hospital to identify patients rehospitalized for suicide attempts or suicidal ideation. For each identified case of suicide, we interviewed relatives or associates of the patient, but those data are not presented in this chapter (instead, see Pokorny & Kaplan, 1976).

RESULTS

Sample Characteristics

Some of the principal characteristics of the sample were as follows:

Characteristics	No. of patients
Sex	
M	4,691
F	109
Race	
Black	1,162
Nonblack	3,638
Marital status on admission	
Single	1,034
Married and together	1,900
Married but separated	566
Widowed	124
Divorced	1,157
Not determined	19
Diagnosis on admission	
Affective disorder	518
Schizophrenia	834
Alcoholism	1,618
Drug abuse	721
Neurosis	400
Personality disorder	428
Organic brain syndrome	281
Age at admission (years)	
<20	98
20–29	1,332
30–39	711
40–49	1,375
50–59	1,039
60–69	178
>70	67

The diagnoses, collapsed into seven principal groups, were those made by the admitting ward physician, according to *Diagnostic and Statistical Manual of Mental Disorders*, second edition (DSM-II) criteria. Because one goal of the project was to see whether suicide could be predicted by the results of a thorough psychiatric examination by treatment of staff at time of admission, we used the admission diagnosis as the offical diagnostic grouping, even though other sources of information might have indicated some other diagnostic category.

Follow-Up

The U.S. death rate from all causes has been about 900 per 100,000 per year in recent years (just under 1% dying annually. The death rate for persons with heart disease has been about 350 per 100,000 per year; for those with malignant neoplasms, about 170 per 1000,000 per year; and for those with stroke, about 100 per 100,000 per year. The death rate from suicide has been around 12 per 100,000 per year. The age- and sex-adjusted suicide rate for all veterans, however, is about 23 per 100,000 per year (Pokorny, 1967). These death rates should be kept in mind as standards against which the reported suicide rates can be evaluated.

During the 5-year follow-up period, we identified 67 suicides within the total group of 4,800 subjects, as well as 179 subsequent suicide attempts. This yields a suicide rate of 279 per 100,000 per year, about 12 times the expected rate for veterans. The high-risk group, which included 803 subjects, had 30 subsequent suicides, giving a suicide rate of 747 per 100,000 per year, about 32 times the expected rate of veterans.

The 67 suicides occurred fairly evenly throughout the 4- to 6-year follow-up period. This observation may appear to contradict the usual finding that most suicides occur soon after release from the hospital. However, many of these subjects were readmitted to the hospital, often more than once. The important duration is the time elapsed since last discharge from the hospital. Analyzed in this way, the 67 cases were grouped as follows: 5 suicides occurred when the patient was still in the hospital; 10, within 1 to 7 days after release; 6, within 8 to 30 days; 8, within 1 to 3 months; 12, within 3 to 6 months; 6, within 6 to 12 months; 8, within 1 to 2 years; and the other 12, within 2 to 6 years after last discharge from the hospital. Excluding the 5 occurring in the hospital, 16 (26%) occurred within 1 month and 36 (58%) within 6 months of hospital discharge, a pattern that resembles the usual experience.

The length of time between last release from the hospital and completed suicide was cross-tabulated against race, age at time of initial admission, marital status, and diagnosis. No striking or significant relationships were observed.

Of the 21 items making up the formula for selecting the "high-risk" subsample, 10 turned out to be significant predictors. Eight of these related to current or past suicidal behavior, one was a diagnosis of affective disorder, and one was not being black (data available from National Auxiliary Publications Services [NAPS]).

Suicide Rates

Table 6.1 shows the age breakdown of the patients who committed suicide and of the total sample. The distributions resemble each other; they are bimodal with peaks in the 20- to 29-year and 40- to 49-year periods. (This age distribution, of course, reflects that of U.S. war veterans in general.) The 20- to 29-year-old group was slightly overrepresented in suicides, but the difference was not statistically significant. In these atypical, high-risk subjects, all of whom had psychiatric disorders requiring hospitalization, the usual principle that suicide rates in men increase progressively with age did not seem to apply. Evidently this "indicator," like many others that are valid in the general population, no longer applies when the rate of suicide is increased greatly; other and stronger risk factors overcome the effect of age.

The bimodal distribution may also represent the recently observed tendency for younger age cohorts in the United States to have higher suicide rates at *all* ages. Within each age cohort, however, suicide rates still increase with age. Combining all age groups results in a bimodal distribution with a first peak in the 20s (Hellon & Solomon, 1980; Murphy & Wetzel, 1980; Solomon & Hellon, 1980).

The bimodal age distribution shown in Table 6.1 was used as a basis for several comparisons. One involved the method of suicide, comparing those under age 40 years with those 40 years old or older at the time of the index admission date. There were no significant differences.

TABLE 6.1. Incidence of Subsequent Suicides by Age at Admission

Age (years)	Total sample, % (n = 4,800)	Suicides, no. (%)
10–19	2	2 (3)
20–29	28	25 (38)
30–39	15	9 (13)
40–49	29	15 (22)
50–59	21	15 (22)
60–69	4	1 (1)
≥ 70	1	0 (0)
Total	100	67 (99)

Note. The mean follow-up period was 5 years. The χ^2 test yielded no significant differences when the 10- to 19-year-old and 60- to 79-year-old categories were collapsed into adjoining groups.

TABLE 6.2. Incidence of Suicide by Diagnosis and Age Group

Diagnosis	Total sample, % (n = 4,800)	Suicides, no. (%)	Age at admission to project (years)	
			<40, No. (%)	≥40, no. (%)
Affective disorder	11	18 (27)	11 (31)	7 (23)
Schizophrenia	17	19 (28)	12 (33)	7 (23)
Alcoholism	34	15 (22)	2 (6)	13 (42)
Drug abuse	15	7 (10)	7 (19)	0 (0)
Neurosis	8	3 (4)	1 (3)	2 (6)
Personality disorder	9	4 (6)	2 (6)	2 (6)
Organic brain syndrome	6	1 (1)	1 (3)	0 (0)
Total	100	67 (98)	36 (101)	31 (100)

Table 6.2 shows the number of suicides by diagnostic group, for the total group and for age subgroups. The distributions show an overrepresentation of patients with affective disorder and schizophrenia in the completed suicide group ($\chi^2 = 24.5$, $p = .001$). All of the drug-abuse-related suicides were in the younger group, whereas most of the alcoholism-related suicides were in the older group.

Table 6.3 gives the same information on diagnostic categories, but expressed as rates. It also gives the total number of deaths from all causes in each diagnostic group. As expected, the death rate for patients with organic brain syndrome was very high, as was the death rate in the alcoholic group. However, the death rate for *all* diagnostic groups was high (2,758 per

TABLE 6.3. Incidence of Death and Suicide by Diagnostic Category

Diagnosis	Total deaths		Suicides		% of total deaths
	No.	Rate/ 100,000/yr	No.	Rate/ 100,000/yr	
Affective disorder (n = 518)	59	2,278	18	695	30.5
Schizophrenia (n = 834)	65	1,559	19	456	29.2
Alcoholism (n = 1,618)	334	4,129	15	187	4.5
Drug abuse (n = 721)	49	1,359	7	194	14.3
Neurosis (n = 400)	30	1,500	3	150	10.0
Personality disorder (n = 428)	21	981	4	187	19.0
Organic brain syndrome (n = 281)	104	7,402	1	71	1.0
Total (n = 4,800)	662	2,758	67	279	10.1

Note. The mean follow-up period was 5 years.

100,000 per year, compared with about 900 per 100,000 per year for the general U.S. population).

Table 6.3 also shows that the suicide rate for the total group of 4,800 subjects was 279 per 100,000 per year, or about 12 times the age- and sex-adjusted rate for male veterans. The completed suicide rate was highest in the affective disorder group, but the schizophrenic group was a close second. Table 6.3 also gives the percentages of deaths that were suicides; for affective disorders and schizophrenia, these percentages were about 30%.

Table 6.4 shows the suicide rates for several special groups. All of the patients who committed suicide were male. The rate for nonblack men was about three times that for black men. The rate for single men was the highest, whereas the marital status group with the lowest rate was "married and together." Our *a priori* "high-risk" group had a suicide rate of 747 per 100,000 per year, compared with 185 per 100,000 per year in the rest of the sample—a ratio of 4.04:1. Therefore, our high-risk formula *did* identify a group with a significantly greater probability of suicide. Finally, patients admitted for a suicide attempt had a subsequent suicide rate of 1,702 per 100,000 per year. On the average, nearly 2% of this group completed suicide during each year of follow-up. This is high as suicide rates go, but in terms of the feasibility of predicting individual cases, it is still relatively low.

Table 6.5 shows the 5-year suicide rates for other special groups. (Some of these rates may have quite broad confidence limits when the base is only a few hundred subjects.) The risk increases progressively as the various lower-risk groups are subtracted, except that in the high-risk subsample the rates do not increase (rather, they drop slightly) when the black subjects are

TABLE 6.4. Incidence of Suicide by Subgroup

Group	No. of subjects	No. of suicides	Suicide rate/ 100,000/yr
Total sample	4,800	67	279
"High-risk" subsample	803	30	747
Rest of sample	3,997	37	185
Women	109	0	0
Men	4,691	67	286
Nonblack	3,549	60	338
Black	1,142	7	123
Single	1,008	23	456
Married	1,860	17	183
Separated, widowed, or divorced	1,823	27	296
Reason for admission			
Suicide attempt	188	16	1,702
Other	4,612	51	221

Note. The mean follow-up period was 5 years.

TABLE 6.5. Incidence of Suicide by Diagnosis and Subgroup

	Affective disorder	Schizophrenia	Alcoholism or drug abuse	Other diagnoses	Total
Total sample					
Suicides/subjects, no.	18/518	19/834	22/2,339	8/1,109	67/4,800
Rate	695	456	188	144	279
Male subjects					
Suicides/subjects, no.	18/498	19/804	22/2,308	8/1,081	67/4,691
Rate	723	473	191	148	286
Nonblack male subjects					
Suicides/subjects, no.	17/429	15/507	21/1,786	7/827	60/3,549
Rate	793	592	235	169	338
High-risk male subjects					
Suicides/subjects, no.	14/200	6/119	7/266	3/194	30/779
Rate	1,400	1,008	526	309	770
Nonblack, high-risk male subjects					
Suicides/subjects, no.	13/187	4/94	7/245	2/171	26/697
Rate	1,380	851	571	234	746

Note. The man follow-up period was 5 years. Rates are given as suicides per 100,000 subjects per year.

removed. Again this illustrates the general point: Although the racial distinction is significant in the general population and even in our total sample, it no longer applies in the high-risk subsample, with its much higher suicide rate.

Cross-Tabulations

Each item from the rating instruments was cross-tabulated against suicide, suicide attempt, or absence of these behaviors during the follow-up period. For the total group of 4,800 subjects there were 153 such cross-tabulations, and 51 showed statistically significant relationships (data available from NAPS). Items that were strongly associated with subsequent suicide included diagnoses of affective disorder or schizophrenia, history of suicide attempt, having been placed on suicide precautions, overt evidence of depression, complaints of insomnia, and presence of guilt feelings, along with 45 others.

The same type of comparison was made for the total group of 4,800 subjects, using 12 factor scores derived from BPRS and NOSIE-30 rating scales. Both the patients who later committed suicide and those who attempted it were rated high on the "depression" factor. The suicide attempters (but not those who actually committed suicide) were rated high on the "personality disorder" and "irritability" factors. The completed suicide group was rated low on "social interest." The suicide groups were not differentiated significantly from each other or from the rest of the sample when cross-tabulated with eight other factor scores: the BPRS factors of "schizophrenia," "somatic symptoms," "deterioration," and "organicity," and the NOSIE-30 factors of "social competence," "personal neatness," "manifest psychosis," and "retardation."

For the 803 high-risk subjects, there were additional ratings and evaluations; those items were examined in 106 additional cross-tabulations, of which 20 showed significant relationships (data available from NAPS). With most of these items, the suicide completers and attempters deviated from the rest of the sample in the same direction, but this was not always true. For example, in response to the item "I have an urge to do harmful, shocking things," the attempters answered "true" more often than did the rest of the sample, but the actual suicides deviated significantly in the other direction.

The additional ratings given to the high-risk group also yielded 10 summary scores (data available from NAPS). Three of them showed significant differences between the two groups. Two of these (the drug abuse and self-derogation scores) were high in both suicide attempters and completers, whereas one (the impulsivity score) was elevated only for the attempters. Seven other summary scores did not differentiate significantly between groups. These were the total scores on the Brief MAST, the internalization-externalization score, the authoritarian score, the score on the Rosenberg "favorable self-presentation" factor (Kaplan & Pokorny, 1969), the guilt score, the anxiety score, and the total score on the Zung Self-Rating Depression Scale (Zung, 1965).

Clearly, we were able to differentiate the groups using any one of a large number of items and summary scores. We had been interested in whether the suicide completers would resemble the suicide attempters. Since the work of Stengel and Cook (1958), it has generally been held that the two groups are basically different, though overlapping. We found, however, that in most respects the two suicidal groups were similar; that is, they were mostly related to the same predictors, and generally in the same direction. Therefore, at least for this population of mostly male adult veterans, suicide attempters do not differ sharply from suicide completers. However, a minority of items were related differently: A prior diagnosis of personality disorder was common in patients who later attempted suicide but not in those who actually succeeded, and the same relationship applied to projection of blame and drug dependency. Therefore, though for the most part the two behaviors involved similar subjects, the suicide attempters did show more personality-disorder-related traits, along with such traits as manipulativeness and hostility.

Of the 281 individual items and factor or summary scores looked at by cross-tabulations, 78 showed statistically significant relationships to subsequent suicide or suicide attempts—almost one of every three predictors examined.

Hence, we did find numerous significant relationships. We confirmed the findings of numerous previous studies by identifying many of the same indicators or "predictors." This kind of information is useful in making clinical judgments; it provides a background for treatment decisions. This is the same kind of information used in patient management in many areas of medicine; physicians make use of trends and correlations to make the best choice of moves, to "play the odds." This approach helps us to adopt a treatment policy that should lead in the long run to the largest proportion of correct decisions. The task is quite different, however, when we attempt to predict for each particular case.

STEPWISE DISCRIMINANT ANALYSIS

We applied the technique of stepwise discriminant analysis (Statistical Package for the Social Sciences) in an attempt to select, from this long list of significantly related items and scores, some weighted combination of variables that could successfully identify at a practical level the patients who would later commit or attempt suicide. As items for use in the discriminant analysis, we chose those that had shown the strongest relationships when looked at individually. Sixty variables were initially selected in this way.

The number of variables was further reduced by running "trial" discriminant-function analyses with 20 variables at a time, and selecting for the final analysis the 20 items with the highest F value in the one-way analysis of variance between groups. For the discriminant analysis, only those variables were retained whose partial multivariate F ratios were larger than 1.00.

Four discriminant-function analyses were performed. In two analyses we attempted to discriminate patients who committed suicide from all the others; this was done separately for the total group of 4,800 subjects and for the high-risk subgroup of 803. The other two analyses, again for both groups, attempted a three-way discrimination: completed suicide versus suicide attempts versus others. There was some loss of cases in these analyses because of incomplete information.

The first discriminant-function analysis was applied to the entire sample and employed the following variables:

Variable	Discriminant coefficient
History of suicide attempt	−.62
Diagnosis of affective disorder or schizophrenia versus other	−.33
Having been on suicidal list at any VA hospital	−.34
Single, widowed, or divorced versus other	−.38

The standardized canonical discriminant-function coefficients are given.

The program was first instructed to disregard prior information concerning the low rate of suicide in the population (i.e., to assume equal base rates). That procedure yielded the following results:

Actual outcome	Prediction		Total
	Suicide	Other	
Suicide	35	28	63
Other	1,206	3,435	4,641
Total	1,241	3,463	4,704

This procedure correctly identified 35 of the 63 subsequent suicides (55.6%), but at the cost of 1,206 false-positive predictions. Of the 1,241 subjects identified as suicides, only 2.8% were identified correctly. Overall, only 73.81% of the cases were classified correctly.

When the program was instructed to use the actual base rates (67 suicides in 4,800 subjects), the results were as follows:

Actual outcome	Prediction		Total
	Suicide	Other	
Suicide	0	63	63
Other	1	4,640	4,641
Total	1	4,703	4,704

The total percentage of cases classified correctly this time was 98.64%. However, a simple prediction that *no one* would commit suicide would have led to a slightly higher percentage.

We also performed a discriminant analysis using only the high-risk subjects, which made available a larger number of predictor items and scores. The following variables were used:

Variable	Discriminant coefficient
History of attempted suicide	.52
Suicidal ideation	.19
Diagnosis of affective disorder or schizophrenia	.27
Recent history of physical violence	−.25
Social interest	.30
Urge to do harmful, shocking thing	.45

Variable	Discriminant coefficient
Fear of losing control	.51
Feeling remorseful	.43
Tendency to become impatient	.34
Sense of being a failure	−.39
Feeling downhearted and blue	.31

When the program was set to disregard the base rates, the results were as follows:

	Prediction		
Actual outcome	Suicide	Other	Total
Suicide	21	8	29
Other	164	550	714
Total	185	558	743

In this high-risk subgroup, the program performed somewhat better in that 72.4% of the actual suicides were correctly identified. However, only 11.4% of 135 classified by the program as suicides were classified correctly. Overall, 76.8% were classified correctly.

When the program was instructed to use the actual base rates, the analysis yielded the following results:

	Prediction		
Actual outcome	Suicide	Other	Total
Suicide	0	29	29
Other	0	714	714
Total	0	743	743

This time, the classification results were the same as if we had simply predicted that no one would commit suicide; 96.1% were classified correctly.

We followed a similar procedure in attempting to separate the suicide completers from the attempters and from the rest of the sample (data available from NAPS). For the total sample of 4,800 patients, 20 of the 63 suicide completers (31.7%) were identified correctly, as were 63 of the 174 attempters (36.2%). Again, there were a large number of false-positive predictions.

The same procedure was applied to 803 high-risk subjects (data available from NAPS). When the program was set to disregard base rates, suicide completers and attempters were identified fairly well, but at the cost of many false-positive identifications. When the program was instructed to use actual base rates, the prediction was extremely conservative, with no subject predicted to commit suicide (thus yielding no true- or false-positive results).

Discriminant analysis was clearly inadequate in correctly classifying the subjects. For a disorder or event as rare as suicide or suicide attempts, our predictive tools and guides are simply not equal to the task.

The general situation regarding the usefulness of a "test" (which could just as well be a suicide prediction scale, a formula, or a discriminant function) is covered thoroughly and clearly in a book by Galen and Gambino (1975). Table 6.6 is adapted from their book and presents the standard definitions of true positives, false positives, and so forth as used in a screening situation. Galen and Gambino define "sensitivity" and "specificity" (paraphrased by them as "positivity in disease" and "negativity in health") as follows:

$$\text{Sensitivity} = \frac{\text{TP}}{\text{TP} + \text{FN}} \times 100$$

$$\text{Specificity} = \frac{\text{TN}}{\text{FP} + \text{TN}} \times 100$$

where TP indicates true positive; FN, false negative; TN, true negative; and FP, false positive.

Galen and Gambino also define the "predictive value" of a test result as follows:

$$\text{Predictive value} = \frac{\text{TP}}{\text{TP} + \text{FP}} \times 100$$

They stress that the predictive value is highly dependent on base rates or prevalence rates of the disorder and define the "efficiency" of a test as the percentage of cases classified correctly. (Sensitivity, specificity, and predictive value are properly *population* measures; the corresponding measures derived from a *sample* are estimates of population values.)

We applied these formulas to the results of the first discriminant analysis, given earlier (total sample, base rates disregarded). As already noted, the "test" or suicide provided by that discriminant function was not very sensitive; only 35 of the 63 subjects who actually committed suicide were correctly identified. Using the formula, we found its sensitivity to be 55.5%, its specificity 74.0%, its predictive value 2.8%, and its efficiency 73.8%. In every-

TABLE 6.6. Predictive Value of a Test When Applied to Healthy and Diseased Populations

	Patients with positive test result	Patients with negative test result	Total
Patients with disease	TP	FN	TP + FN
Patients without disease	FP	TN	FP + TN
Total	TP + FP	TN + FN	TP + FP + TN + FN

Note. TP indicates true-positive classifications; FP, false-positive; TN, true-negative; and FN, false-negative. Adapted from *Beyond Normality: The Predictive Value and Efficiency of Medical Diagnoses* (p. 13) by R. Galen and S. Gambino, 1975, New York: Wiley. Copyright 1975 by Churchill Livingstone. Adapted by permission.

day language, by applying our "test" for suicide we correctly identified just over half of the 63 suicides, but at the cost of 1,206 false-positive identifications. We classified over one-fourth of our subjects as suicidal and still only predicted just over half of the actual suicides. It is not particularly helpful to concentrate our special efforts on one-fourth of the entire group. This level of case identification will not permit any meaningful redirection of effort, because it is simply not feasible to maintain one-fourth of psychiatric inpatients on "suicidal precautions" indefinitely.

Handpicked Predictors

I also assembled a "suicide prediction test" by hand, combining five items that were significantly related to suicide: being in the high-risk group; being nonblack; having a diagnosis either of affective disorder or schizophrenia or of alcoholism or drug abuse; having any marital status other than married and together; and being male. Subjects with all five characteristics had a suicide rate of 1,020 per 100,000 per year, certainly a high rate compared with that of the general population. When this new "formula" was used as a classification tool, 15 of the 67 completed suicides were identified correctly, but there were 279 false-positive predictions. The (estimated) sensitivity was therefore less than half as good as that of the discriminant-function formula, but the specificity was much improved. The predictive value of a positive (completed suicide) score had increased to 5%, and the efficiency was increased to 93%, but neither gain was clinically significant or useful.

In their book, Galen and Gambino (1975) provided a useful set of tables showing the interaction between test sensitivity, specificity, and disease prevalence in influencing the predictive value of positive test results. Table 6.7 gives selected information from their more detailed tables. When the prevalence is as low as 1 per 100,000, even at the unrealistically high levels of 99% sensitivity and 99.9% specificity, the predictive value of a

TABLE 6.7. Predictive Value of a Positive Test Result at Three Prevalence Levels

Specificity, %	Sensitivity, %				
	50	70	90	95	99
A. Prevalence, 1/100,000					
50	0	0	0	0	0
70	0	0	0	0	0
90	0	0	0	0	0
99	0	0	0	0	0
99.9	0	1	1	1	1
B. Prevalence, 10/100,000					
50	0	0	0	0	0
70	0	0	0	0	0
90	0	0	0	0	0
99	0	1	1	1	1
99.9	5	7	8	9	9
C. Prevalence, 500/100,000					
50	1	1	1	1	1
70	1	1	1	2	2
90	2	3	4	5	5
99	20	26	30	32	33
99.9	72	78	82	83	83

Note. Numbers indicate predictive values, given as percentages. See text for further explanation. Adapted from *Beyond Normality: The Predictive Value and Efficiency of Medical Diagnoses* (pp. 167, 170, 174) by R. Galen and S. Gambino, 1975, New York: Wiley. Copyright 1975 by Churchill Livingstone. Adapted by permission.

positive test is only 1%. Table 6.7 gives the corresponding percentages for a situation in which the prevalence is 10 per 100,000, approximately the incidence of suicide in the general population. Again, if both the sensitivity and specificity were 99%, the predictive value of a positive test result would be only 1%.

Given a prevalence of 500 per 100,000, approximately the incidence of suicide found in the population of hospitalized psychiatric patients used in this study, a test with 99% sensitivity and 99% specificity would have a positive predictive value of only 33% (Table 6.7). An actual test, however, is more likely to have only about 50% sensitivity and 90% specificity, reducing the predictive value of a positive test result to only 2%.

Artificial Manipulation of Base Rates

Because of the powerful effect of the low base rates in predicting suicide, we ran a series of discriminant functions using the same predictors, while artificially increasing the proportion of completed suicide cases in the sample. This was done by leaving in the 67 completed suicide cases, but progressively reducing the size of the "other" group by randomly subtracing subjects from it. The size of the "other" group was set so that the proportion of suicide cases would be approximately .01, .05, .10, .20, .30, .40, and .50 (as there was always some loss of cases because of incomplete data, these proportions were only approximated). The results of this series of discriminant-function classifications, with the program instructed each time to use actual base rates, are shown in Table 6.8.

This table shows how our "test" for identifying future suicides would perform if this behavior were less rare. Section A describes the actual situation, and the resulting classification is the same as shown earlier. The subsequent sections of the table, B through G, show how the discriminant-function procedure would perform if completed suicides occurred in a progressively larger proportion of the sample (as shown in the third column). The (estimated) sensitivity improves steadily, but even in section G the procedure identifies only two-thirds of the cases. In conditions B through F, too few of the suicides are identified to make discriminant analysis a very helpful procedure. The false-positive classifications are less of a problem under these artificial conditions; in conditions B through G, the true positives outnumber the false positives, mostly by a 2:1 ratio. The predictive value of a positive prediction does not change appreciably in conditions B through G, and the percentage correctly classified drops steadily. We could probably live with condition G, as two-thirds of the suicide cases are identified, and the number of false-positive predictions is small enough that it might be feasible to treat them all as "suicidal."

This procedure demonstrates that low base rates are not our only problem, but that the "test" or case-identifying procedure we are using is also unequal to the task. We need more sensitive and specific tests or predictive instruments. Our study, which incorporated most of the inquiries, ratings, and measurements previously shown to correlate with suicide, failed to come up with an adequate prediction procedure.

COMMENT

We are attempting to identify cases of a low-incidence disorder with a "test" totally inadequate for that purpose, one that yields too many false-positive and false-negative results to make any clinical use feasible.

False Positives

The false positives are a greater problem than false negatives. We might tolerate 50% false negatives; if we could apply a screening test that would

TABLE 6.8. Discriminant-Function Classifications with Progressively Increased Base Rate of Suicide

Sample employed	No.	Prediction, no. Suicide	Prediction, no. Other	Proportion of suicides in sample	Sensitivity, %	Specificity, %	Predictive value of positive result, %	Subjects correctly classified, %
A.								
Suicide	63	0	63	.013	0.0	99.9	0.0	98.6
Other	4,641	1	4,640					
B.								
Suicide	63	8	55	.046	12.7	99.5	57.1	95.5
Other	1,295	6	1,289					
C.								
Suicide	63	9	54	.105	14.3	98.9	60.0	95.5
Other	535	6	529					
D.								
Suicide	66	13	53	.183	19.7	98.3	72.2	83.9
Other	294	5	289					
E.								
Suicide	63	19	44	.290	30.2	94.2	67.9	75.6
Other	154	9	145					
F.								
Suicide	66	24	42	.370	36.4	90.2	68.6	70.2
Other	112	11	101					
G.								
Suicide	63	43	20	.543	68.6	60.4	67.2	64.7
Other	53	21	32					

125

correctly identify only half of the future suicides without false positives, that would be very helpful. However, with currently known "tests," to identify the actual suicides we will also have to make a great many false-positive identifications, labeling up to a quarter of the total group as "future suicides" when only 1% to 5% actually are. From a cost–benefit standpoint, the application of such a "test" is simply not feasible.

False-positive results are a problem with many screening tests. For example, nationwide mass screening of children for heart disease was said to produce much harm from anxiety-producing false-positive identifications (Golin, 1980). The morbidity in those with false-positive results was greater on follow-up than the morbidity in children with actual organic lesions.

Influence of Base Rates

Galen and Gambino (1975) stress the great influence of base or prevalence rates in determining the usefulness, predictive value, and other characteristics of any test or procedure. They point out that tests are typically developed in an artificial situation, in which the sample is so chosen that the incidence of the disorder is around 50%. The tests are then applied to the screening situation, where the incidence may be very low. Nevertheless, a user may naively expect it to perform as well there as during the "laboratory" standardization.

Error in Predictive Tests

There are several possible sources of error in a test. One source may simply be sloppy application of the test, leading to careless mistakes, which can be minimized by greater care, training, supervision, and motivation.

Even if careless error has been removed, there remains an inevitable residual error characteristic of the test. This, however, is composed of two different elements. First, there is the true chance error in a test, which should be randomly distributed, meaning that a repetition of the same test on the same subjects should make incorrect identifications of *different* subjects, but at about the same rates. Such measurement error can be avoided by repeating the test at least once. If a test has a 10% rate of error, repeating it once should reduce the error to 1%, and repeating it twice should reduce error to 0.1%. This is the logic behind "successive screening" or using two or three different tests designed to measure the same thing.

The second possibility for error lies in the characteristics of a subject that are measured and identified correctly but are in the wrong relation to the predicted state. An example of this condition is a genuine false-positive syphilis test result. The serological response really is reactive, and repeated measurement will repeatedly show it this way. Therefore, repeating the test one or more times is not likely to decrease predictive error.

This type of error applies to many clinical, demographic, and life history predictors of suicide. For example, an elderly, depressed, and alcoholic man who lives alone and has a history of suicide attempt is at increased risk of suicide. If this aggregate of predictors is our "test," then it will predict successfully in some proportion of cases, but wrongly in others. Repeating the test will not change this outcome, as these characteristics remain the same; the procedure will predict wrongly every time. Unfortunately, most of the tests or predictors of suicide fall into this second class, and repeated or successive screenings are therefore of no help.

Limitations of Present Study

In a study such as the one reported here, there is a preset and inevitably limited list of inquiries. Even though we inquired about several hundred items of for each subject, the items were from preset lists, so that there was no follow-up of any lead in greater depth. In the usual clinical situation, by contrast, the clinician is free to pursue each lead or clue at length. From a research standpoint, this is undesirable, as it makes every case study almost unique and thus limits discovery of general truths or relationships. Furthermore, the freehand, artistic method of clinical inquiry makes it almost impossible to eliminate bias, suggestion, and the tendency to find what one expects to find.

There is, however, a more hopeful view of the clinical situation with a "suicidal" patient. Diagnosis in clinical practice (in contrast to a prospective research project) typically consists of a sequence of small decisions. For example, in suicide prediction, the first decision might be based on some altering note or sign, and the decision would be to investigate further. After further investigation, one might stop if no additional alerting or confirming indicators were found, or one might decide to explore the situation even further (perhaps to hospitalize, for example). In each case, the decision is not what to do for all time, but rather what to do next, for the near future. In such a situation, the consequences of "false-positive" identifications early on may be relatively minor, and it may be appropriate for physicians to screen in many cases.

Long-Range versus Short-Range Prediction

The thrust of our project has been long-range prediction of completed suicide during a follow-up period averaging 5 years. The conclusion is inescapable that we do not possess any item of information or any combination of items that permit us to identify to a useful degree the particular persons who will commit suicide, in spite of the fact that we do have scores of items available, each of which is significantly related to suicide.

Yet it seems that psychiatrists do know which patients are highly suicidal, and, on the whole, do an acceptable job of protecting and treating them. This clinical work is in an entirely different time frame, dealing in minutes, hours, or days. It is commonly recognized that a "suicidal crisis" will pass, with or without a suicide attempt, so that after a few days the risk has abated and it may be safe for the patient to be discharged. Such a time frame has not been included in this research, and it may be that suicide risk on this short-term basis is essentially unresearchable, as it would not be ethical to withhold taking appropriate emergency steps to ensure safety. Furthermore, in considering a time frame of minutes, hours, or days with highly disturbed patients, it is not feasible to obtain detailed quantitative ratings or evaluations of mood, or to determine such things as suicide intentionality or the level of hope or despair. In this short-term time frame, the concept of prediction may not even apply; rather, one is required to *identify* a suicidal crisis that is already here, a task involving a different set of concepts and clinical skills.

The negative findings of this study have clear implications. The courts and public opinion seem to expect physicians to be able to pick out the particular persons who will later commit suicide. Although we may reconstruct causal chains and motives after the fact, we do not possess the tools to predict particular suicides before the fact.

REFERENCES

Beck, A. T., Resnik, H. L. P., & Lettieri, D. J. (Eds.). (1974). *The prediction of suicide.* Bowie, MD: Charles Press.

Beck, A. T., Schuyler, D., & Herman, I. (1974). Development of suicide intent scales. In A. T. Beck, H. L. P. Resnik, & D. J. Lettieri (Eds.), *The prediction of suicide.* Bowie, MD: Charles Press.

Beck, A. T., Weissman, A., Lester, D., & Trexler, L. (1974). The measurement of pessimism: The Hopelessness Scale. *Journal of Consulting and Clinical Psychology, 42*, 861–865.

Brown, T., & Sheran, T. (1972). Suicide prediction: A review. *Suicide and Life-Threatening Behavior, 2*, 67–68.

Cohen, E., Motto, J., & Seiden, R. (1966). An instrument for evaluating suicidal potential. *American Journal of Psychiatry, 122*, 886–897.

Diggory, J. (1974). Predicting suicide: Will-o-the-wisp or reasonable challenge? In A. T. Beck, H. L. P. Resnik, & D. J. Lettieri (Eds.), *The prediction of suicide.* Bowie, MD: Charles Press.

Galen, R., & Gambino, S. (1975). *Beyond normality: The predictive value and efficiency of medical diagnoses.* New York: Wiley.

Golin, M. (1980, January 25). Medical computer: Master or servant? *American Medical News* (Impact section), p. 3.

Hellon, C. P., & Solomon, M. I. (1980). Suicide and age in Alberta, Canada, 1951 to 1977: The changing profile. *Archives of General Psychiatry, 37*, 505–510.

Honigfeld, G., & Klett, J. (1965). The Nurses' Observation Scale for Inpatient Evaluation. *Journal of Clinical Psychology, 21*, 65–71.

Kaplan, H. (1975). *Self-attitudes and deviant behavior.* Santa Monica, CA: Goodyear.

Kaplan, H., & Pokorny, A. (1969). Self-derogation and psychosocial adjustment. *Journal of Nervous and Mental Disease, 149*, 421–434.

Lester, D. (1972). *Why people kill themselves: A summary of research findings on suicidal behavior.* Springfield, IL: Charles C Thomas.

Litman, R., Farberow, N., Wold, C., & Brown, T. (1974). Prediction models of suicidal behavior. In A. T. Beck, H. L. P. Resnik, & D. J. Lettieri (Eds.), *The prediction of suicide.* Bowie, MD: Charles Press.

MacKinnon, D., & Farberow, N. (1975). An assessment of the utility of suicide prediction. *Suicide and Life-Threatening Behavior, 6*, 86–91.

Murphy, G. E. (1972). Clinical identification of suicidal risk. *Archives of General Psychiatry, 27*, 356–359.

Murphy, G. E., & Wetzel, R. D. (1980). Suicide risk by birth cohort in the United States, 1949 to 1974. *Archives of General Psychiatry, 37*, 519–523.

Overall, J., & Gorham, D. (1962). The Brief Psychiatric Rating Scale. *Psychology Report, 10*, 799–812.

Pokorny, A. D. (1960). Characteristics of 44 patients who subsequently committed suicide. *Archives of General Psychiatry, 2*, 314–323.

Pokorny, A. D. (1964). Suicide rates in various psychiatric disorders. *Journal of Nervous and Mental Disease, 139*, 499–506.

Pokorny, A. D. (1966). A follow-up of 618 suicidal patients. *American Journal of Psychiatry, 122*, 1109–1116.

Pokorny, A. D. (1967). Suicide in war veterans: Rates and methods. *Journal of Nervous and Mental Disease, 144*, 224–229.

Pokorny, A. D., & Kaplan, H. (1976). Suicide following psychiatric hospitalization: The interaction effects of defenselessness and adverse life events. *Journal of Nervous and Mental Disease, 162*, 119–125.

Pokorny, A. D., Miller, B., & Kaplan, H. (1972). The Brief MAST: A shortened version of the Michigan Alcoholism Screening Test. *American Journal of Psychiatry, 129*, 342–345.

Solomon, M. I., & Hellon, C. P. (1980). Suicide and age in Alberta, Canada, 1951 to 1977: A cohort analysis. *Archives of General Psychiatry, 37*, 511–513.

Stengel, E., & Cook, N. (1958). *Suicide and attempted suicide.* London: Chapman & Hall.

Tuckman, J., & Youngman, W. (1968). A scale for assessing suicide risk of attempted suicides. *Journal of Clinical Psychology, 24*, 17–19.

Zung, W. W. K. (1965). A self-rating depression scale. *Archives of General Psychiatry, 12*, 63–70.

CHAPTER 7

The Clinical Prediction of Adolescent Suicide

Madelyn S. Gould, Ph.D., M.P.H.
David Shaffer, M.D., F.R.C. Psych.
Columbia University
New York State Psychiatric Institute

Prudence Fisher, M.S.
Marjorie Kleinman, M.S.
Alyssa Morishima, M.S.
New York State Psychiatric Institute

The magnitude of the problem of youth suicide warrants its being deemed a major public health problem. Approximately 2,000 youngsters under age 20 killed themselves in 1987 in the United States, representing a rate of approximately 10 per 100,000 of the adolescent population (National Center for Health Statistics, 1990). The suicide rate among teenagers has increased approximately 200% since 1960, moving suicide from the fifth leading cause of death among 15- to 19-year-olds to the second leading cause of death in 1987.

The prediction, identification, and treatment of suicidal behavior pose difficult clinical challenges for mental health professionals. Preventive efforts directed to the general population are likely to reach relatively few teenagers who will eventually commit suicide. A more efficient strategy is to target high-risk groups (Shaffer, Garland, Gould, Fisher, & Trautman, 1988). Knowledge about high-risk groups can be obtained from death certificate data. The suicide rate among teenagers varies considerably by age, sex, and race. Suicide is extremely rare before age 12, is about four times as

Portions of this material were adapted from "Truncated Pathways from Childhood to Adulthood: Attrition in Follow-Up Studies Due to Death" by M. S. Gould, D. Shaffer, and M. Davies, 1990, in L. Robins and M. Rutter (Eds.), *Straight and Devious Pathways from Childhood to Adulthood* (pp. 1–9). Cambridge, England: Cambridge University Press. Copyright 1990 by Cambridge University Press. Adapted by permission.

common in adolescent boys as girls, and is rare in blacks compared to whites. The fact that the age, sex, and race distributions differ for the suicides and the general population shows that age, sex, and race are important risk factors for suicide. Although this information provided by death certificate data is necessary, it is clearly insufficient to form the basis of a specific prediction of suicide risk. Research that provides an adequate and comprehensive description of suicide-specific risk factors and individuals at risk for suicide is critical for preventive and treatment efforts.

RESEARCH STRATEGIES TO IDENTIFY SUICIDE RISK
High-Risk Follow-up Studies

Two basic longitudinal strategies can be used to explore the correlates of suicide: the follow-up of a general population or of a high-risk population. For rare outcomes, such as adolescent suicide, the sample size needed from the general population to yield enough cases to be useful for studying risk factors is daunting. Instead, studying samples stratified to overrepresent high-risk groups is a recommended strategy. Follow-up studies of this kind have been largely confined to psychiatric patients and suicide attempters. Other risk factors for subsequent suicide that have been examined in prospective or retrospective follow-up studies include obstetric complications and biological markers. The majority of the longitudinal studies have dealt primarily with adult attempters, and the studies in this section refer to adults unless otherwise mentioned.

Prior Suicide Attempts

Although only a minority of teenage suicide attempters go on to commit suicide, follow-up studies show that their suicide rate is considerably higher than that of the general population. Observed rates range from approximately 9% of teenage boys admitted to a psychiatric inpatient unit who had been depressed or who had made a suicide attempt (Motto, 1984; Otto, 1972) to fewer than 1% of boys who presented at an emergency room after an overdose but who were not admitted to a psychiatric hospital (Hawton & Goldacre, 1982). Proportions for girls range from 1% for former psychiatric inpatients to 0.1% for those who received no inpatient psychiatric care. In the 5- to 15-year follow-up described by Motto (1984), the symptoms of severe depression (psychomotor retardation, hopelessness, hypersomnia, etc.) best predicted later suicide. The prevalence of the predictors in noncompleters also was high, however, so their specificity was limited. A recent follow-up study of teenagers admitted for self-poisoning has found that death by causes other than suicide is also significantly higher than expected. In this 1- to 6-year follow-up (Sellar, Hawton, & Goldacre, 1990), 14 deaths occurred during the follow-up period, whereas 4.8 deaths were expected. Three of the 14 deaths were suicides, two were from natural causes (both respiratory deaths) and the remaining nine were "violent" or unnatural deaths (e.g., hanging, drowning, road traffic accidents) but had verdicts recorded other than suicide. There are no studies relating suicidal ideation to later suicidal death; however, thinking about suicide is so common among high school students (Smith & Crawford, 1986) that it is unlikely to be a useful or specific predictor of suicide risk.

Mental Illness and Psychiatric Hospitalization

Formerly hospitalized adult psychiatric patients have significantly higher suicide rates than nonpatients (Pokorny, 1964, 1983; Temoche, Pugh, & McMahon, 1964; Winokur & Tsuang, 1975). By contrast, a follow-up study of "control" adults screened to exclude those with psychopathology showed that very few had committed suicide (Winokur & Tsuang, 1975).

Birth History

An excess of obstetric complications among youth suicides was noted by Salk, Sturner, Lipsitt, Reilly, and Levat (1985) in a study that matched consecutive youth suicides to local birth records. This relationship could be mediated in a number of ways. In addition to having complicated obstetric histories, the mothers of the completed suicides had received less prenatal care and were more likely to have smoked and taken alcohol during pregnancy. The excess of suicide in their offspring could reflect such associated factors as the central nervous system consequences of birth complication, exposure to some teratogen during pregnancy, the heritability of psychopathology, or the effects of inappropriate parenting by deviant mothers.

Biological Markers

In the past decade a number of biological correlates of suicide have been identified, all in adult studies (see Stanley & Mann, 1987, for a review). The most frequently replicated finding, first reported by Asberg, Thoren, Traskman, Bertilsson, and Ringberger (1976) in a study of depressed patients, is the presence of low concentrations of the serotonin metabolite 5-hydroxyindoleacetic acid (5-HIAA) in the cerebrospinal fluid (CSF) of suicide attempters and completers. Although CSF 5-HIAA derives from both the brain and the spinal cord, Stanley, Traskman-Bendz, and Dorovini (1985) have reported high correlations between brain and CSF 5-HIAA in autopsy studies. The relationship has been reported in suicidal individuals with a variety of primary diagnoses, specifically in depressed patients (Stanley &

Mann, 1987), borderline and aggressive personality types (Brown et al., 1982), and violent prisoners who have attempted suicide (Linnoila et al., 1983). These studies, although numerous, have in general involved small subject populations. Moreover, the specific behavioral correlates of the abnormal biochemistry have not been established, nor has the distribution of values in nonsuicidal populations been determined. As a result, neither the sensitivity nor the specificity of this measure has been established. Asberg, Nordstrom, and Traskman-Bendz (1986a), however, determined that among 76 hospitalized adult suicide attempters followed over a 1-year period, 21% of those whose CSF 5-HIAA was less than 90 µg/ml went on to commit suicide during the follow-up period, compared with only 2% of those with higher levels. Similar findings have been reported by Roy et al. (1986). The usefulness of CSF 5-HIAA as a predictor of suicide and therefore as an agent of prevention depends on whether or not serotonin indicators are stable over time (i.e., whether they are an index of a suicidal trait or simply of an abnormal state). van Praag (1977) found that low levels in depressed patients remained low in about half of the patients after their recovery. Traskman-Bendz, Asberg, Bertilsson, and Thoren (1984), however, showed that some individuals had stable levels while the levels of others fluctuated. Asberg, Nordstrom, and Traskman-Bendz (1986b) reported on two patients whose levels of CSF 5-HIAA continued to decline after their first attempt; both went on to commit suicide. It would appear that abnormally low levels of CSF 5-HIAA may bring a new level of specificity to the prediction of suicide risk.

High-risk follow-up studies provide reliable baseline information about suicide victims, but their findings cannot be generalized to groups not included in the follow-up. These studies, therefore, may account for only a small fraction of all cases. Moreover, when the risk factors are not known ahead of time, stratification of the sample to overrepresent high- risk groups may still yield small numbers of suicides. When the outcome is rare, as in the case of adolescent suicide, it is preferable to derive descriptive information from retrospective, case–control studies—"psychological autopsies"—because such studies allow for the examination of a wide variety of possible risk factors.

Psychological Autopsies

The term "psychological autopsy" was coined to describe a procedure designed to "reconstruct the lifestyle and personality of the deceased" with details of the circumstances, behaviors, and events that led to the death of that individual" (Shneidman & Farberow, 1961, p. 118; see also Clark & Horton-Deutsch, Chapter 8, this volume). The psychological autopsy method is a retrospective inquiry from one or more surviving informants and/or from contemporary records. It has the potential for obtaining representative, albeit incomplete, information. Psychological autopsy studies of consecutive reported suicides within a predefined geographical area can be assumed to be representative, because suicides are subject to reporting requirements and there is no evidence to suggest that suicides missed are themselves so unrepresentative as to make the identified remainder unrepresentative (Shaffer & Fisher, 1981). The psychological autopsy is an inherently incomplete method, however, because inquiries about the victim's state of mind or early experiences will be confined to the knowledge of the informant(s) and the information in records. Record studies always raise questions about whether missing information was truly absent or simply not noted. Despite these limitations, the psychological autopsy is often the only method available to obtain detailed information about suicide victims (Shaffer et al., 1988). It is a useful approach when applied to a consecutive sample of suicide victims in a geographic area, because information is derived from a more representative sample than the samples that have been followed up in studies of high-risk groups (Shaffer et al., 1988). In addition, prospective studies cannot expect to collect data close to the time of the suicide, so that immediate provoking events will be missed.

Although a number of retrospective psychological autopsy studies of adolescent suicides have been reported, they are generally limited by small sample sizes, the absence of appropriate controls, and/or the absence of comprehensive assessment techniques. Sanborn, Sanborn, and Cimbolic (1973) reported on 10 adolescent suicides in New Hampshire. The number was small; the study was uncontrolled; and standardized instruments were not used. Shaffer (1974) abstracted information from autopsy reports and other pre-existing records of 31 suicides under age 15 who died in England and Wales. The study was uncontrolled, and because survivors were not questioned directly, the information obtained was limited in extent. Jan-Tausch (1964) reported on 41 suicides that occurred in the state of New Jersey. No controls were examined; the sample was confined to pupils in the public school system; and data were confined to school records. Dizmang, Watson, May, and Bopp (1974) reported on 10 Shoshone Indians and utilized a randomly derived normal control group. The numbers were small; the group may not have been broadly representative; and assessment instruments were limited in scope. Shafii, Carrigan, Whittinghill, and Derrick (1985) undertook a controlled psychological autopsy study of 20 suicides aged between 12 and 19 in the Louisville area, using a specifically designed structured interview. Again, the number of cases studied was small, and the use of friendship controls may have minimized differences between the suicides and controls.

Rich, Young, and Fowler (1986) reported on telephone interviews with surviving family members of 204 consecutive suicides of all ages in the San

Diego area. However, of these, only 14 were aged between 10 and 19 at the time of death. The sample was enriched with 79 further suicides aged under 30, but the proportion of these who were aged under 19 was not specified. Although data were contrasted for suicides above and below age 30, they were not presented separately for the adolescents; furthermore, the study was uncontrolled. Brent et al. (1988) reported on a psychological autopsy study of 27 adolescent suicide victims and compared them to a group of 56 suicidal psychiatric inpatients in the Pittsburgh area. Although a broad assessment was carried out using standardized instruments, the total number studied was small, and the absence of nonsuicidal controls precluded the examination of suicide-specific risk factors.

In the next section of this chapter, we describe a geographically based sample of large size that employed both normal and suicidal controls, assessed through multiple informants with standard techniques. The principal goals of the study were as follows:

1. To determine the prevalence and patterns of mental illness among suicide victims.
2. To determine the specificity for suicide of a number of risk factors. These included social class; family structure and early caretaking experiences; educational achievements and history; medical illnesses; sexual orientation and participation; substance use; the availability of firearms; prior suicide attempts or threats; exposure to models of suicidal behavior; the degree and nature of prior stresses, including bereavement and loss; and family history of suicide and other psychiatric disorders.
3. To examine the act of suicide itself. Specifically, we wished to examine evidence of high intent, including planning, isolation, precautions against discovery, and communication of prior intent; the mental state of each suicide victim immediately prior to his or her death; the nature of any external precipitants; the method used; and the extent to which the suicide could be judged to be planned or impulsive—whether it was committed in a "rational" frame of mind or in an apparent state of psychological turmoil (when intoxicated or in a rage or state of despair).
4. To describe how males and females and black and whites differed with respect to all of the factors noted above.
5. To determine whether adolescents who had committed suicide differ from those of the same sex and ethnic group who had made a severe suicide attempt with respect to mental state, risk factors, and characteristics of suicidal behavior.

The following presentation focuses primarily on the examination of patterns of mental illness, substance abuse, prior suicidal behavior, and family history of suicidal behavior.

NEW YORK PSYCHOLOGICAL AUTOPSY STUDY AS AN ILLUSTRATION

Our case–control study of youth suicide illustrates how suicide rates and risk factors can be estimated, in addition to providing predictive information on the risk factors for adolescent suicide. This case–control study was designed to obtain a detailed psychiatric profile of a consecutive series of completed adolescent suicides through the use of the psychological autopsy technique.

Our study conducted psychological autopsies of a consecutive series of the 170 suicides completed by persons under age 20 within a 2-year period in the Greater New York/Tri-State metropolitan region, including New York City and 28 surrounding counties in New York State, New Jersey, and Connecticut. This design was likely to yield representative cases of suicide, a necessity for estimating relative risks for committing suicide. The study included two control groups: a comparison group (matched for age, ethnic group, and sex) of suicide attempters identified from a wide variety of different hospitals within the region, and a stratified random sample of young people of the study region (stratified on the age, ethnic, and sex distribution of the completed suicide cases). The second sample was representative of a population that was demographically similar to the suicide completers. However, it was not representative of the *general* population in the age range studied, because, given the age, ethnic, and sex distribution of suicide completers, the sample overrepresented older ages, whites, and males. Nevertheless, when cases are weighted to make these demographic characteristics like those of the total youth population in this area, the normal controls can provide estimates of the prevalence of risk factors in the general population.

Compilation of Risk Factors

Beyond demographic risk factors, which were ascertainable from death records, data on symptomatic profiles based on 119 "psychological autopsies" were available. The symptom information was derived from a semi-structured clinical interview with multiple informants, which assessed a comprehensive set of symptoms. For the purposes of the present analyses, the diagnostic information was based on a best-estimate DSM-III (*Diagnostic and Statistical Manual of Mental Disorders*, third edition) consensus diagnosis derived from a clinical team conference. Materials covered in the conference included a review and discussion of the narrative summary prepared by the research interviewer, as well as raw interview material and unsummarized documents obtained from relevant clinical sources. Earlier estimates of psychopathological risk factors (Gould, Shaffer, & Davies, 1990) differ from the present estimates, in part because the earlier analyses were derived from symptom counts rather than best-estimate diagnoses; were based on a preliminary subset of the sample; and employed estimates of the prevalence of risk factors in the general population, rather than relying on sample estimates, as currently derived.

The analyses on the best-estimate diagnoses are presented here for three global diagnostic domains—affective disorders, substance abuse, and antisocial behavior—each consisting of several DSM-III diagnoses (see Table 7.1). The domain of affective disorders includes major depression, dysthymic disorder, atypical depression, and adjustment disorder with depressed mood. The domain of substance abuse consists of any substance and/or alcohol abuse diagnosis, and the domain of antisocial behavior encompasses the conduct disorders, oppositional disorder, and adjustment disorder with disturbance of conduct. The analyses revealed the following:

1. Approximately a third of the victims had made a previous suicide attempt, with more girls (48%) than boys (27%) having had a history of previous attempts.
2. Symptoms of any affective disorder, alone or in combination with antisocial behavior and/or substance abuse were found in approximately 40% of the youngsters.

TABLE 7.1. Risk Factors for Suicide in Teenagers

Risk factor	Suicides	Normals	Approximate odds ratio	Approximate suicide rate per 100,000 affected by risk factor
Females (general adolescent population)				4.2[a]
Females (study population)	($n = 25$)	($n = 31$)		
Prior attempt	48.0%	0	—[b]	—[b]
Affective disorders	52.0	6.4	15.7	34
Substance abuse	4.0	0	—[b]	—[b]
Antisocial behavior	16.0	9.7	1.8	7
Family history	36.0	19.4	2.3	8
Males (general adolescent population)				16.2[a]
Males (study population)	($n = 94$)	($n = 116$)		
Prior attempt	26.6	1.7	20.7	250
Affective disorders	41.5	11.2	5.6	60
Substance abuse	30.8	9.5	4.3	53
Antisocial behavior	40.4	19.0	2.9	35
Family history	40.4	26.7	1.9	25

[a]The rates for the general adolescent population are based on unpublished data from the National Center for Health Statistics.
[b]The odds ratio is undefined because the frequency of the risk factor among the nonpsychiatric comparison group is zero.

3. A history of aggressive and antisocial behavior was present in a third of the victims, with boys far exceeding girls in exhibiting this behavior (40% vs. 16%, respectively).
4. Substance abuse, alone or in combination with affective disorders and/or antisocial behavior, was found in approximately a quarter of the completers—about the same as for adult suicides.
5. Approximately 40% of the suicide completers had a first- or second-degree relative who had previously attempted or committed suicide.

Only a small proportion of the suicides (7.5%) appeared to be free of psychiatric symptoms prior to death. Although Brent et al. (1988) and Shafii et al. (1985) found that bipolar symptoms were common in the suicide victims they studied, manic–depressive disorder and schizophrenic psychosis accounted for only a small proportion of teenage suicides in the present study.

Estimation of Risk Rates

Once associations with risk factors such as the ones presented here are determined in a case-control study, the excess risk of suicide for those with these risk factors can be estimated. Longitudinal designs have the advantage over case–control studies of permitting direct calculation of the magnitude of suicide risk for persons with and without hypothesized risk factors. One way of expressing this excess risk is the "relative risk," the ratio of the incidence rate of those with the risk factor to the incidence rate of those without the risk factor (Mausner & Bahn, 1974). In a case-control study such as ours, the proportion of cases and controls with the risk factor can be readily estimated and employed to estimate the relative risk in the population if (1) the outcome is rare; (2) the cases are representative of all cases; and (3) the controls are representative of the general population. If these assumptions are satisfied, the "odds ratio" is a good estimate of the relative risk (Mausner & Bahn, 1974). In addition to the relative risk, one would like to be able to estimate what proportion of people in the population with a particular pattern of risk factors will commit suicide per year. This information is essential to evaluate the predictive value of the risk factor. For this, one needs to know the risk of suicide in the total population; the proportion of the population with the risk factor; and the association between the risk factor and suicide. The overall incidence of suicide is available in published death statistics, and rates of specific risk factors can be estimated from the control group if the controls are "general population" controls. If the control group is matched to the cases on variables that are correlated with the risk, then the prevalence of the risk factors in the general population can be estimated by weighting the cases to represent the general population of adolescents. The odds ratio provides the needed measure of the association between the risk factors and suicide.

In our study, the odds ratio for committing suicide for boys with a previous suicide attempt was 20.7. This odds ratio was calculated from the proportion of the boys in the general population control group with a history of a previous suicide attempt (i.e., exposed). From death records, we ascertained that the annual mortality rate from suicide among boys 15–19 years of age was approximately 16.2 per 100,000. These data permitted an estimation of the incidence among nonattempters as follows (Kelsey, Thompson, & Evans, 1986):

$$\frac{\text{Incidence in total population}}{[(\text{Proportion exposed}) \times (\text{Odds ratio})] + (\text{Proportion nonexposed})}$$

which yielded

$$\frac{16.2 \text{ per } 100,000}{[(.017) \times (20.7)] + (.983)} = 12.1 \text{ per } 100,000 \text{ per year for nonattempters}$$

The estimate of the suicide rate among boys with a history of previous suicide attempts was then $(12.1) \times (20.7) = 251$ per 100,000 for attempters. This would be equivalent to the prediction of a 2% death rate from suicide within a 10-year follow-up of a group of male suicide attempters. A review of the small number of follow-up studies of teenagers who have been treated psychiatrically for suicide attempts or depression (Motto, 1984; Otto, 1972) shows suicide rates much higher than the rates projected from our data on subjects in the New York study, or from Goldacre and Hawton's (1985) study of attempters who for the most part received nonpsychiatric treatment. The most plausible explanation for the difference is one based on selection factors (i.e., more severely disturbed patients are admitted for psychiatric treatment); however, we cannot rule out the possibility that hospital admission worsens the prognosis of attempters (Shaffer et al., 1988).

Applying these procedures to other risk factors that appeared common among the suicide victims yielded the following estimated risks of suicide (see Table 7.1): Among boys, the risk for boys with an affective disorder was 60 per 100,000. A similar risk was found among boys abusing drugs and/or alcohol (53 per 100,000). The risk of suicide among boys with an antisocial disorder was 35 per 100,000, and for boys with family members who had either committed or attempted suicide, the risk of committing suicide was 25 per 100,000. The greatest risk of suicide was among those boys with a history of having made prior suicide attempts (250 per 100,000). Among girls, the rank ordering for risk factors varied slightly, with the greatest risk existing for those girls with an affective disorder (34 per 100,000). The risk of committing suicide for girls with an antisocial disorder was 7 per 100,000. For girls with family members who had either committed or attempted suicide the risk of committing suicide was 8 per 100,000. The risk of suicide among girls who had made a previous suicide attempt or abused drugs and/ or alcohol could not be precisely determined, because the frequency of the disorder was zero among the nonpsychiatric control group (Fleiss, 1981).

The precise estimation of the suicide risk would require weighting the prevalence of risk factors in the control group to account for the stratification of the sample by age and race. Because the prevalence of risk factors in the control group was unweighted for the present analyses, the relative risks have probably been underestimated. Although the presence of multiple risk factors undoubtedly increases the risk of suicide, estimates for samples with multiple risks are not simple sums of risk rates, because these risk factors tend to be intercorrelated. So far, only univariate analyses have been conducted with these data; multivariate analyses will determine whether combinations of risk factors are more powerful predictors of suicide. Nevertheless, the estimates have provided an approximate relative ranking of potential high-risk groups for suicide. The relative ranking of the risk factors among both boys and girls remains essentially unchanged from those derived in preliminary analyses (Gould et al., 1990).

DISCUSSION

Case–control studies are useful for identifying risk factors and can provide annual risk rates by age group, making it possible to estimate risk for suicide among high-risk adolescents. From our study, it appears that previous suicide attempts, depression, substance abuse, antisocial behavior, and suicidal behavior in the family all increase the likelihood of suicide among teenagers. Although the suicide rate is considerably higher among adolescents with these risk factors than in the general population, only a minority will go on to commit suicide. The problem of low specificity (high false-positive rates) makes the task of clinical prediction extremely difficult. The prediction should become more specific when combinations of risk factors are taken into account.

Of the two teenagers described in the case histories provided later in this book (see Chapter 12), Ralph F would appear to have a poorer prognosis because he was depressed, had an alcohol problem, and had a recent example of a suicide in the family—all risk factors that were identified in our psychological autopsy study. His definite plan by a somewhat unusual method would also increase his risk of completing suicide. If Ralph had made a prior suicide attempt, we would unequivocally conclude that he was at extremely high risk for completing suicide. In the absence of a suicide attempt, we have to temper our prediction, because there are no studies relating suicidal death to earlier suicidal ideation. As previously discussed, thinking about suicide is very common among high school students (Smith & Crawford, 1986); therefore, it is not particularly useful as a specific predictor of suicide risk. Nevertheless, given the higher rates of subsequent suicide found in the high-risk follow-up studies among teenage boys admitted to a psychiatric inpatient unit (Motto, 1984; Otto, 1972), and Ralph's constellation of risk factors, we would consider Ralph at high risk for suicidal behavior and advise that he be closely supervised.

The case material presented about Heather B does not describe the profile of a teenage girl that is typical of the majority of suicide victims identified in our psychological autopsy study. Although she was labile and excitable, she did not appear to meet criteria for an affective disorder— one of the strongest risk factors for suicide among teenage girls. Her primary self-destructive symptom, slashing behavior, has not been reported to be predictive of future suicidal behavior. Although her behavior would clearly warrant therapy, it would not appear to us indicative of high suicide risk.

Although errors in the clinical prediction of suicide are inevitable, research data suggest that boys who have made a previous suicide attempt are at particularly high risk for completing suicide, and that it is critical to direct interventions to this group of high-risk teenagers.

ACKNOWLEDGMENTS

The work described in this chapter was partially supported by Research Grant No. R01 MH 38198 from the National Institute of Mental Health, and by Faculty Scholars Award No. 84-0954-84 from the William T. Grant Foundation.

REFERENCES

Asberg, M., Nordstrom, P., & Traskman-Bendz, L. (1986a). Biological factors in suicide. In A. Roy (Ed.), *Suicide* (pp. 47–71). Baltimore: Williams & Wilkins.

Asberg, M., Nordstrom, P., & Traskman-Bendz, L. (1986b). Cerebrospinal fluid studies in suicide. *Annals of the New York Academy of Sciences, 487,* 243–244.

Asberg, M., Thoren, P., Traskman, L., Bertilsson, L., & Ringberger, V. (1976). Serotonin depression: A biochemical subgroup within the affective disorders? *Science, 191,* 478–480.

Brent, D. A., Perper, J. A., Goldstein, C. E., Kolko, D. J., Allan, M. J., Allman, C. J., & Zelenak, J. P. (1988). Risk factors for adolescent suicide: A comparison of adolescent suicide victims with suicidal inpatients. *Archives of General Psychiatry, 45,* 581–588.

Brown, G. L., Ebert, M. H., Boyner, P. F., Jimerson, D. C., Klein, W. J., Bunney,

W. E., & Goodwin, F. K. (1982). Aggression, suicide and serotonin. *American Journal of Psychiatry, 139*, 741-746.

Dizmang, L. H., Watson, J., May, P. A., & Bopp, J. (1974). Adolescent suicide at an Indian reservation. *American Journal of Orthopsychiatry, 44*(1), 43-49.

Fleiss, J. L. (1981). *Statistical methods for rates and proportions*, (2nd ed.). New York: Wiley.

Goldacre, M., & Hawton, K. (1985). Reception of self-poisoning and subsequent death in adolescents who take overdoses. *British Journal of Psychiatry, 146*, 395-398.

Gould, M. S., Shaffer, D., & Davies, M. (1990). Truncated pathways from childhood to adulthood: Attrition in follow-up studies due to death. In L. Robins & M. Rutter, (Eds.), *Straight and devious pathways from childhood to adulthood* (pp. 1-9). Cambridge, England: Cambridge University Press.

Hawton, K., & Goldacre, M. (1982). Hospital admissions for adverse effects of medicinal agents (mainly self-poisoning) among adolescents in the Oxford region. *British Journal of Psychiatry, 141*, 166-170

Jan-Tausch, J. (1964). *Suicide of children 1960-63: New Jersey public school students.* Trenton: State of New Jersey, Department of Education.

Kelsey, J. L., Thompson, W. D., & Evans, A. S. (1986). *Methods in observational epidemiology.* New York: Oxford University Press.

Linnoila, M., Virkkunen, M., Scheinin, M., Nuutila, A., Rimon, R., & Goodwin, F. K. (1983). Low cerebrospinal fluid 5-hydroxyindoleacetic acid concentration differentiates impulsive from nonimpulsive violent behavior. *Life Sciences, 33*, 2609-2614.

Mausner, J. S., & Bahn, A. K. (1974). *Epidemiology: An introductory text.* Philadelphia: W. B. Saunders.

Motto, J. A. (1984). Suicide in male adolescents. In H. S. Sudak, A. B. Ford, & N. B. Rushforth (Eds.), *Suicide in the Young* (pp. 227-244). Boston: John Wright/PSG.

National Center for Health Statistics. (1990). *Vital Statistics of the United States, 1987: Vol. 2. Mortality* (Part A). Washington, DC: U.S. Government Printing Office.

Otto, O. (1972). Suicidal acts by children and adolescents. *Acta Psychiatrica Scandinavica Supplement, 233* (Suppl.), 1-123.

Pokorny, A. D. (1964). Suicide rates in various psychiatric disorders. *Journal of Nervous and Mental Diseases, 139*, 499-506.

Pokorny, A. D. (1983). Prediction of suicide in psychiatric patients: Report of a prospective study. *Archives of General Psychiatry, 40*, 249-257.

Rich, C. L., Young, D., & Fowler, R. C. (1986). San Diego Suicide Study: I. Young vs. old subjects. *Archives of General Psychiatry, 43*, 577-582.

Roy, A., Agren, H., Picker, D., Linnoila, M., Doran, A. R., Cutler, N. R., & Paul, S. M. (1986). Reduced cerebrospinal fluid concentrations of homovanillic acid and homovanillic acid to 5-hydroxyindoleacetic acid ratios in depressed patients. *American Journal of Psychiatry, 143*, 1539-1545.

Salk, L., Sturner, W., Lipsitt, L. P., Reilly, B., & Levat, R. H. (1985). Relationship of maternal and perinatal conditions to eventual adolescent suicide. *Lancet, i*, 624-627.

Sanborn, D. E., Sanborn, C. J., & Cimbolic, P. (1973). Two years of suicide: A study of adolescent suicide in New Hampshire. *Child Psychiatry and Human Development, 3*(4). 234-242.

Sellar, C., Hawton, K., & Goldare, M., (1990). Self-poisoning in adolescents: Hospital admissions and deaths in the Oxford region, 1980-85. *British Journal of Psychiatry, 156,* 866-870.

Shaffer, D. (1974). Suicide in childhood and early adolescence. *Journal of Child Psychology and Psychiatry, 15,* 275-291.

Shaffer, D., & Fisher, P. (1981). The epidemiology of suicide in children and young adolescents. *Journal of the American Academy of Child Psychiatry, 20,* 545-565.

Shaffer, D., Garland, A., Gould, M., Fisher, P., & Trautman, P. (1988). Preventing teenage suicide: A critical review. *Journal of the American Academy of Child and Adolescent Psychiatry, 27,* 675-687.

Shafii, M., Carrigan, S., Whittinghill, J. R., & Derrick, A. (1985). Psychological autopsy of completed suicide in children and adolescents. *American Journal of Psychiatry, 142,* 1061-1064.

Shneidman, E. S., & Farberow, N. L. (1961). Sample investigations of equivocal suicidal deaths. In N. L. Farberow & E. S. Shneidman, *The cry for help* (pp. 118-128). New York: McGraw-Hill.

Smith, K., & Crawford, S. (1986). Suicidal behavior among "normal" high school students. *Suicide and Life Threatening Behavior, 16,* 313-325.

Stanley, M., Traskman-Bendz, L., & Dorovini, K. (1985). Correlations bewteen aminergic metabolites simultaneously obtained from Human CSF and Brain. *LIfe Sciences, 37,* 1279-1286.

Stanley, M., & Mann, J. J. (1987). Biological factors associated with suicide. In A. J. Frances & R. E. Hales (Eds.), *Review of psychiatry* (Vol 7, pp. 334-352). Washington, DC: American Psychiatric Press.

Temoche, A., Pugh, T. F., & McMahon, C. (1964). Suicide rates among current and former mental institution patients. *Journal of Nervous and Mental Diseases, 138,* 124-130.

Traskman-Bendz, L., Asberg, M., Bertilsson, L., & Thoren, P. (1984). CSF monoamine metabolites of depressed patients during illness and after recovery. *Acta Psychiatrica Scandinavica, 69,* 333-342.

van Praag, H. M. (1977). Significance of biochemical parameters in the diagnosis, treatment, and prevention of depressive disorders. *Biological Psychiatry, 12,* 101-131.

Winokur, G., & Tsuang, M. (1975). The Iowa 500: Suicide in mania, depression, and schizophrenia. *American Journal of Psychiatry, 132,* 650-651.

CHAPTER 8

Assessment *in Absentia*:
The Value of the Psychological Autopsy Method for Studying Antecedents of Suicide and Predicting Future Suicides

David C. Clark, Ph.D.
Sara L. Horton-Deutsch, M.S., R.N.
Center for Suicide Research and Prevention
Rush–Presbyterian–St. Luke's Medical Center

The phrase "psychological autopsy" refers to a procedure for reconstructing an individual's psychological life after the fact, particularly the person's lifestyle and those thoughts, feelings, and behaviors manifested during the weeks preceding death, in order to achieve a better understanding of the psychological circumstances contributing to a death. The essential ingredients of the psychological autopsy method include face-to-face interviews with knowledgeable informants within several months of the death, review of all extant records describing the deceased, and comprehensive case formulation by one or more mental health professionals with expertise in postmortem studies.

Why are psychological autopsy studies necessary? Until recently, most clinical studies of suicide risk were based on samples of persons who had made nonfatal attempts (including medically serious or repeated nonfatal attempts), for the simple reason that they remained alive and available for interview, or on samples of persons who were in some form of mental health treatment for an extended period of time before they died by suicide, because detailed observations for the period preceding the suicide were well documented. More recently, however, it has become clear that neither of these types of samples are representative of the kinds of persons who die by suicide (Linehan, 1986). Dahlgren (1945) and Stengel and Cook (1958) were among the first to show that persons who make nonfatal suicide attempts and persons who die by suicide are more different than alike. Community-based psychological autopsy studies conducted in different parts of the world have all converged on the finding that half of the persons who die by suicide never received any mental health treatment in their lifetimes (Barraclough, Bunch, Nelson, & Sainsbury, 1974; Hagnell & Rorsman, 1978, 1979; Beskow, 1979; Rich, Young & Fowler, 1986). Thus only community-based psychological autopsy studies provide investigators with an inclusive or comprehensive overview of the varieties of persons who die by suicide.

Clark and his colleagues have previously argued that prospective studies of suicide are necessary to assess the predictive validity and temporal quality of individual predictor variables (Fawcett et al., 1990). Until the time when psychological autopsy study findings lead investigators to more efficient definitions of groups at high risk for suicide, however, well-controlled prospective studies will remain prohibitive in terms of sample size, personnel, time, and cost. Thus, at present, the well-controlled psychological autopsy study may be the best available window onto the phenomenon of suicide in all its diverse aspects and textures.

The first psychological autopsy study undertaken was probably Zilboorg's unfinished psychoanalytic study of 93 consecutive suicides by police officers in New York City between 1934 and 1940. This interesting but little-known investigation was described by Friedman (1967). The number of police suicides during this period was twice that for the preceding 6 years, probably related to the antiracketeering crusades begun in 1933 following the election of Fiorello LaGuardia as mayor; throughout the 1920s, Tammany Hall politics in New York had fostered rampant gang crime and police corruption. The Zilboorg study was initiated at the request of Mayor LaGuardia in late 1939 (i.e., at the end of the wave of police suicides), and consisted of comprehensive case studies entailing interviews with widows and other family members (years after the deaths) by a research team of psychiatrists, psychologists, social workers, historians, and anthropologists. Zilboorg's investigation focused on psychodynamic motives for suicide, regulation of aggressive impulses, and the role played by gun availability.

The first *completed* psychological autopsy study (1956–1957) was a retrospective community-based study of 134 consecutive cases of suicide in St. Louis (Robins, 1981; Robins, Gassner, Kayes, Wilkinson, & Murphy, 1959; Robins, Murphy, Wilkinson, Gassner, & Kayes, 1959). In the 35 years since, there have been only a handful of other community-based psychological autopsy studies of large size (Barraclough et al., 1974; Beskow, 1979; Chynoweth, Tonge, & Armstrong, 1980; Dorpat & Ripley, 1960; Fowler, Rich, & Young, 1986; Hagnell & Rorsman, 1978, 1979, 1980; Rich, Fowler, Fogarty, & Young, 1988; Rich et al., 1986), but this tradition of research has made unique and significant contributions to the clinician's understanding of completed suicide. In addition, this tradition has fostered important methodological developments in psychological autopsy techniques, leading to a better understanding of the limitations of the method and new conceptual tools for future research.

Close on the heels of the St. Louis study, the Los Angeles Suicide Prevention Center (LASPC) staff coined the phrase "psychological autopsy" to describe a procedure developed in collaboration with the Los Angeles medical examiner's office (Curphey, 1967; Litman, Curphey, Shneidman, Farberow, & Tabachnick, 1963; Shneidman, 1981, 1990). The goal of this collaboration was to help the medical examiner's office decide how to classify deaths in situations where accidental death, suicide, and "death of undetermined causes" were equally viable conclusions, and so were always defined as advisory to the medical examiner's decision-making authority (Curphey, 1961; Litman, 1989; Shneidman, 1990). The method entailed "talking some to key persons—spouse, lover, parent, grown child, friend, colleague, physician, supervisor, coworker—who knew the decedent" (Shneidman, 1981, p. 330). Tactful and systematic inquiries were conducted by trained behavioral scientist/clinicians (Litman, 1987; Litman, et al., 1963). For almost 30 years, beginning in 1960, the LASPC was under contract with the local coroner's office to conduct psychological autopsies in all equivocal cases—about 60 each year (Litman, 1989). This collaboration and accumulation of experience made valuable contributions to knowledge about the validity of coroners' suicide verdicts, as well as about the impact of psychological data on coroners' findings in individual cases. It also spawned several variants of the psychological autopsy method, including the suicide postmortem conference for mental health professionals and the psychological autopsy study for specifically forensic purposes.

In the remainder of this chapter, we highlight some of the findings generated by psychological autopsy research, relying on studies published in English and based for the most part on work done in the United States, Canada, the United Kingdom, Australia, and Sweden. We pay particular attention to significant findings, methodological innovations, alternate definitions of the psychological autopsy method, and implications for predicting or averting suicides. This is followed by recommended criteria for future psychological autopsy studies, and we conclude the chapter with a brief discussion of five clinical case vignettes from the perspective of psychological autopsy research.

THE EARLY COMMUNITY-BASED PSYCHOLOGICAL AUTOPSY STUDIES

Robins and colleagues (Robins, 1981; Robins, Gassner, et al., 1959; Robins, Murphy, et al., 1959) identified 134 consecutive suicides during 1 year in St. Louis County, Missouri, and conducted a structured interview with a *primary* informant (i.e., a close relative or friend) within a few months of death. The interview took more than 2 hours to complete. This was supplemented by an average of 2.3 interviews with *ancillary* informants (other relatives or friends) per case, and by a review of health, police, and postmortem records. Dorpat and Ripley (1960) identified 114 consecutive suicides during 1 year in King County, Washington, and conducted a structured interview with one family member within a few months of death. This was supplemented by review of health, social agency, jail, and postmortem records.

Barraclough et al. (1974) identified 100 consecutive suicides (excluding transients) from 1966 to 1968 in West Sussex and Portsmouth, United Kingdom, and conducted a structured interview with a *main* (i.e., knowledgeable) informant within a few months of death. This was supplemented by an average of 4.5 interviews with other informants per case, interviews with the suicide victim's general practitioner in 94% of cases, and interviews with the victim's mental health care provider in 11% of cases. Barraclough and colleagues were the first to employ a comparison group: They examined the medical records of 150 men from general medical practices in the same regions and matched to the suicide victims by age, sex, and "ever-married" status.

The investigators for all three studies were teams of psychiatrists at university medical centers, and the focus of face-to-face interviews with informants was broadly defined. Information about personality, family and social history, work history, physical health and treatment, alcohol and drug use, psychological symptoms, mental health treatment, communication of suicidal intent, psychological precipitants for the suicidal act, and events leading up to the suicide was systematically collected. Robins (1981) argues that the type of study represented by the "clinical psychological autopsy" method is "inherently more comprehensive than studies limited, for example, to [the domain of] sociology or psychology or anthropology" (p. xiii), because the approach considers individual cases from many different disciplinary perspectives simultaneously and makes an effort to integrate these perspectives in order to recreate the whole person in the real world.

There is considerable agreement among the findings from the studies conducted by Robins and colleagues, Dorpat and Ripley, and Barraclough and colleagues in far-flung regions of the United States and the United Kingdom (Table 8.1). Suicides were more often males by a factor of 2:1. Suicides rarely occurred in the absence of psychiatric pathology; never fewer than 94% of the subjects qualified for a psychiatric diagnosis at the time of the suicide. Major affective disorder, or alcoholism, or both were implicated in 57–86% of all suicides, with affective disorder the more common diagnosis. These diagnostic rates may be conservative underestimates, because most psychological autopsy studies used a hierarchically organized diagnostic scheme permitting a maximum of one psychiatric diagnosis per subject.

TABLE 8.1. Comparison of Findings from Community-Based Psychological Autopsy
Studies, 1959 to 1974

	Robins, Gassner, et al. (1959); Robins, Murphy, et al. (1959)	Dorpat & Ripley (1960)	Barraclough, Bunch, Nelson, & Sainsbury (1974)
Sample size	134	114	100
Comparison group	No	No	Yes
Male (%)	77%	68%	53%
Caucasian (%)	96%	99%	Not reported
Number of families that refused to participate	13	4	Not reported
Cases for which no informants available	2	3	Not reported
Diagnostic classification (%)			
Affective disorder	45%	30%	70%
Alcoholism	23%	27%	15%
(Affective disorder or substance use disorder)	(69%)	(57%)	(86%)
Schizophrenia	2%	12%	3%
Organic brain syndrome	4%	4%	0%
Character pathology and no other diagnosis	0%	9%	0%
Mentally ill but unspecified diagnosis	19%	16%	6%
Mentally well	2% to 6%	0%	1%
Circumstances of suicide (%)			
Living alone	Not reported	Not reported	Not reported
Unemployed	Not reported	Not reported	Not reported
Bereaved in last year	Not reported	~5%	Not reported
Physical illness	Not reported	51%	10%
Terminal illness	4%	Not reported	6%
Communicated intent in broad terms	69%	83%	55%
Communicated intent explicitly	41%	43%	34%
Suicide attempt history	18%	33%	33%
Left a suicide note	34%	38%	39%
Combination murder-suicide	3%	4%	Not reported
Treatment (%)			
Suicide occurred while an inpatient	4%	Not reported	Not reported

(continued)

TABLE 8.1. (*continued*)

	Robins, Gassner, et al. (1959); Robins, Murphy, et al. (1959)	Dorpat & Ripley (1960)	Barraclough, Bunch, Nelson, & Sainsbury (1974)
Suicide occurred within 12 months of discharge	12%	Not reported	Not reported
Professional attention			
Last year	73%	~88%	93%
Last month	—	—	69%
Last week	—	—	48%
Psychiatric attention			
Last year	54%	22%	24%
Last month	31%	—	18%
Last week	—	—	11%
No history of mental health treatment	Not reported	Not reported	48%

Schizophrenia and organic brain syndrome were implicated in a small but consistent fraction of cases. One of the three studies (Dorpat & Ripley, 1960) found that 9% of persons dying by suicide evidenced character pathology but no Axis I (i.e., *Diagnostic and Statistical Manual of Mental Disorders*, third edition, revised [DSM-III-R] definition) psychiatric disorder. The three studies agreed in showing that the fraction of suicide victims struggling with a terminal illness at the time of their death was in the range of only 4–6%.

Two-thirds of the suicide victims communicated their suicidal intent over a period of weeks prior to their death, usually to several different persons, and 40% communicated their suicidal intent in very clear and specific terms (Table 8.1). About 90% of suicide victims had received some kind of health care attention in the year prior to death, but this care was usually not provided by a mental health professional. There is evidence that half of the persons dying by suicide had never been in contact with a mental health professional in their lifetimes, not even once. In one of the studies, 4% of all suicides occurred while the subjects were hospital inpatients, and another 12% occurred within 12 months of psychiatric hospital discharge (Robins, Gassner, et al., 1959; Robins, Murphy, et al., 1959). The three studies all converge on the findings that only a third of persons dying by suicide had previously made a suicide attempt of any kind, and only a third left a suicide note behind.

LATER COMMUNITY-BASED PSYCHOLOGICAL AUTOPSY STUDIES

In 1947, Essen-Moller and colleagues began the Lundby Study, a prospective study of the mental and social conditions of 3,563 persons living in one region of Sweden. All persons in the community were interviewed by psychiatrists in 1947, 1957, and 1972. Hagnell and Rorsman (1978, 1979, 1980) have described the 28 persons who died by suicide during this 25-year period. Because the entire community was interviewed at the beginning of the study and at subsequent intervals, all suicides were preceded by individual psychiatric interviews of the suicide victims on one or two occasions. The Lundby Study represents a small sample of suicides for generalization purposes, but the availability of both prospective and retrospective data on each suicide victim makes it unique. The study is unlike other psychological autopsy studies summarized here, in the sense that information about the circumstances of the suicide was not collected from relatives and other knowledgeable informants until the 1957 or 1972 surveys (i.e., sometimes 15 years later). The investigators point out that "these long intervals naturally meant a certain loss of otherwise available information" (Hagnell & Rorsman, 1979, p. 69). Two control groups were constituted for comparisons: 56 age- and sex-matched persons still alive at follow-up, and 25 persons who died natural deaths at the same ages as those who had committed suicide. Subjects in the suicide group were not more likely to manifest physical illness during the last year of life than those in the control group of subjects still living. The investigators emphasized that among the suicides, negative attitude toward hospital treatment, lack of cooperation with health care providers, and refusal to accept medical help were much more common.

Beskow (1979) identified all male suicides in Stockholm during 1 year and in three rural Swedish counties during a 2-year period, then drew a two-thirds sample of the urban suicides ($n = 161$) and a complete sample of the rural suicides ($n = 110$) for his study. He conducted a semi-structured interview with one relative or close friend of each suicide at an average of 9 months following the death, and supplementary interviews with other relatives, employers, and work colleagues. This information was augmented with data from police and forensic investigations and from medical records. For each suicide victim, a control subject was identified by searching the provincial register for men of the same age from the same parish. Beskow reported that severe and crippling diseases (e.g., cancer, pulmonary tuberculosis, and diseases of the nervous system) were overrepresented among the suicides, but still were not common among them. More men in the suicide group were hospitalized for physical care during the 2 years immediately preceding the suicide, and this overrepresentation was largely due to suicide attempts and accidents.

Chynoweth et al. (1980) identified 135 consecutive suicides during

1 year in Brisbane, Australia, and shortly after death conducted structured interviews with relatives or close friends who had been in recent contact with the subjects. The numbers of informants accessed per subject were one (2%), two (44%), three (37%), and four or more (16%). These interviews were supplemented by contacts with medical practitioners, social workers, psychiatrists, and the police, and by information obtained from medical and psychiatric records and postmortem investigation reports. In their report, Chynoweth et al. compared a subset of the depressed suicide victims with a group of 30 persons who had received treatment for depression during the previous year. They concluded that the large number of younger suicide victims with concomitant physical illness indicates that the relationship between physical illness and suicide is not simply an artifact of the aging process.

Maris (1981) identified a sample of 1,349 suicides (officially designated as such) by white persons in Cook County, Illinois. The suicide victims had been part of a larger, earlier record review study of suicides occurring between 1966 and 1968. From that sample he randomly selected 517 cases, stratified by religion, and contacted the persons who had originally served as coroner's informants from 1 to 3 years following the death. In 65% of cases ($n = 266$), informants were available for a 2-hour interview. On average, two informants were interviewed per case of suicide, and this information was supplemented with psychiatric hospital records, coroner's reports, and police investigation reports. Maris also recruited two comparison groups: a sample of 64 suicide attempters and a sample of 71 persons who died natural deaths, both recruited from the Baltimore area. His multivariate analysis of "suicidal careers" revealed many differences between those who died natural deaths and the others, but few differences between those who made nonfatal attempts and those who completed suicide.

Rich and colleagues (Fowler et al., 1986; Rich et al., 1986, 1988) identified 283 definite or possible suicides during an 18-month period in San Diego County, California, and conducted a structured interview with an average of two family members, friends, employers, or acquaintances per case 1–3 months after the suicide. The 2-hour interviews were supplemented by an average of one phone contact with a health care professional per case, as well as examination of hospital, school, and police records, and postmortem toxicological analyses. Comparing younger to older suicide victims, Rich and colleagues observed that there were fewer affective and organic brain disorders but more drug use and antisocial personality disorders among those aged 30 years and younger.

There have been other, less fully described psychological autopsy studies, but these are difficult to evaluate. Ishii (1985) reported a psychological autopsy study of 143 Japanese university students who died by suicide over a 25-year period, but did not describe his research procedures in much detail. He described a pattern of suicides in response to performance pressures within an achievement-oriented culture, although 72% of subjects exhibited psychopathological disorder in the 2 months prior to suicide. Biro (1987) reported a psychological autopsy study of 200 suicides occurring in a region of Yugoslavia over 3 years, but the study is impossible to evaluate because so little is said about the method. Michel (1987) reported a psychological autopsy study of 50 consecutive cases of suicide in Bern, Switzerland, and compared them to a sample of persons treated for suicide attempts at the local university hospital during the same period. He found that the depressive symptoms of early waking and loss of interest characterized patients in the completed suicide sample significantly more often.

Arato, Demeter, Rihmer, and Somogyi (1988) interviewed one close family member or friend with a structured diagnostic interview to characterize 200 of 217 (92%) consecutive suicides occurring in Budapest, Hungary, during 1985. The prevalence rates for various psychiatric disorders among the suicide victims in the months preceding death, according to Research Diagnostic Criteria, were as follows: major depression, 58%; minor depression, 6%; alcoholism, 20% (8% with alcoholism alone, 12% with alcoholism and major depression); schizophrenia, 8%; schizoaffective disorder, 1%; and no Axis I (DSM-III-R definition) psychiatric disorder, 19%. Only 40% of all subjects had ever made a previous suicide attempt.

The major psychological autopsy studies conducted in the western United States, different regions of Sweden, and Australia after 1974 reinforce the findings of the earlier studies to a surprising degree (Table 8.2). Suicides rarely occurred in the absence of psychiatric pathology; never fewer than 88% of the subjects qualified for a psychiatric diagnosis at the time of the suicide. Major affective disorder, substance use disorders, or both were implicated in 65–89% of all suicides, with affective disorder the more common diagnosis. The studies agreed in showing that the percentage of suicide victims struggling with a terminal illness at the time of their deaths fell in the range of 2–3%. Half the persons dying by suicide had never been in contact with a mental health professional in their lifetimes, not even once (Table 8.2). Ten percent of the suicides occurred while the subjects were hospital inpatients, and another 20–30% occurred within 12 months of psychiatric hospital discharge. Only a third of persons dying by suicide had previously made a suicide attempt of any kind.

With the exception of the study reported by Rich and colleagues, who studied six cases (2%) not adjudicated as suicides by the local coroner and who excluded one case that the coroner adjudicated as a definite suicide, all the psychological autopsy studies summarized thus far have relied on the verdicts of coroners or medical examiners to define cases of suicide. As we discuss below, the empirical evidence suggests that this is a reasonable beginning point for research, but this approach leaves us in the dark about the nature and characteristics of that proportion of suicides (however large or small) not explicitly labeled as suicides by the coroner or medical examiner.

TABLE 8.2. Comparison of Findings from Community-Based Psychological Autopsy Studies after 1974

	Hagnell & Rorsman (1978, 1979, 1980)	Beskow (1979)	Chynoweth, Tonge, & Armstrong (1980)	Fowler, Rich, & Young (1986); Rich, Fowler, Fogarty, & Young (1988); Rich, Young, & Fowler (1986)
Sample size	28	271	135	283
Comparison group	Yes (2)	Yes	Yes	No
Male (%)	82%	100% (by selection)	63%	71%
Caucasian (%)	100%	100%	Not reported	93%
Number of families that refused to participate	0	3%	Not reported	Not reported
Cases for which no informants available	0	6%	Not reported	8%
Diagnostic classification (%)				
Affective disorder	50%	28%	55%	44%
Alcoholism	18%	31%	20%	54%
(Affective disorder or substance use disorder)	(68%)	(65%)	(89%)	(~69%)
Schizophrenia	4%	~3%	4%	3%
Organic brain syndrome	14%	2%	Not reported	4%
Character pathology and no other diagnosis	0%	4%	3%	Not reported
Mentally ill but unspecified diagnosis	0%	0%	Not reported	3%
Mentally well	7%	3%	12%	5%
Circumstances of suicide (%)				
Living alone	Not reported	Not reported	25%	22%
Unemployed	Not reported	Not reported	24%	
Bereaved in last year	0%	Not reported	12%	
Physical illness	57%	26%	52%	16%
Terminal illness	Not reported	3%	2%	Not reported
Communicated intent in broad terms	Not reported	60%	Not reported	66%
Communicated intent in explicit terms	Not reported	49%	Not reported	Not reported
Suicide attempt history	36%	37%	Not reported	38%
Left a suicide note	Not reported	22%	Not reported	40%
Alcohol by toxicology	Not reported	65/161 (40%)	Not reported	Assessed, not reported
Alcohol or drugs by toxicology	Not reported	83/161 (52%)	Not reported	Assessed, not reported
Combination murder-suicide	Not reported	1%	Not reported	Not reported

(*continued*)

TABLE 8.2. (continued)

	Hagnell & Rorsman (1978, 1979, 1980)	Beskow (1979)	Chynoweth, Tonge, & Armstrong (1980)	Fowler, Rich, & Young (1986); Rich, Fowler, Fogarty, & Young (1988); Rich, Young, & Fowler (1986)
Treatment (%)				
Suicide occurred while an inpatient	Not reported	10%	Not reported	Not reported
Suicide occurred within 12 months of discharge	18%	>29%	Not reported	Not reported
Professional attention				
Last year	75%	>55%	—	—
Last month	—	—	44%	—
Last week	—	—	—	—
Psychiatric attention				
Last year	36%	>28%	Not reported	—
Last month	—	15%	—	27%
No history of mental health treatment	43%	44%	Not reported	52%

APPLICATION OF THE PSYCHOLOGICAL AUTOPSY METHOD TO YOUTH SUICIDES

Recently, refinement and extension of the psychological autopsy method has led to its more frequent application to the adolescent age group. Psychological autopsy studies by Shafii and colleagues (Shafii, Carrigan, Whittinghill, & Derrick, 1985; Shafii, Steltz-Lenarsky, Derrick, Beckner, & Whittinghill, 1988), Rich and colleagues (Fowler et al., 1986), Brent and colleagues (Brent, 1989; Brent, Perper, Goldstein, et al., 1988; Brent, Perper, Kolko, & Zelenak, 1988), Shaffer (1988), and Runeson (1989) have examined the prevalence rates of specific types of psychiatric illness—and, in particular, the role of substance abuse—among 10- to 29-year-old suicide victims. Runeson ($n = 58$) and Brent and colleagues ($n = 27$) have reported on the largest samples thus far. Only two of the youth studies have employed comparison groups: Shafii and colleagues compared suicide victims under the age of 20 years with the victims' closest friends, and Brent and colleagues compared adolescent suicide victims with suicidal psychiatric inpatients matched by age.

Shafii and colleagues found that 12- to 19-year-old suicide victims were much more likely than their close friends to evidence two or more psychiatric disorders, usually a mood disorder coexisting with either substance abuse or conduct disorder; this research thus emphasized the high rates of comorbidity among suicide victims. Rich and colleagues demonstrated that 53% of their sample of youths under age 30 years evidenced a substance abuse disorder at the time of death, and that a relatively smaller proportion (39%) evidenced a mood disorder. Only half the subjects with a diagnosis of major depression (16% of the total sample) qualified for a concomitant diagnosis of substance abuse. The implication favored by Rich and colleagues is that profiles of adult suicides developed one or two decades ago do not describe present-day youth suicides well.

Brent and colleagues concluded that adolescent suicide victims differed from psychiatric inpatients in five important ways. The suicide victims were *more* likely to evidence a bipolar disorder, to have a major affective disorder with a concomitant nonaffective disorder, and to have guns in their homes; however, they were *less* likely to have had any prior contact with a mental health professional in their lifetimes and to have been engaged in conflict with their parents. A third of those who died by suicide were legally intoxicated at the time of their deaths. Although 83% of the suicide completers talked about their suicidal state of mind with others within a week of their deaths, half did so only to persons the same age (i.e., siblings or friends). There were no differences between the suicide and comparison groups by psychiatric diagnosis; frequency of common precipitants (e.g., losses, disciplinary problems); history of psychiatric illness prior to the current episode; history of suicidal threats or attempts; family history of psychiatric disorder or suicide; or frequency of exposure to models of suicide. Brent and colleagues speculated that young persons with a major mood disorder and concomitant nonaffective illness have a worse prognosis than peers with an uncomplicated mood disorder, and that in cases of comorbidity the nonaffective illness diverts attention from timely detection and treatment of the mood disorder.

In his sample of 58 suicide victims aged 15 to 29 years, Runeson found that 95% met criteria for a DSM-III-R Axis I disorder, that 3% (two cases) met criteria for an Axis II but not an Axis I disorder, and that only one subject did not qualify for any psychiatric diagnosis. The most prevalent diagnoses were major depression (41%), alcohol use disorder (31%), drug use disorder (16%), and schizophrenia (14%). Only 5% of the suicide victims evidenced a bipolar affective history. Interestingly, there was virtually no overlap between the subsample with affective disorder and the substance-abusing subsample. In 52% of all cases, there was a positive family history for substance abuse.

APPLICATION OF THE PSYCHOLOGICAL AUTOPSY METHOD TO SUICIDES BY ELDERLY PERSONS

It is striking that the psychological autopsy method has not been applied to studies of elderly suicides, despite the fact that the elderly are associated with a higher rate of suicide than any other age group in the United States. (National Center for Health Statistics, 1988). Although a number of record review studies of large community-based samples of elderly suicides have been published (Bock & Webber, 1972; Miller, 1977; Copeland, 1987; Conwell, Rotenberg, & Caine, 1990), we are not aware of any psychological autopsy study of elderly persons that has incorporated informant interviews into the design. Osgood and McIntosh (1986), in their comprehensive bibliography of the literature on geriatric suicide research, emphasize that a rigorous psychological autopsy study of elderly suicides is necessary before research in this field can be expected to progress in the same manner as has been true for other age groups. Perhaps one reason investigators have been slow to undertake a rigorous psychological autopsy study of elderly suicides is the common belief that older adult suicide victims are socially isolated and/or estranged for a long period of time prior to death, so that knowledgeable informants will be difficult or impossible to obtain (Murphy & Robins, 1967).

Younger, Clark, Oehmig-Lindroth, and Stein (1990) reviewed medical examiner's records for 145 persons aged 60 years and over, representing all suicides by elderly people in one metropolitan county for 1 year. Their data suggest that the popular stereotype of the "average, expectable" elderly suicide victim is not justified. Seventy-seven percent of subjects were married at the time of their deaths; moreover, routine police investigative records identified at least one knowledgeable informant who had been in frequent contact with the deceased during the weeks before death in 90% of cases, and two or more knowledgeable informants in almost 50%. This was true although the police had not been asked to make any special effort to discover all possible informants. There were only two cases (1%) of elderly persons dying in institutional settings. The implication is that informant-based psychological autopsy studies of elderly suicides are feasible.

EQUIVOCAL DEATH CONSULTATIONS TO THE LOS ANGELES MEDICAL EXAMINER

One former member of the LASPC staff writes that their first recorded psychological autopsy took place in 1958, when Litman was asked to help the Los Angeles medical examiner's office decide whether the death of a 46-year-old man who drowned after falling from a pier into the ocean should be adjudicated as an accident or a suicide; it was finally ruled an accident (Diller, 1979). Shneidman (1990) writes that the Los Angeles medical examiner invited Farberow, Litman, and Shneidman of the LASPC to help study cases where the evidence for suicide was ambiguous, and that Shneidman was the one who coined the phrase "psychological autopsy," remobilizing a phrase he had used in a different context in one of his earlier books (Shneidman, 1951).

In Los Angeles, the local medical examiner was interested in studying equivocal suicides, or "cases in which suicide is a possibility but in which there could be more than one interpretation and, therefore, the decision is uncertain and doubtful" (Litman et al., 1963, p. 924). The "death investigation team" led by Farberow, Litman, and Shneidman helped him evaluate (1) the clarity of the decedent's conscious intentions or motives, and (2) the decisiveness or medical seriousness of the lethal action. The Los Angeles group believed that these two judgments were crucial to formulations of self-destructiveness and suicide (Litman, 1984, 1987; Litman et al., 1963; Shneidman, 1981). The death investigation team was an advisory body reporting to the medical examiner, who made the final decisions about death verdicts (Curphey, 1961; Litman, 1989; Litman et al., 1963; Farberow & Neuringer, 1971).

The 60–65 cases of equivocal suicide reviewed yearly by the Los Angeles death investigation team were mostly deaths by ingestion (Litman, Curphey, Shneidman, Farberow, & Tabachnick, 1983; Litman, 1989). Data for these determinations were obtained in interviews with persons close to the deceased and persons who had contact with the deceased during the weeks preceding death, including family, friends, work colleagues, and physicians. Interviewers were credentialed as deputy coroners, and they contacted next of kin 4–8 weeks after the death to arrange for face-to-face interviews— usually in an informant's home—that lasted from 45 minutes to 2 hours (Litman et al., 1963). In the course of these interviews, other knowledgeable informants (including other relatives, friends, business associates, physicians, and therapists) were identified and subsequently contacted by phone (Diller, 1979). Next of kin were asked to sign authorizations to release medical and other official records to the psychological autopsy team, and frequently provided access to other relevant materials, including photographs, correspondence, and diaries (Shneidman, 1981).

The major foci of the Los Angeles psychological autopsy study interviews were as follows: (1) deviations from normal routine; (2) expressions of a wish to die; (3) evidence of preparation for death; (4) history of previous suicide attempts or threats; (5) history of a mental disorder; (6) recent depressive symptoms or illness, or any other diagnosable mental disorder; (7) in cases of habitual alcohol and drug abuse, significant deviations from usual practices; (8) important life stressors or changes within the last year; (9) recent refusal of help from a health care professional; and (10) the failure of "expected rescuers" to rescue them (Litman, 1987, 1989; Litman et al., 1963, 1983). The implication was that positive findings in any of these spheres pointed to a greater likelihood of suicide. Similar criteria have been codified as "Operational Criteria for Classification of Suicide" by the Centers for Disease Control and a number of collaborating professional organizations (Jobes, Berman, & Josselson, 1987). Shneidman went even further by hypothesizing a spectrum of intentional deaths that included "subintentional death," by which he meant "demeaned and truncated lives, self-defeating neuroses, obviously inimical behaviors, and even alcoholism and addiction" (Shneidman, 1991, p. 252).

The Los Angeles group was the first to observe that surviving family members' painful emotional states at the time of psychological autopsy interviews inevitably interfered with an *optimal* psychological autopsy study (Litman et al., 1963, 1983). For some informants, anguish, anxiety, public gossip, and/or media attention interfered with their objective judgment or led to pronounced distortions. The conference method for deliberating over cases helped minimize interviewer subjectivity, particularly in cases where an interviewer overidentified with the perspective of the informant. The investigators concluded that most informants ultimately experienced the interview as positive and therapeutic (Litman et al., 1963, 1983; Diller, 1979; Sanborn & Sanborn, 1976; Shneidman, 1969b, 1981). Shneidman (1969a) was among the earliest to recognize that some of the surviving family members of suicide victims needed help to facilitate their adaptive grief, and that some were at risk for suicide in the future. He coined the word "post-vention" to describe the therapeutic impact of the psychological autopsy study and the opportunity it posed for continued preventive and clinical work with them.

The Los Angeles group has applied its psychological autopsy model to scientific studies of deaths by persons using phencyclidine (Heilig, Diller, & Nelson, 1982) and the relationship between Vietnam combat experience and suicide (Farberow, Kang, & Bullman, 1990). The Los Angeles model has spurred other jurisdictions to undertake more detailed and systematic psychological postmortem investigations (e.g., Yanowitch, Mohler, & Nichols, 1972; Jones, 1977; Weston, 1980), although there are only two jurisdictions in the United States where a medical examiner or coroner has routinely made use of psychological autopsy studies for any length of time—St. Louis and Baltimore (where a National Institute of Mental Health [NIMH] suicidology training grant to Johns Hopkins University supported a succession of training fellows and new projects) (Jobes, Berman, & Josselson, 1986).

The Los Angeles model certainly falls within the realm of legitimate psychological autopsy studies, insofar as it is based on structured interviews with knowledgeable informants close to the time of death, but the model has one serious shortcoming. The Los Angeles death investigation team tailored generalizations about suicide proneness and suicide intention to individual cases of equivocal death without reference to a solid foundation of data from large community-based samples of definite suicides where the data was collected in the same manner. That is, can one scientifically evaluate the likelihood that an *equivocal* death represents a suicide, without reference to a large series of *unequivocal* suicides and comparison deaths assessed in precisely the same manner? Can one reach authoritative conclusions about a single case of equivocal suicide when the variety and complexity of un-equivocal suicidal deaths remain to be mapped?

Inferences that the clarity of the decedent's conscious intentions and the decisiveness of the lethal action are key determinants of suicidal tendencies appear straightforward and irrefutable, but these inferences are not easy to apply in individual cases. Litman et al. (1963) observe, for example, that intention is often ambivalent in cases of suicide: A strong wish to live and a strong wish to die can exist side by side, making decisive action appear hesitating or inconclusive. Many investigators are not certain that suicidal intent can be systematically established after a death has occurred (Jobes et al., 1986). There is a tautology inherent in the operational definitions of suicidal intent and decisive action developed by the Los Angeles group: If suicide intent is rated as high and action is rated as decisive, then it follows that the case was a suicide—because suicides are associated with high levels of intent and decisiveness.

The assumptions underlying the Los Angeles theory of suicidal inten-tion may also be wrong. What if systematic psychological autopsy studies were to show that in many cases of definite suicide, victims do *not* tend to reveal suicidal ideation or planning in the months before death? Or that in many cases of definite suicide, the level of acute life stress (whether objec-tively or subjectively defined) does *not* help distinguish between the suicidal and the nonsuicidal? Or that in two-thirds of all cases of definite suicide, the victim had *never* made a prior suicide gesture or attempt in his or her lifetime? Such demonstrations would call into question some of the under-pinnings of the Los Angeles theory of suicidal intention. In fact, the first two counterintuitive arguments are supported by recent studies, though not psychological autopsy studies, of patients with major depression who died by suicide (Fawcett et al., 1987; 1990). The third argument is supported by the psychological autopsy research already summarized (Tables 8.1 and 8.2).

Assumptions underlying the Los Angeles theory of suicidal intention have been not yet been proven true, nor have they been tested against external validity standards. As a result, applications of these formulations to specific cases of death must be considered tentative. As the validated data base about suicide grows over time, aided by findings from large commu-nity-based psychological autopsy studies, clinicians will be equipped with better tools for assessing suicide risk and detecting cases of *genuine* suicide after the fact.

THE ACCURACY OF REPORTED SUICIDE STATISTICS

In the United States, determination of suicide as a mode of death lies in the hands of county medical examiners, coroners, or coroner's juries. These determinations are based on customs and legal procedures that vary widely from county to county. Epidemiological studies of the accuracy of reported suicide rates have consistently suggested that the margin of underreporting is of relatively small consequence (Kleck, 1988; Sainsbury, 1986). What have psychological autopsy studies shown in this regard?

The LASPC group reports that 1,000 deaths in Los Angeles each year are certified as suicides and that another 60–65 are regarded as equivocal cases worthy of special investigation by the death investigation team (Litman 1963; Litman, 1989). Over the last 30 years, 55%–65% of the equivocal cases have finally been certified as suicides. These trends suggest that the medical examiner's initial undercount of true suicides has never been more than 4%. Litman (1989) has written that the death investigation team finds sufficient new information to contradict the original coroner's opinion in about 5% of cases, sometimes changing an accident to a suicide, and sometimes a suicide to an accident.

Jobes et al. (1986) undertook a study of the impact of psychological information on the determination of manner of death. A total of 195 medical examiners and coroners recruited as subjects reviewed factual case descriptions of non-natural deaths; in half the cases, psychological autopsy data supplemented the medical/circumstantial reports presented to all subjects. Case vignettes were divided into two types: those where the mode of death (suicide, accident, or undetermined) was certified as belonging to one category by at least 80% of subjects ("typical"), and those where no more than 60% of subjects agreed on a single category ("equivocal"). The psychological autopsy data had a significant impact on the mode of death determinations in almost all cases of equivocal death, and in several of the cases of unequivocal death: Psychological information generally increased the likelihood that a case would be interpreted as a suicide. The implication is that certification of the manner of death varies as a function of the amount and/or type of salient information available.

SHNEIDMAN'S BROADER VIEW OF THE PSYCHOLOGICAL AUTOPSY

Shneidman (1981) views the psychological autopsy performed in consultation to a medical examiner as only one of several possible purposes of the psychological autopsy. The psychological autopsy can also be used, he argues, to determine *why* a specific instance of suicide occurred, or to explore the "psychosomatics of death" (i.e., psychodynamic forces affecting the timing of natural death); it can also be employed for psychobiographical and literary analyses, and for its therapeutic influence on informant survivors. Shneidman's more expansive sense of the boundaries and value of the psychological autopsy method has ushered in a variety of hybrid autopsy studies, including studies of Herman Melville and Melville's writings (Floyd, 1977; Shneidman, 1976, 1985); suicide postmortem conferences in clinical settings (Krieger, 1968); and postmortem investigations of the psychosocial aspects of death and dying among geriatric patients hospitalized for physical illness (Weisman & Kastenbaum, 1968; Weisman, 1974). In the same vein, Shneidman's studies of genuine and simulated suicide notes are cousins to the psychological autopsy study (Shneidman & Farberow, 1957; Leenaars, 1988), in that they capitalize on suicidal communications of the suicide victims themselves. The position taken here, however, is that the hallmark of the psychological autopsy method is the use of structured face-to-face interviews with knowledgeable informants within several months of death to gather data, and that studies not employing this method should be called something other than "psychological autopsy studies" (e.g., "psychodynamic case explorations," "psychoanalytic case studies," "psychobiographical analyses").

RETROSPECTIVE STUDIES OF PSYCHIATRIC INPATIENT AND JAIL SUICIDES

Despite the fact that only half of all persons who die by suicide ever had any lifetime contact with a mental health professional, and only 12%–30% had access to mental health services in the year prior to their deaths (Tables 8.1 and 8.2), it remains true that hospital-based mental health professionals will come into contact with a greater number of persons soon to die by suicide than anyone else (Black, Warrack, & Winokur, 1985; Copas & Robin, 1982; Crammer, 1984; Flood & Seager, 1968; Rabiner, Wegner, & Kane, 1982; Sletten, Brown, & Evenson, 1972; Temoche, Pugh, & MacMahon, 1964). About 5% of all suicidal deaths each year occur in a hospital inpatient setting (Robins, Gassner, et al., 1959; Beskow, 1979; Crammer, 1984); this statistic highlights the high rate of suicides associated with the first weeks of hospitalization and the first months following discharge (Copas & Robin, 1982), and the inability of good psychiatric facilities to prevent all suicide attempts and all suicidal deaths within their confines (Murphy, 1986). Thus one way to collect large samples of suicide cases for study is to follow large populations of patients admitted for inpatient psychiatric care throughout the hospitalization and for 1 year following discharge. This strategy has the advantage of allowing the investigator to capitalize on extant psychiatric evaluations and treatment records recorded prior to the act of suicide and without foreknowledge of the suicide.

There have been many retrospective record reviews and record linkage studies of psychiatric patients who subsequently died by suicide; strictly speaking, however, these are not psychological autopsy studies, in the sense that the investigators did not interview knowledgeable informants (whether family members or health care providers), within the first months following the suicide. The low base rate of suicide, even among depressed psychiatric patients hospitalized for a suicide attempt, suggests that it would take a decade or more (Modestin & Hoffmann, 1989) or an extraordinary collaboration among a dozen or more large hospitals (Fawcett et al., 1990) to collect a modest-sized sample for purposes of a well-conceived "prospective" psychological autopsy study. In either case, it would be crucial to establish the adequacy of inter-interviewer rating reliability. The same obstacles apply to studies of suicides in detention cells, jails, or prisons, where suicide rates are much higher than among the general population (Dooley, 1990; Salive, Smith, & Brewer, 1989), though Spellman and Heyne (1989) have outlined a psychological autopsy protocol for use in correctional facilities that includes interviews with other inmates, correctional staff, and mental health staff in the weeks immediately following the suicide.

THE SUICIDE POSTMORTEM CONFERENCE AND THE CLINICAL AUDIT

The first postmortem review of a series of hospital suicides for clinical purposes (Krieger, 1968) referred to these reviews as a form of psychological autopsy, and credited Shneidman and Farberow (1961) with having extended the psychological autopsy method to inpatient medical settings. Krieger defined a psychological autopsy conference as an occasion when "medical and paramedical staffs meet to make a retrospective study of each completed [inpatient] suicide, to uncover missed cues or underestimated symptoms" (pp. 218–219). The format had the treatment team from the deceased patient's ward present data about the patient, followed by a candid and reasonably objective discussion of the case by the staff as a whole. The goal of the psychological autopsy conference was to discover treatment decision errors that might have contributed to the suicidal death and patterns or features that might help the staff be more alert to acute suicide risk in the future.

Neill, Benensohn, Farber, and Resnik (1974) similarly described an "autopsy aimed at determining what clues the patient gave [about his or her lethal intentions] and how the clues were handled" (p. 34) in an inpatient psychiatric setting specializing in suicide studies. It is interesting to note Neill et al.'s belief that "the technique does not require special expertise, although it is usually helpful to have an experienced mental health professional available for consultation" (p. 34). Their protocol involved a period of information gathering, wherein treating hospital staff, next of kin, and friends of the patient were interviewed, followed by a multidisciplinary conference of the care-providing staff members.

Although the fundamental idea of the psychological autopsy study has been adapted to the format of mortality conferences at some hospitals in the time since, the technical parameters associated with the classical psychological autopsy study have frequently been neglected. Thus, for example, Salmon, Hajek, Rachut, Mackenzie, and Popkin (1982) reported the proceedings of a mortality conference focusing on a medical service inpatient with an unusual physical illness who died by suicide, but none of the physicians attending the conference had ever seen the patient when he was alive. For them, the goal of the psychological autopsy study was to "reconstruct the patient's life, stresses of physical illness, and his reaction to being sick" (p. 307).

The suicide postmortem conference resembles the psychological autopsy study on several counts: Motives for suicide are reconstructed, and the investigation takes place soon after the death. But in most other respects, the suicide postmortem conference is a different enterprise. In the case of the suicide postmortem conference, the universe of knowledgeable informants is rarely if ever interviewed in preparation for the conference (with the exceptions of Neill et al., 1974; Spellman & Heyne, 1989), and then interviews are rarely standardized. Furthermore, the sample size under consideration in the suicide postmortem conference is one person, making it impossible to evaluate what observations are suicide-specific and what observations are idiosyncratic, given current research knowledge. The plausibility of explanatory formulations is no guarantee of their validity (Shaffer, Perlin, Schmidt, & Himelfarb, 1972).

Once again, the critical question is this: Can one scientifically evaluate the antecedents and psychodynamics of one case of suicide without reference to a large series of suicides and comparison groups assessed in precisely the same manner? Can one reach authoritative conclusions about a single case of suicide when the variety and complexity of suicidal deaths remain to be mapped by the field of suicidology? Single-case studies (particularly well-disciplined psychoanalytic case studies) provide for a deeper, more multidimensional understanding of individual cases of suicide, but this approach is associated with low levels of reliability and validity, and one must be reluctant to generalize from these findings. As we have noted earlier, when such studies are performed in isolation—without reference to a series of other suicides and comparison subjects—they should probably be called something other than "psychological autopsy studies" (e.g., "psychodynamic case explorations," "psychoanalytic case studies," "psychobiographical analyses").

Crammer (1984) has compellingly argued that the primary purpose of suicide postmortem conferences is to review the quality of treatment (i.e., quality assurance in the form of peer review), and recommended that the postmortem conference be called a "medical audit":

Clinical research aims to discover more about illness and prevention of illness; medical audit tests the efficiency of hospital management and the working of the medical–nursing team. Suicide, which is not an intended outcome of treatment, represents an opportunity to review the way the staff is working together using the equipment and building provided. Deficiencies in provision, organization or in training may be revealed. Medical audit asks, "Are we doing our job as well as we could?" and "What would we need to do it better?" This is quite different from the clinical research needed to find out more about suicide. (p. 462)

Perhaps "clinical audit" is a better name than "medical audit," because the former enfranchises psychologists, nurses, social workers, and other mental health professionals, as well as the physicians who work with patients who subsequently die by suicide.

Clinical audits serve one other purpose worth emphasizing. The mental health professional who loses a patient by suicide has the potential to experience a genuine grief reaction that deserves consideration and attention. In addition, the mental health professional who loses a patient by suicide is confronted with his or her human limitations in a sudden and shocking manner that commonly precipitates feelings of personal and professional failure. The experience usually remains on a therapist's mind for decades afterward, and may have a negative impact on that professional's ability to care for other suicidal patients (Brown, 1987a, 1987b; Chemtob, Hamada, Gauer, Kinney, & Torigoe, 1988). A number of investigators have outlined the therapeutic value of the clinical audit, when implemented wisely, for the bereaved mental health professional (Kolodny, Binder, Bronstein, & Friend, 1979; Motto, 1979; Sacks, Kibel, Cohen, Keats, & Turnquist, 1987).

PSYCHOLOGICAL AUTOPSY STUDIES FOR FORENSIC PURPOSES

It is not uncommon for the surviving family members of a suicide victim to press the medical examiner or coroner to remove references to suicide as a mode of death from the death certificate, or to seek compensatory damages from institutions or professionals in situations where human agency might have anticipated or prevented the suicide (Ebert, 1987; Nolan, 1988; Spellman & Heyne, 1989). And sometimes a courtroom defense against charges of homicide leads an attorney to argue that the manner of death was really a suicide (Ebert, 1987). Several types of qualified persons (e.g., suicidologists, mental health professionals, corrections experts) are called upon to testify as expert witnesses in such cases. Should suicide case reviews for courtroom or forensic purposes be considered psychological autopsy studies?

Litman and colleagues at the LASPC have often been called upon to clarify suicidal intentions in the courtroom and to help decide, for example, whether insurance benefits should be paid after a death (Litman, 1987, 1989). In many or most of these cases, the deaths in question were in the series of those routinely investigated by the Los Angeles death investigation team, so that the expert witnesses had access to their own team's interviews with knowledgeable informants that took place soon after the deaths. The situation is markedly different when a consulting expert is not contacted until months or years after a death for an opinion about an unfamiliar case. In these situations, information available to the expert witness is usually in the form of depositions collected many months or years after the suicide. This kind of data is suspect for scientific purposes, because of the passage of time and memory decay. There are no empirical studies documenting the ability of informants to provide valid information about events leading up to a suicide after long delays of time, so the degree of distortion introduced cannot be quantified by any measure currently available.

There are four other serious problems when the primary data base for a case review consists of depositions. First, depositions are elicited in the context of an adversarial, sometimes antagonistic examination and cross-examination. Second, the expert witness is rarely familiar with the interview skills of the deposer, and so is distant from behavioral observations and nuances of the raw data in a way that is not true when the expert or his or her own research team has conducted the interviews. Third, in a deposition informants are not interviewed in a standardized fashion, to optimize investigators' ability to compare and contrast informant responses with results from previous psychological autopsy studies. Fourth and finally, in the deposition process the consulting clinical expert has few means for assessing bias and censorship in the selection of informants, the questions posed, the forms of those questions, and the information made available or not available for case review. Once again, there are no empirical studies quantifying the degree of distortion introduced by these serious confounds.

Thus the expert witness generally finds himself or herself in a situation that absolutely cannot be compared to the psychological autopsy study and its methods. The expert in such cases ordinarily draws on findings from published psychological autopsy studies for comparison purposes and *adapts* psychological autopsy techniques for review of available data, but these superficial drapings do not make the case review a psychological autopsy study. The critical question, once again, is this: How scientifically can one evaluate the likelihood that an equivocal death represents a suicide, or evaluate the antecedents of a specific death by suicide, without reference to a large series of unequivocal suicides assessed in precisely the same manner? In this regard, Shneidman (1991) has opined that the merits of the generic psychological autopsy study tend to be "overstated in the heat of courtroom litigation" (p. 253).

Where the expert has considerable experience in conducting formal community-based psychological autopsy studies involving large sample sizes, the expert is more keenly aware of the ways in which the available data deviate from psychological autopsy study requisites. The expert with psychological autopsy experience is also in a better position than inpatient or correctional facility experts to judge whether an "atypical" inpatient or prison suicide represents a kind of suicide more commonly represented in noninstitutional settings. The only situation where forensic case review truly approximates the psychological autopsy method is that in which the expert undertakes a structured, independent psychological autopsy study of the death in question within a reasonable period of time after the death (i.e., within a year). At the Center for Suicide Research and Prevention in Chicago, for instance, we have worked closely with the Isaac Ray Center for Psychiatry and the Law to establish a preformed psychological autopsy protocol for forensic cases. In this paradigm, the expert witness undertakes a preliminary case review, together with the opposing legal parties, to identify all potential knowledgeable informants; he or she then undertakes structured interviews with identified informants, independently of the deposition process. These interview data, along with other extant medical and legal records, become the basis for case formulation. Other types of expert witness testimony in the courtroom should probably not be represented as psychological autopsy studies or formulations. Expert witnesses can testify knowledgeably about the facts of a case or their opinions about a case without invoking the mantle of the psychological autopsy method.

METHODOLOGICAL CONSIDERATIONS

Too few investigators have reflected on the merits, problems, and limitations of the psychological autopsy method, or discussed the impact of methodological decisions on the conduct of their own studies and on their own results. The few that have attended to these matters have made extremely valuable contributions to the development of the method.

Shaffer et al. (1972), in the course of a psychological autopsy study of 50 suicides and 50 traffic accident victims, outlined what they considered to be some of the primary problems associated with the method. First, they noted that the quest for discovering explanations and causes for specific cases of suicide commonly leads investigators to adopt a "prosecuting attorney" type of approach to data analysis and case formulation, in the sense that investigators are too eager to seize on specific events as sole or principal reasons for the suicide. The plausibility of an explanation, they point out, is no guarantee of its validity. They suggest that comparison groups of persons who die by other causes and living persons are invariably necessary to interpret psychological autopsy findings, and even then the method may not lend itself to verifying *causes* of suicide. Without suitable comparison groups, there can be no conclusions. Shaffer and colleagues also pointed out that unless data from various informants are elicited in the framework of a standardized protocol, (1) the quantity and quality of data will vary as a function of the informant and the interviewer, and (2) reconciling discrepant information from different sources will be fraught with a number of sources of bias. In cases where the psychological autopsy culminates in nothing more than an oral or written narrative, the investigator is deprived of the means for establishing the reliability and validity of the observations.

Rudestam (1979), comparing his experiences in conducting psychological autopsy study interviews in Sweden and the United States, illustrated how crucial the initial procedure for contacting informants is to the success of a study. To this end, he reviewed the differential impact of contacting informants by letter or by phone, depending on the locale and the identity of the research team, and discussed the most effective ways to appeal for participation. Rudestam also emphasized the value of standardized interviews and standardized assessments, albeit in the context of an empathic, flexible semistructured interview that can be translated reliably into quantitative scores to minimize potential biases inherent to the interviewer.

An additional point made by Rudestam was that "if suicidology is to maintain its position as a distinct area in the study of suicidal death, it is advantageous to demonstrate that conclusions about suicidal persons and their survivors are unique to self-destructive deaths by using control groups composed of cases from accidental or natural death" (p. 144). It stands to reason that if the index subjects (suicide victims) have been dead for several weeks or months when the investigator begins interviewing acutely grief-stricken informants, some of the key methodological confounds influencing the amount and quality of data reported include the fact that the proband has died, the time lapse between death and interview, and the bereaved state of the informant. Evaluation of the significance of informant reports about a person who died by suicide in the absence of a comparison group of persons who died by other means seems impossible.

Finally, Rudestam emphasized the special training and experience necessary to prepare an interviewer for psychological autopsy research. He believed that because many grieving informants are "uniquely anguished, guilty, angry, and perplexed about the deaths of those close to them, . . . they have, for the most part, a need to vindicate themselves in the eyes of the world as represented by the interviewer" (p. 142). Rudestam recommended that interviewers in training rehearse interviews by means of role-playing situations; that they accompany senior interviewers on some interviews; and eventually that they be accompanied by observing senior interviewers on the early interviews they conduct themselves.

Brent, Perper, Kolko, and Zelenak (1988) posed three questions about methodological issues that complicate any psychological autopsy study, and brought data from their own psychological autopsy study of 27 adolescent suicides to bear on each. The questions were as follows: (1) Since the informants for a psychological autopsy study are almost invariably grief-stricken, how do the mood symptoms associated with bereavement influence the information reported by the informants? (2) Since informants are typically interviewed weeks to months after a death, how does the time lag influence the information reported? and (3) Since comparison samples are almost invariably composed of living subjects, how does differential access to data about living and dead subjects influence the overall results of a psychological autopsy study (the problem of asymmetry of information)?

Brent and colleagues found, in answer to their first question, that parents of adolescent suicide victims who manifested an affective disorder at the time of study interviews were not more likely to describe their deceased adolescents as depressed or suicidal, or to attribute psychiatric diagnoses to their adolescents, when compared to the parents of suicidal inpatients. In response to the second question, the length of time between the suicidal death and the informant interview (from 2 to 10 months) was not associated with a greater or less likelihood of ascribing depressive features, suicidal features, or psychiatric diagnosis to the suicide victim. Finally, Brent and colleagues found that parental informants contributed a greater proportion of information to final diagnostic decisions than did other informants for the sample of adolescents who died by suicide, and that parents of suicidal inpatients underestimated mood disorder in their offspring more than the parents of suicide victims did. They hypothesized that for the suicide cases, "adjunctive data sources (e.g., teachers, peers, and siblings) are likely to *confirm* parental report . . . [but they] do not appear to contribute much additional information to the . . . [final] diagnoses" (p. 365, italics in original). In this context, "not much additional information" meant less information than direct interview with a living adolescent subject added to the information provided by his or her parents. The investigators concluded that for purposes of psychological autopsy studies, parental reports provide more accurate diagnostic information than a combination of reports from other informants and sources.

Cowles (1988), after completing a study of the experiences of adult survivors of murder victims during the first 4 months following the murder, has provided a thoughtful discussion of some of the clinically sensitive issues raised by interviews with the acutely bereaved. These include the question of how long interviews should last, techniques for responding to emotional flooding in the informant, the need for the interviewer to maintain objectivity, and techniques for managing the interviewer's emotional reactions to the interviews.

In their overview of some of the methodological issues raised by the psychological autopsy method, Beskow, Runeson, and Asgard (1990) emphasize the need to specify how informants were initially contacted; to interview informants soon after the subject's death, to minimize the impact of time delay on the quality of information; to specify who the informants were and how they were selected; to recruit meaningful comparison groups;

to employ explicit and well-accepted diagnostic classification schemes; to employ experienced clinicians as interviewers; and to monitor and report on tests of interviewer reliability. The complex ethical issues discussed include protecting the confidentiality of the deceased and surviving family members, respecting the right of family members to refuse participation in the study, and monitoring the emotional demands of the interviews on both informants and the interviewers. Investigators might consider sharing this paper by Beskow et al. (1990), particularly the discussion of ethical considerations, with their local human investigations and/or medical ethics committees. Such committees are often asked to approve or oversee psychological autopsy study research, despite little prior knowledge of or acquaintance with the method.

RESEARCH ASSESSMENT INSTRUMENTS

What are the optimal assessment instruments for psychological autopsy research? Our position is that no one yet knows the best way to plumb the breadth and depth of any specific case of suicide, given the limitations on current knowledge, and that no one can deliver an authoritative conclusion about why a given case of suicide occurred. An investigator can, however, spell out a limited number of hypotheses, recruit an appropriate sample with appropriate comparison groups, and design a structured or semistructured protocol for informant interviews that will elicit information bearing on those hypotheses. As is true for all other types of research, the adequacy of findings from a psychological autopsy study is limited by the adequacy of the sample and comparison groups, the adequacy of the questions posed, the adequacy of the data analysis, and the care and logic shown in drawing conclusions. Among the critical variables in this equation, then, are the nature and quality of the assessment instrument.

If the principal questions posed by a given psychological autopsy study concern phenomenological diagnosis, the problem of selecting a clinical assessment instrument can be addressed with the help of recent psychometric advances in the study of psychiatric diagnosis. In a paper published at the beginning of the DSM-III era, Spitzer and Fleiss (1974) reported that reliability studies of psychiatric diagnoses made by senior clinical investigators at the most respected psychiatric research centers in the United States and the United Kingdom showed extremely poor agreement. In a companion paper, Spitzer, Endicott, and Robins (1975) demonstrated that the two principal reasons expert clinicians disagreed in their diagnostic formulations were "information variance" and "criterion variance." "Information variance" refers to the situation where clinicians have different kinds of information about the same patient. "Criterion variance" refers to the situation where clinicians use different formal inclusion and exclusion criteria to translate available information into one or more psychiatric diagnoses. By far the largest source of variance in diagnostic reliability found by Spitzer et al. was criterion variance.

Since the validity of any psychiatric diagnostic scheme is limited at its foundation by the reliability of that scheme, Spitzer and colleagues reasoned, studies of psychiatric classification must necessarily employ structured interviews (wherein the types and forms of questions to be covered are laid out in a predetermined sequence) and companion diagnostic criteria (including both formal inclusion and exclusion criteria for each diagnosis) if they are to lay any claims to good replicability and (ultimately) validity. There are only three widely recognized clinical interview protocols that meet these criteria: the Present State Exam (PSE) with accompanying CATEGO diagnostic criteria (Wing, Cooper, & Sartorius, 1974); the Schedule for Affective Disorders and Schizophrenia (SADS; Endicott & Spitzer, 1978) with accompanying Research Diagnostic Criteria (Spitzer, Endicott, & Robins, 1978); and the Structured Clinical Interview for DSM-III (SCID) (Riskind, Beck, Berchick, Brown, & Steer, 1987).

Epidemiological interviews (such as the NIMH Diagnostic Interview Schedule; Robins, Helzer, Croughan, & Ratcliff, 1981) are probably much less appropriate for purposes of psychological autopsy studies, because they were designed for administration by lay interviewers and designed for large-scale surveys wherein the modal subject has no history of psychopathology. The clinical difficulties of eliciting clear and objective information from grieving informants weeks to months following a suicide requires the attention of an experienced clinician using a psychometric instrument that integrates both clinician judgment and informant report. Nevertheless, it is important to note that all of the instruments recommended here (i.e., the PSE, SADS, and SCID) were developed to incorporate information from direct patient interviews and all available ancillary sources. The limitations on diagnostic validity introduced when the index subject (i.e., the suicide victim) cannot be directly interviewed remains to be mapped in future studies. It is also important to note that there is a version of the SADS designed for use with 9- to 16-year-old children (Orvaschel & Puig-Antich, 1986).

THE EXPERIENCE OF BEING INTERVIEWED FOR A PSYCHOLOGICAL AUTOPSY STUDY

Before going on to suggest standards for future psychological autopsy studies, we believe it may be helpful to pause and consider what the experience of a psychological autopsy study is like for the spouse, parent, child, sibling, or friend of the person who has died by suicide. Approaching family members soon after a loss by suicide is a delicate social and clinical problem, and raises important ethical issues as well. Shafii et al. (1985), for instance, obtained names and phone numbers for the family of youthful suicide victims from the local coroner's office, contacted the parents by telephone, and asked permission to visit with them within days of the death—"most often the first contact was made during visitation hours at the funeral home" (p. 1062). Is it right to approach family members and solicit informed consent for a research study in the earliest weeks of acute grief? Are there guidelines for estimating when is too early or too late to contact bereaved family members?

Our experience and that of many other investigators has been that more than three-quarters of all families willingly volunteer to participate in psychological autopsy studies that are well conducted and well explained (Tables 8.1 and 8.2). Most investigators contacted the family 1 to 6 months after the suicidal death (Beskow et al., 1990). Reasons surviving family members commonly give for participating include the opportunity to talk with a professional who listens intently and does not judge, to ask questions of a professional who has become acquainted with many other cases of suicide, and to share personal experiences with scientists in the altruistic hope that what can be learned will someday spare another family from experiencing the same tragedy.

It is incumbent on investigators to respect the rights and life situation of the bereaved by conducting interviews in a manner that is considerate to each individual informant. Informants ought to be allowed to decide when they are ready to be interviewed; to dictate the duration of each interview session and the location of interviews; and to change or cancel interviews on short notice as their mood dictates. Psychological autopsy investigators have an obligation to protect bereaved family members from all but the most experienced, knowledgeable, skillful, and empathic interviewers. The ability of interviewers to tolerate the distress of reminiscing informants often differs in a positive sense from the informants' experiences with well-intended friends, many of whom mistakenly believe that the informants "should not let themselves get so upset." Most surviving informants, adults and adolescents alike, describe study participation as a positive and useful experience (Shneidman & Farberow, 1961; Litman et al., 1963, 1983; Diller, 1979; Sanborn & Sanborn, 1976; Shneidman, 1969b, 1981; Beskow et al., 1990), and we have found that most spontaneously maintain some form of contact with the research group after their task is finished, to follow the course of the study or to share new family developments.

STANDARDS FOR FUTURE PSYCHOLOGICAL AUTOPSY STUDIES

There is not yet any consensual scientific definition of a psychological autopsy study, though considerable progress has been made in this direction (Shaffer et al., 1972; Rudestam, 1979; Robins, 1981; Brent, Perper, Kolko, &

Zelenak, 1988; Brent, 1989; Beskow et al., 1990). The essential ingredients of the psychological autopsy method include face-to-face interviews with knowledgeable informants within several months of the death, review of all extant records describing the deceased, and comprehensive case formulation by one or more mental health professionals with expertise in postmortem studies. We have taken the position that knowledge about suicide generated by psychological autopsy studies to date is limited and addresses only a few important clinical and research questions that follow from the design of the study. For these reasons, we continue to view the psychological autopsy method as a research method and not a clinical tool. And for these reasons, we believe that psychological autopsy studies should aim to include sample sizes of 60 or more completed cases (i.e., cases with complete data), so that there is sufficient variance to warrant some generalization and sufficient power to test the principal hypotheses posed by the study.

We recommend the following standards for defining and/or constituting a good psychological autopsy study:

1. Delineation of the primary hypotheses that guide the study.
2. Definition of the geographical and temporal boundaries of the catchment area.
3. Precise definition of what constitutes a case of suicide.
4. Description of the clinical qualifications and training of the interviewers.
5. A standardized interview protocol for eliciting data, including a statistical report of inter-interviewer reliability using that protocol.
6. Formal definition of what constitutes a "knowledgeable informant" and documentation of the number of knowledgeable informants potentially available.
7. Description of how potential informants are introduced to the nature of the study and report of the proportion who refuse to be interviewed.
8. Specification of a time frame (i.e., time from the suicide in question to the interview) that will be adhered to for all cases, or report of the distribution of time lapses from death to interview for the sample.
9. A detailed discussion of the way in which discrepant information from different sources is reconciled as it bears on an individual case.
10. A formal plan for how to deal with the validity of data in cases where the minimum specified number of knowledgeable informants cannot be interviewed or where key knowledgeable informants refuse to participate.
11. If diagnostic judgments are rendered, reference to the formal diagnostic criteria applied.

12. Selection of one or more matched comparison groups, accompanied by a rationale for those choices; choice of an appropriate comparison group hinges on the principal hypotheses being tested.

Criteria 1, 5, 11, and 12 make clear what questions the investigator has posed and what questions the investigator is capable of answering or not answering. Criteria 2 and 3 define the population of suicides under study. Criteria 7 and 10 help clarify the degree to which the study sample is representative of the population of all suicides under study, and thus whether it is fair to generalize from the findings. Criteria 4, 6, 9, and 10 allow the reader to evaluate the adequacy of the critical data in a psychological autopsy study—those provided by the informants in face-to-face interviews.

A psychological autopsy study of completed adolescent suicide, now in progress at the Center for Suicide Research and Prevention in Chicago, has included an exploration of some of the methodological parameters of the autopsy technique. One line of study has suggested to us that the number and relationship of informants available for interview have a profound influence on the kind of information elicited, and ultimately on the final autopsy conclusions. Our preliminary findings lead us to believe that a psychological autopsy diagnosis may not be optimal unless *all* available informants (i.e., parents, siblings, other family members, and close friends of both sexes) can be interviewed (Beskow et al., 1990). Close friends of adolescent suicide victims often supply information about the decedents' drug use or abuse history that is not known to parents or siblings. Clinical studies suggest that parents are often unaware of their children's recent or prior suicide attempts (Walker, Moreau, & Weisman, 1990). Our experience with adolescents suggests that four or more informant interviews are necessary for valid conclusions; however, there is a critical need for empirical studies of the degree to which the *number* of informants per case, and the relationship of those informants to the suicide victim, influence the reliability and validity of psychological autopsy study conclusions.

The central task of the psychological autopsy study is to minimize the inevitable distortions that will be introduced, particularly unconscious distortions, by the informants and the interviewers. Such distortions may be the results of the passage of time since death; acute grief or post-traumatic stress syndrome affecting an informant; premorbid characteristics or experiences of the informant; the informant's personal theory about why this suicide occurred; communal explanations or myths about why this suicide occurred; qualities inherent to the interviewer (including intellectual theories about suicidal behavior); the nature of the relationship between the informant and the suicide victim; and the nature of the relationship between the informant and the interviewer. The relationship that develops between each informant–interviewer dyad is critical to the quality of the information obtained by the psychological autopsy study. For this reason, interviewers must be well grounded in suicidology and interview techniques, and should conduct their work under the close and continuous supervision of the principal investigator.

It is surprising that none of the major psychological autopsy studies published to date have employed comparison groups consisting of dead subjects (i.e., persons who have died as a result of accidents, homicide, or natural causes). Although we agree with those who believe that persons afflicted with major psychiatric disorders or those in a life situation similar to that of the suicide victims constitute meaningful comparison groups, depending on the kind of study contemplated, no one type of comparison group is demonstrably optimal or sufficient. We suggest that the unique aspects of the psychological autopsy study—namely, the facts that the subjects are all dead; that relevant information must be recalled and formulated retrospectively; that the principal informants are acutely bereaved; and that the recall and judgment of principal informants are profoundly influenced by after-the-fact knowledge that a suicide did finally occur—are all likely to bias or confound the data available to the investigator. Therefore, we believe it will be important for some psychological autopsy investigators to undertake comparisons between persons who have died by suicide and persons who have died by other means, using identical research protocols and procedures, in attempts to demonstrate that hypothesized differences are not artifacts of the psychological autopsy method.

Finally, we recommend that clinicians conceive of the clinical formulations and psychiatric diagnoses resulting from psychological autopsy studies as *research* formulations and *research* diagnoses. From the time of its introduction by Robins and colleagues (Robins, Gassner, et al., 1959; Robins, Murphy, et al., 1959), the psychological autopsy has almost always been used as a research method. Where mental health experts have worked with medical examiners to conduct psychological autopsies, the findings and formulations of the mental health experts have always been considered *advisory* to a medical examiner's final decisions (Curphey, 1961; Litman, 1989; Litman et al., 1963; Farberow & Neuringer, 1971), and not conclusive in their own right.

Although the psychological autopsy method generates psychological formulations and psychiatric diagnoses that outwardly resemble clinical diagnoses, the investigators conducting and reporting those studies have almost always presented their formulations and diagnoses as *research* diagnoses. Research diagnoses, such as those rendered in large-scale epidemiological surveys, cannot be considered equivalent to clinical diagnoses unless a clinician has validated them by means of face-to-face clinical evaluations. In large-scale epidemiological surveys, one sometimes has the opportunity to send a clinician back to interview individuals who were "diagnosed" by lay raters using a screening instrument of good sensitivity and specificity. In psychological autopsy studies, however, one can never send a clinician back to interview the deceased in an attempt to validate the research diagnosis. Another example of the difference between research and clinical diagnoses can be borrowed from prevailing methods employed to diagnosis familial psychopathology. The "family history method" is designed to elicit data about first- and second-degree family members of a subject from one or two designated informants, and generates *research* diagnoses about persons not directly interviewed. The "family study method," which can be used to evaluate the validity of the family history method, entails face-to-face clinical interviews with individual family members to make the appropriate *clinical* diagnoses (Andreasen, Rice, Endicott, Spitzer, & Winokur, 1977; Andreasen, Endicott, Reich, & Coryell, 1986).

By referring to the clinical formulations and psychiatric diagnoses resulting from psychological autopsy studies of individual cases as *research* formulations and diagnoses, we simply wish to emphasize that there is a critical limit on how much information we can reconstruct about the person who has died by suicide, and emphasize that external validation of our formulations and diagnoses is difficult if not impossible.

CASE VIGNETTES FROM THE PERSPECTIVE OF PSYCHOLOGICAL AUTOPSY RESEARCH

1. *Heather B, age 13.* Although young white females are demographically at relatively low risk for suicide, Heather (see Chapter 12 for full details on this and the other four cases) should be considered at high risk for the following reasons: (a) suicidal wishes, both written and spoken; (b) recent history of self-injury; (c) severe psychological anguish ("my mentality is severely corrupted, distorted, and disturbed"); (d) marked anhedonia ("I stopped caring about a lot of things"); (e) a current episode of major depression; (f) concomitant affective and nonaffective (i.e., conduct) disorders; (g) important questions about drug use (not adequately explored); (h) parental minimization of the seriousness of suicide risk; and (i) severe functional impairment (i.e., social and academic).

2. *Ralph F, age 16.* Ralph should be considered at extremely high risk for the following reasons: (a) persistent suicidal ideation with a recently developed plan; (b) current homicidal impulses; (c) anhedonia; (d) despair (i.e., hopelessness); (e) a current episode of major depression; (f) concomitant affective and substance use disorders (i.e., severe alcohol abuse and drug use); (g) mood-congruent auditory hallucinations; (h) a close family member's death by suicide 8 weeks earlier, apparently in Ralph's home; and (i) increasing marital conflict between parents, lessening the amount of

parental support available to Ralph. Family history of suicidal behavior probably does not help estimate acute risk of completed suicide in clinical situations (Scheftner et al., 1988).

3. *John Z, age 39.* John should be considered at extremely high risk for the following reasons: (a) two extremely serious suicide attempts in recent weeks, albeit interrupted; (b) loss of libido (i.e., anhedonia); (c) a current episode of major depression; (d) apparent panic attacks complicating current depression; and (e) help negation (i.e., dropping out of treatment for 2 months after slight improvement, agreeing to emergency hospitalization and then changing his mind). He should be hospitalized immediately.

4. *Faye C, age 49.* Faye should be considered at moderate risk for suicide for the following reasons: (a) no suicidal thoughts or recent suicidal behavior noted; (b) hyperanxiety, trembling, and fear; (c) insomnia; (d) a current episode of delusional disorder associated with delusions of control, delusions of mind reading, and thought disorder (probably a schizophrenic disorder); (e) history of a major depressive episode; (f) temporal lobe epilepsy, which is associated with higher rates of suicide (Barraclough, 1981); and (g) poverty of interpersonal relationships. Schizophrenic persons are most likely to make fatal suicide attempts during periods when their florid psychotic symptoms abate and depressive symptoms come to the fore (Drake, Gates, Whitaker, & Cotton, 1985).

5. *José G, age 64.* José should be considered at extremely high risk for suicide for the following reasons: (a) being "especially sad about no longer being able to hold a gun firmly"; (b) acute anxiety and restlessness; (c) diminished concentration; (d) early morning awakening; (e) hopelessness; (f) no interest in sex (i.e., anhedonia); (g) a current episode of major depression; (h) long history of heavy alcohol use, several arrests for drunk driving, and increased drinking for the last month; (i) significant psychological losses in last 6 months (i.e., loss of livelihood following wrist injury, permanently disabled wrist); and (j) impending psychological losses (i.e., recently diagnosed diabetic retinopathy threatening his eyesight, recently diagnosed emphysema threatening his activity level and mobility).

ACKNOWLEDGMENT

This review was supported in part by a grant from the NIMH (USPHS MH-45501, "Affective disorder, substance abuse, teen suicide, and health care utilization").

REFERENCES

Andreasen, N. C., Endicott, J., Spitzer, R. L., & Winokur, G. (1977). The family history method using diagnostic criteria. *Archives of General Psychiatry, 34,* 1229–1235.

Andreasen, N. C., Rice, J., Endicott, J., Reich, T., & Coryell, W. (1986). The family history approach to diagnosis. *Archives of General Psychiatry, 43,* 421–429.

Arato, M., Demeter, E., Rihmer, Z., & Somogyi, E. (1988). Retrospective psychiatric assessment of 200 suicides in Budapest. *Acta Psychiatrica Scandinavica, 77,* 454–456.

Barraclough, B. M. (1981). Suicide and epilepsy. In E. H. Reynolds & M. R. Trimble (Eds.), *Epilepsy and Psychiatry* (pp. 72–76). Edinburgh: Churchill Livingstone.

Barraclough, B. M., Bunch, J., Nelson, B., & Sainsbury, P. (1974). A hundred cases of suicide: Clinical aspects. *British Journal of Psychiatry, 125,* 355–373.

Beskow, J. (1979). Suicide and mental disorder in Swedish men. *Acta Psychiatrica Scandinavica, 277*(Suppl. 277), 1–138.

Beskow, J., Runeson, B., & Asgard, U. (1990). Psychological autopsies: Methods and ethics. *Suicide and Life-Threatening Behavior, 20,* 307–323.

Biro, M. (1987). Factor analytic study of suicidal behavior. *Crisis, 8,* 62–68.

Black, D. W., Warrack, G., & Winokur, G. (1985). The Iowa record-linkage study: Suicides and accidental deaths among psychiatric patients. *Archives of General Psychiatry, 42,* 71–75.

Bock, E. W., & Webber, I. L. (1972). Suicide among the elderly: Isolating widowhood and mitigating alternatives. *Journal of Marriage and the Family, 34,* 24–31.

Brent, D. A. (1989). The psychological autopsy: Methodological considerations for the study of adolescent suicide. *Suicide and Life-Threatening Behavior, 19,* 43–57.

Brent, D. A., Perper, J. A., Goldstein, C. E., Kolko, D. J., Allan, M. J., Allman, C. J., & Zelenak, J. P. (1988). Risk factors for adolescent suicide: A comparison of adolescent suicide victims with suicidal inpatients. *Archives of General Psychiatry, 45,* 581–588.

Brent, D. A., Perper, J. A., Kolko, D. J. & Zelenak, J. P. (1988). The psychological autopsy: Methodological considerations for the study of adolescent suicide. *Journal of the American Academy of Child and Adolescent Psychiatry, 27,* 362–366.

Brown, H. N. (1987a). The impact of suicide on therapists in training. *Comprehensive Psychiatry, 28,* 101–112.

Brown, H. N. (1987b). Patient suicide during residency training: I. Incidence, implications, and program response. *Journal of Psychiatric Education, 11,* 201–216.

Chemtob, C. M., Hamada, R. S., Gauer, G., Kinney, B., & Torigoe, R. Y. (1988). Patients' suicides: Frequency and impact on psychiatrists. *American Journal of Psychiatry, 145,* 224–228.

Chynoweth, R., Tonge, J. I., & Armstrong, J. (1980). Suicide in Brisbane—a retrospective psychosocial study. *Australian and New Zealand Journal of Psychiatry, 14,* 37–45.

Conwell, Y., Rotenberg, M., & Caine, E. D. (1990). Completed suicide at age 50 and over. *Journal of the American Geriatrics Society, 38,* 640–644.

Copas, J. B., & Robin, A. (1982). Suicide in psychiatric inpatients. *British Journal of Psychiatry, 141,* 503–511.

Copeland, A. (1987). Suicide among the elderly—the Metro-Dade County experience, 1981–1983. *Medical Sciences and the Law, 27,* 32–36.

Cowles, K. V. (1988). Issues in qualitative research on sensitive topics. *Western Journal of Nursing Research, 10*, 163–179.

Crammer, J. L. (1984). The special characteristics of suicide in hospital inpatients. *British Journal of Psychiatry, 145*, 460–476.

Curphey, T. (1961). The role of the social scientist in the medicolegal certification of death from suicide. In N. L. Farberow & E. S. Shneidman (Eds.), *The cry for help* (pp. 110–117). New York: McGraw-Hill.

Curphey, T. (1967). The forensic pathologist and the multi-disciplinary approach to death. In E. S. Shneidman (Ed.), *Essays in self-destruction* (pp. 463–474). New York: Science House.

Dahlgren, K. G. (1945). [*On suicide and attempted suicide*]. Lund, Sweden: A.-B. PH. Lindstedts Universitat-Bokhandel. (In Swedish)

Diller, J. (1979). The psychological autopsy in equivocal deaths. *Perspectives in Psychiatric Care, 17*, 156–161.

Dooley, E. (1990). Prison suicide in England and Wales, 1972–1987. *British Journal of Psychiatry, 156*, 40–45.

Dorpat, T. L., & Ripley, H. S. (1960). A study of suicide in the Seattle area. *Comprehensive Psychiatry, 1*, 349–359.

Drake, R. E., Gates, C., Whitaker, A., & Cotton, P. G. (1985). Suicide among schizophrenics: A review. *Comprehensive Psychiatry, 26*, 90–100.

Ebert, B. W. (1987). Guide to conducting a psychological autopsy. *Professional Psychology: Research and Practice, 18*, 52–56.

Endicott, J. & Spitzer, R. L. (1978). A diagnostic interview: The Schedule for Affective Disorders and Schizophrenia. *Archives of General Psychiatry, 35*, 837–844.

Farberow, N. L., Kang, H. K., & Bullman, T. A. (1990). Combat experience and postservice psychosocial status as predictors of suicide in Vietnam veterans. *Journal of Nervous and Mental Disease, 178*, 32–37.

Farberow, N. L., & Neuringer, C. (1971). The social scientist as coroner's deputy. *Journal of Forensic Sciences, 16*, 15–39.

Fawcett, J., Scheftner, W. A., Clark, D. C., Hedeker, D., Gibbons, R., & Coryell, W. (1987). Clinical predictors of suicide in patients with major affective disorders: A controlled prospective study. *American Journal of Psychiatry, 144*, 35–40.

Fawcett, J., Scheftner, W. A., Fogg, L., Clark, D. C., Young, M. A., Hedeker, D., & Gibbons, R. (1990). Time-related predictors of suicide in major affective disorder. *American Journal of Psychiatry, 147*, 1189–1194.

Flood, R. A., & Seager, C. P. (1968). A retrospective examination of psychiatric case records of patients who subsequently committed suicide. *British Journal of Psychiatry, 114*, 443–450.

Floyd, N. M. (1977). Billy Budd: A psychological autopsy. *American Imago, 34*, 28–49.

Fowler, R. C., Rich, C. L., & Young, D. (1986). San Diego Suicide Study: II. Substance abuse in young cases. *Archives of General Psychiatry, 43*, 962–965.

Friedman, P. (1967). Suicide among police: A study of ninety-three suicides among New York City policemen, 1934–1940. In E. S. Shneidman (Ed.), *Essays in self-destruction* (pp. 414–449). New York: Science House.

Hagnell, O., & Rorsman, B. (1978). Suicide and endogenous depression with somatic symptoms in the Lundby Study. *Neuropsychobiology, 4,* 180-187.

Hagnell, O., & Rorsman, B. (1979). Suicide in the Lundby Study: A comparative investigation of clinical aspects. *Neuropsychobiology, 5,* 61-73.

Hagnell, O., & Rorsman, B. (1980). Suicide in the Lundby Study: A controlled prospective investigation of stressful life events. *Neuropsychobiology, 6,* 319-332.

Heilig, S. M., Diller, J., & Nelson, F. L. (1982). A study of 44 PCP-related deaths. *International Journal of the Addictions, 17,* 1175-1184.

Ishii, K. (1985). Backgrounds of higher suicide rates among "name university" students: A retrospective study of the past 25 years. *Suicide and Life-Threatening Behavior, 15,* 56-68.

Jobes, D. A., Berman, A. L., & Josselson, A. R. (1986). The impact of psychological autopsies on medical examiners' determination of manner of death. *Journal of Forensic Sciences, 31,* 177-189.

Jobes, D. A., Berman, A. L., & Josselson, A. R. (1987). Improving the validity and reliability of medical-legal certifications of suicide. *Suicide and Life-Threatening Behavior, 17,* 310-325.

Jones, D. R. (1977). Suicide by aircraft: A case report. *Aviation, Space, and Environmental Medicine, 48,* 454-459.

Kleck, G. (1988). Miscounting suicides. *Suicide and Life-Threatening Behavior, 18,* 219-236.

Kolodny, S., Binder, R., Bronstein, A., & Friend, R. (1979). The working through of patients' suicides by four therapists. *Suicide and Life-Threatening Behavior, 9,* 33-46.

Krieger, G. (1968). Psychological autopsies of hospital suicides. *Hospital and Community Psychiatry, 19,* 218-220.

Leenaars, A. A. (1988). *Suicide notes.* New York: Human Sciences Press.

Linehan, M. M. (1986). Suicidal people: One population or two? *Annals of the New York Academy of Sciences, 487,* 16-33.

Litman, R. E. (1984). Psychological autopsies in court. *Suicide and Life-Threatening Behavior, 14,* 88-95.

Litman, R. E. (1987). Mental disorders and suicidal intention. *Suicide and Life-Threatening Behavior, 17,* 85-92.

Litman, R. E. (1989). 500 psychological autopsies. *Journal of Forensic Sciences, 34,* 638-646.

Litman, R. E., Curphey, T., Shneidman, E. S., Farberow, N. L., & Tabachnick, N. (1963). Investigations of equivocal suicides. *Journal of the American Medical Association, 184,* 924-929.

Litman, R. E., Curphey, T., Shneidman, E. S., Farberow, N. L., & Tabachnick, N. (1983). The psychological autopsy of equivocal deaths. In E. S. Shneidman, N. L. Farberow, & R. E. Litman (Eds.), *The psychology of suicide* (pp. 485-496). New York: Jason Aronson.

Maris, R. (1981). *Pathways to suicide: A survey of self-destructive behaviors.* Baltimore: John Hopkins University Press.

Michel, K. (1987). Suicide risk factors: A comparison of suicide attempters with suicide completers. *British Journal of Psychiatry, 150,* 78-82.

Miller, M. (1977). A psychological autopsy of a geriatric suicide. *Journal of Geriatric Psychiatry, 10*, 229–242.

Modestin, J., & Hoffmann, H. (1989). Completed suicide in psychiatric patients and former inpatients: A comparative study. *Acta Psychiatrica Scandinavica, 79*, 229–234.

Motto, J. A. (1979). The impact of patient suicide on the therapist's feelings. *Weekly Psychiatry Update Series, 3*(21), pp. 2–7.

Murphy, G. E. (1986). Suicide and attempted suicide. In G. Winokur & P. Clayton (Eds.), *The medical basis of psychiatry* (pp. 562–579). Philadelphia: W. B. Saunders.

Murphy, G. E., & Robins, E. (1967). Social factors in suicide. *Journal of the American Medical Association, 199*, 303–308.

National Center for Health Statistics. (1988). *NCHS monthly vital statistics report* (Vol. 37, Suppl. 6). Rockville, MD: Author.

Neill, K., Benensohn, H. S., Farber, A. N., & Resnik, H. L. P. (1974). The psychological autopsy: A technique for investigating a hospital suicide. *Hospital and Community Psychiatry, 25*, 33–36.

Nolan, J. T. (1988). *The suicide case: Investigation and trial of insurance claims.* Chicago: American Bar Association.

Orvaschel, H. & Puig-Antich, J. (1986). *Schedule for Affective Disorders and Schizophrenia for School-Aged Children* (4th ed.). Pittsburgh: Western Psychiatric Institute and Clinic.

Osgood, N., & McIntosh, J. (1986). *Suicide in the elderly: An annotated bibliography and review.* New York: Greenwood Press.

Rabiner, C. J., Wegner, J. T., & Kane, J. M. (1982). Suicide in a psychiatric population. *Psychiatric Hospital, 13*, 55–59.

Rich, C. L., Fowler, R. C., Fogarty, L. A., & Young, D. (1988). San Diego Suicide Study: III. Relationships between diagnoses and stressors. *Archives of General Psychiatry, 45*, 589–594.

Rich, C. L., Young, D., & Fowler, R. C. (1986). San Diego Suicide Study: I. Young vs. old subjects. *Archives of General Psychiatry, 43*, 577–582.

Riskind, J. H., Beck, A. T., Berchick, R. J., Brown, G., & Steer, R. A. (1987). Reliability of DSM-III diagnoses for Major Depression and Generalized Anxiety Disorder using the Structured Clinical Interview for DSM-III. *Archives of General Psychiatry, 44*, pp. 817–820.

Robins, E. (1981). *The final months: A study of the lives of 134 persons who committed suicide.* New York: Oxford University Press.

Robins, E., Gassner, S., Kayes, J., Wilkinson, R. H., & Murphy, G. E. (1959). The communication of suicidal intent: A study of 134 consecutive cases of successful (completed) suicide. *American Journal of Psychiatry, 115*, 724–733.

Robins, E., Murphy, G. E., Wilkinson, R. H., Gassner, S., & Kayes, J. (1959). Some clinical considerations in the prevention of suicide based on a study of 134 successful suicides. *American Journal of Public Health, 49*, 888–899.

Robins, L. N., Helzer, J. E., Croughan, J., & Ratcliff, K. S. (1981). National Institute of Mental Health Diagnostic Interview Schedule: Its history, characteristics, and validity. *Archives of General Psychiatry, 38*, 381–389.

Rudestam, K. E. (1979). Some notes on conducting a psychological autopsy. *Suicide and Life-Threatening Behavior, 9,* 141-144.

Runeson, B. (1989). Mental disorders in youth suicide: DSM-III-R Axes I and II. *Acta Psychiatrica Scandinavica, 79,* 490-497.

Sacks, M. H., Kibel, H. D., Cohen, A. M., Keats, M., & Turnquist, K. N. (1987). Resident response to patient suicide. *Journal of Psychiatric Education, 11,* 217-226.

Sainsbury, P. (1986). The epidemiology of suicide. In A. Roy (Ed.), *Suicide* (pp. 17-40). Baltimore: Williams & Wilkins.

Salive, M. E., Smith, G. S., & Brewer, T. F. (1989). Suicide mortality in the Maryland state prison system, 1979 through 1987. *Journal of the American Medical Association, 262,* 365-369.

Salmon, J. A., Hajek, P. T., Rachut, E., Mackenzie, T. B., & Popkin, M. K. (1982). Mortality conference: Suicide of an "appropriately" depressed medical inpatient. *General Hospital Psychiatry, 4,* 307-313.

Sanborn, D. E., & Sanborn, C. J. (1976). The psychological autopsy as a therapeutic tool. *Diseases of the Nervous System, 37,* 4-8.

Scheftner, W. A., Young, M. A., Endicott, J., Coryell, W., Fogg, L., Clark, D. C., & Fawcett, J. (1988). Family history and five-year suicide risk. *British Journal of Psychiatry, 153,* 805-809.

Shaffer, D. (1988). The epidemiology of teen suicide: An examination of risk factors. *Journal of Clinical Psychiatry, 49,* (Suppl.), 36-41.

Shaffer, J. W., Perlin, S., Schmidt, C. W., & Himelfarb, M. (1972). Assessment in absentia: New directions in the psychological autopsy. *John Hopkins Medical Journal, 130,* 308-316.

Shafii, M., Carrigan, S., Whittinghill, J. R., & Derrick, A. (1985). Psychological autopsy of completed suicide in children and adolescents. *American Journal of Psychiatry, 142,* 1061-1064.

Shafii, M., Steltz-Lenarsky, J., Derrick, A. M., Beckner, C., & Whittinghill, R. (1988). Comorbidity of mental disorders in the post-mortem diagnosis of completed suicide in children and adolescents. *Journal of Affective Disorders, 15,* 227-233.

Shneidman, E. S. (Ed.). (1951). *Thematic test analysis.* New York: Grune & Stratton.

Shneidman, E. S. (1969a). *On the nature of suicide.* San Francisco: Jossey-Bass.

Shneidman, E. S. (1969b). Suicide, lethality, and the psychological autopsy. *International Psychiatry Clinics, 6,* 225-250.

Shneidman, E. S. (1976). Some psychological reflections on the death of Malcolm Melville. *Suicide and Life-Threatening Behavior, 6,* 231-242.

Shneidman, E. S. (1981). The psychological autopsy. *Suicide and Life-Threatening Behavior, 11,* 325-340.

Shneidman, E. S. (1985). Some psychological reflections on Herman Melville. *Melville Society Extracts, 64,* 7-9.

Shneidman, E. S. (1991). A life in death: Notes of a committed suicidologist. An epistolary autobiography. In C. E. Walker (Ed.), *The history of clinical psychology in autobiography* (pp. 225-292). Pacific Grove, CA: Brooks/Cole.

Shneidman, E. S., & Farberow, N. (1957). Some comparisons between genuine and simulated suicide notes. *Journal of General Psychology, 56,* 251-256.

Shneidman, E. S., & Farberow, N. (1961). Sample investigation of equivocal suicidal deaths. In N. L. Farberow & E. S. Shneidman (Eds.), *The cry for help* (pp. 118-128). New York: McGraw-Hill.

Sletten, J. W., Brown, M. L., & Evenson, R. C. (1972). Suicide in mental hospital patients. *Diseases of the Nervous System, 33*, 328-335.

Spellman, A., & Heyne, B. (1989). Suicide? Accident? Predictable? Avoidable? The psychological autopsy in jail suicides. *Psychiatric Quarterly, 60*, 173- 183.

Spitzer, R. L., Endicott, J., & Robins, E. (1975). Clinical criteria for psychiatric diagnosis and DSM-III. *American Journal of Psychiatry, 132*, 1187-1192.

Spitzer, R. L., Endicott, J., & Robins, E. (1978). Research Diagnostic Criteria: Rationale and reliability. *Archives of General Psychiatry, 35*, 773-782.

Spitzer, R. L., & Fleiss, J. L. (1974). A reanalysis of the reliability of psychiatric diagnosis. *British Journal of Psychiatry, 125*, 341-347.

Stengel, E., Cook, N. G. (1958). *Attempted suicide.* (Maudsley Monograph No. 4). London: Chapman and Hall.

Temoche, A., Pugh, T. F., & MacMahon, B. (1964). Suicide rates among current and former mental institution patients. *Journal of Nervous and Mental Disease, 138*, 124-130.

Walker, M., Moreau, D., & Weissman, M. M. (1990). Parents' awareness of children's suicide attempts. *American Journal of Psychiatry, 147*, 1364-1366.

Weisman, A. D. (1974). *The realization of death: A guide for the psychological autopsy.* New York: Jason Aronson.

Weisman, A. D., & Kastenbaum, R. (1968). The psychological autopsy: A study of the terminal phase of life. *Community Mental Health Journal* (Monograph 4), 1-59.

Weston, J. T. (1980). Alcohol's impact on man's activities: Its role in unnatural death. *American Journal of Clinical Pathology, 74*, 755-758.

Wing, J. K., Cooper, J. E., & Sartorius, N. (1974). *The measurement and classification of psychiatric symptoms: An instruction manual for the PSE and CATEGO program.* London: Cambridge University Press.

Yanowitch, R. E., Mohler, S. R., & Nichols, E. A. (1972). The Psychosocial Reconstructive Inventory: A postdictal instrument in aircraft accident investigation. *Aerospace Medicine, 43*, 551-554.

Younger, S. C., Clark, D. C., Oehmig-Lindroth, R., & Stein, R. J. (1990). Availability of knowledgeable informants for a psychological autopsy study of suicides committed by elderly people. *Journal of the American Geriatrics Society, 38*, 1169-1175.

CHAPTER 9

Personality Assessment in Suicide Prediction

James R. Eyman, Ph.D.
The Menninger Clinic, Topeka, Kansas
Susanne Kohn Eyman, Ph.D.
Mental Health Associates, Manhattan, Kansas

One way to ascertain whether someone is contemplating suicide is to interview that person. A variety of suicide scales can also aid the assessment process (Eyman & Eyman, 1990; Eyman, Mikawa, & Eyman, 1990). Where, then, lies the usefulness of personality assessment in the evaluation of suicide risk? To answer this question requires a review of the research related to using the Rorschach, the Thematic Apperception Test (TAT), and the Minnesota Multiphasic Personality Inventory (MMPI) in the assessment of suicidality. A case illustration shows how a battery of psychological tests can be used to identify characteristics that make an individual vulnerable to suicidal behavior.

THE RORSCHACH

The Rorschach has been widely used in clinical settings to assess suicide potential. However, studies evaluating the Rorschach's success at predicting suicide have yielded variable results (Eyman, Mikawa, & Eyman, 1990; Exner & Wylie, 1977; Farberow, 1981; Neuringer, 1974). A number of approaches using the Rorschach to evaluate suicidal potential have been attempted, including the use of a single sign, the use of multiple signs or a configurational approach, and evaluation of content. The most widely researched of these various approaches are reviewed here.

Single Sign Approach

Sapolsky (1963) believed that suicidal ideation is guided by the wish to return to the womb. On the basis of this theory, he suggested that individuals with suicidal motivation may give responses to the lower center portion on Card VII (this card is typically regarded as the "mother card," and the area of response is the "vaginal" area). Although he found significantly more suicidal histories among psychiatric patients who gave some type of response to the "vaginal" area than among nonsuicidal psychiatric patients, no other research has been able to confirm Sapolsky's findings (Cooper, Bernstein, & Hart, 1965; Cutter, Jorgenson, & Farberow, 1968; Drake & Rusnak, 1966). This lack of validation is not surprising, given the narrowness of this sign and the infrequency of subjects' responding to this area.

Blatt and Ritzler (1974) investigated the relationship between suicide potential and "transparency" responses (e.g., a room divided by two glass partitions, a woman with a see-through dress) and cross-sectional responses. A suicidal group gave significantly more transparency and cross-sectional responses than did a matched nonsuicidal group. The authors warned that the absence of transparency and cross-sectional responses should not be taken as an indication of low suicide potential. They suggested that a transparency or cross-sectional response is indicative of a loss of self–object differentiation, and that suicide becomes likely when there is a merging of the self with a hated object. In addition, this merging can also represent a loss of the sense of self, with resultant feelings of emptiness, and a loss of the sense of the future, which can exacerbate feelings of hopelessness.

Rierdan, Lang, and Eddy (1978) attempted to cross-validate Blatt and Ritzler's findings. Although the findings were confirmatory, in that the suicidal group gave more transparency responses than the nonsuicidal group, Rierdan et al. proposed a different understanding of the relationship between the transparency response and suicide. They suggested that the process of giving a transparency response is similar to the suicidal individual's fantasy of remaining alive after death; that is, both a transparency response and the view of death represent a transitional phase rather than a definite end.

Kestenbaum and Lynch (1978) did not find that transparency responses differentiated between psychiatric patients who later committed suicide and matched nonsuicidal psychiatric patients. Hansell, Lerner, Milden, and Ludolph (1988) administered the Rorschach and the Hamilton Rating Scale for Depression to depressed psychiatric inpatients. The transparency response was found to be unrelated to current suicidal risk, as measured by the Suicide subscale of the Hamilton Rating Scale for Depression, but was significantly related to a history of more than one previous suicide attempt. The transparency responses were seen consistently by the same subjects over time, whether or not they were in a depressive episode—a finding suggesting that this sign may reflect a permanent characterological state, rather than an immediate and time-limited proneness to suicidal behavior. The theoretical explanations for why the transparency response is related to suicide most likely apply to some, but not all, suicidal individuals. There is some empirical support for the use of the variable to assess suicide risk; however, three studies are insufficient to allow a clinician to feel confident in its use.

Other single-sign approaches using the Rorschach to predict suicidal behavior have focused on color and color-shading responses. Hertz (1948) found that suicidal subjects gave significantly fewer color responses than did nonsuicidal individuals, which she felt reflected a repression of emotional responsiveness to the environment. However, Fisher (1951) found no significant differences in color responses between suicidal and nonsuicidal paranoid schizophrenics.

Appelbaum and Holzman (1962) investigated the relationship between the color-shading response and suicide potential. A "color-shading response" is the use of shading within a colored area—for example, the response "animal tissue" to the pink area of Card X, in which the color pink and the differing darknesses or shading of the pink make it look like tissue. Appelbaum and Holzman found that the color-shading determinant occurred with significantly greater frequency in a suicidal group than in a control group. They also found a greater incidence of the color-shading determinant among completed suicidal patients than among a group of suicide attempters. The authors believed that the color-shading response reflects a sensitivity to nuances of feelings and experiences, which, in a person who is functioning problematically, may lead to excessive anxiety and preoccupation.

Appelbaum and Colson (1968) also found that color-shading responses were more frequent among a suicidal group than among a nonsuicidal patient group. The determinant correctly identified 88% of the suicidal group; however, 49% of the nonsuicidal group also gave one or more of these responses, thereby reducing the discriminant validity of the sign. The authors assumed that some of the nonsuicidal subjects might make a suicide attempt in the future, although no evidence was presented to support this assumption. The authors suggested that color-shading responses represent an aspect of suicidality—that is, being immersed in affect and feeling overwhelmed by perturbation.

Colson and Hurwitz (1973) devised the Color-Shading Technique to facilitate further investigation of the relationship between color-shading responses and suicide potential. They constructed 10 cards similar to the Rorschach, in which three were achromatic and seven chromatic with a broad range of color and hue. The cards were administered to hospitalized psychiatric patients who had made previous suicide attempts and hospitalized psychiatric patients who had never made any attempt or expressed any suicidal ideation. Color-shading responses again emerged as significantly related to suicidal behavior.

Several studies have found no relationship between color-shading responses and suicide lethality (Blatt & Ritzler, 1974; Cutter et al., 1968; Hansell et al., 1988; Neuringer, McEvoy, & Schlesinger, 1965). Despite the contradictory findings, however, it seems worthwhile to pursue these responses, particularly in conjunction with other Rorschach indicators. For example, it might be interesting to look at the relationship between form level, or the degree of realism in a response, and color-shading responses. The ability to be keenly aware of affect and to immerse oneself easily in one's internal state is something that can be an asset and a desirable quality in psychologically healthier individuals, yet quite a problem in individuals who are more disturbed. Assessing indicators of overall ego organization such as form level may help to further elucidate the possible relationship between color-shading responses and suicide potential.

Although there is some support for the single signs described here, we feel strongly that they should be used with great caution. The presence of one of these signs should be a signal to the tester to be alert to other evidence of potential suicidality, yet their absence should not be interpreted as obviating the need for concern.

Configurational or Constellational Approach

Proponents of a multiple-sign or configurational approach believe that suicidality is too complex a phenomenon to be captured reliably by a single Rorschach indicator—a point of view with which we agree. From this perspective, the presence of a certain number of signs from a constellation or configuration is necessary to determine whether or not an individual is suicidal. Cutoff scores reflecting the number of indicators present in a protocol are used to make inferences about suicide potential.

Hertz (1948, 1949) described 14 psychological variables that, on the basis of her extensive clinical experience and of reports in the literature, she felt reflected suicidal tendencies. Each psychological variable is operationally defined by a long list of Rorschach criteria. In a study involving suicidal and nonsuicidal individuals, 10 of the 14 psychological variables were found to differentiate reliably between the two groups: neurotic structure, depressed states, active conflict and deep inner struggle, deep anxiety, constriction, ideational symptomatology, sudden and/or inappropriate emotional outbursts, withdrawal from the world, resignation trends, and agitation. Seventy-four percent of the suicidal group showed 6 or more of the signs, whereas only 5% of the nonsuicidal psychiatric group and none of the normal subjects showed 6 or more signs. Ninety-four percent of the suicidal group, 22% of the nonsuicidal psychiatric group, and 1% of the normal subjects showed 5 or more of the signs. In a validation study, Hertz (1949), using a cutoff score of 5 or more signs, correctly identified 84% of the cases. Hertz concluded that 6 or more of the 10 signs point to suicidal trends and that 5 are highly suggestive of a proneness to suicide.

Fisher (1951) applied the Hertz criteria and failed to discriminate between suicidal and nonsuicidal schizophrenics. A greater proportion of the suicidal patients manifested 6 or more of the signs; however, 25% of the nonsuicidal patients showed 6 or more and 80% gave 5 or more of the signs. Conversely, Sakheim (1955) found that 5 signs differentiated significantly between a suicidal and a nonsuicidal group: deep anxiety, depressed states, withdrawal from the world, agitation, and resignation trends. Hertz's suicidal configuration has not been investigated further, largely because of the enormous amount of time involved in calculating the presence of each psychological variable, as well as the lack of clear definition as to how many Rorschach indices need to be present before one of the psychological variables can be judged to have appeared in a protocol. Nevertheless, Hertz's configuration shows promising discriminant utility, and certainly warrants further research. The negative findings may indicate that the suicide configuration may only be appropriate for certain diagnostic groups. Given the current use of computers, the variables should be less cumbersome to calculate than in the past.

Martin (1951, 1960) empirically derived 16 Rorschach signs that differentiated significantly between a group of suicide attempters and a matched nonsuicidal group at the .10 level or better. In a cross-validation study (Martin, 1960), he tried to replicate his earlier finding using two new groups of matched subjects. Only 5 variables differed significantly between the two groups at the .05 level. However, Martin suggested retaining all 16 signs and adding a 17th sign. When this was done, 7 or more of these signs correctly identified 69% of the suicidal patients. Martin speculated that since a great number of the signs involve color and/or shading, they reflect the suicidal person's high affective arousal, poor affect control, and insensitivity to internal and external control. In another cross validation study, Daston and Sakheim (1960) added a group of individuals who had committed suicide to the two groups used by Martin and failed to differentiate between the two suicidal groups but could differentiate between the group of suicide completers and the nonsuicidal control group. Seven or more of the signs correctly identified 62% of the completed suicides.

Weiner (1961) examined the Rorschach protocols of 42 psychiatric hospital patients and 29 outpatients. Twenty-four of the subjects had made prior suicide attempts. The author concluded that the Martin checklist was useful for identifying suicidal persons and that the best cutoff score for predictive use was 8 or more signs, which correctly classified 79% of the suicide attempters and 60% of the controls. Cutter et al. (1968) found that as the level of suicidal intent increased, there was a corresponding increase in the number of Martin constellation signs in the Rorschach protocols. However, Neuringer et al. (1965) found that the Martin checklist did not differentiate suicidal from nonsuicidal females. Nevertheless, the majority of the research indicates that the Martin suicide checklist seems promising and deserves further investigation.

Exner developed an Adult Suicide Constellation and a Children's Suicide Constellation, based on his Comprehensive System for Scoring the Rorschach (Exner & Wylie, 1977; Exner, 1978, 1986; Exner & Weiner, 1982). In the empirical derivation of the Adult Suicide Constellation, the Rorschach protocols of individuals who completed suicide and individuals who attempted suicide within 60 days of completing the Rorschach were compared to three control groups: depressed inpatients with no history of a suicide attempt, inpatient schizophrenics with no history of a suicide attempt, and nonpsychiatric patients with no history of suicidal behavior. The suicidal subjects were classified into three broad lethality classes: (1) subjects using methods that appeared to have the greatest probability of producing death, (2) subjects using methods with great probability of producing death but with a greater time interval for rescue, and (3) subjects using methods with the lowest probability of producing death and the greatest time interval available for rescue. Various combinations of 12 variables were found to appear with a higher frequency among the completed suicides and the patients who were tested before their suicide attempts. A composite of 8 or more of the variables correctly identified 75% of the suicide completers and 45% of the suicide attempters, while identifying only 20% of the depressed inpatient control group, 12% of the inpatient schizophrenic control group, and none of the nonpatient control group. When the lethality of the act was reviewed, 74% of class 1 subjects were correctly identified, 83% of class 2 subjects were classified correctly, and 63% of class 3 subjects were correctly identified. In a validation study, Exner (1986) analyzed the Rorschach protocols of individuals who committed suicide within 60 days of being administered the Rorschach. Eight of the variables correctly identified 74% of the suicide completers, and correctly identified as nonsuicidal 88% of the inpatient depressive group, 94% of the schizophrenics, and 100% of the nonpsychiatric control group.

We (Eyman & Eyman, 1987) analyzed the Rorschach protocols of individuals who had completed suicide and individuals who had made three or more mild, nonlethal suicide attempts. Only two subjects, one completer and one mild-attempt individual, met the established criterion of eight or more suicide constellation variables. Contrary to expectation, the mild-attempt group had significantly more suicide constellation variables than the suicide completers. Furthermore, the suicide constellation was no more accurate for individuals who commmited suicide shortly after taking the Rorschach (within 90 days) than for those who completed suicide after much longer periods of time. We concluded that the Adult Suicide Constellation was ineffective in predicting suicidal behavior.

Exner and his colleagues (Exner, 1978, 1986, 1987; Exner & Weiner, 1982) also developed the Children's Suicide Constellation for children aged 8–18 after it was discovered that the Adult Suicide Constellation contained many variables that were developmentally normative for children and adolescents. None of the studies supported the scale's ability to discriminate suicidal from nonsuicidal children, and Exner and Weiner (1982) concluded that the Children's Suicide Constellation has limited clinical utility.

The Rorschach can be useful in assessing suicide risk if it is used with appropriate clinical judgment. The configurational approaches have the best discriminant validity, and the variables of Hertz (1948, 1949) and Martin (1951, 1960) seem promising. Although we believe that suicide is too complex a behavior to be captured adequately by a single sign, the transparency response (Blatt & Ritzler, 1974) and color-shading responses (Appelbaum & Colson, 1968; Appelbaum & Holtzman, 1962; Colsen & Hurwitz, 1973) have some support. These signs may be clinically useful if they are corroborated by other clinical data.

THE THEMATIC APPERCEPTION TEST

Little research has been conducted using the TAT to assess suicidal risk. The few studies using only the TAT all failed to differentiate suicidal from nonsuicidal groups (McEvoy, 1974). These studies are reviewed briefly here.

When Broida (1954) analyzed the themes given to Card 3BM, known as one of the cards that elicit suicidal themes, he failed to find a difference between a psychotic suicidal group and a nonsuicidal group. Shneidman and Farberow (1958) used a Q-sort technique to determine the characteristics of the TAT heroes of suicidal and nonsuicidal subjects. Judges could not differentiate suicidal from nonsuicidal individuals on the basis of the characteristics of the TAT heroes. Fisher and Hinds (1951), McEvoy (1974), and Lester (1970) all failed to find a difference in aggressive content between suicidal and nonsuicidal groups.

THE MINNESOTA MULTIPHASIC
PERSONALITY INVENTORY

The MMPI is one of the most frequently used clinical assessment instruments. Various studies have attempted to use MMPI data to assess suicide potential, and to discriminate between suicidal and nonsuicidal individuals or between those individuals who commit suicide and those who make unsuccessful attempts. Investigation of the MMPI to determine suicide potential has included the examination of individual items, single scales, and profiles.

Individual Item Analysis

The success of special MMPI scales led researchers (Clopton, 1979) to examine the possibility that individual MMPI items differentiating between suicidal and nonsuicidal individuals might be used in developing a suicide scale. Without success, Simon and Gilberstadt (1958) and Clopton and Jones (1975) attempted to isolate MMPI items related to suicidal behavior. Farberow and Devries (1967) developed the Suicide Threat scale, consisting of 52 MMPI items that significantly differentiated a male psychiatric suicide threat group from a nonsuicidal psychiatric control group. The scale correctly classified 80% of the suicide threateners and 68% of the nonsuicidal subjects. In a replication study, the scale correctly classified 72% of the suicide threateners but only 42% of a nonsuicidal group, which is too low a percentage to be relied on in clinical settings. Further studies (Clopton & Jones, 1975; Ravensborg & Foss, 1969; Watson, Klett, Walters, & Vassar, 1984) failed to find significant differences between groups, clearly indicating the lack of validity of the Suicide Threat scale.

Two studies have reported positive results with MMPI individual items. Controlling for age, education, occupation, marital status, and number of hospital admissions, Devries (1967) found that 16 items significantly differentiated between a nonsuicidal control group and psychiatric patients who had made some type of suicide attempt. However, the item numbers were not reported. Koss, Butcher, and Hoffman (1976) examined the items endorsed by male psychiatric patients in six crisis states: acute anxiety, depressed–suicidal ideation, mental confusion, persecutory ideas, situational stress due to alcoholism, and threatened assault. Unfortunately, the authors did not specify exactly who was in the depressed–suicidal group (i.e., patients with suicidal ideation, patients who had made suicide attempts, or both). The item responses of these depressed–suicidal patients were compared to a control sample of male subjects. Eighty-nine MMPI items were found to differentiate significantly between the two groups. All the items that discriminated a crisis group from the control group at a probability of less than .001 and that were unique to only one crisis group were formed into the 67-item Koss and Butcher Critical Items scale. Twenty-five of these items relate to depressed–suicidal ideas (Greene, 1980).

Neither the Devries nor the Koss and Butcher study has been replicated, and the authors present insufficient information to permit any evaluation of the usefulness of these items. From the research conducted to this point, one must conclude that individual-item analysis of the MMPI is not worthwhile to pursue.

Individual-Scale Differences

Studies investigating the difference in elevation of individual MMPI scales between suicidal and nonsuicidal individuals have produced contradictory results. The two scales most consistently related to suicidal ideation or behavior are the Depression (D) and Masculinity–Femininity (Mf) scales. Simon (1950) found a peak on the D scale to be particularly characteristic of male patients who attempted suicide by hanging. However, most of the literature that supports an elevation on the D scale associated with suicide risk is based solely on case study. These clinical formulations suggest that elevations of T-scores greater than 70 on the D scale, in subjects who are denying a depressive state and depressive thoughts and feelings, do indicate an increased risk of suicide (Dahlstrom, 1972). However, several studies have found that elevations on the D scale do not differentiate significantly between suicide attempters and nonattempters (Clopton & Jones, 1975; Tarter, Templer, & Perley, 1975; Watson et al., 1984).

A few studies have concluded that a high score for males and a low score for females on the Mf scale is associated with increased risk for suicidal behavior (Sendbuehler, Kincel, Nemeth, & Oertel, 1979; Simon & Gilberstadt, 1958). For example, Waters et al. (1982) correctly classified 72.5% of male suicide attempters and nonsuicidal depressed subjects and 80% of the female subjects with a discriminant analysis of the Mf scores. Simon and Gilberstadt (1958) discussed the finding of poor masculine identification as an important variable in the personalities of males vulnerable to suicide, especially when coupled with narcissism and impairment in psychosocial development. However, several studies have failed to find differences between attempters and nonattempters on the Mf scale (Clopton & Jones, 1975; Watson et al., 1984). Several studies have identified gender differences, but the various results are not consistent (Leonard, 1977; Tarter et al., 1975; Waters, Sendbuehler, Kincel, Boodoosingh, & Marchenko, 1982). The confusing array of results suggests that the various findings might be related to sampling differences.

Two studies have investigated the relationship of individual MMPI scales to suicide in an adolescent population. Marks and Haller (1977) found gender differences. MMPI scale scores for Hypochondriasis (Hs) and Mf were significantly higher for those adolescent boys who attempted suicide than for adolescent male nonattempters. The suicidal adolescent girls who attempted suicide had significantly higher scale scores on D and Hysteria (Hy) than did the adolescent female nonattempters. Spirito, Faust, Myers, and Bechtel (1988) analyzed the MMPIs of adolescent females hospitalized on a general pediatrics unit after a suicide attempt and the MMPIs of adolescent females referred for psychiatric evaluation. Using a univariate analysis of variance, they found that only the Correction (K) scale was significantly different between the two groups, with nonsuicidal female adolescents obtaining a higher mean score.

Profile Analysis

Meyer (1983) asserts that the prototypical profile for a suicidal individual is an elevation of the D and Psychasthenia (Pt) scales. The likelihood of someone's acting on suicidal anger increases as the Paranoia (Pa), Schizophrenia (Sc), and Hypomania (Ma) scale scores rise. In addition to the suicidal urges accounted for by the D and Pt scales, elevations on Pa, Sc, and Ma reflect a loss of control over impulses, impaired reality testing, a sense of isolation, and the energy available to engage in a suicidal act. Although the logic and rationale behind Meyer's clinical observations are sound, he presents no empirical data to support his claims.

Studies have investigated MMPI high-point profiles to determine those that might be related to suicidal symptomatology. A few researchers have found MMPI profiles related to suicidal behavior, but the profiles have been different in each study. Marks and Seeman (1963) analyzed the MMPIs of psychiatric inpatients and outpatients and found profiles related to combined suicidal behavior, threats, and ideation. However, Watson et al. (1984) and Clopton and Jones (1975) found that few of the Marks and Seeman profiles were present in truly suicidal subjects; thus, the validity of these profiles was not supported. Some studies (Clopton, Pallis, & Birtchnell, 1979; Clopton & Jones, 1975; Waters et al., 1982) have found limited differences in profiles between suicidal and nonsuicidal subjects, but none of the differences discriminate sufficiently between groups to be useful clinically. Several studies have failed to find differences in MMPI profiles between suicidal and nonsuicidal individuals (Clopton & Baucom, 1974; Clopton, Post, & Larde, 1983; Ravensborg & Foss, 1969; Spirito et al., 1988).

The MMPI has been recently restandardized (Hathaway et al., 1989) and is now called the MMPI-2. A total of 2,600 subjects (1,138 males and 1,462 females aged 18–90) were matched according to 1980 U.S. Census data in terms of geographic distribution, ethnic and racial composition, age and educational levels, and marital status. Unfortunately, Hispanics and Asian-Americans were underrepresented in this restandardization sample. These subjects were given a research form of the MMPI, containing 550 items from the current MMPI (with some editorial modifications and without the 16 duplicated items), plus an additional 154 items. Some of the new items were revised versions of existing items, but the majority were designed to provide better coverage of topical areas, including suicide.

The goal of the restandardization was not to revise the original validity and clinical scales. These scales were therefore kept relatively intact in the MMPI-2. The new national norms are more representative of the general population in the United States; uniform T-scores are used; and objectionable wording has been eliminated. In addition, 15 new content scales were developed for the MMPI-2 by Butcher, Graham, Williams, and Ben-Porath

(1989). Among these new scales is a new 37-item content scale on Depression. Elevation on this scale is believed characteristic of individuals with significant depressive thoughts and possible suicidal thoughts or wishes for death. No study has examined the validity of the Depression content scale for assessing suicide wish. The Koss–Butcher Critical Items scale has been retained in the MMPI-2. All but five of the depressed suicidal ideation questions of the Koss-Butcher Critical Items are found in the Depression content scale.

An experimental adolescent version of the MMPI-2, Form TX, is currently being evaluated to determine whether there will be an MMPI-2 form specifically for adolescents (Williams, 1990). The experimental form contains both the original MMPI items and new items to evaluate specific adolescent problems such as peer group influence, family relations, substance abuse, and sexuality. Also, 16 new content scales are being developed.

Despite considerable research effort, no MMPI item, scale, or profile configuration has been found to differentiate consistently between suicidal and nonsuicidal individuals. The MMPI thus cannot be recommended as a tool for assessing suicide risk. Perhaps the restandardized MMPI-2 will provide more valid indicators of suicidality.

PSYCHOLOGICAL TEST BATTERY

Smith and Eyman (1988) used evaluation of Rorschach and TAT content to assess characterological features thought to exist in suicidal individuals. They compared groups of male and female psychiatric patients who had made very serious suicide attempts with groups who had made mild, nonlethal attempts with little chance of death. Constructs were rated by the two authors as "present," "not present," or "undetermined." Male serious attempters and mild attempters were significantly differentiated by four characteristics. The first, overcontrol of aggressive ideation, was seen in percepts such as "attacking animals, growling, but they have heads like raccoons," or "missile with outrageous fins for better control." Some schizophrenic patients showed unmodulated aggressive ideation outstripping their ability to control affect. The second characteristic, high expectations of self, was evident in percepts such as "a crown," "statue on a pedestal," and "the Eiffel Tower." Third, conflictual dependent yearnings were seen in responses such as "a torn-up teddy bear." Finally, an ambivalent and nonfrivolous attitude toward death was seen in themes of death described with anxiety, pauses, and a great deal of reworking.

Different results were found for the females in the study. Only one characteristic, overcontrolled aggression, was found to differentiate the groups. Female serious attempters were significantly more overcontrolled in their expression of affect. It may be that different content scales need to be developed for females. For example, it is well known in the psychological literature that women's achievement expectations tend to be directed toward relationships, as opposed to the typical male emphasis on career success and fame. Thus, a "crown" or "tower" may not reflect high expectations of self for a woman. Nevertheless, the results of this study support the notion that some characterological features may differentiate seriously suicidal individuals from mild attempters, and that these characteristics can be assessed by means of the Rorschach and TAT.

CASE ANALYSIS

We have chosen to discuss the case of Heather B because of the detailed psychological test data available (see Chapter 12 for complete details). Heather, a 13-year-old student, showed affective and behavioral instability. At age 7, when her father died, she showed no emotional reaction. She had few friends at school and fantasized that the 33-year-old president of a rock star's fan club was her boyfriend. Her schoolwork had been deteriorating, and she began to express suicidal ideation in letters and other writings.

Heather's Rorschach protocol suggests that a single-sign approach would not be fruitful. For example, she gave no transparency or cross-sectional responses, nor any response to the lower center portion of Card VII. There may have been one color-shading response, on Card IX ("the collision of two alien worlds . . . looks like it's exploding"); however, there was insufficient inquiry to establish this. Exner's Children's Suicide Constellation could not be used, because it is not a valid indicator of suicidality. The test data do lend themselves to an analysis following the approach that we and our colleagues have described elsewhere (Smith, 1985; Smith & Eyman, 1988; Eyman et al., 1990; Richman & Eyman, 1990). As noted earlier, this model uses psychological testing to assess an individual's tendency toward suicidal behavior by identifying four variables: a defensive stance toward aggression, high self-expectations, conflicted dependent yearnings, and an ambivalent yet serious attitude about death. The reader will recall that, for females only, the defensive stance toward aggressive ideation significantly differentiated serious and nonserious attempters. However, the failure of the other variables to distinguish between the two groups was suspected to be due to the scales' having been composed without adequate attention to female psychological characteristics. For the purpose of analyzing this case, we now explore Heather's Rorschach and TAT protocols for the presence of any of these variables, with particular attention to how they might be presented by a female adolescent.

Defensive Stance toward Aggression

The establishment of the first construct, a defensive stance toward aggression, depends on the level of ego organization of the individual. Among individuals with a midborderline to neurotic level of organization, lethality is believed to increase with evidence of withholding and constricting aggressive ideation. Aggressive responses are quickly defused and minimized. Individuals with a low borderline or psychotic ego organization show an increased lethality in aggressive ideation that is graphic and embellished. Such persons ineffectively control aggressive ideation and are instead captivated by it (Smith & Eyman, 1988).

It is clear from Heather's Rorschach that she was quite angry, but that she was uncomfortable with her aggressive feelings. Her discomfort was most apparent in the process of her responses. Each particularly aggressive response was followed by an emotionally distant one that often minimized any threat. For example, "Two dogs tearing something" was followed by "On a road to something far away." "Arguing faces" preceded "They're warming their hands over the fire." Similarly, "a dragon" was followed by "a butterfly," and "The collision of two alien worlds" came immediately before "pink . . . cabbages."

Several individual responses also demonstrate Heather's attempts to control and minimize affect, particularly aggression. For example, on Card III Heather said, "The red comes in; it just doesn't mean anything to me. It's just there." Here, her affect was clearly coming into awareness, demonstrated by her noting the color, but she quickly discounted its impact and meaning. Heather's lack of ease in handling her emotions during the psychological testing was also apparent in her writing. She wrote about her father's death, "I should have cried. But I didn't." Her anger over her father's death and her subsequent feelings of guilt were poignantly expressed in this journal entry: "For seven years and what do I get? A grave and a photo? . . . I'm sorry, Daddy."

High Expectations of Self

Lethality is felt to increase as a person exhibits a striving for and a longing to accomplish a sense of self-importance, an overvaluation of the self. Goals for the self typically far exceed actual capabilities. Although these individuals have quite low self-esteem, many are driven always to expect more from themselves, so are rarely satisfied. There is a gulf between their dismal experience of themselves in reality and their often unrealistic wish to be different (Smith & Eyman, 1988; Richman & Eyman, 1990).

In two TAT stories, Heather revealed her longing to achieve and to be recognized for her creativity and artistic talent, as well as a sense of inadequacy. For Card 1, she described a boy who wants to play a beautiful violin but is not old enough: "he wants to but he can't." For Card 8GF, which is a picture of a woman sitting at a table, Heather told of the woman's having completed "a really great sculpture." We find shortly that the sculpture is not as great or as complete as the woman wants; it is only "in clay right now," not yet "into marble."

In Heather's and her mother's recital of historical information, other areas of unreachable self-expectations and inevitable disappointment can be seen. Heather fantasized about popularity and social acceptance, only to feel unaccepted and alienated. She defined herself as an "anarchist" and "weirdo," and showed disdain for the prevailing "preppy" styles, but was bitterly disappointed and angry when not invited to a party. Similarly, she referred to the 33-year-old president of a rock star's fan club as her "boyfriend," a relationship that was unlikely to exist outside her imagination.

Conflictual Dependent Yearnings

Many seriously suicidal individuals have an unconscious and desperate desire to be passively nurtured, taken care of, and totally gratified by others. These individuals seem to be searching for an all-powerful, perfectly attuned "mother" who will supply them with endless comfort, gratification, and a feeling of completeness. However, because they are conflicted about such strong dependency wishes, these individuals often act in counterdependent ways (Smith & Eyman, 1988; Richman & Eyman, 1990).

There are no indications in Heather's test data that she either wished or expected to be taken care of without any effort on her part. What was evident was her belief that the world is unsafe, alongside a feeling that she must fend for herself because strong, nurturing, and validating others are not available. Heather's TAT stories revealed her unrelinquished longings for a reunion with lost loved ones, most likely her dead father. It is noteworthy that in those TAT stories (Cards 2, 3GF, 5) some other male relative is always the one missing, never a father. Heather was evidently unable to acknowledge and work through her mourning for her father.

Anxious but Serious Attitude about Death

Lethality is heightened by a serious but anxious attitude about death, as if the individual has thought about death as a real solution. Such individuals do not take death lightly or frivolously (Smith & Eyman, 1988; Richman & Eyman, 1990). In the two TAT stories in which Heather spoke directly about death (Cards 3GF and 13MF), she gave no indications of a wish to escape intolerable pain. Rather, the stories revealed the sadness of those who had lost someone dear. Thus, the stories seem to express an unresolved mourning process instead of a real wish to die. In her writing, Heather clearly expressed her self-destructive tendencies, but again her motivation seemed to be a wish for retaliation and communication of distress, rather than a clear intention to kill herself.

Summary of the Case

In Heather's Rorschach and TAT protocols, we see at least two characteristics common to suicidally vulnerable people: a striving to gain a sense of self-importance, and a discomfort with aggressive ideation. Although she showed no signs of passive dependency yearnings, she was in conflict between wanting closeness and missing lost relationships, yet believing that she needed to function without depending on others. Her attitude toward death and self-injury was flamboyant, and she paraded it for its impact on others, rather than because she felt serious and anxious. However, among adolescents (unlike adults), this parading attitude does not necessarily lessen suicide risk. Thus, Heather should be considered to be at risk for some type of suicidal behavior.

In contrast to these risk factors, certain aspects of Heather's functioning would appear to mitigate against serious likelihood of suicide at this time. Most importantly, Heather did not seem to want to die. Her thoughts about death seemed to revolve around perceived social rebuffs and her own unresolved mourning for her father. She also appeared to harbor some hope that the future might bring a sense of accomplishment, positive relatedness, and accompanying self-esteem. Nevertheless, any situations or circumstances intensifying her feelings of rejection and abandonment might lead her to entertain the idea that suicide could solve her painful inner turmoil.

CONCLUSION

Even though each individual psychological test's ability to predict immediate suicidal risk has not consistently been supported by research, personality assessment can still be of aid in evaluating suicidal risk. The Rorschach, TAT, and MMPI are not particularly useful instruments for the assessment of acute, immediate risk. Many components important in determining immediate lethality are not obtainable by psychological tests, such as the pervasiveness and severity of suicidal ideation, and aspects of intent such as specific plans to kill oneself. Personality tests are best used in delineating the ego capacities and self-other representations that may predispose a person toward responding to major life crises with suicidal behavior. The richness of projective test data also lends itself to gathering information about what circumstances may lead a person to consider suicide as a viable option.

In assessing suicidal vulnerability, it is important to use a battery of psychological tests and not to rely on only one instrument. For example, the

Rorschach and TAT supply different types of psychological information, although, of course, they overlap considerably. The Rorschach more directly elicits information about a person's reality testing, ability to integrate and modulate affect, and defensive maneuvers around conflicts. The TAT pulls for a more conscious experience of self and the world, and is a measure of the individual's efforts to deal with problems of living. Thus, using more than one psychological test supplies information that leads to a fuller and more enriched view of a person's psychological functioning than would be gained by reliance on only one test. In addition, using a battery of psychological tests allows one to confirm hypotheses with data from a variety of sources.

REFERENCES

Appelbaum, S. A., & Colson, D. B. (1968). A reexamination of the color-shading Rorschach test response and suicide attempts. *Journal of Projective Techniques and Personality Assessment, 32,* 160-164.

Appelbaum, S. A., & Holzman, P. S. (1962). The color-shading response and suicide. *Journal of Projective Techniques, 26,* 155-161.

Blatt, S. J., & Ritzler, D. A. (1974). Suicide and the representation of transparency and cross-sections on the Rorschach. *Journal of Consulting and Clinical Psychology, 42*(2), 280-287.

Broida, D. C. (1954). An investigation of certain psychodiagnostic indications of suicidal tendencies and depression in mental hospital patients. *Psychiatric Quarterly, 28,* 453-464.

Butcher, J. N., Graham, J. R., Williams, C. L., & Ben-Porath, Y. (1989). *Development and use of the MMPI-2 content scales.* Minneapolis: University of Minnesota Press.

Clopton, J. R. (1979). The MMPI and suicide. In C. S. Newmark (Ed.), *MMPI: Clinical and research trends* (pp. 149-166). New York: Praeger.

Clopton, J. R., & Baucom, D. H. (1979). MMPI ratings of suicide risk. *Journal of Personality Assessment, 43*(3), 293-296.

Clopton, J. R., & Jones, W. C. (1975). Use of the MMPI in the prediction of suicide. *Journal of Clinical Psychology, 31*(1), 52-54.

Clopton, J. R., Pallis, D. J., & Birtchnell, J. (1979). Minnesota Multiphasic Personality Inventory profile patterns of suicide attempters. *Journal of Consulting and Clinical Psychology, 47*(1), 135-139.

Clopton, J. R., Post, R. D., & Larde, J. (1983). Identification of suicide attempters by means of MMPI profiles. *Journal of Clinical Psychology, 39*(6), 868-871.

Colson, D. B., & Hurwitz, B. A. (1973). A new experimental approach to the relationship between color-shading and suicide attempts. *Journal of Personality Assessment, 37*(3), 237-241.

Cooper, G. W., Bernstein, L., & Hart, C. (1965). Predicting suicidal ideation from the Rorschach: An attempt to cross-validate. *Journal of Projective Techniques and Personality Assessment, 29*(2), 168-170.

Cutter, F., Jorgensen, M., & Farberow, N. L. (1968). Replicability of Rorschach signs with known degrees of suicidal intent. *Journal of Projective Techniques and Personality Assessment, 32*, 428-434.

Dahlstrom, W. G. (1972). *An MMPI handbook: Vol. 1. Clinical interpretation* (rev. ed.). Minneapolis: University of Minnesota Press.

Daston, P. G., & Sakheim, G. A. (1960). Prediction of successful suicide from the Rorschach test using a sign approach. *Journal of Projective Techniques, 24*, 355-361.

Devries, A. G. (1967). Control variables in the identification of suicidal behavior. *Psychological Reports, 20*, 1131-1135.

Drake, A. K., & Rusnak, A. W. (1966). An indicator of suicidal ideation on the Rorschach: A replication. *Journal of Projective Techniques and Personality Assessment, 30*(6), 543-544.

Exner, J. E. (1978). *The Rorschach: A comprehensive system. Vol. 2.* New York: John Wiley & Sons.

Exner, J. E. (1986). Structural data IV—special indices. In J. E. Exner, *The Rorschach: A comprehensive system. Vol. 1. Basic foundation* (2nd ed., pp. 411-428). New York: Wiley.

Exner, J. E. (1987, June). Children's suicide constellation. *Rorschach Workshops Alumni Newsletter*, p. 6.

Exner, J. E., & Weiner, I. (1982). *The Rorschach: A comprehensive system* (Vol. 3). New York: Wiley.

Exner, J. E., & Wylie, J. (1977). Some Rorschach data concerning suicide. *Journal of Personality Assessment, 41*(4), 339-348.

Eyman, J. R., & Eyman, S. K. (1990). Suicide risk and assessment instruments. In P. Cimbolic and D. Jobes (Eds.), *Youth suicide: Issues, assessment and intervention* (pp. 9-32). Springfield, IL: Charles C Thomas.

Eyman, J. R., Mikawa, J. K., & Eyman, S. K. (1990). The problem of adolescent suicide: Issues and assessments. In P. McReynolds, J. C. Rosen, & G. Chelune (Eds.), *Advances in psychological assessment* (Vol. 7, pp. 165-202). New York: Plenum.

Eyman, S. K., & Eyman, J. R. (1987, August). *An investigation of Exner's suicide constellation.* Paper presented at the meeting of the American Psychological Association, New York.

Farberow, N. L. (1981). Assessment of suicide. In P. McReynolds (Ed.), *Advances in psychological assessment* (Vol. 5, pp. 124-190). San Francisco: Jossey-Bass.

Farberow, N. L., & Devries, A. G. (1967). An item differentiation analysis of MMPIs of suicidal neuropsychiatric hospital patients. *Psychological Reports, 20*, 607-617.

Fisher, S. (1951). The value of the Rorschach for detecting suicidal trends. *Journal of Projective Techniques, 15*, 250-254.

Fisher, S., & Hinds, E. (1951). The organization of hostility controls in various personality structures. *Genetic Psychology Monographs, 44*, 3-68.

Greene, R. (1980). *The MMPI: An interpretive manual.* New York: Grune & Stratton.

Hansell, A. G., Lerner, H. D., Milden, R. S., & Ludolph, P. S. (1988). Single-sign Rorschach suicide indicators: A validity study using a depressed inpatient population. *Journal of Personality Assessment, 52*(4), 658-669.

Hathaway, S. R., McKinley, C. K., Butcher, J. N., Dahlstrom, W. G., Graham, J., Tellegen, A., & Kaemmer, B. (1989). *Manual for administration and scoring on the Minnesota Multiphasic Personality Inventory-2 (MMPI-2)*. Minneapolis: University of Minnesota Press.

Hertz, M. R. (1948). Suicidal configurations in Rorschach records. *Rorschach Research Exchange, 12*, 1–56.

Hertz, M. R. (1949). Further study of "suicidal" configurations in Rorschach records. *Rorschach Research Exchange, 13*, 44–73.

Kestenbaum, J. M., & Lynch, D. (1978). Rorschach suicide predictors: A cross validational study. *Journal of Clinical Psychology, 34*(3), 754–758.

Koss, M. P., Butcher, J. N., & Hoffmann, N. G. (1976). The MMPI critical items: How well do they work? *Journal of Consulting and Clinical Psychology, 44*(6), 921–928.

Leonard, C. V. (1977). The MMPI as a suicide predictor. *Journal of Consulting and Clinical Psychology, 45*(3), 367–377.

Lester, D. (1970). Factors affecting choice of methods of suicide. *Journal of Clinical Psychology, 26*, 437.

Marks, P. A., & Haller, D. (1977). Now I lay me down for keeps: A study of adolescent suicide attempts. *Journal of Clinical Psychology, 33*(2), 390–400.

Marks, P. A., & Seeman, W. (1963). *The actuarial description of abnormal personality*. Baltimore: Williams & Wilkins.

Martin, H. A. (1951). *A Rorschach study of suicide*. Unpublished doctoral dissertation, University of Kentucky.

Martin, H. A. (1960). A Rorschach study of suicide. *Dissertation Abstracts, 20*, 37–38.

McEvoy, T. L. (1974). Suicidal risk via the Thematic Apperception Test. In C. Neuringer (Ed.), *Psychological assessment of suicidal risk* (pp. 95–117). Springfield, IL: Charles C Thomas.

Meyer, R. G. (1983). *The clinician's handbook: The psychopathology of adulthood and late adolescence*. Boston: Allyn & Bacon.

Neuringer, C. (1974). Rorschach ink blot test assessment of suicidal risk. In C. Neuringer (Ed.), *Psychological assessment of suicidal risk* (pp. 74–94). Springfield, IL: Charles C Thomas.

Neuringer, C., McEvoy, T. L., & Schlesinger, R. J. (1965). The identification of suicidal behavior in females by the use of the Rorschach. *Journal of General Psychology, 72*, 127–133.

Ravensborg, M. R., & Foss, A. (1969). Suicide and natural death in a state hospital population: A comparison of admission complaints, MMPI profiles, and social competence factors. *Journal of Consulting and Clinical Psychology, 33*(4), 466–471.

Richman, J., & Eyman, J. R. (1990). Psychotherapy of suicide: Individual, group, and family approaches. In D. Lester (Ed.), *Current concepts of suicide* (pp. 139–158). Philadelphia: Charles Press.

Rierdan, J., Lang, E., & Eddy, S. (1978). Suicide and transparency responses on the Rorschach: A replication. *Journal of Consulting and Clinical Psychology, 46*(5), 1162–1163.

Sakheim, G. A. (1955). Suicidal responses on the Rorschach test: A validation study. *Journal of Nervous and Mental Disease, 122*, 332–334.

Sapolsky, A. (1963). An indicator of suicidal ideation on the Rorschach test. *Journal of Projective Techniques and Personality Assessment, 27*(3), 332–335.

Sendbuehler, J. N., Kincel, R. L., Nemeth, G., & Oertel, J. (1979). Dimension of seriousness in attempted suicide: Significance of the MF scale in suicidal MMPI profiles. *Psychological Reports, 44,* 343–361.

Shneidman, E. S., & Farberow, N. L. (1958). TAT hostility and psychopathology. *Journal of Projective Techniques, 22,* 211–228.

Simon, W. (1950). Attempted suicide among veterans. *Journal of Nervous and Mental Disease, 111,* 451–468.

Simon, W., & Gilberstadt, H. (1958). Analysis of a personality structure of 26 actual suicides. *Journal of Nervous and Mental Disease, 127,* 555–557.

Smith, K. (1985). An ego vulnerabilities approach to suicide assessment. *Bulletin of the Menninger Clinic, 49,* 489–499.

Smith, K., & Eyman, J. R. (1988). Ego structure and object differentiation. In H. Lerner & P. Lerner (Eds.), *Primitive mental states and the Rorschach* (pp. 175–202). Madison, CT: International Universities Press.

Spirito, A., Faust, D., Myers, B., & Bechtel, D. (1988). Clinical utility of the MMPI in the evaluation of adolescent suicide attempters. *Journal of Personality Assessment, 52*(2), 204–211.

Tarter, R. E., Templer, D. I., & Perley, R. L. (1975). Social role orientation and pathological factors in suicide attempts of varying lethality. *Journal of Community Psychology, 3,* 295–299.

Waters, G. H., Sendbuehler, J. M., Kincel, R. L., Boodoosingh, L. A., & Marchenko, I. (1982). The use of the MMPI for the differentiation of suicidal and non-suicidal depressions. *Canadian Journal of Psychiatry, 27,* 663–667.

Watson, C. G., Klett, W. G., Walters, C., & Vassar, P. (1984). Suicide and the MMPI: A cross-validation of predictors. *Journal of Clinical Psychology, 40*(1), 115–119.

Weiner, I. B. (1961). Cross-validation of a Rorschach checklist associated with suicidal tendencies. *Journal of Consulting and Clinical Psychology, 25*(4), 312–315.

Williams, C. (1990). Adolescents and the MMPI: Present and future. *MMPI-2 News and Profiles, 1*(1), p. 5.

A Comparison and Review of Suicide Prediction Scales

Joseph M. Rothberg, Ph.D.
*Walter Reed Army Institute of Research, and
Uniformed Services University of the Health Sciences*
Carol Geer-Williams, Ph.D.
National Rehabilitation Hospital

Suicide prediction scales are explicit psychological test instruments that are designed to standardize information transfer from the potentially suicidal person to the clinician. Because of the low frequency of suicide and the dire consequences of an error in the judgment that a person is not suicidal, the development and evaluation of such scales are not standard psychometric exercises. Indeed, even the possibility of prediction of this form of violent behavior continues to be debated (Monahan, 1984; Balon, 1987). However, Motto's (Motto, Heilbron, & Juster, 1985; see also Chapter 31, this volume) approach of focusing on the prediction of the *risk* of the behavior, rather than prediction of the behavior itself, justifies the continuing interest in this area.

The evaluations[1] of suicide prediction scales have focused on those that serve the clinician's need to make decisions about the probable future actions of the distressed patient. The widespread use of such scales requires that they do not identify too many subjects when administered in a screen-

---

This chapter reports work done while Joseph M. Rothberg was an employee of the U. S. Federal Government. Our views do not purport to reflect the position of the Department of the Army or the Department of Defense.

1. Within the present context, the evaluation of a suicide prediction scale is assumed to proceed according to the following paradigm: The scale is initially administered to a group of individuals (a "test" that can be scored dichotomously as indicating high risk, a "positive screening test result," or low risk, a "negative screening test result"). The suicide status of these individuals is then determined during some subsequent follow-up period. The term "sensitivity" is defined to

ing mode (e.g., MacKinnon & Farberow, 1976). Bassuk's (1982) checklist for assessment, which incorporates suicide prediction scales, is a typical description of the general principles of clinical assessment for the mental health clinician and illustrates the usual role for such scales.

This chapter describes previous reviews of suicide scales, some psychometric concepts important to test evaluation, some of the attributes of documented suicide prediction scales, and the application of the scales to the five clinical cases used as examples throughout this book.

REVIEWS OF SUICIDE PREDICTION SCALES

Reviews of suicide prediction scales are relatively rare. In an early critical review, Lester (1970) intensively investigated the use of psychological tests in identifying and predicting suicidal behavior. He discussed seven psychological assessment scales with some documented success at suicide prediction, and described four scales explicitly designed for suicide prediction. He concluded, "The tests devised to utilize admissions data and data from the personal history of the individual appear to be the most useful [ones] available at the present time" (p. 16.) A few years later, Beck, Resnik, and Lettieri (1974) edited the material presented at a conference on the measurement of suicidal behaviors into a multifaceted discussion of the predictors of suicide. This volume is the source for several frequently cited scales.

Farberow (1981) reviewed the assessment of suicide in the 1970s. His comprehensive work included an annotated description of 11 clinical and hospital scales, and he provided access to a large amount of assessment literature in his citation of 150 references. Burk, Kurz, and Moller (1985) reviewed 15 rating scales for the estimation of suicide risk published between 1966 and 1984, and concluded that the scales are clinically useful, though their statistical accuracy is not satisfactory. Finally, Lewinsohn, Garrison, Langhinrichsen, and Marsteller (1989) reported on a survey of scales that are suitable for epidemiological and clinical research on suicidal behavior in adolescents. They identified 25 assessment instruments for which reliability, validity, and/or normative data are available, and they described an additional dozen instruments. Among the problem areas they noted are that current instruments pay insufficient attention to validity and that the intended purpose of many of the instruments is unclear.

---

mean the fraction of the total who commit suicide (cases) during the follow-up period and whom the scale has correctly scored as being at high risk; the term "specificity" refers to the fraction of those who do not commit suicide and whom the scale has correctly scored as being at low risk. This is equivalent to the epidemiological definitions (of "sensitivity" as the fraction of truly diseased individuals who test positive, and "specificity" as the fraction of truly disease-free individuals who test negative), with the time sequence reversed (Last, 1988).

PSYCHOMETRICS

An application of the decision-theoretical aspects of suicide prediction appeared as "An Assessment of the Utility of Suicide Prediction" (MacKinnon & Farberow, 1976). The authors calculated the "usefulness" of a suicide prediction scale, which they defined as the proportion of those who were predicted to kill themselves who actually did so. This definition is the "posterior probability" in decision-theoretical terms and the "positive predictive value" in epidemiological terms.

Suicide prediction scales can be objectively assessed by the same psychometric approaches (Nunnally, 1978) used for measures of other human behaviors or states (Korchin, 1976). Cohen (1986) has described the statistical pitfalls of evaluating scales on the same sample that was used to develop the scales, as well as the problems of statistically distinguishing correlation and causation. Future approaches to the analysis of suicidal risk factors and future scale development will benefit from his thoughtful analysis, particularly his caution on the base rate dependence of the use of the epidemiological constructs.

A scale can be psychometrically evaluated for the extent to which it possesses three qualities: cogency, reliability, and validity. "Cogency," an unquantified construct, is the extent to which the scale is developed from an analysis of the problem (i.e., was the scale developed from a theoretical base, using operational concepts?). A scale may not be cogent for one of several reasons. Spurious items may have been inadvertently correlated in some unique sample, or the scale may be measuring something else and its only failing is that it is not titled properly. The "reliability" of a scale may be defined as the proportion of a measurement's variance that is due to the error component (see Kerlinger, 1973, for the derivation). It can be evaluated by measures of "internal consistency"—that is, the extent to which items or factors that seem to "go together" actually covary when the scale is administered to multiple individuals. Cronbach's alpha and the Kuder–Richardson formulae are internal-consistency measures of reliability. Reliability can also be measured as "test–retest reliability," or the extent to which an individual's scores at two different times are similar.

"Validity" is the third dimension on which a scale can be evaluated, and this term is commonly used in three ways. "Concurrent validity," an indirect measure, refers to the agreement of the scale with some other instrument (administered to the same individual at the same time). "Predictive validity," a direct measure, refers to the scale's current ability to include all of the subjects' future behaviors of interest (and sometimes makes the implicit assumption that false positives are of no consequence). "Discriminant validity" refers to the scale's ability to exclude the subjects' behaviors that are not of interest. In some usage, "predictive validity" is used with a continuous scale and/or outcome, while "discriminant validity" is used for discrete predictions and/or outcomes.

ATTRIBUTES OF PUBLISHED SUICIDE PREDICTION SCALES

Our criterion for inclusion of a suicide prediction scale in the present review was that the scale itself or an assessment of the scale had been published in the professional literature. Several scales that measure only the presence and extent of suicidal ideation have been omitted (e.g., Beck, Kovacs, & Weissman, 1979; Reynolds, 1987), although we recognize that they may be particularly useful in some situations. We have used the authors' categories and spelling in briefly describing the research. The reader is encouraged to refer to the original sources, since the brevity of this review has required us to omit a large amount of useful information about the scales.

We have imposed a functional division, based on our judgment of how information is obtained: Those for which the subject must be the informant are contrasted with those for which another person (a "second party") can be the informant. The first type of scale gathers information directly from the potentially suicidal person. It may be either a self-administered questionnaire completed by the subject or a structured interview completed by the interviewer. The second type of suicide scale gathers information indirectly, such as by chart review.

We report all the information that we have located on each scale in the following order: format, development, usage, reliability, and validity.

Scales Relying on Subject as Informant

Hopelessness Scale

The Hopelessness Scale (Beck, Weissman, Lester, & Trexler, 1974) consists of 20 true–false self-report statements, which were developed from statements by psychiatric patients regarding the past and future. The scale was found to differentiate among threateners, attempters, and controls. The authors report that the scale has three factors and an internal consistency of .93 (Kuder–Richardson). The scale results have been found to be related to social desirability responses (Mendonca, Holden, Mazmanian, & Dolan, 1983; Holden & Mendonca, 1984). A 10-year follow-up for eventual suicide showed 91% sensitivity for inpatients (Beck, Steer, Kovacs, & Garrison, 1985), and a 3½-year follow-up showed 94% sensitivity for outpatients (Beck, Brown, Berchick, Stewart, & Steer, 1990). Kazdin, French, Unis, Esveldt-Dawson, and Sherick (1983) have developed a children's version. For this version, Spirito, Williams, Stark and Hart (1988) reported a Spearman-

Brown split-half reliability of .75 on 834 high school students and .91 on 89 adolescent suicide attempters. A mean item–total correlation of .43 was recorded for the students and .53 for the attempters. A 10-week test–retest reliability of .49 was observed on a subsample of high school students.

Index of Potential Suicide

The Index of Potential Suicide (Zung, 1974) consists of 19 social and 50 clinical items scored on a 0–4 Likert scale, with three versions for clinician report, significant other report, and self-report, which were developed by experts from other scales. The scale is intended for adults with suicidal ideation and was found to differentiate between attempters and nonattempters. The correlations between versions were reported by the authors to be .82 for self–clinician, .33 for clinician–other, and .34 for self–other. The scale was reported to differentiate normal controls from an inpatient suicidal psychiatric population (Zung & Moore, 1976). Petrie and Chamberlain (1985) reported a Cronbach's alpha of .84 in a 6-month follow-up study, but the scale showed very poor predictive power and was unrelated to future suicide attempts or ideation in their 46 patients.

Reasons for Living Inventory

The Reasons for Living Inventory (Linehan, Goodstein, Nielsen, & Chiles, 1983) consists of 48 true–false statements developed from a survey of college students, workers, and senior citizens who were asked about their reasons for living. The self-report scale is intended for adults and was found to differentiate among nonsuicidal individuals, suicide ideators, and parasuicides. The authors report a factor analysis of six factors and an internal consistency of .72–.89 for the subscales. Cole (1989) has reported two validation studies for adolescents.

Rorschach Suicide Constellation

The Rorschach Suicide Constellation (Exner & Wylie, 1977) consists of 12 ratios summarized from the complete Rorschach protocol and was developed from psychiatric patients who committed suicide within 60 days of testing. The test is intended for adults and adolescents aged 12 and above, and was found to differentiate among suicidal patients, depressed patients, and nonpatients. It is based on professionally administered and scored patient responses. The authors report the classification accuracy (predictive validity) as 75%, with 20% misclassification for depressives, 12% for schizophrenics, and 0% for nonpatients. (For a fuller discussion of the use of the Rorschach in suicide prediction, see Eyman & Eyman, Chapter 9, this volume.)

Suicide Probability Scale

The Suicide Probability Scale (Cull & Gill, 1982) consists of 36 items scored on a 1–4 Likert scale; items were retained on the basis of their ability to differentiate adult attempters from nonattempters. The scale was developed to be self-administered by adults on a proprietary, easy-to-score form, and was found to differentiate normals, psychiatric patients, and attempters. The authors report an internal consistency of .93, a test–retest reliability of .92, a split-half reliability of .93, and four factors. Eisenberg, Hubbard, and Epstein (1989) reported 100% sensitivity and 50% specificity in 1,397 Veterans Administration patients. These same authors (Eisenberg, Hubbard, & Epstein, 1990) reported the inability of the scale to determine the lethality of intent.

Suicide Risk Measure

The Suicide Risk Measure (Plutchik, van Praag, Conte, & Picard, 1989) consists of 14 yes–no items, derived from 219 psychiatric patients and 83 college student controls. The scale has been found to discriminate suicide attempters from controls. The internal reliability was .84 as measured by the split-half correlation coefficient. The sensitivity and specificity were 60% each for patient versus controls, and 68% each for normal college students versus attempters.

Scales Relying on Second Party as Informant

Clinical Instrument to Estimate Suicide Risk

The Clinical Instrument to Estimate Suicide Risk (CIESR; Motto et al., 1985) is a 15-item checklist of demographic variables and clinical symptoms. The checklist is intended for adults aged 18–70 who have been hospitalized for depression or suicidal states; its aim is to differentiate high-risk from low-risk individuals during the 2 years following hospitalization. It was derived from an initial 101-variable assessment of 2,753 subjects and is based on the subjective judgment of the interviewer. The authors' scaling of the transformed scores gives 10 deciles of risk from "very low" through "very high." The approximate expectation of suicide ranges from less than 1% for the lowest decile to over 10% for the highest decile. The authors report the predictive validity from a 2-year follow-up by risk group. Clark, Young, Scheftner, Fawcett, and Fogg (1987) were unable to replicate Motto et al.'s finding, though they did not definitively invalidate it.

Instrument for the Evaluation of Suicide Potential

The Instrument for the Evaluation of Suicide Potential (IESP; Cohen, Motto, & Seiden, 1966) consists of 14 yes–no items, derived from a 5- to

8-year follow-up of 193 subjects who were given a 22-item instrument to predict subsequent suicides among hospitalized attempters. The authors' categories are "low-risk" (0–3), "moderate-risk" (4–6), and "suicide-prone" (7+). The presence of one or more items gave a sensitivity of 68% and specificity of 96.5% when evaluated on the subjects used to develop the criteria.

Intent Scale

The Intent Scale (Pierce, 1977) consists of 12 circumstantial and clinical items scored on a 0–2 Likert scale; the items were developed from responses of deliberate self-injury patients on a psychiatric ward. The scale is intended as a measure of suicidal intent for adults and is scored from combined self-report, situational, and medical data. The author reports an interrater reliability of .97, internal consistency ranging from .64 to .77 for subscale and total scale scores, and a correlation with the Suicide Intent Scale (see below) of .93. Good predictive validity was reported for a 5-year follow-up (Pierce, 1981).

Los Angeles Suicide Prevention Center Scale

The Los Angeles Suicide Prevention Center (LASPC) Scale (Beck, Resnik, & Lettieri, 1974) consists of 65 items in 10 categories; each item is scored 0–9 for severity. The average score across categories is rated as indicating "low risk" (0–3), "medium risk" (4–6), or "high risk" (7–9). The scale was developed for use at the LASPC Hotline with data scored by counselors from telephone conversation. It is widely used by many phone centers and served as the source for the Suicidal Death Prediction Scale (see below).

Neuropsychiatric Hospital Suicide Prediction Schedule

The Neuropsychiatric Hospital Suicide Prediction Schedule (Farberow & MacKinnon, 1974a, 1974b) consists of 11 items weighted for severity; it was developed from items of other scales that differentiated hospitalized suicide attempters who later committed suicide from those who did not. The scale is intended for adults who are currently hospitalized for a suicide attempt. It was designed to predict future suicidal behavior of those patients and is scored from staff ratings of patient behavior and emotional status. The authors report interrater reliability ranging from .81 to .99 and the establishment of cutoff points. The authors also found that the scale correctly identified 79% of the attempters who later committed suicide and misidentified 25%. A replication study (Farberow & MacKinnon, 1975) found predictive validity of 95% for a high-risk group and 80% for nonsuicidal controls.

Scale for Assessing Suicide Risk

The Scale for Assessing Suicide Risk (Tuckman & Youngman, 1968) is a 14-item checklist of demographic variables derived from police reports of attempters who eventually committed suicide. It was developed for adult attempters and found to differentiate between low-risk and high-risk groups, based on the subjective judgment of the initial interviewer. The authors tabulate the risk-related items that comprise the high-risk category. Resnick and Kendra (1973) added three more demographic variables and reported a nine-item subscale that differentiated completers from attempters.

Suicidal Death Prediction Scale, Long and Short Forms

The Suicidal Death Prediction Scale (Lettieri, 1974) has a long form (SDPS-L) and a short form (SDPS-S, which uses a subset of the SDPS-L items). Items are scored 0–2 for severity, based on data gathered during a telephone conversation. There are versions for each of four major demographic categories: over 40/male, under 40/male, over 40/female, and under 40/female. The numbers of items in the long and short forms are 13 and 7, 9 and 5, 10 and 4, and 8 and 3 for these categories, respectively. The forms use demographic variables derived from the hospital records of suicidal patients who later completed suicide. Each of the four versions of the long and short forms uses a different weighting of the response categories, but the resulting scores are all scaled to deciles of risk. The deciles of risk are then grouped into "low risk" (1–3), "moderate risk" (4–6), or "high risk" (7–9), with "high risk" suggesting that the person will commit suicide within the next few years. These scales were developed to be used by suicide hotlines and were found to differentiate suicides from attempters.

Short Risk Scale

The Short Risk Scale (SRS; Pallis, Barraclough, Levey, Jenkins, & Sainsbury, 1982) consists of six items developed from work with 151 attempters (Pallis & Sainsbury, 1976) to discriminate future suicide from future suicide attempts. It was validated on 1,187 subjects using discriminant analysis. After weighting by the appropriate value, scores exceeding 0.25 predicted suicide, while lower values predicted suicide attempts. A sensitivity of 83% and a specificity of 74% were reported for a 1-year follow-up; a replication found sensitivity and specificity to be 83% and 67%, respectively (Pallis, Gibbons, & Pierce, 1984).

Suicide Intent Scale

The Suicide Intent Scale (Beck, Schuyler, & Herman, 1974) consists of 20 items scored 0–2 for severity; the items were derived from clinical experience and expert judgment. The scale is intended to be used with adults following a suicide attempt. It was found to differentiate suicide completers from attempters, based on interviews and data about the circumstances of the attempt. The authors report an internal consistency of .82 and an interrater reliability of .95. Four factors have been reported by Wetzel (1977) and by Beck, Weissman, Lester, and Trexler (1976). Predictive validity has been demonstrated in a 1-year follow-up (R. W. Beck, Morris, & Beck, 1974) and by higher scores just before suicide completion (Lester, Beck, & Narrett, 1978).

SAD PERSONS

SAD PERSONS (SP; Patterson, Dohn, Bird, & Patterson, 1983) is a 10-item checklist of demographic variables found in the literature. The scale is meant for adult psychiatric patients and is based on the subjective judgment of the evaluator. It is reported to be useful in helping medical students to differentiate between high-risk and low-risk patients (as compared to un-aided clinical judgment). The authors' guidelines for proposed clinical actions based on the scores are as follows: "send home with follow-up" (0–2); "close follow-up: consider hospitalization" (3–4); "strongly consider hospitalization, depending on confidence in follow-up arrangement" (5–6); and "hospitalize or commit" (7–10). A modified version of the scale had a sensitivity of 94% and a specificity of 74% in identifying the need for hospi-talization (Hockberger & Rothstein, 1988).

Suicide Potential Scale

The Suicide Potential Scale (SPS; Dean, Miskimins, DeCook, Wilson, & Maley, 1967) is a 26-item checklist of demographic variables drawn from hospital records that were found to differentiate suicides from nonsuicidal patients. It was developed for adults in hospitals, crisis centers, or suicide prevention centers, and is based on the subjective judgment of the inter-viewer. The authors have tabulated the probability of suicide, based on the weighted scores, as "low" (0–24), "moderate" (25–32), or "high" (33–60). A predictive validity of 58% was reported for an 8-year follow-up subsequent to psychiatric hospitalization (Braught & Wilson, 1970). A revised version of 16 items was developed by Miskimins and Wilson (1969).

Scale for Predicting Subsequent Suicidal Behavior

The Scale for Predicting Subsequent Suicidal Behavior (SPSSB; Buglas & Horton, 1974) uses six present–absent items, developed from work with patients admitted to a regional poisoning treatment center. The presence of one or more items was found to predict suicide repetition with 88% sensitivity and 44% specificity. A 1-year follow-up of 147 first-time attempters reported a sensitivity of 61% and a specificity of 43% (Siani, Garzotto, Zimmerman-Tarsella, & Tarsella, 1979). Wilmotte, Charles, and Depauw (1983) surveyed several replications and reported a sensitivity range of 63–73% and a specificity range of 63–78%.

GENERAL COMMENTS ON THE SCALES

The publications dealing with the 19 suicide prediction scales discussed above are variable in their coverage of the scales' psychometric properties. We have not been able to locate comparable reports for every study. Many of the publications did not report any data on internal consistency, test–retest reliability, prediction, or concurrent validity. The clinical community would certainly benefit if full sets of psychometric descriptions were available for these and other contemporary suicide scales. Another area of interest for future description is the utility of the scales—that is, their ease of use, the amount of information gained from them, and the confidence that can be placed in the results. A scale that may be acceptable as an emergency room screening instrument may not be appropriate for inpatient treatment planning.

Among the publications that we have located, there are some conflicting results. Both the incomplete information and the contradictory information suggest that further work in the area of suicide prediction is indicated. There is a large body of day-to-day clinical experience with suicide prediction scales that could be assembled and published. Such an evaluation would constitute a useful scientific contribution, and we encourage our colleagues to share their experience with suicide scales.

APPLICATION OF SOME SECOND-PARTY INFORMANT SCALES TO THE FIVE CLINICAL CASES

We have reviewed the five case summaries presented in Chapter 12 of this book and have applied nine of the second-party-informant scales to the cases without benefit of ancillary information. This mimics the role of a consultant applying the scales to another clinician's case reports. Additional information might have been gathered from one or more of the six subject-informant scales had those scales been administered to the subjects in the vignettes. Four second-party scales have not been included here because they require information about a current hospitalization or a current self-injury event that is not available from the vignettes.

The scores and the associated suicide risk estimates appear in Table 10.1 and are described below.

TABLE 10.1. Second-Party Suicide Prediction Scale Scores and Risk
Categories for the Five Clinical Cases

Scale	Heather B	Ralph F	John Z	Faye C	José G
CIESR	219	490	697	644	349
	Low	Hi	VHi	VHi	Mod
IESP	2	5	3	4	6
	Low	Mod	Low	Mod	Mod
LASPC Scale	32	56	64	45	48
	Low	Mod	Mod	Mod	Mod
SDPS-L	21.5	44.7	42.8	59.5	94.9
	Low	Mod	Mod	Hi	Mod
SDPS-S	1.1	22.0	22.0	10.0	31.7
	Low	Hi	Hi	Hi	Hi
SRS	−0.72	0.19	0.95	1.75	0.21
	Low[a]	Low[a]	Hi[a]	Hi[a]	Low[a]
SP	2	8	6	6	5
	Low	Hi	Mod	Mod	Mod
SPS	16	34	38	29	23
	Low	Hi	Hi	Mod	Low
SPSSB	0	1	1	3	1
	Low	Some	Some	Some	Some

Note. Low, low risk; Some, some risk; Mod, moderate risk; Hi, high risk; VHi, very high risk.
[a]Risk of suicide relative to risk of suicide attempt.

1. *Heather B.* None of the scales places Heather above the lowest
category for immediate suicide risk.

2. *Ralph F.* The scales place Ralph in the medium long-term risk and
high short-term risk categories. The SP score is in the "hospitalize or
commit" range. The CIESR suggests that the risk of death by suicide within
the next 2 years is as high as 5–10%. The SDPS-S score is in the high range,
with death as the predicted outcome; the SDPS-L score is slightly lower,
predicting moderate risk with survival expected. The SPS score of 34 is in
the high-risk category. The SRS indicates suicide as less likely than a suicide
attempt.

3. *John Z.* The scales place John in the medium short-term risk and
high long-term risk categories. The SP score of 6 is in the "strongly consider
hospitalization" range. The CIESR of 697 places him in the very high long-
term risk category (a risk greater than 10% of death by suicide in the next
2 years). The SDPS-S score is in the high range, with an expectation of a
fatal outcome; the SDPS-L score is in the moderate range, with the expectation of survival. The SPS score of 38 places him in the high-risk category.

4. *Faye C.* The CIESR score of 644 is in the very high-risk category,
with greater than a 10% expectation of death within 2 years. The SP score is

in the "strongly consider hospitalization" range. Both the SDPS-L and SDPS-S scores indicate high risk, with an expected fatal outcome. The SPS score suggests a moderate risk of suicide.

5. *José G.* The LASPC scale score indicates moderate risk. The CIESR rating suggests moderate to low risk, with a 2.5–5% chance of mortality within 2 years. The SP score is in the "strongly consider hospitalization" range. The SDPS-L score indicates moderate risk without a fatal outcome, but the SDPS-S score suggests high risk and failure to survive. The SPS score of 23, however, is in the low-risk range.

We have applied the scales to these five cases, despite the differences between the cases and the populations on which the scales were developed (inpatients, hotline callers, or self-poisoners). The result has been a wide range of estimates for each case (except for the uniformly low estimates of suicide risk for Heather, the 13-year-old white female). Some of the variability may come from the limited information in the brief case summaries, although we feel that the major limitation lies in the scales themselves and the lack of operational definitions for many of the items. An additional reason for caution is found in the recent work of Stelmachers and Sherman (1990), who demonstrated considerable variability among experienced crisis workers in assigning a simple 7-point rating of short- and long-term suicide risk to sample case vignettes.

CONCLUSION

In summary, we have discussed some issues related to suicide risk prediction scales, with emphasis on the need to consider the psychometric properties of cogency, reliability, and validity. After surveying previous reviews, we have presented the details of 19 scales, divided into 6 subject-informant and 13 second-party-informant instruments. We have then applied the 9 relevant second-party scales to the five clinical cases discussed throughout this book, and found considerable variation in the risk estimates for the subjects.

One of the major findings of this review is the relative absence of information on the psychometric properties of the suicide prediction scales. Without such documentation, the proper application of the scales is limited. Further work characterizing suicide risk assessment instruments seems to be indicated.

REFERENCES

Balon, R. (1987). Suicide: Can we predict it? *Comprehensive Psychiatry, 28,* 236–241.
Bassuk, E. L. (1982). General principles of assessment. In E. L. Bassuk, S. C.

Schoonover, & A. D. Gill (Eds.), *Lifelines: Clinical perspectives on suicide* (pp. 17–46). New York: Plenum Press.

Beck, A. T., Brown, G., Berchick, R. J., Stewart, B. L., & Steer, R. A. (1990). Relationship between hopelessness and ultimate suicide: A replication with psychiatric outpatients. *American Journal of Psychiatry, 147,* 190–195.

Beck, A. T., Kovacs, M., & Weissman, A. (1979). Assessment of suicidal intent: The Scale for Suicide Ideation. *Journal of Consulting and Clinical Psychology, 47,* 343–352.

Beck, A. T., Resnik, H. L. P., & Lettieri, D. J. (Eds.) (1974). *The prediction of suicide.* Bowie, MD: Charles Press.

Beck, A. T., Schuyler, D., & Herman, I. (1974) Development of suicidal intent scales. In A. T. Beck, H. L. P. Resnik, & D. J. Lettieri (Eds.), *The prediction of suicide* (pp. 45–56) Bowie, MD: Charles Press.

Beck, A. T., Steer, R. A., Kovacs, M., & Garrison, B. (1985). Hopelessness and eventual suicide: A ten year prospective study of patients hospitalized with suicide ideation. *American Journal of Psychiatry, 142,* 559–563.

Beck, A. T., Weissman, A., Lester, D., & Trexler, L. (1974). The measurement of pessimism: The Hopelessness Scale. *Journal of Consulting and Clinical Psychology, 42,* 861–865.

Beck, A. T., Weissman, A., Lester, D., & Trexler, L. (1976).Classification of suicidal behaviors: II. Dimensions of suicidal intent. *Archives of General Psychiatry, 33,* 835–837.

Beck, R. W., Morris, J. B., & Beck, A. T. (1974). Cross-validation of the Suicide Intent Scale. *Psychological Reports, 34,* 445–446.

Braught, G. N., & Wilson, W. S. (1970). Predictive utility of the revised Suicide Potential Scale. *Journal of Consulting and Clinical Psychology, 35,* 426.

Buglas, D., & Horton, J. (1974). A scale for predicting subsequent suicidal behavior. *British Journal of Psychiatry, 124,* 573–578.

Burk, F., Kurz, A., & Moller, H.-J. (1985). Suicide risk scales: Do they help to predict suicidal behavior? *European Archives of Psychiatry and Neurological Science, 235,* 153–157.

Clark, D. C., Young, M. A., Scheftner, W. A., Fawcett, J., & Fogg, L. (1987). A field test of Motto's risk estimator for suicide. *American Journal of Psychiatry, 144,* 923–926.

Cohen, E., Motto, J. A., & Seiden, R. H. (1966). An instrument for evaluating suicide potential: A preliminary study. *American Journal of Psychiatry, 122,* 886–891.

Cohen, J. (1986). Statistical approaches to suicide risk factor analysis. *Annals of the New York Academy of Sciences, 487,* 34–41.

Cole, D. A. (1989). Validation of the Reasons for Living Inventory in general and delinquent adolescent samples. *Journal of Abnormal Child Psychology, 17,* 13–27.

Cull, J. G., & Gill, W. S. (1982). *Suicide Probability Scale manual.* Los Angeles: Western Psychological Services.

Dean, R. A., Miskimins, W., DeCook, R., Wilson, L. T., & Maley, R. F. (1967). Prediction of suicide in a psychiatric hospital. *Journal of Clinical Psychology, 23,* 296–301.

Eisenberg, M. G., Hubbard, K. M., & Epstein, D. (1989). Efficacy of a suicide detection scale in determining lethality of ideation among hospitalized veterans: A case study. *Military Medicine, 154*, 246-249.

Eisenberg, M. G., Hubbard, K. M., & Epstein, D. (1990). Detection of suicidal risk among hospitalized veterans: Preliminary experiences with a suicide prediction scale. *Journal of Rehabilitation, 56*, 63-68.

Exner, J. E., & Wylie, J. (1977). Some Rorschach data concerning suicide. *Journal of Personality Assessment, 41*, 339-348.

Farberow, N. L. (1981). Assessment of suicide. In P. McReynolds (Ed.), *Advances in psychological assessment* (Vol. 5, pp. 124-190). San Francisco: Jossey-Bass.

Farberow, N. L., & MacKinnon, D. R. (1974a). A suicide prediction schedule for neuropsychiatric hospital patients. *Journal of Nervous and Mental Disease, 158*, 408-419.

Farberow, N. L., & MacKinnon, D. R. (1974b). Prediction of suicide in neuropsychiatric hospital patients. In C. Neuringer (Ed.), *Psychological assessment of suicidal risk.* (pp. 186-224). Springfield, IL: Charles C. Thomas.

Farberow, N. L., & MacKinnon, D. R. (1975). Prediction of suicide: A replication study. *Journal of Personality Assessment, 39*, 497-501.

Hockberger, R. S., & Rothstein, R. J. (1988). Assessment of suicide potential by nonpsychiatrists using the SAD PERSONS score. *Journal of Emergency Medicine, 6*, 99-107.

Holden, R. R., & Mendonca, J. D. (1984). Hopelessness, social desirability, and suicidal behavior: A need for conceptual and empirical disentanglement. *Journal of Clinical Psychology, 40*, 1342-1345.

Kazdin, A. E., French, N. H., Unis, A. S., Esveldt-Dawson, K., & Sherick, R. B. (1983). Hopelessness, depression, and suicidal intent among psychiatrically disturbed inpatient children. *Journal of Consulting and Clinical Psychology, 51*, 504-510.

Kerlinger, F. S. (1973). *Foundations of behavioral research.* New York: Holt, Rinehart & Winston.

Korchin, S. J.(1976). *Modern clinical psychology.* New York: Basic Books.

Last, J. M. (1988). *A dictionary of epidemiology.* New York: Oxford University Press.

Lester, D. (1970). Attempts to predict suicidal risk using psychological tests. *Psychological Bulletin, 74*, 1-17.

Lester, D., Beck, A. T., & Narrett, S. (1978). Suicidal intent in successive suicidal actions. *Psychological Reports, 43*, 110.

Lettieri, D. J. (1974). Research issues in developing prediction scales. In C. Neuringer (Ed.), *Psychological assessment of suicidal risk.* (pp. 43-73). Springfield, IL: Charles C. Thomas.

Lewinsohn, P.M., Garrison, C. Z., Langhinrichsen, J., & Marsteller, F. (1989). *The assessment of suicidal behavior in adolescents: A review of scales suitable for epidemiological and clinical research.* (Contract Report No. 316774-76, Child and Adolescent Disorders Research Branch), Rockville, MD: National Institute of Mental Health.

Linehan, M. M., Goodstein, J. L., Nielsen, S. L., & Chiles, J. K. (1983). Reasons for staying alive when you are thinking of killing yourself: The Reasons for Living Inventory. *Journal of Consulting and Clinical Psychology, 51*, 276-286.

MacKinnon, D. R., & Farberow, N. L. (1976). An assessment of the utility of suicide prediction. *Suicide and Life-Threatening Behavior, 6,* 86–91.

Mendonca, J. D., Holden, R. R., Mazmanian, D., & Dolan, J. (1983). The influence of response style on the Beck Hopelessness Scale. *Canadian Journal of Behavioral Science, 15,* 237–247.

Miskimins, R. W., & Wilson, L. T. (1969). Revised Suicide Potential Scale. *Journal of Consulting and Clinical Psychology, 33,* 258.

Monahan, J. (1984). The prediction of violent behavior: Toward a second generation of theory and policy. *American Journal of Psychiatry, 141,* 10–15.

Motto, J. A., Heilbron, D. C., & Juster, R. P. (1985). Development of a clinical instrument to estimate suicide risk. *American Journal of Psychiatry, 142,* 680–686.

Nunnally, J. C. (1978). *Psychometric theory.* New York: McGraw-Hill.

Pallis, D. J., Barraclough, B. M., Levey, A.B., Jenkins, J. S., & Sainsbury, P. (1982). Estimating suicide risk among attempted suicides: I. The development of new clinical scales. *British Journal of Psychiatry, 141,* 37–44.

Pallis, D. J., Gibbons, J. S., & Pierce, D. W. (1984). Estimating suicide risk among attempted suicides: II. Efficiency of predictive scales after the attempt. *British Journal of Psychiatry, 144,* 139–148.

Pallis, D. J., & Sainsbury, P. (1976). The value of assessing intent in attempted suicide. *Psychological Medicine, 6,* 487–492.

Patterson, W. M., Dohn, H. H., Bird, J., & Patterson, G. A. (1983). Evaluation of suicide patients: The SAD PERSONS scale. *Psychosomatics, 24,* 343–352.

Petrie, K., & Chamberlain, K. (1985). The predictive validity of the Zung Index of Potential Suicide. *Journal of Personality Assessment, 49,* 100–102.

Pierce, D. W. (1977). Suicidal intent in self-injury. *British Journal of Psychiatry, 130,* 377–385.

Pierce, D. W. (1981). The predictive validity of a suicide intent scale: A five year follow-up. *British Journal of Psychiatry, 139,* 391–396.

Plutchik, R., van Praag, H. M., Conte, H. R. & Picard, S. (1989). Correlates of suicide and violence risk: 1. The Suicide Risk Measure. *Comprehensive Psychiatry, 30,* 296–302.

Resnick, J. H., & Kendra, J. M. (1973). Predictive value of the "Scale for Assessing Suicide Risk" (SASR) with hospitalized psychiatric patients. *Journal of Clinical Psychology, 29,* 187–190.

Reynolds, W. M. (1987). *The Suicidal Ideation Questionnaire.* Odessa, FL: Psychological Assessment Resources.

Siani, R., Garzotto, N., Zimmerman-Tarsella, C., & Tarsella, M. (1979). Predictive scales for parasuicide repetition: Further results. *Acta Psychiatrica Scandanavica, 59,* 17–23.

Spirito, A., Williams, C. A., Stark, L. J., & Hart, K. J. (1988). The Hopelessness Scale for Children: Psychometric properties with normal and emotionally disturbed adolescents. *Journal of Abnormal Child Psychology, 16,* 445–458.

Stelmachers, Z. T. & Sherman, R. E. (1990). Use of case vignettes in suicide risk assessment. *Suicide and Life-Threatening Behavior, 20,* 65–84.

Tuckman, J., & Youngman, W. F. (1968). Assessment of suicide risk in attempted suicides. In H. L. P. Resnik (Ed.), *Suicidal behaviors: Diagnosis and management* (pp. 190–197). Boston: Little, Brown.

Wetzel, R. D. (1977). Factor structures of Beck's suicide intent scales. *Psychological Reports, 40,* 295-302.

Wilmotte, J., Charles, G., & Depauw, Y. (1983). [Detection of new suicide attempters within a year]. *Acta Psychiatrica Belgica, 83,* 558-568. (In French).

Zung, W. W. K. (1974). Index of Potential Suicide (IPS): A rating scale for suicide prevention. In A. T. Beck, H. L. P. Resnik, & D. J. Lettieri (Eds.), *The Prediction of Suicide.* Bowie, MD: Charles Press. (pp. 221-249).

Zung, W. W. K., & Moore, J. (1976). Suicide potential in a normal adult population. *Psychosomatics, 17*(1), 37-41.

CHAPTER 11

Statistical Concepts of Prediction

Cheryl L. Addy, Ph.D.
University of South Carolina

Probabilistic prediction of any rare event is a difficult task. The prediction of many such events, including suicidal behaviors and suicidal ideation, is complicated by the existence of many different etiological or influential factors and by a lack of complete knowledge and understanding of these factors. Various potential predictors of suicide—and their appropriateness and validity—are discussed in other chapters. This chapter focuses on the statistical methodology of using these variables to predict an outcome (such as suicide attempt or completion) and to predict a continuous response (such as some degree of suicidal tendency).

The difficulty of accurately predicting suicide or any rare event is summarized by Maltsberger (1986):

> Predicting suicide at present is an insuperable task. We cannot do it. The challenge to identify those who at some time in the future will commit suicide is essentially a statistical one—the difficulties are immense. Suicide remains a comparatively rare event; as case frequency diminishes, prediction becomes more uncertain because of the decreasing probability that any given case will be positive (Murphy, 1985). Statistical methods will identify high risk groups readily enough, and that is a valuable aid. But they cannot do more; selecting the particular patient in the high risk group who is sure to commit suicide is beyond this approach. Absolute prediction is impossible by any method. Alerted by known probabilities, however, the clinician may make informed judgments about individual patients in the high risk group with the help of psychodynamic formulation. (p. 50)

Thus, although this chapter discusses some methodology to predict the probability that a person with a given set of risk factors will commit suicide, much of the discussion evolves around predicting suicide ideation or high-risk groups.

Collection of data is an important issue in the construction of a predictive model. To be useful, such statistical models must be based on reasonably large samples, rather than on smaller selective samples or case studies. Because of the difficulty of following a large enough population-based sample to observe a substantial number of any rare event, data are often collected in such a manner that an absolute probability of the event is not estimable; instead, a relative probability or risk is calculated. Appropriate application and interpretation of models incorporating this type of data, typically arising from case–control studies, are discussed.

GENERAL LINEAR MODEL
Description

A common statistical model seen with a wide variety of applications is the general linear model. This model, along with its many variations, is discussed in most basic statistical methodology textbooks (e.g., Neter, Wasserman, & Kutner, 1985; Zar, 1984). This model assumes that the dependent variable is continuous and follows a normal or Gaussian distribution. It also assumes that there is a linear relationship between a dependent variable Y and a set of independent or predictor variables $X_1, \ldots, X_p$. For the ith observation, the model can thus be written as follows:

$$Y_i = \beta_0 + \beta_1 X_{1i} + \ldots + \beta_p X_{pi} + \epsilon_i \tag{1}$$

where $\beta_0, \ldots, \beta_p$ are regression coefficients and ϵ_i is an unknown error term.

Estimation of the regression coefficients and any statistical inference related to the model depend on several assumptions: that the linear structure of model is appropriate; that the observations on which estimation and inference are based are independent; and that the dependent variable follows a normal distribution with constant variance for any combination of levels of the predictor variables. The predictor variables are typically assumed to be known constants, to avoid introducing additional distributional assumptions and sources of variability. These variables can be continuous or discrete variables; the latter are represented by indicator variables, and either can be transformations or combinations of directly measured variables.

The regression coefficients in equation 1 are estimated using the method of least-squares estimation, widely available in computer software packages for statistical analysis. Statistical inference is primarily based on analysis of the various sources of variability in the response variable: each of the predictor variables and the random error term. The statistical importance of each of the predictor variables, and the overall significance of the model, are measured by F statistics. Each F statistic is the ratio of two mean-square error terms, each of which is an adjusted average of the squared deviations of the observed values of the dependent variable about an appropriate mean value of that variable.

Two other uses of the linear model are estimating the value of the dependent variable for an observation in the data set used to estimate model parameters, and predicting the value for some observation not in the data set. For either of these purposes, the point estimate of the dependent variable is the same:

$$\hat{Y} = \hat{\beta}_0 + \hat{\beta}_1 X_1 + \ldots + \hat{\beta}_p X_p \tag{2}$$

where $\hat{\beta}_0, \hat{\beta}_1, \ldots, \hat{\beta}_p$ are the least-squares estimates of the regression coefficients and $X_1, \ldots, X_p$ are the values of the independent variables for the observation for which the dependent variable is being estimated or predicted. The difference in estimation and prediction is the variance of the point estimator. The variance of an estimated value for an observation already in the data set is simply the variance of the linear combination given in equation 2, where the regression coefficients have variances and covariances calculated as part of the estimation procedure and the independent variables are regarded as constants. The variance of a predicted value for an unobserved individual, however, includes this term plus the estimated variance of the random error term.

Example 1

To illustrate a linear regression model and prediction of the dependent variable for a new observation, let us consider a set of school screening data described elsewhere (Garrison, Jackson, Addy, McKeown, & Waller, 1991). These data were collected from seventh- and eighth-graders in a Southeastern school district as the first stage of a longitudinal study of adolescent depression. A minimum score of 0 on the suicide scale used in this study indicates rare or no thoughts of self-injury, thoughts of suicide, or feelings that life is not worth living; a maximum score of 9 indicates that a student has such thoughts or feelings most or all of the time. Of the 1,525 students with valid data, 4.6% scored 6 or above on the suicide scale; the mean score was 0.94. Ages ranged from 11 to 16 years, with a large majority of the subjects (96%) being 12 to 14 years old. Approximately half the students were male, and 53% of the students lived with both natural parents. Another scale included in the screening protocol was the Center for Epidemiologic Studies Depression Scale (CES-D), a 20-item self-report instrument for measuring depressive symptomatology during the previous week (Radloff, 1977). Possible scores range from 0 to 60, with a higher score indicating more depressive symptomatology; in this screening sample, scores ranged from 0 to 54, with a mean of 15.10.

When only the demographic variables were used, the least-squares estimates of the regression coefficients were $\hat{\beta}_0 = -2.2221$, $\hat{\beta}_{age} = 0.2123$, $\hat{\beta}_{gender} = 0.5555$, and $\hat{\beta}_{guardian} = 0.3286$. Thus older students, females, and those who did not live with both natural parents tended to have higher suicide scores. The estimated variance of the random error terms, the mean-square error of the model, was 3.37955. The complete analysis-of-variance table is shown in Table 11.1.

The estimated response for a 16-year-old male living with both parents would be $-2.2221 + 16 \cdot 0.2123 = 1.175$. The variance for an estimated value, calculated with the variance–covariance matrix of the regression coefficients, would be 0.04332; or, equivalently, the estimated value above would have a standard error of 0.20814. These demographic variables describe the case of Ralph F (see Chapter 12 for full details). If one were predicting a suicide score for Ralph, the variance of this estimate would be $3.37955 + 0.04332 = 3.42287$. Similarly, the estimated suicide score for a 13-year-old female not living with both parents would be $-2.2221 + 13 \cdot 0.2123 + 0.5555 + 0.3286 = 1.4220$. These variables describe the case of Heather B (see Chapter 12); the predicted value would have a variance of 3.38656.

When the CES-D scale was added to the regression model, the results summarized in Table 11.2 were attained. Clearly, this measure of depressive symptomatology was a strong predictor of the suicide score. Also, the CES-D score was strongly associated with the demographic variables in the smaller model, as evidenced by the changes in magnitude and significance of the other regression coefficients.

A caveat in using a linear regression model for predicting a new value is that one must assume that the new observation is from the same population as the original sample on which the model is based—that is, that the linear model is appropriate for the prediction requested. In the example given

TABLE 11.1. Summary of Analysis of Variance for Linear Regression of Demographic Variables on Suicide Score

Source of variation	SS	df	MS	R^2
Regression	195.037	3	65.012	0.037
Error	5,140.291	1,521	3.380	
Total	5,335.329	1,524		

Parameter	Estimate	Std. error	Probability
Intercept	−2.2221	0.7816	0.0045
Age	0.2123	0.0606	0.0005
Gender	0.5555	0.0947	0.0001
Guardian status	0.3286	0.0950	0.0006

TABLE 11.2. Summary of Analysis of Variance for Linear Regression of Demographic Variables and CES-D Score on Suicide Score

Source of variation	SS	df	MS	R^2
Regression	2,128.693	4	532.173	0.339
Error	3,200.855	1,514	2.114	
Total	5,329.548	1,518		

Parameter	Estimate	Std. error	Probability
Intercept	−2.3437	0.6195	0.0002
Age	0.1067	0.0481	0.0268
Gender	0.0981	0.0766	0.2002
Guardian status	0.0616	0.0758	0.4167
CES-D	0.1215	0.0040	0.0000

here, a suicide score could not be predicted for an adult, since the sample was composed only of adolescents. In fact, the prediction for Ralph might be suspect; although there were two 16-year-olds in the sample, they were in seventh or eighth grade, in contrast with Ralph's being in the 11th grade. Also, one must be confident that the linear model is appropriate for the associations being modeled—that is, that the assumptions of the model are met reasonably well by the data being analyzed. In the present example, the assumption of normality was certainly violated, since almost 70% of the students screened had a suicide score of 0. The large sample size and robustness of multiple linear regression somewhat justified this violation of the assumption, however.

Although the general linear model can stand up to mild violations of the assumptions of normality and homoscedasticity, these assumptions and the linear association forced by the model must be evaluated for appropriateness before the results can be meaningfully interpreted. Transformation of either the independent or the dependent variables is possible to attain a model more closely satisfying the linearity or the normality assumption. Certainly, if a model is not appropriate for the observed data, it cannot yield valid predictions for new observations.

Several methods are available to assess the appropriateness of a linear model. A crude indication of the goodness of a model is the coefficient of multiple determination, R^2, or the ratio of the regression sum of squares to the total sum of squares. In the first model of the present example, $R^2 = 0.0366$, indicating that virtually none of the variability in the suicide score was explained by its linear relationships with the demographic variables in the model. (These predictor variables were selected because they were in the screening data set and were known for the two adolescent case studies, rather than for any expected strong predictive ability; race was found to have no impact on suicide scores in this sample.) However, when the CES-D score was added to the model, 40% of the variability was explained. A better evaluation of the appropriateness of a model might involve a graphical assessment of the estimated error terms for normality and homoscedasticity, in addition to the assumption of linearity.

The general linear model is far more flexible than the present discussion indicates. For the applications presented, there are no restrictions on the distributions of the independent variables. Therefore, these variables can reflect any combination of continuous and categorical variables. The variables can also represent more complex study designs, such as a blocked design or a repeated-measures design. The application of the general linear model to prediction of suicide may not be immediately obvious, since the distribution of a suicide outcome such as completion or attempt clearly does not satisfy the assumption of normality. However, a linear model may be useful in predicting a related continuous variable, such as a score on a scale that measures suicidal ideation and thus is itself a predictor of a suicidal outcome. The linear model also provides a basis for developing other models that are more appropriate for categorical response variables.

LOGISTIC REGRESSION

Description

Logistic regression is a mathematical modeling technique appropriate for a dichotomous outcome such as suicide. The logistic model is discussed in numerous textbooks on epidemiological methods (e.g., Schlesselman, 1982; Kleinbaum, Kupper, & Morgenstern, 1982). A more detailed treatment is provided by Hosmer and Lemeshow (1989). The quantity actually estimated by the model is the probability that the event occurs. Theoretically, if one is willing to rely on the robustness of linear regression, the model of the preceding section could be applied to these probabilities. However, an immediate problem that arises is the range of predicted values. Although probabilities are restricted to the range 0 to 1, the linear model incorporates no such restrictions; it thus may predict a negative probability or a probability greater than unity. The estimated probabilities of the logistic model, however, must fall in the range 0 to 1 because of the structure of the model.

The basic logistic model can include both categorical and continuous independent (predictor) variables and can incorporate interactions among these variables. To state the general model, let us assume that the response variable Y has a value of 1 for response (suicide) and a value of 0 for no response (no suicide). Also, let us assume that $X_1, X_2, \ldots, X_p$ is an arbitrary set of independent variables for the response. Then, for the ith observation, the model is as follows:

$$\text{logit} \, (\Pr(Y_i = 1)) = \log \frac{\Pr(Y_i = 1)}{(\Pr(Y_i = 0)} = \beta_0 + \beta_1 X_{1i} + \beta_2 X_{2i} + \ldots + \beta_p X_{pi} \quad (3)$$

or, equivalently,

$$\Pr(Y_i = 1) = \frac{1}{1 + \exp[-(\beta_0 + \beta_1 X_{1i} + \beta_2 X_{2i} + \ldots + \beta_p X_{pi})]} \quad (4)$$

Each coefficient β_j can be interpreted as a log odds ratio for a one-unit increase in the corresponding independent variable. The association between any independent variable in the model and the response can be evaluated, in contrast to the more traditional methods such as Mantel-Haenszel adjustment after stratification by confounding variables.

The model specified in equation 3 or 4 above is predicting a probability of response, but the model is applicable to research designs in which the probability is not estimable. In a prospective study of a representative study population, the probability of the response can theoretically be estimated; however, a prospective study for a rare event such as suicide is unusual. Much more common for studies of rare events are case–control series. With a typical case–control study, data are collected on all cases (i.e., suicide completions or attempts) occurring during a specified period of time and on a representative sample of controls during the same period of time. The controls may be selected to force the distributions of variables to be the same among the cases and controls, or to force each case to match uniquely with one or more controls. Technically, the probability of the response's occurring is not estimable because the estimate of the intercept β_0 is a function of the log odds of disease among those with all independent variables simultaneously 0 and the sampling fractions of cases and controls, the latter of which is typically unknown.

The parameters from the logistic model that are typically of more interest than the probabilities are the odds ratios measuring the association of one of the independent variables and the response variable. Algebraically, the ratio of the odds of disease among "exposed" and "nonexposed" groups is the same as the ratio of the odds of exposure among cases and controls. Therefore, the odds ratios can be estimated from a prospective or a retrospective study design. When a rare event such as suicide is being studied, the odds ratio is a good estimate of the relative risk, or the ratio of the probabilities of disease among "exposed" and "nonexposed" groups.

Estimates of the logistic regression parameters are calculated by an iterative procedure called "maximum-likelihood estimation." For a matched design, estimates of the model parameters are calculated by conditional maximum-likelihood estimation. Either maximum-likelihood procedure yields asymptotic standard errors of the estimates of the model parameters. The log likelihood functions can be used as crude indicators of the predictive ability of a logistic model. The statistic R^2, defined as

$$R^2 = \frac{2(\log L_F - \log L_0)}{-2 \log L_0} \, ,$$

where L_F is the likelihood function for the full model (with independent variables) and L_0 is the likelihood model for the model with no independent variables, can be interpreted as the proportion of the log likelihood explained by the model; the numerator of this statistic is often adjusted for the number of independent variables in the model. Individual R statistics can also be calculated for separate variables in the model.

As in any statistical analysis incorporating multiple variables, strong correlations among independent variables can cause difficulties in both estimation and interpretation of a logistic model. Therefore, only subsets of all the independent variables can typically be used in any particular model. The logistic model as presented in equations 3 and 4 assumes no interaction among the independent variables. That is, the association between any independent variable and suicide is the same, regardless of the levels of the other independent variables in the model.

Example 2

The data in Table 11.3 represent a hypothetical case–control study. The response variable was suicide completion. The independent variables were age (index of five 5-year categories was treated as a continuous variable); prior suicide attempt; and awareness of a suicide completion by a friend or relative (no awareness of a suicide, suicide by an acquaintance or distant relative, suicide by a close friend or relative).

The maximum-likelihood estimates of the logistic regression parameters are displayed in Table 11.4. From these estimates, the odds ratios measuring the association between suicide and the independent variables could be calculated. For example, the odds of a suicide completer's having made a prior suicide attempt would be $\exp(1.4159) = 4.12$ times the same odds for a control, adjusting for the confounding effects of age and awareness of a suicide attempt. The odds of a suicide completer's knowing about the suicide of an acquaintance or distant family member, relative to his or her not knowing anyone who had recently committed suicide, would be 2.13 times the same odds for a control, adjusting for the confounding effects of age and prior suicide attempt.

TABLE 11.3. Data for Illustration of Logistic Regression Estimation and Prediction of Suicide Completion

		Age groups[a]								
		25–29		30–34		35–39		40–44		45–49	
Awareness of suicide	Previous attempt	Case	Ctl.	Case	Ctl.	Case	Ctl.	Case	Ctl.	Case	Ctl.
None	Yes	6	24	4	16	3	6	4	19	4	9
	No	5	99	5	75	9	80	8	172	6	74
Distant	Yes	18	56	8	23	5	13	5	12	8	4
	No	6	78	14	165	17	164	26	195	37	65
Close	Yes	7	13	18	21	23	19	15	13	9	4
	No	8	59	17	69	20	74	43	134	41	87

[a]Age is coded as 1, 2, 3, 4, or 5, in logistic model.

These data are derived from a case-control study, but if they were derived from a prospective study, the probability of a suicide completion could be calculated as follows. John (see Chapter 12) was 39 years old and thus in the third age group; he had made a prior suicide attempt, but did not know of a friend or relative who had committed suicide. Thus, the predicted probability of his committing suicide would be

$$\frac{1}{1 + \exp[-(-3.6522 + 0.2987 \cdot 3 + 1.4159)]} = 0.2075.$$

The predicted probability for Faye (see Chapter 12), in the oldest age group with no other risk factors, could be similarly calculated as

$$\frac{1}{1 + \exp[-(-3.6522 + 0.2987 \cdot 5)]} = 0.1035.$$

Thus a prior attempt was seen as a stronger predictor of suicide than older age in this hypothetical data set. Probabilities cannot be calculated for other cases described in Chapter 12 because of the ages, but Ralph, for example, would have a higher probability because of his aunt's suicide. These probabilities would be much higher than those that would be attained from a true prospective study because suicide completers were overrepresented in the sample, thus inflating the estimated probability of completing a suicide.

To determine the relative predictive value of the independent variables, a stepwise procedure may be followed in which any of the measured independent variables may be included in the model. Although a backward-elimination stepwise procedure is in general more desirable, the large number of variables in many studies may necessitate either a forward-selection procedure or a combination of the two. The primary method of inference for this logistic model with either estimation procedure is the likelihood ratio test. This test compares the likelihoods of a reduced model (L_R) and a general model (L_G). The statistic $-2 \log L_R - (-2 \log L_G)$ has an asymptotic chi-square distribution with degrees of freedom equal to the difference in the numbers of parameters estimated in the reduced and general models. A large test statistic indicates that the general model is significantly better than the reduced model, and thus that the additional variables in the general model are needed.

Note that interactions can be included in the model built in this manner, with only one additional assumption: If an interaction represented as the cross-product of two or more independent variables is included in the model, all component parts of that cross-product must also be included in the model. Also, at any step in the selection procedure, if a variable previously added to the model loses its statistical significance with the addition of other variables, it may be deleted.

ALTERNATIVES TO LOGISTIC REGRESSION

One common alternative to logistic regression appropriate for a dichotomous response is the "probit" model (probability integral transformation). In this model, the probability of a response is calculated as follows:

TABLE 11.4. Logistic Regression Coefficients for Suicide Completion Data in Table 11.3

Variable	β	Std. error	χ^2	OR
Intercept	−3.6522	0.2302	251.80	
Age	0.2987	0.0472	40.11	1.35
Prior attempt	1.4159	0.1379	105.48	4.12
Awareness of suicide				
Distant	0.7545	0.1737	18.87	2.13
Close	1.4149	0.1700	69.27	4.12

$$P(Y = 1) = \frac{1}{2\pi} \int_{-\infty}^{\beta_0 + \beta_1 X_1 + \ldots + \beta_p X_p} \exp(-u^2/2) \, du$$

That is, the probabilities are transformed to the cumulative standard normal distribution. The curvilinear response function of this model is almost the same as that of the logistic model, differing primarily in the tails of the distribution. Estimation for the probit model is somewhat more complicated than for the logistic model, but inferences can be made about the model more easily (Neter et al., 1985). This probit model has been used often to model dose–response relationships in biological assays (Schlesselman, 1982). The model is discussed in detail by Finney (1971).

Another approach to predicting a response such as suicide is to use discriminant analysis. This multivariate technique, along with the related procedures of classification, involves separating two or more sets of observations (say, suicidal and nonsuicidal individuals) according to other variables and allocating new observations into these groups. The goals of discrimination and classification are summarized by Johnson and Wichern (1982):

> 1. To describe either graphically or algebraically, the differential features of objects (observations) from several known collections (populations). We try to find "discriminants" whose numerical values are such that the collections are separated as much as possible.
> 2. To sort objects (observations) into two or more labeled classes. The emphasis is on deriving a rule that can be used to optimally assign a new object to the labeled classes. (p. 461)

Since the introduction of discriminant analysis (Fisher, 1936), it has been known that calculating the discriminant function can be formulated as a multivariate linear regression problem. If two populations have some vectors μ_1 and μ_2 of mean values for p discriminant variables, then the linear discriminant function is a function of the difference in these two mean vectors and the common variance–covariance matrix of the p random discriminant variables in the two populations. Essentially, this function reduces the set of random variables to a single random variable by taking a linear combination of those variables based on the discriminant function. Classification (or prediction) involves calculating the linear discriminant function for a set of random variables and comparing it to the midpoint of the mean discriminant function for the two populations.

Discriminant analysis is typically exploratory in nature. Evaluation of the error rates for misclassification requires the specification of the distribution of the random variables in the two populations. Often the two populations are assumed to be multivariate normal—a supposition that may or may not be realistic.

LOG-LINEAR MODELS
Description

A final class of statistical models that may be considered for prediction of suicide events is that of log-linear models. Log-linear models can be considered together with virtually all the models discussed in this chapter as part of a broad class of models called "generalized linear models" (McCullagh & Nelder, 1989). Thus all of the models (excluding discriminant analysis, which cannot properly be called a model) can be written as linear models after appropriate transformation of the dependent variable. However, generalized linear models do not necessarily depend on the assumptions of normality and homoscedasticity.

Log-linear models are part of a rapidly growing area of statistical methodology for analyzing categorical data. The logistic regression model discussed earlier is actually a special case of a log-linear model. The more general log-linear model, however, is suitable for a dependent variable having multiple responses, rather than just two. Log-linear models are a primary focus of many books and articles on categorical data analysis (e.g., Agresti, 1990; Fienberg, 1980; Bishop, Fienberg, & Holland, 1975).

The basic idea of a log-linear model is that the categorical response variable follows a multinomial distribution. The logarithms of the probabilities of this multinomial distribution are linear functions of the independent variables. The log-linear model typically uses categorical independent variables, but it is possible to incorporate continuous variables, as has been seen in the logistic regression model. When categorical variables are used, the log-linear model looks much like a traditional analysis-of-variance model.

The maximum-likelihood procedure is commonly used to estimate the parameters of a log-linear model. This method allows the use of continuous independent variables, directly provides estimates of standard errors of the parameters, and allows the use of likelihood ratio testing for statistical inference. The other procedure commonly used for estimating the parameters of a log-linear model is the weighted least-squares method. This procedure, as the name indicates, is similar to the ordinary least-squares method used in the general linear model, but is weighted by the inverse of the variance–covariance matrix of the responses. The estimation thus accounts for the lack of homoscedasticity required in the general linear model and for the covariances among the multiple responses. Weighted least-squares estimation can be applied to more general models than maximum-likelihood estimation, such as models of marginal probabilities or repeated-measures analyses. A major disadvantage is that it cannot be applied when there are any zero frequencies without making some arbitrary adjustment to the frequencies.

Like the logistic regression, the log-linear model can be interpreted as predicting the probability of a specific outcome (such as a suicide event) as a function of several independent variables. The interpretation of this probability must include assessment of the variables included in the model and an awareness that it is not possible to identify an individual who will definitely have a particular response.

Example 3

In Example 1, a significant problem with the assumption of normality was noted. These school screening data (Garrison et al., 1991) were analyzed again as a log-linear model, with the suicide score dichotomized as high (6 or above) versus low (0–5). Age was also dichotomized as 12 and younger versus 13 and older. CES-D scores were treated as a continuous variable in this example. The two sets of variables used as predictor variables in Example 1 were used in comparable log-linear models. The results are summarized in Table 11.5.

The conclusions that might be drawn from the log-linear models are similar to those from the linear models: The proportion of high suicide scores was higher among older adolescents, females, and those students who did not live with both natural parents. Also, CES-D score was a strong predictor of a high suicide score. In log-linear models, however, the distributional assumption of normality is unnecessary, so the results may be viewed less skeptically.

To illustrate prediction with a log-linear model, let us again consider the case studies of Ralph and Heather. With the smaller model, the proba-

TABLE 11.5. Summary of Log-Linear Models of Demographic Variables and CES-D Score on Suicide Score

Parameter	Estimate	Std. error	Probability
Intercept	−4.4300	0.3562	0.0001
Age	0.6698	0.2929	0.0222
Gender	1.0682	0.2751	0.0001
Guardian status	0.4985	0.2523	0.0482

Parameter	Estimate	Std. error	Probability
Intercept	−7.1859	0.5227	0.0001
Age	0.4059	0.3279	0.2158
Gender	0.2749	0.3144	0.3820
Guardian status	0.0441	0.2906	0.8793
CES-D	0.1612	0.0148	0.0001

bility of Ralph's having a high suicide score would be estimated as $\exp(-4.4300 + 0.6698) = 0.0233$. The probability of Heather's having a high suicide score would be $\exp(-4.4300 + 0.6698 + 1.0682 + 0.4985) = 0.1115$. As in the linear model, these predicted probabilities would be much more reliable with additional predictor variables. Also, probabilities are generally considered more meaningful when applied to a group rather than to an individual.

CONCLUSION

Absolute probabilistic prediction of any rare event, such as suicide, is difficult if not impossible. This chapter surveys some of the statistical methodology available for purposes of estimation and prediction. The methodology is perhaps more useful in identifying groups that are at higher risk than in attempting to predict the suicide of a specific individual. Such groups can be identified by variables that are most strongly associated with a suicidal outcome, and individuals in such groups can then be targeted with more intensive suicide prevention intervention.

REFERENCES

Agresti, A. (1990). *Categorical data analysis.* New York: Wiley.

Bishop, Y. V. V., Fienberg, S. E., & Holland, P. W. (1975). *Discrete multivariate analysis.* Cambridge, MA: MIT Press.

Fienberg, S. E. (1980). *The analysis of cross-classified data* (2nd ed.). Cambridge, MA: MIT Press.

Finney, D. J. (1971). *Probit analysis* (3rd ed.). Cambridge, England: Cambridge University Press.

Fisher, R. A. (1936). The use of multiple measurements in taxonomic problems. *Annals of Eugenics, 7,* 179-188.

Garrison, C. Z., Jackson, K. L., Addy, C. L., McKeown, R. E., & Waller, J. L. (1991). Suicidal behaviors in young adolescents. *American Journal of Epidemiology, 133,* 1005-1014.

Hosmer, D. W., & Lemeshow, S. (1989). *Applied logistic regression.* New York: Wiley.

Johnson, R. A., & Wichern, D. W. (1982). *Applied multivariate statistical analysis.* Englewood Cliffs, NJ: Prentice-Hall.

Kleinbaum, D. G., Kupper, L. L., & Morgenstern, H. (1982). *Epidemiologic research: Principles and quantitative methods.* Belmont, CA: Lifetime Learning.

Maltsberger, J. T. (1986). *Suicide risk: The formulation of clinical judgment.* New York: New York University Press.

McCullagh, P., & Nelder, J. A. (1989). *Generalized linear models* (2nd ed.). London: Chapman & Hall.

Murphy, G. E. (1985). The prediction of suicide—why is it so difficult? *American Journal of Psychotherapy, 38,* 341–349.

Neter, J., Wasserman, W., & Kutner, M. H. (1985). *Applied linear statistical models* (2nd ed.). Homewood, IL: Richard D. Irwin.

Radloff, L. S. (1977). The CES-D scale: A self-report depression scale for research in the general population. *Applied Psychological Measurement, 1,* 385–401.

Schlesselman, J. J. (1982). *Case–control studies: Design, conduct, analysis.* New York: Oxford University Press.

Zar, J. H. (1984). *Biostatistical analysis* (2nd ed.). Englewood Cliffs, NJ: Prentice-Hall.

PART IV

The Cases

Five Potential Suicide Cases

Alan L. Berman, Ph.D.
Washington Psychological Center
National Center for the Study and Prevention of Suicide
Washington School of Psychiatry

The empirical base from which we derive risk factors sufficient to help discriminate suicidal from nonsuicidal individuals has been written with the nomothetic pen. Suicidal individuals collectively provide us with epidemiological snapshots. These macroscopic views provide estimates of prevalence and incidence, which in turn point us toward demographic, temporal, and cross-cultural trends. Out of these nomothetic nets we have traditionally built theories, established hypotheses, and developed models of early detection, intervention, and prevention. With regard to prevention in particular, various models of intervention are entirely dependent upon the descriptions of high-risk groups developed through these methods (Lorion, Price, & Eaton, 1989). In suicidology, this is in the Durkheimian tradition.

As valuable and important as these statistical profiles are to suicidology, they paint with such a broad brush that they may inadvertently mislead the clinician/caregiver. Checklists, scales, and profiles describe the modal suicide. These predictive tools are extraordinarily helpful in large-scale screenings of potentially at-risk individuals; however, they may obscure discriminations necessary to translate into clinically relevant cues. For this reason, models of triage are often designed to incorporate a series of screenings, beginning with the use of scales and checklists and ending with the clinical interview (see, e.g., Rotheram-Borus & Bradley, 1991). Test makers understand this well, as they typically publish their scales with a stated caveat that they are meant to guide the clinician and should not replace clinical judgment. However, this warning probably has the most impact on those least in need. By analogy, warnings about the dangers of smoking are placed on packages of cigarettes being bought only by smokers! Users of these scales must constantly be reminded that, given the low base rate of both completed suicides and nonfatal suicide attempts, scales and tests will invariably produce unacceptably high rates of false positives when not used in conjunction with intensive clinical observation (Eyman & Eyman, 1990).

Consider, for example, what we have learned about the suicidal adolescent. How well would any profile of risk have led us to predict the following suicide?

Brenda was a 15-year-old black female. The seventh child in a family of nine and the only one adopted, Brenda's death was planned and intended. She wrote about death in her journal. She told her mother that she wanted "to die a slow death and experience all the pain." Already in her brief life she had been hospitalized five times for suicide attempts (by overdose, cutting, and scorching herself with an iron). Although she was diagnosed as having borderline personality disorder, she was known to be hearing voices; she had first heard them when she was 12, but until recently the symptoms had been controlled by imipramine (Tofranil) and thioridazine (Mellaril). It was with these medications, apparently hoarded over several weeks, that she overdosed.

Brenda is an actuarial exception. The typical completed suicide is an elderly white male. The typical completed suicide in adolescence is a white male victim of a gunshot wound. The typical nonfatal attempter is a young white female who overdoses with little intent to die and uses methods with low lethality. As a black female completed suicide who overdosed with intent to die, Brenda fits none of these profiles very well. But auditory hallucinations (perhaps command hallucinations) and a history of repeat attempts should dramatically shift our expectations of possible suicide, leading us to rely more on clinical intuition of danger for potentially lethal outcomes. Let me illustrate in another way the difference between statistical and clinical realities.

A young adult male schizophrenic patient, with a 5-year chronic history of symptoms and related hospitalizations, bought a gun and 24 hours later used it to kill himself. At the time of his suicide, he was an outpatient at a community mental health center (CMHC); he was being seen twice a month in supportive therapy by a master's-level caseworker and was being medicated by a psychiatrist. Upon his death, the CMHC and the caseworker were sued for malpractice by the patient's surviving family.

Counsel for the plaintiffs hired an expert witness who in a written report waxed eloquent about the suicide risk among chronic schizophrenics. She quoted statistics about lifetime risk and about associated risk factors. Her position was exceedingly clear: Schizophrenics are dangerous folk, "at *constant* risk for suicide." Acknowledging that "case managers are the primary mental health providers for suicide-vulnerable populations in settings such as the CMHC," she then presented the following: "[T]he chronically ill patient is *seven* times more likely to [complete] suicide than a person in the general population. In my opinion, the case manager is not the appropriate professional to deal with a suicidal population." This expert reasoned that (1) case managers are assigned chronic patients; (2) chronic patients are more suicidal than normal patients; (3) because of that suicide risk, case managers should not be assigned to work with chronic patients; and (4) assigning a case manager to a chronic patient, therefore, is evidence of malpractice. I believe that this is a good example of how an academic understanding of suicide risk can be too far removed from the realities of clinical work.

Suicidology is the study of things suicidal. The core datum of study, ultimately, is the suicidal individual. The clinician must come to understand suicidal behavior on both nomothetic and idiographic levels. It is only through the intensive study of the suicidal "case"—the realities presented by that case, and the reasons why it fits and/or does not fit modal descriptors of risk factors—that the macroscopic view of suicide risk has clinical relevance.[1] No one set of risk factors will apply to all suicidal individuals. Not all individuals sharing known risk factors will be suicidal. In this sense, each case serves to illustrate what we know about the suicidal individual and, at the same time, confirms the rule that there is an exception to every rule. In this sense, also, the case should be the primary object of our teaching in suicidology. In psychological and psychiatric education, this is in the Freudian tradition.

THE CASE METHOD

The case method of teaching has long been used in other fields of graduate study, notably the law and business.[2] In medicine, it might be considered a derivative of "grand rounds." In suicidology, however, extended cases are rare, the more common presentation being that of a paragraph or two of case information (the "case vignette") illustrative of a point of text.[3] More extended presentations have been given by Litman and Diller (1985), who

---

1. The reader will understand that the use of the word "case" is not meant to dehumanize the suicidal person. Rather, it is chosen to collectively describe that which is of clinical interest about the person, specifically here with regard to the problem of understanding risk and assessing probable future behavior.

2. The case method was first used at the Harvard Business School in 1909 (Lawrence, 1953).

3. Pfeffer's (1986) *The Suicidal Child* is a good example of the liberal use of case vignettes (there are 86 of them) as illustrations in a text. Berman and Jobes (1991) provide some 40 vignettes in a book half as long. For a discussion in the present volume of the use of case vignettes, see Stelmachers and Sherman, Chapter 13.

describe 12 cases (six youthful suicide completers and six controls), and Niswander, Casey, and Humphrey (1973), who have provided nine cases in a casebook of psychological autopsies. In 1988, the American Association of Suicidology presented the first case conferences at its annual meetings. These have subsequently been transcribed, edited, and published in book form (Berman, 1990). In addition, the journal *Suicide and Life-Threatening Behavior* began a series of "case consultations" with its Winter 1989 issue. And now, the case method serves in the present volume as a unifying focus and source of illustrations for most chapters.

Cases, well described, bring a concrete reality into our teaching. As Lawrence (1953) put it, they provide an "anchor on academic flights of speculation" (p. 215). Theory and research come to life in the presentation of case material, each being given the opportunity to be tested against clinical practice. A case simply presents a factual outline, posing issues requiring judgment and the application of principles. Ideally, the student of this volume will first study each case closely, form his or her own opinions, and then compare them to those of each of the authors of other chapters. In this way, the reader will become a problem solver, applying his or her knowledge to the clinical case with the opportunity to validate and affirm or apply corrective reasoning to these opinions.

In this book, only five cases are presented. These cases were chosen with a few simple criteria in mind. First, they were intended to cover as much as possible of the spectrum of suicidal individuals (e.g., in regard to the factors of age, race, gender, etc.). Of course, the reader should keep in mind that we cannot hope to cover the entire spectrum of suicidal individuals in five cases. Second, as much as possible, these cases were chosen to give the chapter authors something to illustrate their arguments with. There is sufficient information in each case to which to apply either scales or intuition. From a discussion of suicidal methods to issues of modeling, from influences of economics to the role of physical illness, there is something for almost everyone. Again, of course, there are some notable gaps with only five cases. For example, there is no case illustrative of a jail or prison suicide. Information on biological markers (levels of serotonin, cortisol, etc.) was not available to allow case illustrations of the potential influence of such markers. Only one case is presented with more than the minimum of psychological test data. Personal documents are also provided only for this case. For those used to applying aggregate data to the prediction of suicide risk (e.g., sociologists), each and every case poses a potential exception to the rule.

Each case is presented to the reader from a different vantage point, referral source, and context. In the case of Heather B, the youngest person in this series, her mother sought an outpatient consultation. A consultation was requested in the case of Ralph F, who had been on inpatient status for a week. John Z had been in outpatient treatment for over 4 months when his wife sought a second opinion regarding his need for hospitalization. Faye C presented at the emergency room, brought there by her landlady. Lastly, José G was referred for an evaluation by his physician. The decisions requested in each case involved the risk for suicide and the need for hospitalization.

Most importantly, all of these cases are presented without prior knowledge of the suicide outcome. Chapter authors have been asked to make their assessments and predictions in ignorance of whether a subject died by suicide or some other manner, made an attempt and survived, or had not (at the time of writing) engaged in any self-harm behavior. Because each case was chosen with the intent of providing sufficient discussable risk factors, it may be fair to assume that each case was at least at some risk for suicidal behavior.

It may be instructive for the reader to make a global assessment of risk and a prediction of outcome of each case before leaving this chapter. If we assume that each of the case subjects was a *possible* suicide, then subsequent discussion must address whether each was a *probable* suicide and, if so, when and with what consequences. Three simple questions may serve to guide the assessment of each case:

1. Is this person likely to have engaged in a suicidal behavior?
2. If yes, is this person likely to have attempted or completed suicide?
3. Temporally, would the risk for this behavior be likely to be long-term or imminent?

The reader will note that this list does not include the more typical questions suggesting a continuum of risk (e.g., from low risk to high risk), although such a rating is implied in both questions 1 and 3 above. For both the reader and the chapter authors, the outcomes of each case (and feedback regarding follow-up, where applicable) are presented in the final chapter of this book.

Lastly, before presenting the cases, I should highlight for the reader some of the more evident problems with the case method. The case is essentially static. It lacks the dynamism of a live person interacting with the interviewer or assessor. It does not provide the reader with the opportunity to ask unasked questions or to follow up on information that has been presented. It also lacks the life of that interaction over the minutes, hours, days, or weeks we may have available to us in dealing with suicidal individuals. Unavailable as well are the nonverbal cues that often lead to our more organismic response—the intuitive "gut feeling" that often differentiates the actuarial from the clinical approach to risk assessment. And, most powerfully, these cases are necessarily brief; thus, they invite projection. In this sense, we may learn more about ourselves as we attempt to understand each of these possibly suicidal individuals.

In the ideal case available to us for interview and assessment, we would have considerably more data at our disposal. For example, family history would be extensively developed; corroborative interviews might be held with family members; more psychometric evaluations might be sought; and more personal documents would be available for our scrutiny. In the ideal case, furthermore, each of the specific predictors outlined in the chapters that follow would be explored and presented as present or absent, and if present would be delineated more fully. In addition, the interpersonal impact of the patient on the interviewer could be experienced as well as described. The result of that experience is often the more visceral response described above, difficult to encode as a risk factor but known to most clinicians as a "gut response."

In addition, as a method of teaching, the case method requires over time an accumulation and presentation of a large body of cases from which the student can derive common factors of clinical importance. In this sense, the idiographic approach ultimately must mimic the nomothetic. This is what clinicians mean when they credit their knowledge base to that of "experience" (i.e., a sequential accumulation of common observations leading to our more personalized definitions of suicide risk). Large numbers of new cases must continually be developed, presented, and studied if the case method is to succeed in educating us about suicidal individuals.

With this preface and frame, I now introduce to the reader the cases presented to each of our chapter authors.

CASE 1: HEATHER B

Heather B, a latency-age early adolescent, presented with problems of mood and behavior, the latter illustrative of both provocation and conflict. Her cognitions were self-deprecatory and expressive of self-harmful thoughts and behaviors. Her interpersonal world showed signs of alienation reflective of her more personal concerns of identity and acceptability. Presented with her case information are her unanalyzed responses to a psychological test battery and selected writings and drawings (personal documents).

Background Information

Heather, a 13-year-old white female, the older of two sisters, was referred by her mother for consultation and psychological evaluation. Her mother stated that Heather's moods and behavior were becoming increasingly problematic. She illustrated her concerns with stories of Heather's lying, violating restrictions and curfews, sneaking out of the house past midnight, and making a number of unapproved long-distance telephone calls to various rock stars' "1-900" numbers. (In particular, Heather was placing calls with great frequency to the "33-year-old president of some rock star's fan club whom she considers to be like a boyfriend.") The mother did not believe that Heather was using drugs. She further stated, however, that Heather was isolating herself in her room (ostensibly reading and listening to "heavy metal" music); in addition, her writings and drawings had depressed themes, reflected thoughts of suicide, and contained suggestions that she was "maiming" herself. (However, in other writings and drawings she disavowed suicidal intent; see Figure 12.1 for an example.) Furthermore, the mother reported that Heather frequently talked about herself as a "manic-depressive" and was constantly saying "I'm sorry" or "I'm stupid . . . I hate

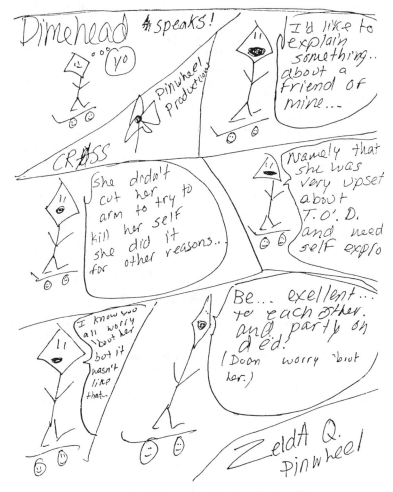

FIGURE 12.1. A drawing by Heather B.

myself." Recently, she was talking more about wanting to hurt herself, although she denied any plan to do so. She did not want to talk about her suicidal thoughts; she merely told her mother that she was "sad and confused." Her mother reported that Heather had a history of being provocative—of saying things "for shock value."

Heather's school behavior was also of some concern. Her grades had dropped over the past three terms from a straight B average, with only one C included, to last term's three C's and two D's out of seven grades. Heather talked of "hating school and of being bored with and disliking her classmates, other than one or two who shared her self-definition as an "anarchist" and a "weirdo." The boys she was hanging out with all were out of school and older than 20; Heather's mother expressed some concern about her daughter's being sexually precocious. Heather was especially antagonistic to the "preppy" norm of dress at school and purposely dressed herself in "dramatic, eccentric, sloppy, and unflattering" outfits. She was making it quite clear to her mother that she wished to transfer to another school.

Heather's mother stated that Heather's appetite, eating behavior, and sleeping were fine. Her attention and concentration were also reported to be unproblematic. As for Heather's developmental history, her birth and early childhood were without incident. The first and only major trauma in her childhood had occured at the age of 7, when her father died of cancer, 11 months after diagnosis. Heather's response to his death was to go outside and play in the snow, showing no strong emotional reaction. Heather's mother had remarried 1 year ago after a 10-month courtship. However, the marriage had lasted only 8 months because, according to Heather's mother, "he had a Madonna complex about sex, he was irresponsible, he was hyperreligious, and he drank a lot!" Heather had fought a fair amount with her stepfather and seemed relieved at the impending divorce.

Psychological Test Results Summary

Wechsler Intelligence Scale for Children–Revised

Heather's Wechsler Intelligence Scale for Children—Revised (WISC-R) IQ scores were as follows: Verbal, 118; Performance 112; and Full Scale, 118. Her subtest scaled scores were as follows: Information, 13; Similarities, 13; Arithmetic, 13; Vocabulary, 15; Comprehension, 11; Digit Span, 11; Picture Completion, 9; Picture Arrangement, 12; Block Design, 11; Object Assembly, 15; and Coding, 12.

Rorschach

All of Heather's reaction times on the Rorschach were within 8 seconds; there were no rotations. Her responses were as follows:

Card I. Two dogs (W) tearing (?: biting) something (?: don't know) up.

Card II. 1. On a road (W, S) to something far away; 2. Arguing faces (?: human).

Card III. Thye're warming their hands over the fire. The red comes in; it just doesn't mean anything to me. It's just there.

Card IV. A dragon with its head bending down (?: facing me).

Card V. A butterfly, upside down.

Card VI. I don't know.

Card VII. Dancing rabbits . . . facing each other. Their ears and paws are out.

Card VIII. The two pink things look like bears or some kind of animal climbing on stuff, like an iceberg.

Card IX. The collision of two alien worlds or something like that (?: Top D) . . . looks like it's exploding. The pink looks like cabbages.

Card X. Sea animals. The blue are crabs or crayfish, the green and pink are seahorses, and the gray are sea lice.

Thematic Apperception Test

Heather's Thematic Apperception Test (TAT) responses were as follows:

Card 1 (boy with violin). This little boy, named Billy, wants to learn to play the violin, but he can't. He likes it, thinks it's beautiful. Maybe he'll learn it later. He can't learn it right now because he's not old enough. He's 8 and needs to be 10. [Feel?] Sad . . . he wants to but he can't.

Card 2 (farm family). . . . It's a farm on St. Stephen's Creek in Illinois. A mother, brother, and sister. Sis teaches school. The boy helps out on the farm. Mother helps on the farm, too. There's another little brother . . . he's not here . . . he's in the barn feeding the pigs. The husband's off in World War II. Mom misses him. She's thinking of him and wants him to come back. Sis, the teacher, is waiting for her beau to come back. [Feel?] Lonely.

Card 3GF (woman, hand on bowed head, at door). [There was a 64-second lag with distractibility to drawing on her hand.] Her name is Eleanor. She's crying because she just got a notice that her brother in France is missing and presumed dead. [How?] In World War II.

Card 5 (older woman peering in room). . . . Grandma was in the kitchen. She was cooking breakfast and heard a noise. She went to look in the front room and found out her three sons were visiting. She's surprised because they never visit. [Why?] Because they're busy. [Feel?] Happy.

Card 6BM (young man, older woman looking away). They're worried because they might not have enough money to keep their farm. They had a bad corn crop . . . not enough rain. The son is angry because the landlord is trying to take away the farm. The mother is worried about where they will go. But the landlord has to go to Chicago for a business meeting. While there, his daughter gets married and he's preoccupied and forgets about wanting to take away the farm.

Card 8GF (woman, hand on chin looking pensive). She's a sculptor and she lives by herself in a home in England. She did a really great sculpture and she likes it a lot. She's happy to have finished it. It's in clay right now; she can't wait to get it into marble.

Card 9GF (woman behind tree, woman below running by). There was a boat wrecked near a lighthouse. They are running to see what happened because they knew some people who went out boating and wanted to see if everybody was all right. When they got there, all were OK, except for a fish that got caught between a rock and the boat. [Appears anxious to end testing.]

Card 13MF (woman in bed, man standing arm across eyes looking away). He's very sad, because she died. It's his sister and he's the big brother. There's another brother in between. She had pneumonia. And now he has to tell his mom what happened.

Card 14 (silhouette of man at window). A man . . . he's looking outside. He sees the moon and stars. He lives on a beach in Ireland. He's a writer and he's content.

Selected Writings

Letter to Classmate

Robin,

I know the reason I'm not invited to the party. . . . I wouldn't go if I wanted to. You used to be my friend. I'm not sure when you decided I was such a bitch but you obviously have. Whenever I like a boy . . . you seem to hang all over him or talk about me behind my back. . . . You've hurt me too much for me to care any more. Leave me alone to inflict self pain (ask anyone about my arm) in peace.

Letter to Friend

Babs,

OK, the newest big deal: I belong in a mental hospital. My mentality is so severely corrupted, distorted, and disturbed. . . . I need to become unattached. . . . If I told my mom this she would freak. She thinks I am normal, well, partly normal. But I don't care. I've stopped caring about a lot of things. . . . This is a mongo big problem. . . . I need serious mental help.

Journal Entry

School [is] so stupid I could puke on the floor. . . . Lots of things are really wrong. I have a suicide risk life. . . . I want to run away, not come back. . . . I need some air. Self-confidence = Q[?]. I hate myself and I'm stupid. Most people could add to that list and about half the school already has. I need some serious help. How do you tell your mom you're suicidal and mentally . . . crazy?

Journal Entry

I'm sorry . . . When you told me he was dead, I didn't believe you. How could I? My dad was always there. For seven years and what do I get? A grave and a photo? What else? Broken conscious [sic]. I should have cried. But I didn't. I'm sorry, Daddy. I miss you.

CASE 2: RALPH F

Ralph F, a middle adolescent, was currently hospitalized as a dual-diagnosis (viz., depression and alcoholism) patient. His case material includes more extensive family background information than that available for Heather, as well as a mental status exam, a summary of his psychological evaluation, and progress summaries over the course of his hospital treatment.

Background Information

Ralph, a 16-year-old white male, was referred for consultation and suicide risk assessment 1 week into his first inpatient psychiatric hospitalization. Ralph was originally referred for voluntary emergency hospitalization "for treatment of depression and alcohol problems" by a local mental health center psychologist. On intake he complained of sleep problems (with frequent awakening and reduced total sleep time), rapid fluctuations in appetite (with a recent 5-pound weight loss), increased anhedonia, anergia, and social isolation. In addition, he stated that he had had persistent suicide ideation with a recently developed plan (i.e., jumping from a local bridge). Ralph stated that he was afraid of suicide, although he appeared to romanticize death.

Ralph had also considered committing suicide by drinking several fifths of alcohol and consuming drugs. He denied abusing other substances, although he admitted to smoking cigarettes daily (about a pack) and having experimented with marijuana. His alcohol use, which had begun at the age of 12 when his parents were separated, was reported by Ralph to average a fifth of bourbon, vodka, or gin each day at present. In addition, he described an increasing tolerance for alcohol, with no reported passing out, vomiting, or hangovers. However, he admitted to having visual hallucinations of insects when coming off alcohol.

Ralph attributed the onset of these symptoms and exacerbation of his drinking to the recent death of his aunt. Her death followed a significantly stressful period for Ralph's family. Two years earlier, the patient's maternal grandfather had been accused by Ralph's younger sister (then aged 12) and cousin of sexual molestation. With these accusations, Ralph's mother and aunt (the two girls' mothers) revealed that they too had been molested by their father when they were children. The maternal aunt proceeded to bring charges against her father; however, 3 months ago the charges had been dropped. During the ensuing weeks his aunt became depressed, left her husband to live in Ralph's house, and, 8 weeks ago, killed herself with a shotgun. From that point on, Ralph became increasingly depressed and homicidal toward his grandfather. He stated that he was trying to handle his anger at his grandfather by turning it toward himself when he thought of suicide.

At the time of admission, Ralph lived at home with both natural parents and his sister. His mother had had an earlier, first marriage. His parents' marriage had suffered through several (by Ralph's count, eight) separations in a 1-year period (4 years ago), but had been intact over the past year. Within the past 2 months, however, marital conflict had increased coincident with Ralph's depression. Both natural parents and the paternal grandfather had a history of alcoholism. His mother had had a "breakdown," with an attempted suicide by overdose, when Ralph was 5. She was hospitalized for 2 weeks. At present she had diagnosed hypertension; the father had heart disease.

Little additional significant history was elicited, as Ralph was more guarded in discussing his own background. He claimed to have almost electrocuted himself as a toddler (by placing a utensil in an electrical outlet). At age 13 he had been diagnosed as having juvenile rheumatoid arthritis. Currently, his arthritis was in remission, with only some morning stiffness noted. There was no clear-cut fusiform swelling or joint deformation. Furthermore, Ralph suffered from stress-induced asthma. He claimed to be very sexually active, and stated that he currently had herpes and had had syphilis in the past. The former was verified upon physical examination; the latter could not be confirmed. At the time of admission, Ralph was an 11th-grade student with a B+ average. Some slippage in his academic performance was reported since his aunt's death. Ralph named several friends from school, mostly "drinking buddies." Raised as a Lutheran, Ralph expressed little interest in religion.

Mental Status Exam

Ralph was a tall, well-nourished male, casually dressed and groomed. His mannerisms were very expressive, almost histrionic. His responses to questions were appropriate to questioning with elaboration. He was cooperative with good eye contact, except when discussing his family history. His mood was dysphoric, especially during the discussion of his aunt's death. He denied visual or auditory hallucinations, but appeared obsessed with the notion of suicide. He related feelings of hopelessness and fatalism. As noted above, he spoke about his childhood guardedly, with nonchalance and near-apathy. His memory appeared intact for recent and remote events. Concentration, insight, and judgment were fair. He was oriented to time, place, and person.

Psychological Results

Ralph's Wechsler Adult Intelligence Scale—Revised (WAIS-R) Full Scale IQ was 102 (Verbal IQ = 114; Performance IQ = 85). His Bender–Gestalt was unremarkable; he recalled four of nine designs correctly. Neuropsychological screening tests showed no significant localized or diffuse organic involvement. On the Rorschach, he gave 15 responses with no card rejections. Form level was adequate, and a number of populars were given. Small details were avoided; a limited use of movement was noted. On the Minnesota Multiphasic Personality Inventory (MMPI), he obtained a T-score of 120 on the F scale with associated lower scores on both the L and K scales, invalidating the clinical scale profile.

Course in Hospital Over 7 Days

Assessment of Ralph's alcohol abuse suggested that, although substantial, it was probably overstated. Significant signs of depression were noted. His response to desipramine (Norpramin) was moderate. He began developing mood-congruent auditory hallucinations, which persisted and became increasingly self-deprecatory and attacking. These appeared to disappear in response to small doses of thiothixene (Navane). In group and individual therapy, he seemed obsessed with existential despair and expressed considerable ambivalence about suicide. He maintained a strong histrionic quality.

Diagnoses

Ralph's DSM-III-R (*Diagnostic and Statistical Manual of Mental Disorders*, third edition, revised) diagnoses were as follows:

Axis I.   Major depression, single episode
          Alcohol abuse, episodic, secondary
Axis II. None
Axis III. Juvenile rheumatoid arthritis, in remission
Axis IV. 5 (extreme)
Axis V.   Current Global Assessment of Functioning (GAF) score: 25
          Highest GAF past year: 60

CASE 3: JOHN Z

The case material for John Z provides us with a 4½-month summary of his outpatient psychotherapy, in addition to his presenting symptoms and history. In this case, the added interactive picture (between therapist and patient) serves as the basis for his risk assessment, coupled with the demand to consider involuntary hospitalization.

Background Information

John, a 39-year-old white male who was married and the father of three sons, was laid off from his supervisory job of 11 years because of a massive cutback in personnel. With his salary went all his benefits (health insurance, etc.). Devastated, he chose to enroll immediately in a master's degree program at the university in order to upgrade his skills and marketability; however, he dropped out within 3 weeks when he realized that it would take 2 years to complete his degree and that he could not live off his savings and his wife Mary's meager salary (Mary was a schoolteacher) in the meantime. He became increasingly depressed and sought help from a psychiatrist, Dr. Smith, who saw him initially on March 21.

Dr. Smith's intake revealed an unremarkable history, except for one sister (of four) who had been hospitalized as an anorexic with two suicide attempts. John himself had no prior episodes of depression and no known hospitalizations. He had served one tour of duty in the Army, which included combat in Vietnam. On this tour there was one incident in which he was ordered by his commanding officer during a sniper attack to mount a tank in open view of the sniper, and he refused; instead, the officer took the tank position, only to be killed instantly. Dr. Smith described John as "intelligent, gregarious, competent, devoted [to family], and cocky." The doctor noted that John complained of the following symptoms: weight loss, early morning insomnia, a loss of libido, shakiness, inability to concentrate, fatigue, low self-esteem, and constant tearfulness.

Outpatient Psychotherapy

John was diagnosed as having a major depression, single episode; Dr. Smith prescribed an antidepressant and scheduled a second session in 2 weeks. Follow-up appointments were held on April 4, April 14, and May 5, during which Dr. Smith documented a slight weight gain (6 pounds), improved sleep, and the beginnings of a job search. An appointment was scheduled but canceled by John on May 12. No further appointments were scheduled or held until July 12. During May and June, according to Mary, John's depression increased as his job applications turned into rejections. At one point he told her that he was so depressed that he put a plastic bag over his head, but was so uncomfortable that he stopped. On July 12, Dr. Smith noted that John was doing better but that signs of depression continued. On July 16, Mary telephoned Dr. Smith's office in order to get a prescription to control her husband's "panic attacks." Because Dr. Smith was out of town, the call was responded to by his partner, who prescribed alprazolam (Xanax) to John.

John did not keep his next appointment (July 26) with Dr. Smith. About this time, the Z family moved in with Mary's mother because their house had been sold, and John received word that he would have at least some part-time employment beginning August 1. Instead of going to work on August 1, however, John went to the basement of his mother-in-law's house and allegedly attempted to hang himself. He did not complete the attempt and reported his action to his wife, who called Dr. Smith. A session was scheduled for the following day to evaluate John. At that session, Dr. Smith could not confirm the patient's alleged hanging attempt, because he found no abrasions on John's neck. However, he did recommend that John be hospitalized for observation and treatment. John agreed to go to the hospital that night, and Dr. Smith wrote up an admission note and orders, including mention that the patient was "very depressed" and "in need of a secure room."

The next day, August 3, Dr. Smith learned upon making his hospital rounds that John had never been admitted the evening before. He immediately called the Z home and, upon speaking with Mary, learned that John had "refused to go last night." She further reported that her husband was calmer now and not in apparent distress. Dr. Smith changed John's medication to imipramine (Tofranil). On August 6, in response to a report by telephone from Mary that John was "not tolerating the Tofranil well," new prescriptions for amoxapine (Asendin) and desipramine (Norpramin) were ordered.

Frustrated with her husband's lack of response to either the medication or Dr. Smith's treatment, Mary now sought a consultation for a second opinion. She was concerned that there had been no change in John's condition, and documented a 20-pound weight loss in the past 2 months, his decreased ability to concentrate, and his "obsession with trivia." Fearful that he might again attempt suicide and this time be successful, she asked also whether her husband should not now be involuntarily hospitalized.

CASE 4: FAYE C

Faye C was a middle-aged female who presented to the emergency room with florid symptoms of a thought disorder and panic. Thirty years had passed since her first and only inpatient hospitalization, the consequences of which were evident as part of her currently presenting dynamics.

Background Information

Faye was a 49-year-old, unmarried white female who was brought to the hospital emergency room by her landlady. A tall, ungainly woman, Faye complained that she had been up all night except for about 2 hours' sleep, feeling hyperanxious, tremulous, and scared. She stated that she could not distinguish the real from the unreal and that her thoughts were uncontrollable. She spoke of radio waves that were controlling her thinking and of others' being able to tell what was going on in her head. On intake she said to the intake interviewer, "I see you as a magician!" and stated that people and books "are telling me to remove my inhibitions." Furthermore, she remarked, "What makes me so uncomfortable is knowing I have free will. I can bend the world to suit my fancy. . . . I create what is happening around me by what I choose to believe or not believe. . . . I can see an infinity of universes moving away from me into the future." In addition, she described feelings of depersonalization, "strange and unreal feelings . . . I'm not really where I am. . . . I'm watching myself."

She described being terrified of hospitalization, equating being a mental patient with being a robot. "Therapists are the enemies," she exclaimed. Immediately thereafter, she screamed, "You're not going to let me kill myself, are you?" In spite of her irrationality, Faye was able to give a reasonably coherent account of her life history. She was delivered by Caesarian section because of a breech presentation. She remembered her childhood as one in which she felt clumsy and dull-witted; she recalled her adolescence as marked by awkwardness, a negative self-image, loneliness, and social isolation. She had never had a sexual relationship with a man. Rather, she idolized men, never coming close enough to relate to them, and harbored obsessional, erotic fantasies to which she masturbated with both frequency and consequent guilt.

Faye described herself as greatly overprotected as an adolescent: "I never had any experiences associated with youth." She blamed her mother for this, describing her as old and tired (she suffered from some unnamed disease), always at home, always tense, and closed off from any expression of love. The mother, according to Faye, equated food with love, alternated between expressions of great worry and rage, and frequently made jokes about urination and defecation. In contrast, Faye stated that she was very close to her father: "I love my father more than any man in the world." He was described as "gentle, humorous, caring, bright, thoughtful, and sympathetic." Her home life was characterized as quiet, passive, and intellectual. She had no recollection of any physical contact between her parents. Rather, evenings were spent watching television, reading, or playing solitaire. In spite of her family life, Faye now described a great fear of her parents' dying from old age.

Earlier Treatment

Faye left home to attend college, only to have her freshman year interrupted by her first hospitalization for a depressive episode. She reported nothing in the way of precipitating events for this 3-week inpatient stay, but had very strong reactions to her treatment, which included electroconvulsive therapy (ECT). She described this experience as "torture" and remembered her therapist as the "torturer." Subsequent to this hospitalization, Faye was diagnosed as having temporal lobe epilepsy, for which she was receiving carbamazepine (Tegretol). She blamed her epilepsy on her ECT. She was able to complete college and earned a master's degree in public health. With this degree in hand, she went on to "reform the mental health system," only to have her idealism met with further evidence of her powerlessness. Having failed at this, she now felt depressed and confused; she felt that she herself was worthless and that life was not worthwhile. Fearing another breakdown and rehospitalization, Faye had entered outpatient treatment 6 years ago. After 4 months, however, she terminated therapy abruptly over a dispute in her fee. Within 6 months she re-entered treatment and stayed 3 years, primarily to deal with her "depression, social isolation, low self-concept, and obsessional style." To the present admission, Faye brought a copy of an MMPI taken at entry into that treatment. The Welsh Code on her MMPI profile (dated approximately 5 years earlier) was 2*875"34'.

CASE 5: JOSÉ G

José G, a man at the threshold of being classified as "young–old," was in involuntary retirement because of a job-related disability. The consequences of that disability and his lack of recovery from it were resulting in more and more deterioration in his psychological well-being and level of functioning. As we often observe, trouble comes in bunches: More recently, José had been given two additional medical diagnoses. It was through the attention of his primary physician, alert to his patient's style of coping, that a psychological consultation was requested.

Background Information

José, a 64-year-old Hispanic male, was seen on referral from his physician for evaluation and treatment. The referral noted José's "increasing depression" subsequent to an injury sustained on the job 6 months earlier. Employed for 29 years on the railroad, Mr. Garcia had fractured his wrist in a fall off a flatcar while helping unload rails. The wrist injury was severe and required surgery. Although initially optimistic about returning to work,

José became frustrated by his lack of recovery and the extended medical leave required for physical therapy. After a couple of months of rehabilitative effort, it became clear to his doctor that only minimal progress was being made. José continued to have no strength in his hand and to complain of swelling, numbness, and pain. He was frustrated at the lack of healing and his consequent inability both to return to his job and to work around the house. Having no ability to grasp objects "as small as a broom handle," he felt reduced to "puttering and tinkering around the house—just busy work." He was especially sad about no longer being able to hold a gun firmly, which meant that he could never go hunting again with his sons and grandchildren. After 5 months of treatment, he was informed a month ago that he was being placed on permanent disability, because he was not seen as capable of returning to his old job.

José lived with his wife of 42 years and his mother-in-law, who was disabled and for whom he had been caring since he had been on leave. He had two married sons (aged 41 and 37), each of whom also worked on the railroad, and six grandchildren. He described his marriage as "OK." He had married 4 years after meeting his wife; his courtship had been interrupted by military service from which he was honorably discharged. His early employment was as a ranch laborer—an occupation he frequently returned to when laid off by the railroad in short-term reductions in force. He began his employment with the railroad as a gang laborer, later earning promotions to machine operator and ultimately to foreman. His employment record was free of any disciplinary actions throughout his years of service.

Mental Status Exam and Medical History

José was cooperative in the interview, responsive although not elaborative to questions. His mood was dysphoric and anxious. Although he was husky and muscular, his gait and demeanor were characteristic of a defeated man. José related that he had always been an outgoing, jovial, "happy-go-lucky" guy. Although neither a great socializer nor a very gregarious individual, he was well liked by those he managed on the job, and often would go out for a beer or two with them after work. He prided himself on being responsible, helping others, and never asking anything for himself. He saw himself as self-contained, self-sufficient, and not one to talk about or share problems with others.

José described feeling trapped by his injury, frustrated that he could not do something to solve it, and increasingly hopeless about the future. He felt himself to be a burden. His frustration showed in increased restlessness, aimlessness, and irritability. Some of his feelings were externalized in anger toward the railroad. He felt that he was being blamed for causing his injury (by the kind of questions asked by the claims agent), and he also felt betrayed that the railroad did not appear to value his years of loyalty. Above all, he felt that he had failed to fulfill his responsibility to make it to 30 years of service before he retired—that, somehow, he was "cheating." All he wanted to do was work. "The railroad is in my blood," he said. "I've worked and slept railroads all my life!"

In the last several weeks, José reported increasing feelings of worthlessness ("I'm not worth anything to anybody"). He described feeling preoccupied ("in a daze . . . my mind is somewhere else . . . I'm spacey . . . I keep forgetting pieces of conversations"). For the past several months he had shown no interest in sex, his appetite had changed, and he was awakening early from sleep. He stated that he had nothing to look forward to, and wished aloud that "the rail should have hit me on the head and ended it."

Medically, José suffered from adult-onset diabetes mellitus that required self-administered insulin. José reported that he had adapted well to this routine without complication for many years. However, 2 months earlier he had been diagnosed as having "widespread diabetic retinopathy." In addition, 1 month earlier he had been diagnosed as having emphysema. He immediately gave up a 40-year cigarette habit. Complicating this was a history of alcohol use. Mr. Garcia admitted to having a long history of heavy alcohol use, including two charges of driving under the influence and careless driving, both of which were associated with single-car accidents. In the last month, his drinking had increased "a lot."

CONCLUSION

The application of empirically derived factors of risk to the individual case makes the assessment and prediction of future suicidal behavior more than gazing into a crystal ball. The goal of this exercise is not simply to be right in our predictions, although honing our skills toward that end ought to be an unending effort for us as suicidologists. Rather, the goal is to achieve a better understanding of the suicidal individual through both the fit and lack of fit between this individual's case and modal descriptors of risk. In this context, it is perhaps a truism that as we become more expert at something, we are increasingly likely to encounter the exceptions to the rule.

Furthermore, although clinical experience does appear to affect our ratings of risk by making us into better observers of risk, there is some question as to how our assessments may be reflected in our behavioral responses. Recent research (Engleman, 1990) suggests that a higher rating of risk (e.g., "danger to self") does not necessarily have a direct effect on decisions to detain a patient evaluated as being at high risk. Instead, such decisions may be more strongly influenced by personal characteristics of the decision maker (e.g., a historical tendency to detain or not to detain) and by the availability of hospital beds. When characteristics of the clinician and/or of the environment exert more control over clinical decision making than characteristics of the patient do, something is amiss with our model. To the extent that the suicidal individual becomes our mentor, let us hope that such variability in clinician behavior can be minimized as a contributor to effective treatment decisions. Ultimately, the goal of better prediction of risk is better intervention. The consequences of this process, then, should include a more effective help-giving system and more effectively functioning individuals.

REFERENCES

Berman, A. L. (1990). (Ed.). *Suicide prevention: Case consultations.* New York: Springer.

Berman, A. L., & Jobes, D. A. (1991). *Adolescent suicide: Assessment and intervention.* Washington, DC: American Psychological Association.

Engleman, N. B. (1990). *Involuntary commitment: An investigation of the clinician's decision-making.* Unpublished doctoral dissertation, American University.

Eyman, J. R., & Eyman, S. K. (1990). Suicide risk assessment instruments. In P. Cimbolic & D. A. Jobes (Eds.), *Youth suicide: Issues, assessment, and intervention* (pp. 9–32). Springfield, IL: Charles C Thomas.

Lawrence, P. R. (1953). The preparation of case material. In K. R. Andrews (Ed.), *The case method of teaching human relations and administration* (pp. 215–224). Cambridge, MA: Harvard University Press.

Litman, R. E., & Diller, J. (1985). Case studies in suicide. In M. L. Peck, N. L. Farberow, & R. E. Litman (Eds.), *Youth suicide* (pp. 48–70). New York: Springer.

Lorion, R. P., Price, R. H., & Eaton, W. W. (1989). The prevention of child and adolescent disorders: From theory to research. In D. Shaffer, I. Phillips, & N. B. Enzer (Eds.), *Prevention of mental disorders, alcohol, and other drug use in children and adolescents* (Office of Substance Abuse Prevention Monograph No. 2, DHHS Publication No. ADM-1646, pp. 55–98). Washington, DC: U.S. Government Printing Office.

Niswander, G. D., Casey, T. M., & Humphrey, J. A. (1973). *A panorama of suicide.* Springfield, IL: Charles C Thomas.

Rotheram-Borus, M. J., & Bradley, J. (1991). Triage model for suicidal runaways. *American Journal of Orthopsychiatry, 61,* 122–127.

Pfeffer, C. R. (1986). *The suicidal child.* New York: Guilford Press.

The Case Vignette Method of Suicide Assessment

Zigfrids T. Stelmachers, Ph.D.
University of Minnesota
Crisis Intervention Center, Minneapolis
Hennepin County, Minnesota, Medical Center
Robert E. Sherman, Ph.D.
Hennepin County, Minnesota, Office of Planning
and Development

This chapter summarizes the findings of two studies applying a case vignette method to suicide risk assessment. The impetus for these studies came mainly from a dissatisfaction with the day-by-day clinical utility of most suicide potential rating scales (Brown & Sheran, 1972; Litman, Farberow, Wold, & Brown, 1974; MacKinnon & Farberow, 1976; Motto, 1985). Most measuring instruments have the following shortcomings:

1. They are based on a *prediction* rather than an *assessment* model, despite the well-established fact that in most instances prediction of individual suicidal behavior is nearly impossible to achieve by the existing instruments (Pokorny, 1983; see Chapter 6, this volume). Also, the use of an actual suicidal event as a criterion of antecedent suicide risk is questionable, because very high-risk individuals sometimes survive suicide attempts and low-risk persons end up committing suicide. Furthermore, those who eventually attempt or commit suicide may do so many years later, in a state of mind and under circumstances that may have little relationship to the situation at the time suicide risk was assessed. Finally, a prediction based mainly on the characteristics of the suicidal person is made more difficult because we often lack knowledge and control over such variables as precipitating events, opportunity to act out a suicidal impulse, availability of the chosen method, and the effectiveness of intervening treatment.

2. Most rating scales are specific to certain defined populations, and therefore cannot be validly applied to very different groups of individuals or clinical settings (Brown & Sheran, 1972; Litman et al., 1974; Motto, 1985). The same measuring instrument is not likely to have the same applicability in a school, a prison, a psychiatric emergency service, or a medical–surgical hospital ward.

3. With few exceptions, the risk factors in suicide potential rating scales are not weighted. Two rating scales have used a rationally derived weighting system: a scale developed by the Los Angeles Suicide Prevention Center (Beck, Resnik, & Lettieri, 1974), and, more recently, one developed by Robert Yufit (Yufit, 1989). The only scale with an empirically derived weighting system is the Suicide Risk Assessment Scale developed by Motto (1985). The various response categories receive scores ranging from 0 to 100, in recognition of the differential contribution to suicide risk made by the various items.

4. Hardly any existing rating scale permits an interaction effect among the risk factors. Obviously, the meaning of any one risk factor may change, depending on the context of other factors, which may have a potentiating or an ameliorating effect.

5. The very nature of constructing rating scales by isolating the most powerful predictors of suicide does not permit the inclusion of microcosmic factors, situations, and events that may make a significant difference in individual cases.

6. Most writers advocate a subjective, global suicide risk assessment based on all available information, in addition to rating scales. In fact, clinical judgment is viewed as more important than scores derived from even the best empirically constructed instruments. To quote one group "the scales should supplement but not replace the clinical judgment of people with experience in any particular setting" (Litman et al., 1974, p. 157). Motto (1985, p. 147) states that his rating scale "is intended as a supplement to, not a substitute for, clinical judgment" and that "when the scale is not consistent with clinical judgment, clinical judgment should be given precedence" (p. 148).

If such clinical judgment is always indicated, it is important to make it as reliable as possible. In the first of the two studies to be reported here, an attempt was made to select certain vignettes as anchoring points for levels of suicide risk. These vignettes were intended to guide clinicians in their future judgments.

STUDY 1

In our first study, (Stelmachers & Sherman, 1990b) 33 charts containing recent global suicide risk ratings were selected from a crisis intervention center's active files. One of us (Stelmachers) summarized the record, attempting to include most of the data relevant to the assessment of suicide risk. The case summaries were then given to 19 crisis workers for 7-point short-term and long-term suicide risk ratings. The raters were, for the most part, very experienced mental health professionals, with more than half of them having in excess of 10 years' crisis intervention experience.

Means and standard deviations were computed for both the short-term and long-term suicide risk ratings. The mean risk ratings, as expected, differed significantly among the vignettes, but the variation in ratings within a given vignette across raters was also quite large (there were even instances when one staff member rated a vignette 1 [minimum risk], while another staff member gave the same vignette a 7 [maximum risk]). This within-vignette rating error represents a substantial level of unreliability. The intraclass correlation coefficient for the short-term risk ratings was found to be .49, and for long-term risk ratings it was a mere .22. Neither reliability would be considered very satisfactory for clinical purposes.

Short- and long-term risk ratings were always positively correlated across raters (.44) and across vignettes (.55). Although positive, these correlation coefficients support the widely held opinion that separate judgments need to be made for short-term and long-term risk. Perhaps the most encouraging finding was that the variation for the ratings of short-term high risk was considerably smaller than the variation for ratings of either short-term mild and moderate risk or long-term risk.

Not only did certain crisis workers tend to give consistently high or low ratings across vignettes, but they also differed considerably on the spread of their ratings. They also differed significantly in their willingness to rate the case histories. Some found all vignettes rateable, whereas others rejected as many as 10! Long-term risk was apparently harder to rate, as judged by the higher mean number of rejections (5.1 vs. 2.8 for short-term risk). The most common element in the content of vignettes rejected by most raters was the inability to complete a comprehensive evaluation at the time of the index visit (because the patient was intoxicated, uncooperative, incoherent, or otherwise difficult to interview).

Some methodological shortcomings of the study should be mentioned: (1) The numbers of case histories and raters were rather small; (2) the case histories were summarized by one individual using subjective judgment in the selection of relevant clinical material; (3) it is unknown which aspects of the case histories determined the ratings; (4) the case summaries were quite brief, and the kind of clues one may observe in face-to-face situations were not available to the raters; (5) the average age of the selected patients was quite low, and therefore the study did not adequately cover older individuals; (6) the issue of validity was not addressed; (7) there was a high number of females among the cases.

In the final phase of this study, five case histories with the lowest standard deviations were selected to represent each of three categories: "low," "moderate," and "high" short-term risk (see Appendix 13.1). These vignettes were intended to guide clinicians in their future ratings of suicidal individuals. In this admittedly rather cumbersome process, the crisis worker has to read the case histories, somehow integrate them, and establish some similarity among common elements in the vignettes and characteristics of the case to be judged. This process is quite similar to the one used by psychologists to interpret the Minnesota Multiphasic Personality Inventory (MMPI) by means of comparing a given profile to a collection of profiles with brief case histories attached. The clinicians must select profiles of sufficient similarity to the index profile and use the content of case histories common to them in their test interpretation. Rating scales that emphasize commonalities to begin with avoid this extra step, and, at the very least, are more convenient to use.

STUDY 2

In our second study (Stelmachers & Sherman, 1990a), the following questions were addressed: (1) Would the use of anchoring vignettes increase the reliability of clinicians' judgments of short-term suicide risk? (2) What was the case history content that led to the ratings? (3) Would the raters show greater agreement on their preference for the clinical disposition of these cases than on their suicide risk ratings? (4) To what extent would the suicide risk ratings be correlated with clinical disposition preferences?

Usefulness of the Vignettes in Making Ratings

Of the original 19 raters, 17 were available 2 years after the original study to perform a second short-term risk rating on 15 sample vignettes (the ones not used as anchor points from the original sample of 33 case histories). It should be remembered that the raters made judgments of relatively lower reliability on these 15 vignettes in the earlier study; that is why they were not selected as anchor points. Therefore, one can conclude that these vignettes must have been more difficult to rate.

As predicted, with the use of the benchmark vignettes as a guide, the raters were able to reduce the variability in the ratings. This reduction was modest but statistically significant at the .01 level. When asked whether the anchor vignettes influenced their subsequent ratings, the great majority of crisis workers indicated that they were "somewhat" guided by them (a mean score of 5.2 on a scale of 1 to 10, 10 denoting "considerable influence" and 1 "no influence").

Content Determining Ratings

In addition to rating the suicide risk, the clinicians were also asked to identify the content in each vignette that mainly determined the rating.

Vignettes with low and high suicide risk ratings were selected. For "low" suicide risk, five vignettes were identified. Some raters listed as few as 1 factor, some as many as 4 (mean of 2.1). Three cases were selected to represent high suicide risk. The number of factors listed ranged from 2 to 8 (mean of 4.8). Although the mean number of factors for high-risk cases was somewhat higher, it is interesting to note that the number of factors listed as determining suicide risk ratings was very small, even considering the brevity of the case histories. One possible explanation is that even with more extensive knowledge about patients, we may base our judgments on a few items that, in a particular context, assume special significance. Such an approach would be more similar to a "critical item" methodology, as compared to responding to every item on a standard rating scale.

The results were not particularly surprising; certainly most of the high-risk factors listed could be easily found in most rating scales. Of course, if case histories could be *completely* summarized by a list of risk factors, the latter would represent an equally valid and more convenient method of assessment. The advantage of the former, if any, lies in the power of idiosyncratic content to shape the final judgment. The raters may or may not be able to identify such content explicitly, assign weight to it, or describe the process by which it is combined with other and more universally accepted risk factors. The following case vignette factors were judged to contribute to low short-term suicide risk ratings (with decreasing frequency): patient described as manipulative; absence of concrete suicide plan; problem chronic, patient at baseline; explicit denial of suicide intent; diagnoses of personality or adjustment disorder; patient currently in treatment; history of suicide gestures with high rescuability. Case vignette factors contributing to high short-term suicide risk ratings (also with decreasing frequency) were as follows: prior serious suicide attempt; depression, with vegetative signs; lethal suicide plan; feelings of hopelessness and worthlessness; symptoms of schizophrenia and/or paranoia; significant other's suicide; persistent suicidal thoughts; recent breakup of marriage; impulsivity; out-of-control feeling; sleep deprivation; physical illness.

Perhaps one of the more interesting findings was the use of an interaction effect among factors, which one typically does not find in instruments measuring suicide potential. For one of the cases, five raters combined a previous serious attempt with a particular precipitant—namely, the breakup of the patient's marriage—because a similar precipitant had led to an earlier suicide attempt.

Crisis Management Procedures and Clinical Dispositions

The clinicians were also asked to make judgments about the appropriateness of the following interventions for each case vignette: legal holds, seclusion, physical restraint, psychiatric consultation, and psychotropic medications. In addition, they rank-ordered the following dispositions in terms of their desirability, as long as they were considered to be within clinically acceptable range: hospitalization, inpatient detoxification, crisis home program, outpatient referral, and crisis intervention and release.

Tables 13.1 and 13.2 show the interrater agreement across 17 raters and 15 vignettes for crisis management procedure choices and proposed clinical dispositions. The kappa statistic (which may be interpreted as an intraclass correlation coefficient) was selected because it takes into account chance agreement and is generalizable to the use of multiple raters (Fliess, 1981). The kappa values we obtained, however, would be considered to indicate very poor agreement (e.g., less than .40), often in cases where our intuitive inspection of the data suggested very good agreement. A good example of the apparent discrepancy is seen in the results for the item "Would you request a psychiatric consultation?" Across raters and vignettes, this item was rated "yes" 91% of the time. In four of the vignettes, the "yes" was unanimous. In another seven vignettes, there was only one "no." This looked like a high order of agreement, yet the kappa statistic turned out to be a miniscule .07. How should this be interpreted?

What the kappa statistic did not take into account in this case was the evident fact that there was a high order of agreement in requesting a psychiatric consultation, *regardless of case history content*. Instead, the kappa emphasized the fact that the (22) instances where psychiatric consultation was not thought desirable were not focused on a few cases, but were scattered around among 11 different vignettes. Thus, although raters seemed to agree that psychiatric consultation was indicated for all but one or two of the vignettes, they did not agree well on which one or two vignettes to exclude.

The kappa statistic effectively discounted the amount of agreement that would occur by chance alone if raters all used the same base rate in making

TABLE 13.1. Reliability of Crisis Management Procedure Choices (across 17 Raters and 15 Vignettes)

Crisis management procedures	Average rate of choice (%)	Reliability of choice	
		κ	κ^*
Legal hold	68%	.22	.38
Medications	22%	.22	.49
Seclusion	69%	.23	.38
Restraints	53%	.24	.28
Psychiatric Consultation	91%	.07	.71

Note. From *Clinical Consequences of Suicide Risk Ratings* by Z. T. Stelmachers and R. E. Sherman, 1990, paper presented at the annual meeting of the American Association of Suicidology, New Orleans.

TABLE 13.2. Reliability of Proposed Clinical Dispositions (across 17 Raters and 15 Vignettes)

Preferred clinical disposition	First or second preference (%)	Reliability κ	κ^*
Hospitalization	64%	.15	.27
Inpatient detoxification	15%	.81	.92
Crisis home program	26%	.43	.60
Outpatient referral	34%	.15	.27
Crisis intervention and release	35%	.23	.35

Note. From *Clinical Consequences of Suicide Risk Ratings* by Z. T. Stelmachers and R. E. Sherman, 1990, paper presented at the annual meeting of the American Association of Suicidology, New Orleans.

their judgments. To correct this problem, we computed a modified form of kappa, kappa*. This statistic assumes minimal prior knowledge and base rate choices that are expected to be equally likely. The kappa* gives credit to clinicians for using a common base rate (which, after all, can be viewed as some form of clinical knowledge of the patient population characteristics). The difference between the outcomes of using kappa and kappa* demonstrates the importance of conceptual clarity in discussing the reliability of these measures.

As one can readily see from Table 13.1, just as in the case of suicide risk ratings, overall agreement on the clinical desirability of various crisis management procedures must be considered poor. Even when kappa* was used, the highest agreement was on obtaining psychiatric consultation. This is a rather "cheap" agreement, since such consultation is readily available, certainly does no harm, and could benefit almost everyone seen at a crisis center. The next highest agreement was on *not* giving psychotropic medications. Again, relatively few patients at the crisis center in question receive medications, and there is a general philosophy that discourages use of medications as a means of crisis management. It is likely that this philosophy, to a large extent, would override individual patient characteristics as described in the case histories.

Table 13.2 shows that the best agreement on clinical dispositions was obtained for inpatient detoxification, though this option was infrequently chosen. This is not surprising, since the presence of significant current intoxication was clearly mentioned in only two vignettes. Thus, if someone needed to be in a safe place and was also intoxicated, inpatient detoxification would be the logical choice, and it would not make much sense otherwise.

In sum, there was considerable variation across vignettes and across procedures and dispositions. There was good agreement on *some* procedures and dispositions, but not on others. Also, as might be expected, some vignettes were rated more consistently than others. From the current analysis, it is difficult to determine which factor contributed most significantly to the variance: the content of the case vignettes, the characteristics of raters, or the content of the ratings (i.e., suicide risk, hospitalization, need for legal holds, etc.). A more detailed analysis of variance seems futile in the light of the considerable variability of the ratings.

When the relationship of suicide risk ratings with crisis management procedures was examined, it turned out that, as expected, there was a strong and significant relationship between suicide risk and legal holds (.83), seclusion (.81), and restraint (.80). (These crisis management procedures themselves were also highly intercorrelated.) There were also substantial correlations between suicide risk ratings and such clinical dispositions as hospitalization (.64) and a preference for crisis intervention and release (−.63), although these latter correlations did not achieve statistical significance.

Another way to look at the relationship between suicide risk ratings and clinical decision making is to subdivide clinical dispositions into groups of low and high "restrictiveness." Low-restrictiveness dispositions included outpatient referral and crisis intervention and release; high-restrictiveness dispositions included hospitalization and inpatient detoxification. Table 13.3 again demonstrates that clinical dispositions are related to the perceived suicide risk. As one would expect, the clinicians in this study were more apt to indicate preference for low-restrictiveness dispositions for low-risk patients, and high-restrictiveness dispositions for high-risk patients; moderate-risk patients occupied an intermediate position. The product–moment correlation between suicide risk ratings and restrictiveness of clinical dispositions was found to be .81, which was statistically significant at the .001 level. It is clear that perceived suicide risk plays a very significant role in determining clinicians' treatment choices.

Since the best agreement in the first study was on *high* short-term suicide risk, it seemed possible that there might be greater agreement also on procedures and dispositions for these high-risk cases. To examine this hypothesis, we selected vignettes on which there was good agreement among raters for individual procedures and dispositions. Good agreement was defined as 80% of raters or more endorsing or not endorsing a certain procedure or disposition. Three vignettes were identified that showed *generally* higher overall agreement, and four vignettes were identified with *generally* poorer agreement. The data indeed confirmed the hypothesis: When we examined the mean suicide risk ratings across raters, the high-agreement vignettes had a higher mean suicide risk rating (5.13) than the low-agreement vignettes (3.79). The mean suicide risk rating for all 15 vignettes was 4.25. Thus, the high-risk suicide cases showed a higher degree of agreement on crisis management procedures to be used and clinical

TABLE 13.3. Relationship of Suicide Risk with Restrictiveness
of Clinical Disposition

Suicide risk[a]	Percentage of total	Restrictiveness[b]	
		Low	High
Low	14	28	6
Moderate	59	55	84
High	27	2	61

Note. From *Clinical Consequences of Suicide Risk Ratings* by Z. T. Stelmachers and R. E. Sherman, 1990, paper presented at the annual meeting of the American Association of Suicidology, New Orleans.
[a]"Low" equals ratings of 1 and 2; "moderate" equals ratings of 3, 4, and 5; and "high" equals ratings of 6 and 7 (on a 1-to-7 scale).
[b]The numbers represent rater-vignette combinations, i.e., 28 low/low = 28 such combinations with risk ratings of 1 or 2 combined with outpatient referral or crisis intervention. "Low" equals outpatient referral or crisis intervention and release. "High" equals hospitalization or inpatient detoxification. Crisis home program is scored "high" if it is second choice to either hospitalization or detoxification; it is called "low" if it is second choice to outpatient referral or crisis intervention and release.

dispositions to be made. One reasonable conclusion would be that there is higher consistency in judgments about cases that are more emergent, critical, or extreme.

One of the original questions asked was this: "Are judgments about preferred crisis management procedures and clinical dispositions more reliable than judgments about suicide risk?" One way to answer the question is to compare the intraclass correlation coefficients, as measured by kappa, for all these variables. For this comparison, kappa rather than kappa* was selected because it is statistically more rigorous. Kappa for suicide risk was found to be .42. The only kappas larger than that were for inpatient detoxification (.80) and the crisis home program (.44). None of the other procedures or dispositions reached a kappa higher than .25. Thus, with the exception of inpatient detoxification and the crisis home program, there was better agreement on the suicide risk ratings than on the clinical procedures and dispositions. The hoped-for improvement in clinicians' reliability in making clinical dispositions over assessing suicide risk did not materialize.

SUMMARY OF THE TWO STUDIES

The findings indicate disappointingly low reliability of clinical judgments about the selection of crisis management procedures and clinical dispositions. This is most disturbing when it comes to such important clinical dispositions as hospitalization. For the most part, judgments about the desirability of various procedures and dispositions were not significantly more reliable than judgments about suicide risk. However, there was a quite significant relationship, as expected, between short-term suicide risk ratings on the one hand, and the choice of certain clinical procedures and dispositions (e.g., legal holds, seclusion, and restraints) on the other. The relationship was also relatively strong between suicide risk ratings and preference for hospitalization, but it did not reach statistical significance.

How can we explain the poor reliability of clinicians' judgments? One possible answer is that the vignettes were very short, with highly selected content, and the clinicians did not have an opportunity either to hear or to see the patients. On the other hand, in a crisis center setting, the information obtained about patients is often very scanty; extensive social histories, results from batteries of psychological tests, or even the results of a single test are typically not available. Furthermore, the literature suggests that clinical judgments crystallize very quickly and are based predominantly on information obtained early during the evaluation process. Nor is there a strong proven relationship between the *amount* of information provided and the accuracy of clinical judgment.

The five case histories provided in Chapter 12 of this book are somewhat longer and contain significantly more social history data, but the relevance of this type of information for suicide assessment and clinical decision making is largely unknown. Mental status may be more important than social history, but this has not been convincingly demonstrated. In any case, what is available to the therapist is typically not available to the crisis worker (and this, by the way, is a good reason to develop different evaluation techniques for both settings).

The two studies certainly indicate that when good agreement among clinicians exists, it seems to be based mainly on general response tendencies, which in turn are generated by knowledge about base rates in a given population or by adherence to prevailing clinical philosophy, policies, and traditional practice. Some earlier studies about clinical judgment have amply demonstrated that social perceptions are more a function of internal frames of reference than of specific stimuli (Gage, 1951); that global dispositions appear to account for much of the variance in accuracy scores (Gage & Cronbach, 1955; and that social perception is dominated far more by what the judge brings to it than by what he takes in during it (Gage & Cronbach, 1955).

When clinicians attempt to be more differential in their judgments and to depart from these global response tendencies, they may gain a few points for *some* subjects, but lose accuracy for others. Whatever the clinicians gain by having access to more detailed and specific information is almost balanced out by losses in accuracy, probably caused by a partial abandonment of their more global and powerful response tendencies (Stelmachers & McHugh, 1964). If all this is true, one avenue of improving our judgments as clinicians would be to study our population norms and base rates, and to use this knowledge explicitly and deliberately in our decision making. In addition, we should study in greater detail which *critical content*—not just a cluster of risk factors—sets off such responses as "This is a high-risk patient who should be hospitalized."

THE FIVE CASE HISTORIES

Whether the knowledge of more detailed information in fact leads to more reliable or valid judgments, it certainly is clinically richer than a list of risk factors. At least intuitively, one feels that such clinical detail is superior to the bloodless content of a rating scale. The only difference between the two methods may end up being the method by which the critical content is generated—either by empirical studies or in the clinician's mind. To judge by the very small number of risk factors listed by the clinicians we studied as determining their ratings of suicide risk, it appears that some abstraction takes place to reduce complex clinical pictures to a manageable number of variables.

Still, if we agree that subjective clinical judgments are always indicated, we cannot entirely rely on even the best available rating scales. This brings us right back to a case history approach. John Z, for instance, would receive positive scores on only 6 out of the 16 clearly scorable risk factors listed by Berman in Chapter 12. A case can be made for him as the most imminently suicidal individual among the five, but he would receive the lowest rating if only a rating scale approach were used. John's case illustrates other advantages of the case history method. Even empirically derived *normative* weights for various risk factors cannot achieve the more refined *idiosyncratic* weights for such factors when it comes to individual cases. For instance, John's depression was of a particular quality and severity. It was described by his therapist as "major" and was accompanied by rather severe vegetative signs, including a 20-pound weight loss in 2 months. Also, the *sequence* or *progression* of events may be significant, such as the increase of John's depression during May and June. Finally, the serious concern of a significant other would not be typically found as an item in a rating scale (John's wife, Mary, sought a second opinion and requested involuntary hospitalization for her husband).

The "suicide ideation" is qualitatively quite different between Heather B and Faye C, although both would receive only 1 point if a rating scale were used. Although Heather described herself as having a "suicide risk life," and her writings and drawings "reflected thoughts of suicide," she denied any suicide plan, had no vegetative signs of depression, and seemed more self-injurious than suicidal. Faye, on the other hand, was suffering from severe mental illness, was floridly psychotic, and was scared of what would happen to her; suicide might appear to her to be an escape from future torment.

The case of José G illustrates the importance of context. To note simply that he suffered a physical injury and became unemployed would miss the essence of his predicament. José was a self-sufficient, independent, responsible, and proud man who became a "defeated man," reduced to "puttering and tinkering around the house"; he felt that he was becoming a burden, whereas he used to derive his sense of self-worth from helping others in the past. In a dependent, passive individual, the same injury and unemployment would very likely not produce such a psychologically devastating response.

If the individual path of a potentially suicidal individual is unpredictable; if existing rating scales do not provide the necessary clinical detail; if clinicians base their judgments mostly on internal response tendencies, even if given such detail; if subjective judgment always enters (and should enter) the evaluation process, in addition to whatever measuring instrument one uses; and if such judgments are shown to be quite unreliable, apart from validity—how are we to proceed in improving our assessment skills? We certainly need instruments with weighted factors, and the weights should ideally be idiosyncratic for each individual. We have to take into account interaction effects among factors and the context in which these factors operate. There may even be potentiating effects on top of the additive effects of a cluster of risk factors. Perhaps we should also study individual sequences of events, taking into account the progression of one psychological state or situation to another.

CHAOS THEORY: A DIRECTION FOR THE FUTURE?

At this point, it seems that we should stop concentrating our efforts on developing more and more refined assessment instruments. We have probably gone as far as we can with such instruments, especially if they are based on a linear prediction model, and only minor advances can be expected by further methodological refinement. Instead, we should probably concentrate on studying the entire assessment enterprise and its component parts. Otherwise, there seems to be little chance for a significant breakthrough. Sequential patterns, in addition to cross-sectional patterns, would enable us to propose intervention strategies appropriate to various points in the paths of suicidal individuals.

Chaos theory, which is becoming more and more widely accepted as an alternative to a strictly deterministic Newtonian science, may provide a radically different approach (Gleick, 1987). Many processes in nature are discovered to be chaotic (i.e., fundamentally irregular and unpredictable), and yet, when taken in the aggregate, show underlying repeatable and fixed patterns that can be geometrically represented. Such "chaos" is thus not completely random or disorganized, but has been described as "deterministic chaos," with a kind of constrained randomness that permits the coexistence of Newtonian determinism and unpredictability. The patterns that are detected in chaotic processes may suggest relationships where none were previously suspected, but chaos also imposes fundamental and absolute limits on prediction. Therefore, precise predictability cannot *in principle* be achieved by further gathering of information or reductionistic breaking down of a system into smaller and smaller parts.

One reason for this essential unpredictability is something called "the butterfly effect" (Lorenz, 1963). This effect postulates that small differences in a microcosm at the point of impact are amplified as the process unfolds, and eventually can lead to major macrocosmic changes that cannot be deduced from the knowledge of the initial event. Thus, Lorenz concluded that accurate long-range weather forecasts are impossible because the meteorological system is too sensitive to minor changes (e.g., a butterfly flapping its wings) in a system's component parts (temperature, in this case).

It may be this butterfly effect, in addition to the well-known base rate problem, that hampers our ability to predict suicidal events. In that way, it is similar to predicting a tornado's formation and path, a heart attack, the shape of clouds, or the motion of water in a stream. Tiny random events, in the context of other relevant component parts of the system (such as general risk factors for suicide), can in time become critical events with the power to lead sequentially to very magnified outcomes (such as suicide). Perhaps we should study these sequences and try to isolate the patterns that govern deterministically the random surface behaviors.

Nonlinear deterministic chaos is observed as a normal feature in the functioning of the heart and the nervous system, for instance. As a matter of fact, irregularities are found to be associated with health, whereas states of illness seem to decrease variability (Goldberger, Rigney, & West, 1990). It is indeed intriguing to view chaos as a universal condition of nature that allows for progress to take place. The following quotation exemplifies this kind of theorizing:

> Even the process of intellectual progress relies on the injection of new ideas and on new ways of connecting old ideas. Innate creativity may have an underlying chaotic process that selectively amplifies small fluctuations and models them into macroscopic coherent mental states that are experienced as thoughts. In some cases, the thoughts may be decisions, or what are perceived to be the exercise of will. In this light, chaos provides a mechanism that allows for free will within a world governed by deterministic laws. (Crutchfield, Farmer, Packard, & Shaw, 1986, p. 57).

One quite disturbing thought emerges from these considerations. If chaos exists to allow adaptability, flexibility, and creativity, and moreover is associated with health, suicide itself may be an aberrant consequence of such a system because it does allow the human organism to cope with the exigencies of an unpredictable and changing environment. Like evil, suicide may be the price we have to pay for the constructive use by nature of chaos. The only way to eliminate suicide would be to reduce chaos and the creativity that flows from it. This philosophical analysis is of little help at the clinical level, but it may challenge some of our basic assumptions about suicide prevention, as well as suicide assessment.

REFERENCES

Beck, A. T., Resnik, H. L. P., & Lettieri, D. J. (Eds.). (1974). *The prediction of suicide.* Bowie, MD: Charles Press.

Brown, T. R., & Sheran, T. J. (1972). Suicide prediction: A review. *Suicide and Life-Threatening Behavior, 2,* 67–98.

Crutchfield, J. P., Farmer, J. D., Packard, N. H., & Shaw, R. S. (1986). Chaos. *Scientific American, 255*(6), 45–57.

Fliess, J. L. (1981). *Statistical methods for rates and proportions* (2nd ed.). New York: Wiley.

Gage, N. L. (1951). *Explorations in the understanding of others.* Paper presented at the 16th Annual Guidance Conference, Purdue University, West Lafayette, Indiana.

Gage, N. L., & Cronbach, L. J. (1955). Conceptual and methodological problems in interpersonal perception. *Psychology Review, 62,* 411–422.

Gleick, J. (1987). *Chaos: Making a new science.* New York: Viking Penguin.

Goldberger, A. L., Rigney, D. R., & West, B. J. (1990). Chaos and fractals in human physiology. *Scientific American, 262*(2), 43–49.

Litman, E. L., Farberow, N. L., Wold, C. I., & Brown, T. R. (1974). Prediction models of suicidal behaviors. In A. T. Beck, H. L. P. Resnik, & D. J. Lettieri (Eds.), *The prediction of suicide* (pp. 141–159). Bowie, MD: Charles Press.

Lorenz, E. N. (1963). Deterministic nonperiodic flow. *Journal of Atmospheric Sciences, 20,* 130–141.

MacKinnon, D. R., & Farberow, N. L. (1976). An assessment of the utility of suicide prediction. *Suicide and Life-Threatening Behavior, 6,* 86–91.

Motto, J. A. (1985). Preliminary field-testing of a risk estimator of suicide. *Suicide and Life-Threatening Behavior, 15,* 139–150.

Pokorny, A. D. (1983). Prediction of suicide in psychiatric patients: Report of a prospective study. *Archives of General Psychiatry, 40,* 249–257.

Stelmachers, Z. T., & McHugh, R. B. (1964). Contribution of stereotyped and individualized information to predictive accuracy. *Journal of Consulting Psychology, 28,* 234–242.

Stelmachers, Z. T., & Sherman, R. E. (1990a). *Clinical consequences of suicide risk ratings.* Paper presented at the annual meeting of the American Association of Suicidology, New Orleans.

Stelmachers, Z. T., & Sherman, R. E. (1990b). Use of case vignettes in suicide risk assessment. *Suicide and Life-Threatening Behavior, 20*(1), 65–84.

Yufit, R. (1989). Developing a suicide screening instrument for adolescents and young adults. In M. Rosenberg & K. Baer (Eds.), *Report of the Secretary's Task Force on Youth Suicide. Volume 4: Strategies for the Prevention of Youth Suicide.* Washington, DC: U.S. Department of Health and Human Services.

APPENDIX 13.1

SELECTED REPRESENTATIVE SHORT-TERM RISK VIGNETTES

LOW RISK

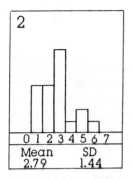

26-year-old white female phoned her counselor, stated that she "might take pills," then hung up and kept phone off the hook. Counselor called police, and patient was brought to the Crisis Intervention Center (CIC) on a transportation hold. Patient angry, denies suicidal intent, refused evaluation. Described as "selectively mute." Diagnostic impression: dependent and/or borderline personality.

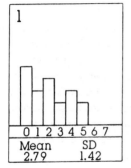

37-year-old white female, self-referred. Stated plan is to drive her car off a bridge. Precipitant seems to be verbal abuse by her boss; after talking to her nightly for hours, he suddenly refused to talk to her. As a result, patient feels angry and hurt, threatened to kill herself. She is also angry at her mother, who will not let patient smoke or bring men to their home. Current alcohol level is .15; patient is confused, repetitive, and ataxic. History reveals a previous suicide attempt (overdose) 7 years ago, which resulted in hospitalization. After spending the night at CIC and sobering, patient denies further suicidal intent.

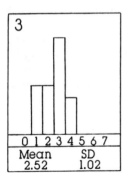

17-year-old Native American female, referred from a detoxification center for an evaluation of suicide risk. Patient lacerated her wrist with a piece of glass while intoxicated. Now regrets the attempt and denies being suicidal. Has been depressed for approximately 1 month, but there are no vegetative signs of depression. Self-esteem is impaired, however. Patient recently lost boyfriend and has difficulties coping with it; did not finish school and is unable to provide for herself. There was one previous suicide attempt *exactly* 1 year ago (cut wrist); this attempt also occurred following the loss of a boyfriend. Patient is dependent on alcohol and marijuana and has had chemical dependency treatment in the past. She also received 1 month of counseling following the previous suicide attempt. Diagnostic impression: atypical depression.

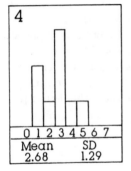

19-year-old female, Native American, referred from the Emergency Room with lacerations on both forearms requiring 26 stitches. Patient calls her suicide attempt a "mistake" and a "gesture." Denies being depressed and having any further suicidal impulses ("It's not worth it"). Precipitant: argument with boyfriend (jealousy). Patient cut herself "to hurt him." Patient is cooperative in the interview, and her cousin confirms the patient's story.

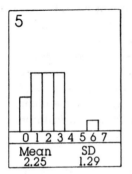

16-year-old Native American female, self-referred following an overdose of 12 aspirins. Precipitant: could not tolerate rumors at school that she and another girl are sharing the same boyfriend. Denies being suicidal at this time ("I won't do it again; I learned my lesson"). Reports that she has always had difficulty expressing her feelings. In the interview, is quiet, guarded, and initially quite reluctant to talk. Diagnostic impression: adjustment disorder.

MODERATE RISK

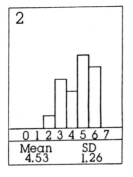

0 1 2 3 4 5 6 7
Mean SD
4.05 1.31

49-year-old white female brought by police on a transportation hold following threats to overdose on aspirin (initially telephoned CIC and was willing to give her address). Patient feels trapped and abused, can't cope at home with her schizophrenic sister. Wants to be in the hospital and continues to feel like killing herself. Husband indicates that the patient has been threatening to shoot him and her daughter but probably has no gun. Recent arrest for disorderly conduct (threatened police with a butcher knife). History of aspirin overdose 3 years ago. In the interview, patient is cooperative; appears depressed, anxious, helpless, and hopeless. Appetite and sleep are down, and so is her self-esteem. Is described as "anhedonic." Alcohol level: .12.

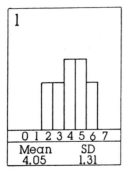

0 1 2 3 4 5 6 7
Mean SD
4.53 1.26

27-year-old Cambodian female called the suicide line after ingesting 20 sleeping pills last night. Following the ingestion, she induced vomiting, slept until morning, and then called CIC. Patient still feels suicidal, refused to give identifying information. Phone call was traced, and police brought the patient to CIC. Patient still feels frustrated and hopeless, but states that the attempt was impulsive. Stress: has been recently fired from her job, broke up with boyfriend, and has chronic painful back injury. Patient was pregnant by her boyfriend and had a recent abortion. He has abused her physically. There is a history of two previous suicide attempts, one at age 18, the other 18 months ago. Currently in treatment in two groups (one of them for sexual assault). Poison Control Center informed CIC that patient is medically safe.

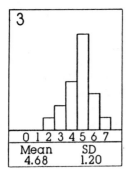

0 1 2 3 4 5 6 7
Mean SD
4.68 1.20

23-year-old white male, self-referred. Patient bought a gun 2 months ago to kill himself and claims to have the gun and four shells in his car (police found the gun but no shells). Patient reports having planned time and place for suicide several times in the past. States that he cannot live any more with his "emotional pain" since his wife left him 3 years ago. This pain has increased during the last week, but the patient cannot pinpoint any precipitant. Patient has a history of chemical dependency, but has been sober for 20 months and currently goes to AA.

There is one previous psychiatric admission. During the marriage, the patient beat his wife severely several times a week. She is currently in another relationship, and there is little likelihood of her returning to the patient. In the interview, patient appears depressed and irritable. Is angry, hostile, and threatening ("You bitch, I hate women"). Reports no sleep or appetite disturbance.

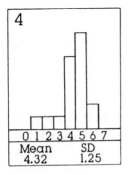

22-year-old black male referred to CIC from the Emergency Room on a transportation hold. He referred himself to the Emergency Room after making fairly deep cuts on his wrists requiring nine stitches. Current stress is recent breakup with his girlfriend and loss of job. Has developed depressive symptoms for the last 2 months, including social withdrawal, insomnia, anhedonia, and decreased appetite. Blames his sister for the breakup with girlfriend. Makes threats to sister ("I will slice up that bitch, she is dead when I get out"). Patient is an alcoholic who just completed court-ordered chemical dependency treatment lasting 3 weeks. He is also on parole for attempted rape. There is a history of previous suicide attempts and assaultive behavior, which led to the patient being jailed. In the interview, patient is vague regarding recent events and history. He denies intent to kill himself but admits to still being quite ambivalent about it. Diagnostic impression: antisocial personality.

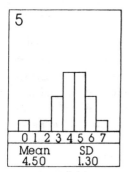

24-year-old white female brought by police on hold. Patient was found "hanging from a bridge." Precipitant was an argument with her husband. Has been married for 9 months; relationship is abusive, with daily arguments and partners pulling each other's hair. Patient just hitchhiked here from Florida. Patient states, "If I can't be with my husband, I don't want to live." In the interview, is described as impulsive, immature, histrionic, angry, hostile, and demanding. Shouts at the interviewer. Also appears to have low self-esteem. Diagnostic impression: mixed personality disorder.

HIGH RISK

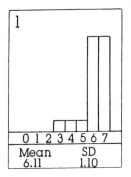

Mean 6.11   SD 1.10

19-year-old white male found by roommate in a "sluggish" state following the ingestion of 10 sleeping pills (Sominex) and one bottle of whiskey. Recently has been giving away his possessions and has written a suicide note. After being brought to the Emergency Room, declares that he will do it again. Blood alcohol level: .23. For the last 3 or 4 weeks there has been sleep and appetite disturbance, with a 15-pound weight loss and subjective feelings of depression. Diagnostic impression: adjustment disorder with depressed mood versus major depressive episode. Patient refused hospitalization.

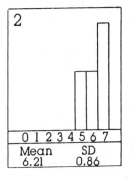

Mean 6.21   SD 0.86

21-year-old male, foreign graduate student, brought to CIC by friends and pastor. After informing his friends that he planned to jump off a bridge, he actually went there and had to be physically restrained from jumping. Had written several suicide notes, one willing his computer to a friend, another to a different friend stating that the patient would be dead by the time his note would be opened. Describes himself as being quite depressed, with low energy, poor sleep and appetite, and persistent suicidal ideation. Precipitant seems to have been his girlfriend's breaking off their engagement 4 days ago. He has a psychiatric history of several years, but refuses to reveal details about it. Exhibits some grandiosity, paranoid mentation, anger, agitation, and irritability. Appears to be somewhat manic but not depressed. Denies acute plan to commit suicide and is threatening to sue CIC for being detained.

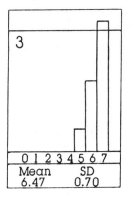

Mean 6.47   SD 0.70

25-year-old white male referred from the Emergency Room following a suicide attempt with gas and strangulation. Patient turned on the gas and tied a towel around his neck until he turned blue and passed out. His roommate was present while he turned on the gas. Emergency Room classifies this medically as a high-lethality suicide attempt. At CIC patient maintains that he will still hang himself, given the opportunity. Precipitant seems to be the patient finding out 1 week ago that his girlfriend was dating his friend. Other stressors include a recent move, financial problems, and being on probation at work for absenteeism. History reveals an overdose at the age of 15, which led to psychiatric hospitalization. Diagnostic impression: adjustment disorder with depression, plus questionable alcohol abuse.

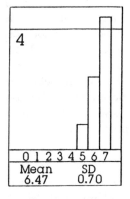

30-year-old white male brought from his place of employment by a personnel representative. Patient has been thinking of suicide "all the time" because he "can't cope." Has a knot in his stomach; sleep and appetite are down (sleeps only 3 hours per night); and plans either to shoot himself, jump off a bridge, or drive recklessly. Precipitant: constant fighting with his wife leading to a recent breakup (there is a long history of mutual verbal/physical abuse). There is a history of a serious suicide attempt: patient jumped off a ledge and fractured both legs; the precipitant for that attempt was a previous divorce. There is a history of chemical dependency with two courses of treatment. There is no current problem with alcohol or drugs. Patient is tearful, shaking, frightened, feeling hopeless, and at high risk for impulsive acting out. He states that life isn't worthwhile.

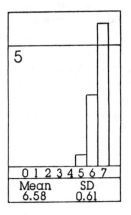

32-year-old white male referred from the Emergency Room. Patient was in the process of overdosing when he was called by a friend, who arranged for the ambulance to bring patient to CIC. The patient took 72 over-the-counter sleeping pills and 10 or 15 aspirin tablets. Patient wrote a long suicide note bequeathing belongings, expressing guilt about not doing well on his job, feeling hopeless about a "hereditary thinking disorder." Feels that no one can help him; suffers from low self-esteem ("I'm a misfit"). Three nights ago, made a suicide attempt with Navane and aspirin but woke up by himself in the morning. Lives by himself. No obvious immediate precipitant, but the patient's mother died 6 months ago. Currently in therapy and also has a psychiatrist.

Specific Predictors
of Suicide

CHAPTER 14

Mental Disorders, Psychiatric Patients, and Suicide

Bryan L. Tanney,
M.D., F.R.C.P.(C.)
University of Calgary

In the later years of the 17th century, the legal and religious proscriptions against "self-death" began to decline (MacDonald, 1977). This marked an important change in society's understanding of suicide. In place of such concepts as "willful badness" or "possession by spirits," "unreasoning passion" and "idiotic incomprehension" were recognized as possible explanations for self-destruction. Various authors even proposed some subtypes of insanity that might be associated with suicide. This move toward madness as the explanation for suicide allowed social institutions and caring persons to usher in the "age of Bedlam." For the next three centuries, with the exception of a few authors like Hales and Donne who contemplated the rationality of suicide, suicidal persons would by definition be considered insane.

In 1897 Durkheim (1897/1951) proposed an alternative explanation: Suicide is not a process, but an accident of the social-societal situation of the person. From this perspective, suicide is *not* correlated with the prevalence of mental disorders, nor is there any clear relationship with different forms of mental disorder. These beliefs—in suicide as insanity or in suicide as an outcome of our place in society—are most readily identified with either medicine (psychiatry) or sociology. These very different perspectives have dominated and dichotomized our thinking about the relationship between psychiatric disorders and suicide throughout the 20th century. Increasingly, researchers, clinicians, and caregivers have recognized that the framework for study and for treatment of this often preventable cause of death must accommodate both perspectives.

This chapter explores the value of psychiatric disorders as a predictive variable for suicide by addressing recent evidence concerning the relationship between psychiatric disorders and suicide. This approach is not unique, and the chapter freely cites existing works that summarize various aspects of the topic. Specifically, it builds from Miles's (1977) overview of the literature by reviewing studies since that date and by considering other works not covered in that review. A general discussion of the definition and classification of psychiatric disorders and of suicidal behaviors is provided at the outset. Then recent studies investigating a link or association between psychiatric disorders and suicide are summarized, with special attention to the relationships between specific disorders and suicide. Various explanations addressing the nature of the association or relationship are proposed. Finally, some broad conclusions about the value of psychiatric information in the assessment and prediction of suicide are offered.

THE DIAGNOSIS OF MENTAL DISORDERS
Definition and Classification

Because many disciplines are active in the study and treatment of persons at risk of suicide, the more generic term "mental disorder" and not "psychiatric disorder" is preferred. Mental disorders are clinically significant behavioral or psychological syndromes or patterns that are a manifestation of behavioral, psychological, or biological dysfunction (American Psychiatric Association, 1987). They are associated with present distress or disability, or with an increased risk of suffering death, pain, or disability. They are more severe than McWhinney's "disorders of living." "Disorders" are only one of a number of ways in which psychopathology can be described; other approaches involve "signs," "symptoms," "syndromes," or "diseases." Mental disorders are more than a collection of the signs and symptoms that constitute a syndrome, and are more than syndromes in having somewhat more predictable courses, outcomes, and prognoses. Because the causes and mechanisms that disable the person are not fully understood, however, disorders cannot be considered diseases.

Mental disorders are defined and classified for the purposes of studying, communicating about, and treating/helping persons distressed by them. A mental disorder describes an entity, not a person. Labeling of the person *as* the disorder, through terms such as "schizophrenic" or "suicidal," is avoided in this chapter.

Process and Procedures for Diagnosing

Deciding about the presence of a mental disorder and *distinguishing* among the types of such disorders involves the process and procedures of diagnosis. This is a clinical skill that requires specialized training. Signs and symptoms are assessed and evaluated within the framework of the mental status examination. Information about the context of present events, and about past psychological, developmental, and social history, is actively gathered both from the distressed person and from collateral others. This data base of personal information is compared or matched to known, or consensus-developed, templates describing each of the mental disorders. In the most recent classification systems, this matching process is standardized by specifying observable criteria of behavior and history for each unique disorder. Each disorder is described according to a multiaxial system that recognizes the multiple facets of mental disorder. This approach emphasizes that the process of distinguishing among mental disorder diagnoses is based on the description of observable behaviors and not an etiology. For present purposes, the revised third edition of the *Diagnostic and Statistical Manual of Mental Disorders* DSM-III-R; American Psychiatric Association, 1987) is used, although the terminology of previous versions is recalled in discussing neurotic and homosexual disorders. Another major classification system is widely used outside of North America: The *International Classification of Diseases* is in its ninth edition (World Health Organization, 1978), and the Clinical Modifications of this alternative system (ICD-9-CM; Commission on Professional & Hospital Activities, 1978) are broadly equivalent to DSM-III-R categories.

A definition of suicide itself is also needed. The umbrella term "suicidal behaviors" (Beck et al., 1973) is preferred. It refers to both completed suicide (suicide) and nonfatal suicidal behaviors, with the latter term including suicide attempts and parasuicide.

DSM-III-R Diagnoses for the Five Clinical Cases

Only Axes I and II of the multiaxial framework are provided unless Axis III offers relevant information. This is compatible with the suggestion in DSM-III-R that these axes provide adequate diagnostic information. Axes IV and V supply only research or specialized information at this time. Numerical codes link the DSM-III-R classification with similar codes in the ICD-9-CM. The best-fitting DSM-III-R codes for the five clinical cases described in Chapter 12 of this book are as follows:

Heather B
    Axis I: Adjustment disorder with mixed disturbances of emotions and conduct (309.40)
    Axis II: Deferred
Ralph F
    Axis I: (a) Major depressive disorder, single episode, with mood-congruent psychotic features (296.24)
            (b) Alcohol dependence, mild (303.90)
            (c) Other specified family circumstances (V 61.80)
    Axis II: Deferred

Axis III: Juvenile rheumatoid arthritis
Sexually transmitted disease (herpes)
Asthma (stress-induced)

John Z
Axis I: Major depressive disorder, single episode, severe (296.23)
Axis II: Deferred

José G
Axis I: (a) Major depressive disorder, single episode, moderate (296.22)
(b) Alcohol dependence, moderate (303.90)
Consider organic mental syndrome not otherwise specified (294.80)
Axis II: Deferred
Axis III: Diabetes mellitus (adult-onset, insulin-dependent, with vascular complications)
Chronic obstructive pulmonary disease (emphysema)

Faye C
Axis I: Schizophrenia, paranoid type, subchronic with acute exacerbation (295.33)
Consider schizoaffective disorder (295.70)
Consider atypical psychosis (298.90) in schizotypal personality disorder (301.22) (Axis II principal diagnosis)
Axis II: Obsessional traits
Axis III: Temporal lobe epilepsy

THE LINK BETWEEN MENTAL DISORDERS AND SUICIDE

Diagnosis is not only the process of assessment, evaluation, and matching, but also the outcome that is decided in that process. This diagnosis of a specific mental disorder becomes part of a data base of information about a person. It conveys information about the person's mental state and psychiatric history in a succinct format, and comprises one of many variables describing that person. It is then possible to look for relationships among these variables. Our particular interest at present is in the existence of any links between the variables "mental disorder diagnosis" and "suicidal behaviors." If such a link can be established beyond chance expectations in the data bases of many individuals, it suggests that a diagnosis of mental disorder may mark or signal an increased likelihood of suicidal behavior. With this knowledge, the presence of mental disorder in another person whose risk of suicidal behavior is unknown suggests an increased likelihood of that behavior even before it occurs. Along with other variables, information about mental disorder diagnoses can thus contribute to the prediction of future suicidal behavior. This section reviews the methods and measures that are used to establish this potential link, and presents results from recent investigations.

Completed Suicide (Suicide)

Methodological Issues

The methodology and results of the "psychological autopsy" (reviewed by Clark & Horton-Deutsch, Chapter 8, this volume) have strongly influenced our understanding of the linkage between mental disorders and suicide. In adults, numerous studies have emphasized the importance of affective disorders and substance abuse disorders. In children, these investigations have identified conduct disorders, "neurotic" or anxiety disorders, and substance abuse as common diagnoses in adolescents and youths who kill themselves (Kovacs & Puig-Antich, 1989).

There are severe criticisms of this methodology: (1) The data base for understanding the self-destructive act will always be incomplete without the opportunity to appreciate the event from the perspective of the deceased person; (2) interviewer bias is alleged because the outcome of suicide is already known; (3) whether consciously or unconsciously motivated, informant bias with distortion of information by the bereaved is possible; and (4) because retrospective studies can only identify correlations and associations between events, it is inappropriate to conclude from psychological autopsies that a causal mechanism links the presence of mental disorder and the decision for suicide. The concerns about the validity of this method of investigation are realistic, but can be addressed. The objections based on faulty or incomplete observation seem less relevant with the behavioral criteria used in DSM-III-R for diagnosing mental disorders. The ability of the psychological autopsy to identify links and associations, even if they are not causal relations, is important because our present interest is in learning about indicators that precede suicide and not about rationales for treatment. Within these limitations, psychological autopsy studies have produced consistent results that appear to support a link between mental disorders and suicide.

To avoid the issue of observer and informant bias, other researchers have examined this linkage through retrospective review of the medical, psychological, and social records of persons who have completed suicide. To avoid concerns about sampling bias in situations where the selection criteria for the group of suicides to be studied might affect the generalizability of the results, large samples and comprehensive coverage of all suicides in a population under study are needed. These goals are achieved most effectively through studies using patient or case registers. Where the records of the same individual appear in different registers, the recorded information within each register can be merged to increase the data base for further study of that particular person. Record and registry linkage studies are well established in Scandinavia and have been recently developed in Missouri and Iowa (Black & Winokur, 1986). In this way, record linkage is used to discover the mental disorder care history of completed suicides. In reverse linkage, it can also establish the outcome of suicide as a proportion of all mortality in prospective follow-ups of mental disordered clinical populations. Groups whose records have been linked using this method have included hospital patient populations, and both inpatient and mixed (inpatient–outpatient) psychiatric patient populations.

There are a number of restrictions to be appreciated in interpreting the results of record linkage studies. First, suicide occurs early in those patients diagnosed with affective disorders and schizophrenias, and late in those with substance abuse/dependent disorders, as Box Score A indicates.

Box Score A. Suicide during the Course of Different Mental Disorders

Disorder	Numbers of studies with suicide occurring:		
	Early	Throughout	Late
Affective disorders	5	0	0
Schizophrenias	3	1	2
Anxiety disorders	1	0	1
Alcohol or other substance abuse/dependence	0	0	3

In estimating the frequency of either mental disorder in completed suicides or suicide outcome in psychiatric patients, the length of the follow-up period in which such linkages are sought or examined will be important. Second, inpatient suicides are more likely to be diagnosed with schizophrenia, and outpatient suicides are more likely to carry diagnoses of substance abuse (Fernando & Storm, 1984; Beskow, 1987; Barner-Rasmussen, Dupont, & Bille, 1986; Modestin & Kopp, 1988). Comparisons are best made to similar samples and populations. If this is not possible, the nature of the population being studied and the process used to establish the sample itself should be specified as fully as possible. Goldney, Positano, Spence, and Rosenman (1985) and Hirschfeld and Davidson (1988) provide tables that describe and summarize the major features of many recent studies examining suicide in mental disorders. The present work lies between their descriptive approach and a formal meta-analysis of the studies. Whenever appropriate, a "Box Score" review (to borrow a term from baseball) of studies addressing a particular topic is used to support conclusions. In summarizing data from a number of studies, median and range measures are preferred to account for sample bias and to discount outlier data points.

Before I review the recent data using these linkage approaches, the Lundby Study deserves special mention. Over many years, the 3,563 inhabitants of the Swedish community of Lundby have been interviewed regularly by an ongoing team of psychiatrists. As of this writing, 28 suicides have been reported in this population, and the longitudinal data base offers a unique opportunity to uncover any associations to mental disorders and other problems that were known before the event. Fifty-seven percent of the individuals committing suicide had been in psychiatric care, as opposed to 20% and 11% of matched control groups from the same community (Hagnell, Lanke, & Rorsman, 1981). Because most (23) of the Lundby suicides have been male, comparison between suicides of those persons with a history of mental disorder diagnosis and the general population have involved only the male population. The rate of suicide among males with a mental disorder diagnosis was at least 2.5 times that of the general male population (Rorsman, Hagnell, & Lanke, 1985).

Linkage Evidence

Table 14.1 summarizes 15 studies that reported the history of known psychiatric disorder or psychiatric care in a series of suicides in the general population. Thirty-eight percent of completed suicides (range = 11.9–92%) had a known history of mental disorder. In most of these investigations, the mental disorder was found to have been present well in advance of the time of death. In Borg and Stahl's (1982) study, for example, fully two-thirds of the suicides with a history of psychiatric disorder had been diagnosed more than one year before the suicide. Modestin and Kopp (1988) reported that 24% of inpatient suicides in Berne between 1971 and 1981 had been hospitalized as inpatients for more than 1 year.

Table 14.2 presents three investigations of suicides in hospital populations. Again, it is clear that a large majority of the suicide deaths were known to a psychiatric or mental health care delivery system. Because most suicidal patients today are treated within psychiatric care settings, this finding may seem self-evident. Hesso (1977) cited six European studies of suicide rates in psychiatric hospitals prior to 1950, with a range of 40–91.7 suicides per 100,000 patients. The median rate of slightly greater than 50 per 100,000 was approximately five times that of the general population. Levy and Southcombe (1953) reported a much higher suicide rate of 350 per 100,000 for hospitalized psychiatric patients in their American sample during the same time period. In another estimation of the number of suicides in hospital populations, inpatient suicides among psychiatric patients were noted to comprise 5.5% of all suicides in Helsinki between 1964 and 1972

TABLE 14.1. The Role of Mental Disorders in Suicide: General Populations

Study	Number of suicides	% with known psychiatric disorder or history of care
Barner-Rasmussen (1986)	~13,475	27.6[a]
		29.47[b]
Nuttall, Evenson, & Cho (1980)	1,761	12
Temoche, Pugh, & MacMahon (1964)	1,457	12.6
Kullgren (1988)	693	49
Hoberman & Garfinkel (1988)	656[c]	47
James & Levin (1964)	629	11.9
Flood & Seager (1968)	325	30
Robin, Brooke, & Freeman-Browne (1968)	315	29
Beskow (1979)	271	50
Myers & Neal (1978)	260	38
Kraft & Babigian (1976)	179	45
Retterstol, Hesso, & Ekeland (1985)	148[c]	28
Borg & Stahl (1982)	85	39
Hagnell & Rorsmann (1979)	28	57
Egeland & Sussex (1985)	26	92

[a]Known disorder.
[b]History of care.
[c]Youth suicides.

(Niskanen, Lonnqvist, & Rinta-Manty, 1974), and 1.8% of all suicides in Norway from 1950 to 1962 (Odegard, 1967).

Figure 14.1 displays the results of 15 studies concerning overall mortality and deaths by suicide in psychiatric patient samples (Barner-Rasmussen et al., 1986; Black, Warrack, & Winokur, 1985a, 1985b; Burke, 1983; Ciompi, 1976; Eastwood, Stiashy, Meier, & Woogh, 1982; Forssman & Jansson, 1960; Haugland, Craig, Goodman, & Siegel, 1983; Innes & Millar, 1970; Martin, Cloninger, Guze, & Clayton, 1985; Pokorny, 1964, 1983; Rorsman et al.,

TABLE 14.2. The Role of Mental Disorders in Suicide: Clinical Populations in Hospitals

Study	Number of suicides	% with clear psychiatric disorder or history of care
Farberow, Ganzler, Cutter, & Reynolds (1971)	966	67
Beskow (1987)	579	96
Pokorny (1960)	44	89

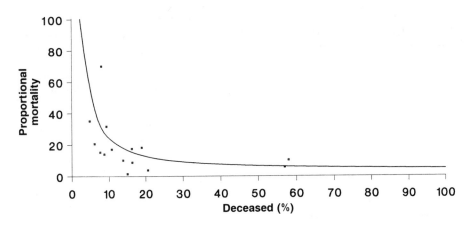

FIGURE 14.1. Proportional mortality by suicide among psychiatric patients in 15 studies. ($y = 3.021 + 174.016/x$; $r^2 = 0.297$; $p = 0.036$)

1985; Winokur & Tsuang, 1975; Zilber, Schufman, & Lerner, 1989). Fitting a curve to these data indicates that 4.75% of all psychiatric patients will eventually die by suicide. Although no direct comparison can be made to lifetime mortality from suicide in a cohort of the general population, 1.3–1.5% of all deaths in the United States each year are attributed to suicide. Despite its apparent slightness, this difference in suicide mortality between psychiatric patients and the general population is significant, the more so because the general population figure includes the suicides of those who have been psychiatric patients. The shape of the curve also indicates that most of the suicide deaths occur early in the follow-up period, when only a small fraction of the total patient sample have actually died.

Table 14.3 summarizes other studies of suicide in psychiatric patient populations. The frequency of suicide is measured in one of two ways: "rate of suicide" or "risk of suicide relative to the general population." The median suicide rate is 167 (range = 37–452) per 100,000 for mixed (inpatient and outpatient) study samples. The risk of suicide in such samples clusters at about five times that of the general population. Both the rate and the comparative risk measurements point clearly to increased suicide among psychiatric patients. More exact comparisons to the general population, with adjustment for age and sex, use standardized mortality ratios (SMRs): the ratio of observed to expected suicides for a given sample. These data, although variable for study locations in Israel, the midwestern United States, and the United Kingdom, also support higher-than-expected suicide frequencies in persons with a psychiatric care history (Table 14.4).

TABLE 14.3. The Role of Mental Disorders in Suicide: Clinical Populations—Psychiatric Inpatients and Outpatients

Study	Number of suicides	Suicide rate[a]	Risk relative to that of general population
Inpatient only			
Copas & Robin (1982)	375	56 male 33 female	4.6 times
Hesso (1977)	108	247	
Ritzel (cited in Hesso, 1977)	—	100	
Koester (cited in Hesso, 1977)	—	98	
Outpatient only			
Morrison (1982)	48	120	15 times
Hillard, Ramm, Zung, & Holland (1983)	22	111	
Mixed			
De Graaf (1982)	776	234	19.5 times
Farberow et al. (1971)	650	72	6 times
Evenson, Wood, Nuttall, & Cho (1982)	207	169[b] 99[b]	5.7 times (male) 10–11 times (female)
Modestin & Hoffmann (1989)	72	209	
	102	452	20 times
Pokorny (1964)	117	165	4.5 times
Ciompi (1976)	107	—	4.7 times
Sletten, Brown, Evenson, & Altman (1972)	97	90	
James & Levin (1964)	75	119	5.3 times
Niskanen, Lohnqvist, & Rinta-Manty (1974)	71	140	
Pokorny (1983)	67 male	279	
Temoche et al. (1964)	66	37	3.9 times
Goldney, Positano, Spence, & Rosenman (1985)	46	222	
Borg & Stahl (1982)	34	—	4–5 times
Bolin, Wright, Wilkinson, & Lindner (1968)	27	177	
Fernando & Storm (1984)	22	333	
Haugland, Craig, Goodman, & Siegel (1983)	12[c]	—	> expected

[a]Per 100,000 patients admitted/treated/at risk.
[b]Inpatient subsample only ($n = 154$).
[c]Accidents and suicides.

TABLE 14.4. The Role of Mental Disorders in Suicide: Clinical Populations—
Psychiatric Patients (SMRs)

Study	Number of suicides	SMRs Overall	Male	Female
Copas & Robin (1982)	696	—	5.46	4.79
Black, Warrack, & Winokur (1985b)	68	—	14.98	41.33
Zilber, Schufman, & Lerner (1989)	35	3.98	3.20	5.38

Nonfatal Suicidal Behaviors

The studies in Table 14.5 investigated the presence of mental disorders and suicidal behaviors in two populations: suicide-attempting patients identified in the community, and clinical samples of deliberate self-harm patients. For suicide attempters identified during large surveys of overall mental health in a community, a history of lifetime psychiatric disorder is registered much more frequently (2.6–8.4 times more often) than in nonattempters. Of persons identified with mental disorders in these surveys, 6.7% had a history of suicide attempts, compared to 2.9–4.3% in the general population. In the clinical studies, persons with nonfatal suicidal behaviors usually had a prior psychiatric history, or achieved scores on standardized measures comparable to those of mentally disordered populations. Four controlled studies indicated that suicide attempters resembled psychiatric, and especially depressive, patients in the pattern and frequency of their presenting signs and symptoms.

Conclusions

The conclusions are unequivocal: (1) Mental disorders are more common in populations of persons completing suicide, and (2) suicide and suicidal behaviors occur much more frequently than expected in populations of psychiatric patients. The presence of a mental disorder diagnosis does increase the likelihood that suicidal behavior may occur. This is not the same as saying that "psychiatric patienthood" increases the likelihood of suicidal behavior. Many persons who seek mental health support resources must be assigned a diagnosis only in order to meet the requirements of statistical data bases or third-party payment. They should not automatically be considered at increased risk of self-harm. DSM-III-R has clarified this distinction between seeking help for mental distress and being diagnosed with what have been called the major mental disorders by introducing "V codes." These describe a group of mental disorders under the heading "conditions not attributable to mental disorder."

TABLE 14.5. The Role of Mental Disorders in Nonfatal Suicidal Behaviors

Study	Number of suicide attempters	Measure	Results
General population			
Mościcki et al. (1988)	~550	DIS	Rate of lifetime psychiatric disorder 8.4 times that of general population
			For all diagnoses, 6.7% had history of suicide attempts
Dyck, Bland, Newman, & Orn (1988)	146	DIS, GHQ	Rate of lifetime psychiatric disorder 2.6 times that of general population; ~85% had disorder history
Deliberate self-harm patients			
Morgan, Burns-Cox, Pocock, & Pottle (1975)	338	Clinical record	90% had psychiatric history
Urwin & Gibbons (1979)	539	Clinical record	70% had psychiatric history
Eastwood, Henderson, & Montgomery (1972)	92	GHQ	Scores 2 times cutoff for mental illness
Newson-Smith & Hirsch (1979)	79	GHQ	90% had scores exceeding cutoff for mental illness
		PSE	61% had scores exceeding threshold for diagnosis
Comparison studies			
Vinoda (1966)	50	Symptom–Sign Inventory	Similar to psychiatric controls in symptom frequency, patterns
Birtchnell & Alarcon (1971)	68	Zung	Severity and rank order of symptoms similar to those of depressed ECT patients
Silver, Bohnert, Beck, & Marcus (1971)	45	Beck	80% had clinically depressed pattern of moderate depressive symptoms like that of outpatient depressive controls
New Haven (in Weissman, 1974)	NA	NA	Pattern of moderate depressive symptoms like that of outpatient depressive controls

Note. DIS, Diagnostic Interview Schedule; GHQ, General Health Questionnaire; PSE, Present State Examination; Zung, Zung Self-Rating Scale for Depression; Beck, Beck Depression Inventory; ECT, electroconvulsive therapy, NA, not available.

THE RELATIVE IMPORTANCE OF
DIFFERENT DIAGNOSES

Suicide

If a person's receiving a mental disorder diagnosis is sufficient to enable us to predict an increased risk of suicide for that person, this association does not mean that mental disorders *cause* suicide. In fact, it can be argued that the label and sometimes the accompanying stigma of psychiatric patient-hood may itself lead to suicide in a reversed causal link. A stronger conclusion regarding the importance of mental disorders in suicide can be argued if different mental disorders can be shown to have a unique relationship to the likelihood of suicide, whether the differences are qualitative or quantitative. In this section, the evidence for a difference in the magnitude of the relationship between different mental disorders and suicide is presented, and specific points for each disorder are briefly noted.

Following Durkheim (1897/1951), and as recently as 1965, few efforts (e.g., Lipschutz, 1942) were made in North America to demonstrate the linkages between specific mental disorders and suicide. Zilboorg (1936) stated that the suicidal drive neither depends on nor derives from any entity in psychiatric nosology. With psychological autopsy data, and the studies reported here and in Miles (1977), this opinion has changed.

Three studies have attempted to quantify the importance of mental disorders in predicting suicide. Evenson, Wood, Nuttall, and Cho (1982) reported that 57% of the variance derived from diagnosis, the most important among their three variables. Pokorny (1983; see Chapter 6, this volume) found psychiatric diagnosis to be the second largest coefficient in a discriminant-function analysis. The third study (Modestin & Kopp, 1988) noted significant differences in the distribution of mental disorder diagnoses in their suicide and control groups, but diagnosis was not among the six most useful discriminants in their stepwise logistic regression on 57 variables.

Summarizing studies about diagnoses and suicide is difficult, because there are two major classification systems and each of these has undergone planned revisions. In addition, several different measures for establishing the linkages between diagnoses and suicide, and for estimating the size and importance of those relationships for different disorders, have been used.

Summed Rank Scores

Table 14.6 presents data on the relative frequencies of mental disorders among those who end their own lives. The 28 studies are divided into four groups, according to the type of population studied and the classification system used. A rank score has been assigned to each diagnosis in each study, according to the frequency of that diagnosis among the suicides in the study. Diagnosis rank scores for all studies in a group have then been

TABLE 14.6. Mental Disorder Diagnoses in Suicide: Frequency by Rank Score

	Diagnostic classification used			
	ICD		DSM	
Frequency (total rank score)[a]	General population (2 studies)	Clinical psychiatric patients (mixed) (19 studies)	Clinical psychiatric patients (mixed) (4 studies)	Clinical psychiatric outpatients (3 studies)
1				
2				
3	AD			
4		AD	AD, Sc	AD, Sc
5				
6				SA
7		Sc	SA, A	
	N	PD		PD
8	OP, SA, PD	SA, N		OP
9	Sc		OP, OMS PD	A, OMS
10		OMS		
		OP		
11				
12				
13	OMS			
14				
15				

Note. AD, affective disorders; Sc, Schizophrenias; OP, other psychoses; SA, substance abuse; N, neuroses; A, anxiety disorders; PD, personality disorders; OMS, organic mental syndromes (brain disorders, in ICD).
[a]Rank: 1, most frequent; 2, next most frequent; etc.

summed as a measure of the relative frequency of different mental disorders among the suicides in that group. In all four groups, mood (affective) disorders are the most frequent diagnosis. In those studies using the DSM classification, the schizophrenic disorders appear as frequently as the mood disorders. In earlier versions of the DSM system, which were used in almost all of the studies summarized here, a much broader and more inclusive definition of schizophrenia was in vogue. As a result, the association of a schizophrenic diagnosis with suicide may have been overestimated in these studies. With the exception of organic mental syndromes, most other mental disorders appear to be clustered with almost equal frequency. In the DSM groups, it is notable that organic mental syndromes appear in the less frequent portion of the cluster. In the ICD groups, these diagnoses appear less often among suicides than the other diagnoses.

Percentage and Rate

The amount of association can also be estimated by comparing the frequency of different diagnoses among samples of completed suicides. The studies are the same as those employed in the calculation of the summed rank score. Both percentage and rate measures of the frequency of suicide have been used. Figure 14.2 presents the median value for both percentage of suicides and rate of suicide in the diagnostic groups found associated with suicide. Rates of suicide for all of these disorders, except organic mental syndromes, are considerably elevated above those for the general population. When the frequency of suicide is compared between diagnostic groups, similar trends are noted with both measures. Mood disorders are the most frequent and organic mental disorders the least frequent diagnoses; as in the summed rank score measurement, the majority of the other diagnoses cluster with little discrimination. For both personality disorders and substance abuse disorders, however, the measures of rate and percentage give different results. Explaining the difference is a complex matter; it probably relates to inconsistencies, in studies using either measure, in their consideration of multiple and coexisting diagnoses. The diagnosing of multiple disorders has a disproportionately large impact on personality and substance abuse disorders. Personality disorders on Axis II may not even be considered unless they are the Axis I principal diagnosis. Because substance abuse disorders are the most common disorders present as coexisting or dual disorders, their numbers may not be properly counted, depending upon the study's protocol for assigning diagnoses. In general, the "rate of suicide" measure is regarded as more accurate than that using percentages. The lower rate of suicide associated with both personality and substance abuse disorders relative to other diagnostic groups is in agreement with other studies to be presented in the next section.

Standardized Mortality Ratios

SMRs are again the most accurate measurement tool. SMRs for suicide are significantly increased for a number of diagnoses. There are very few studies, and they have little consistency in estimating the order of importance of different diagnoses. Again, mood disorders are strongly associated with a

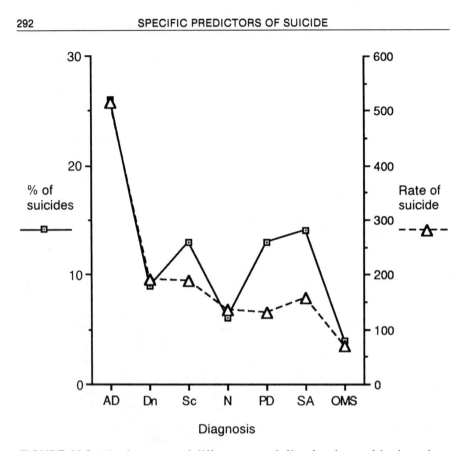

FIGURE 14.2. The frequency of different mental disorders in psychiatric patients who die by suicide. AD, affective disorders; Dn, depressive neuroses; Sc, schizophrenias; N, neuroses; PD, personality disorders; SA, substance abuse; OMS, organic mental syndromes.

suicide outcome, as are neuroses. This latter group of disorders includes the category of depressive neurosis—a diagnosis that the present DSM system includes in the mood disorder category as dysthymic disorder. Confusion about the allocation of this diagnosis to the category of mood or anxiety disorder (or sometimes personality disorder) may explain some of the inconsistency in the results of SMR studies.

Controlled Studies

A further perspective on the relative importance of different mental disorders in suicide can be derived from controlled studies. The diagnoses of persons dying by suicide are compared with those of control psychiatric subjects who have been matched to the sample of suicides on a number of variables. Box Score B summarizes studies that estimate either the number of suicides in affectively disordered patients versus controls or the frequency of affective disorder diagnoses in suicides versus natural deaths; Box Score C does the same for studies of schizophrenic patients. The strong association of both diagnoses with suicide is clear.

Box Score B. Affective Disorders and the Frequency of Suicide: Controlled Studies

Greater in affective disorders	No difference	Greater in matched controls
Flood & Seager (1968)	Bolin,	—
Goldney et al. (1985)	Wright,	
Robin, Brooke, &	Wilkinson, &	
Freeman-Browne (1968)	Lindner	
Roy (1982)	(1968)	
Fernando & Storm	Burke (1983)	
(1984) (n.s.)		
Myers & Neal (1978) (n.s.)		
Pokorny (1960) (n.s.)		

Note. (n.s.), greater but not statistically significant.

Box Score C. Schizophrenias and the Frequency of Suicide: Controlled Studies

Greater in schizophrenias	No difference	Greater in matched controls
Goldney et al. (1985)	Bolin et al. (1968)	Fernando & Storm (1984)
Roy (1986)	Beisser & Blanchette (1961)	
Wilson (1968)		

Summary

It appears that different mental disorders are associated with suicide to different extents. A number of measures confirm the variation of this relationship with diagnosis. Affective disorders are most often associated; schizophrenias are less closely linked; and organic mental disorders seem to have little presence in those who commit suicide. Studies utilizing matched controls further affirm the importance of affective disorders and schizo-phrenias. Miles's (1977) conclusions about studies published prior to 1977 are supported by those reviewed here. The only notable difference is that the association of alcohol and other substance abuse disorders with sui-cide appears less important in the present review. This finding is also confirmed by Murphy and Wetzel (1990). A possible explanation for this difference has been offered in Box Score A and elaborated in the dis-cussion of restrictions on the interpretation of data from record linkage studies.

Nonfatal Suicidal Behaviors

Different mental disorders are also associated with nonfatal suicidal behav-iors to differing extents. Not surprisingly, the diagnoses assuming more important associations are not identical to those found linked with suicide. In samples of suicide attempters, depressive neuroses (dysthymic disorders), personality disorders, and substance abuse appear most frequently. In some unselected studies investigating the frequency of suicidal behaviors in these disorders, 22.5% of subjects with nonpsychotic depressions (d'Elia, von Knorring, & Perris, 1974), 20–50% of subjects with substance abuse disorders, and a significant minority of subjects with personality disorders (21%, 29%, and 48% in three studies) had histories of self-destructive behavior. Again, comparison can be made to the general population, in which fewer than 5% report any history of suicidal behaviors.

SPECIFIC MENTAL DISORDERS
AND SUICIDAL BEHAVIORS

Using the DSM-III-R hierarchy to order the discussion, this section presents brief comments about suicidal behaviors in specific mental disorders. In-itially, the associations with suicide of the broad historical categories of psychosis and neurosis are addressed.

Psychosis and Neurosis

Gordon (1929) stated that more serious suicidal behavior accompanies psy-chosis than neurosis. In general terms, this was a restatement of the assump-tion that more severe psychopathology leads to greater likelihood of suicide. Dorpat and Boswell (1963) affirmed this relationship, but Lester and Beck's (1976) study of psychopathology in suicide attempters disconfirmed it. Six of the 12 studies in Box Score D support a contention that suicide is more frequent in psychotic conditions. It is notable that 8 of the 12 studies involve samples of patients with affective disorders.

Box Score D. Psychotic versus Neurotic Disorders and the Frequency of Suicide

Study population	More likely in psychosis	No difference	More likely in neurosis
Mixed diagnoses	Borg & Stahl (1982) Flood & Seager (1968)	Beskow (1979)	Westermeyer & Harrow (1989)
Affective disorders	Brent, Kupfer, Bromet, & Dew (1988) Evenson et al. (1982) Roose, Glassman, Walsh, Woodring, & Vital-Herne (1983) Sletten, Brown, Evenson, & Altman (1972)	McDowall, Brooke, Freeman-Browne, & Robin (1968) Tsuang, Dempsey, & Fleming (1979)	Black, Winokur, & Nasrallah (1988) Copas & Robin (1982)

Mental Retardation

The proportional mortality due to completed suicide among individuals with mental retardation is only slightly greater than that in the general population (Bryan & Herjanic, 1980), and a single study suggested that the rate of suicidal behaviors approximates that of the general population (Sternlicht, Pastel, & Deutsch, 1970). Data are available only because persons with this diagnosis were present in large numbers in the institutions that provided patient data for such studies.

Developmental Disorders

Hayes and Sloat (1988) reported an increase in suicide occurrences among learning-disabled students in the educational systems of four Texas counties. An argument for a nonverbal learning disorder whose clinical presentation resembles that of patients exhibiting suicidal behaviors (Rourke, Young, & Leenaars, 1987; Bigler, 1989) has been put forward. Suicidal behaviors as part of a maladaptive response to developmental disorders appears a more promising explanation (Kowalchuk & King, 1989).

Eating Disorders

A review (Gardner & Rich, 1988) of 33 studies concludes that 1.5% of patients with eating disorders commit suicide, and that 18–29% of overall mortality in this population can be attributed to self-destruction. The importance of these figures is hard to assess, because most of these patients are young and it is known that suicide already accounts for a large proportion of mortality in this age group. Nonfatal suicidal behaviors are common, and Viesselman and Roig (1985) note that these may be more lethal or serious in action and intent than usual for this age and sex group. Persons with eating disorders often have comorbid diagnoses of borderline personality disorder, substance abuse, or major depression, or these may be recognized later in the persons' development (Hatsukami, Eckert, Mitchell, & Pyle, 1984). Each of these latter diagnoses is itself clearly associated with suicide and nonfatal suicidal behaviors.

Organic Mental Disorders

Organic mental disorders make little contribution to an increasing likelihood of suicide (Black, Warrack, & Winokur, 1985c). It is likely that their association was considered in many studies only because they represented a significant proportion of the psychiatric inpatient populations available for study. The association of epilepsy and increased suicide (Matthews & Barabas, 1982; Brent, 1986; Barraclough, 1987) must be noted. AIDS and the possible preclinical diagnosis of Huntington's chorea have reinitiated interest in the thorny issue of assisted or rational suicide in organic mental disorders.

Substance Abuse Disorders

In a number of toxicological investigations, it appears that about 20% of suicides are legally intoxicated at the time of their deaths (references in Brent et al., 1988). This association does not demonstrate that alcohol abuse or dependence is linked to suicide, but does warn us that the disinhibiting or depressant effects of ethanol as a drug may contribute to the likelihood of suicide. Other studies affirm that abuse/dependence disorders involving both alcohol and other substances are linked to suicidal behaviors (Lester & Beck, 1975; Weissman, Beck, & Kovacs, 1979). Scheftner et al. (1988) and Rich Fowler, and Young (1989) further suggest an additive effect if ethanol and other drugs are being abused. Hirschfeld and Davidson (1988) provide an excellent summary of recent studies. Murphy and Wetzel (1990) have calculated that the lifetime risk of suicide in alcoholism is 2.0–3.4%. This is much less than Miles's (1977) estimate of 10%, but still significantly higher than that of the general population.

Because 47% of substance abuse disorder diagnoses have been found to co-occur with another mental disorder diagnosis (Helzer & Przybeck, 1988), the effect of these concurrent diagnoses and especially depression on the likelihood of suicidal behavior cannot be ignored. In comparisons of ethanol-dependent/abusing persons with and without nonfatal suicidal behaviors, four of five studies indicate that depression is more common in the suicide attempt group (Black, Yates, Petty, Noyes, & Brown, 1986; Hasin, Grant, & Endicott, 1988; Morrison, 1982; Murphy, Rounsaville, Eyre, & Kleber, 1983; Schuckit, 1985), and three of four studies (Whitters, Cadoret, & Widmer, 1985; Hasin et al., 1988; Murphy et al., 1983; Rich, Fowler, & Young, 1986) affirm the presence of more psychopathology in this group. Among completed suicides in alcoholic patients, two studies reported that suicide was more likely with concurrent depressive disorder (Whitters et al., 1985; Berglund, 1984). In those with alcohol abuse and depression, Berglund (1984) argues that suicide is even more likely with increasing severity of the depression component. Scheftner et al. (1988) suggest that a history of alcohol and drug abuse can distinguish those who may commit suicide among a population of depressed patients.

Substance abuse disorder in adolescents, in Native Americans, in military personnel, and in those with concurrent mental disorders should be considered a clear predictor of increased risk of suicide. All deaths involving motor vehicle accidents, violence, and undetermined causes where alcohol or other drug dependence or abuse is involved should be examined closely for the possibility of a disguised or "subintentioned" suicide.

Schizophrenias

Roy (1986) and Virkkunen (1974) offer excellent literature reviews of both the history and present state of knowledge concerning suicide in schizophrenias. Young male schizophrenics appear to be exceptionally at risk. Shneidman, Farberow, and Leonard (1962) suggested that suicide in a patient with schizophrenia is "a somewhat organized and planned action . . . in an apparent attempt to extricate himself from . . . an intolerable life situation" (p. 10). This has been reiterated by recent work (various chapters in Williams & Dalby, 1989; Prasad & Kumar, 1968; Dassori, Mezzich, & Keshavan, 1990) pointing out that depression and hopelessness are important factors in the suicide of those with schizophrenia. Whether this mood state is part of the illness process or a secondary/ reactive depression occurring as an adaptation to this chronic illness is not known.

The distressing idea that suicide may occur in those with schizophrenias as an iatrogenically induced complication of antipsychotic medications (Drake & Ehrlich, 1985) or of the treatment milieu (Perris, Beskow, & Jacobsson, 1980) continues to appear. These are irregular and isolated case reports with much accompanying speculation. Recently, three reports have noted an increased suicide risk among those experiencing atypical psychoses (Buda, Tsuang, & Fleming, 1988; Westermeyer & Harrow, 1989; Rich et al. 1986).

Affective Disorders

With the adoption of the term "affective disorder" and then "mood disorder," DSM-III and DSM-III-R recognized the important distinction that must be made between depression as a symptom or syndrome and depression as a disorder or possibly a disease. In their study, Beisser and Blanchette (1961) observed that 83% of their suicide sample versus 28% of controls were depressed. Achté, Stenback, and Teravainen's (1966) study of 57 Helsinki suicides reported depression in 65%. Both studies, however, referred to the presence of depressive symptoms or syndromes, and not necessarily to the presence of depressive (affective/mood) mental disorders. Confusion about this overlap and about the definition of affective or mood disorders continues, and has made it difficult to reach definite conclusions about the association between suicidal behaviors and these disorders. Despite these difficulties, psychological autopsy studies consistently find that affective disorders are the most important diagnoses related to suicide. In addition, Jamison's (1986) update of the Guze and Robins (1970) review of this relationship lists 27 studies that found death by suicide as a significant and frequent outcome in depressed/affectively disordered patients. More recent studies to be added to this list include those by Black, Winokur, and Nasrallah (1987), Berglund and Nilsson (1987), Coryell, Noyes, and Clancy (1982), and Fawcett et al. (1987), with proportional mortalities by suicide of 26.1%, 22%, 16.2%, and only 2.6% respectively, in their affectively disordered patients. Studies using matched control groups (see Box Score B, above) further confirm the important association of affective disorders with an increased likelihood of suicide.

For nonfatal suicidal behaviors in affectively disordered patients, Jamison (1986) also reports eight follow-up studies in which their frequency was well above that reported in the general population. The confusion surrounding depression as a symptom/syndrome versus depression as a disorder reappears even more strongly in studies of nonfatal suicidal behaviors. Weissman (1974) concluded that 35-75% of suicide attempters are depressed, but acknowledged that these are mostly individuals with secondary depressions. Schuckit (1989) suggests similarly high proportions of depression (as either a symptom/syndrome or a disorder) in 50-60% of adults and 55-95% of adolescents and children who are identified as suicide attempters.

Because classification of the group of mood disorders has been especially difficult, it is important to clarify the relationship of different subtypes to suicide.

Psychotic versus Neurotic Depressions

Four of eight studies found that suicide was more frequently associated with psychotic than with neurotic depressions (see Box Score D, above).

Unipolar versus Bipolar Disorders

Only one of nine studies in Box Score E contends that suicide is more likely in bipolar than in unipolar affective disorders. Although Modestin and Kopp (1988) supported this conclusion in comparing the percentages and absolute number of each of these disorders, only bipolar disorders appeared significantly more often in their suicide group than in their control group. Although a robust conclusion is warranted from the box score approach, concerns about the differing definitions for bipolar and unipolar disorders in these studies suggest a need for further examination of the original data.

Box Score E. Unipolar versus Bipolar Disorders and the Frequency of Suicide

More likley in unipolar	More likely in bipolar
Angst (1980)	Egeland & Sussex (1985)
Barner-Rasmussen (1986)	
Berglund Krantz, Lundqvist, & Therup (1987)	
Black et al. (1987)	
Kullgren, Renberg, & Jacobsson (1986)	
Modestin & Kopp (1988)	
Morrison (1982)	
Weeke, Vaeth, & Juel (1985)	
Winokur & Tsuang (1975)	

Several authors point out that box score or meta-analytic conclusions that psychotic depressions are more frequently associated with suicide than neurotic depressions, and that unipolar disorders are more frequently associated with suicide than bipolar disorders, do not mean that neurotic depressions or bipolar disorders are not significantly associated with suicide. Odegard (1967), Ciompi (1976), Sletten et al. (1972), Barner-Rasmussen (1986), d'Elia et al. (1974), and Modestin and Kopp (1988) all clearly document the frequent presence of depressive neuroses in psychiatric patients who die by suicide. (For cross-comparison, a diagnosis of "depressive neurosis" is broadly equivalent to or includes dysthymic disorder, adjustment disorder with depressed mood, and reactive depression.) Roy (1982) found that recurrent affective disorders were associated with an increased likelihood of suicide. Within the strict sense of their original definitions, recurrence is a characteristic both of bipolar and of unipolar disorders.

Primary versus Secondary Depression

"Secondary depression" is the appearance of a depressive mood disorder when the presence of another mental disorder diagnosis has already been established. Its importance in association with suicide is emphasized in all five studies that have introduced this subtype (Berglund & Smith, 1988; Black et al., 1987; Hagnell & Rorsman, 1979; Khuri and Akiskal, 1983; Martin et al., 1985). All five stressed that suicide occurred as often or more often in the disorders with secondary mood disturbance. Again, comorbidity is an important consideration, and it is possible that the severity of the overall distress or disability is additive when two disorders are present. The association of suicide outcome with "double depression" (in which an episode of major depression overlies a dysthymic disorder) is an example of this possibility.

Other Issues

The increase in the likelihood of suicide with the simultaneous presence of affective and substance abuse disorders has already been described. Several studies also suggest that increasing severity of psychopathology is a guide to increased suicide risk (Modestin & Kopp, 1988; Berglund, 1984; Farberow, Shneidman, & Neuringer, 1966; Hagnell et al., 1981). Because severity is a nonspecific measure, and possible effects of the subtypes of mood disorder described above were not specified in these studies, it is difficult to be sure that severity offers the most parsimonious explanation for the differences observed.

   In a number of controlled studies, there was little agreement concerning which, if any, specific symptoms of depressive disorder could be linked to suicide (Barraclough & Pallis, 1975; McDowall et al., 1968; Farberow & McEvoy, 1966; Birtchnell & Alarcon, 1971). These controlled studies also found that depressives who committed suicide were more alike than different from depressives who did not. Considering other reports (Burke, 1983; Martin et al., 1985; Copas & Robin, 1982) that affective disorders by themselves do not constitute a useful predictor of suicide, the assessment of the relationship between mood disorders and suicide becomes even more complicated. Differences in suicidal outcome within subtypes may account for some of these findings, but it is impossible to reach any assured conclusions. For example, Khuri and Akiskal's (1983) conclusion that depressions are insufficient and not necessarily necessary for suicide seems to deny mood disorders any major role in the matrix of suicide causation. Their apparent expectation that any single factor (such as depression) would meet the conditions of being necessary and sufficient to cause suicide, when suicide is accepted to be multifactorial and multidetermined in its origins, goes too far. In addition, their assertion is literally not true, for suicides do occur in which a biologically induced depression appears to have been the sufficient and solitary cause. Although the mechanism of this relationship remains a puzzle, the fact remains that suicide occurs more often in association with mood disorders than with any other type of mental disorder.

Anxiety Disorders

In earlier DSM classifications, and in the present ICD system, discrimination between anxiety disorders (previously called "neuroses" in DSM II) and personality disorders is difficult. Comparison across classification systems for this group of disorders is also complicated by the allocation of the depressive neuroses to the affective disorder category of dysthymia in DSM-III.

In nine follow-up studies reporting the mortality of patients with anxiety disorder, 16.7% (range = 2.12–40%) of the deaths were due to suicide (Coryell et al., 1982; Harris, 1938; Kerr, Schapira, & Roth, 1969; Martin et al., 1985; Noyes, Clancy, Moenk, & Slymur, 1978; Rosenberg, 1968; Sims & Prior, 1978; Tyrer, Remington, & Alexander, 1987; Wheeler, White, Reed, & Cohen, 1950). Some of these studies included neuroses (and depressive neuroses) in the sample population, but the author of the largest study reported in a later publication (Sims, 1984) that mortality by suicide remained high in anxiety disorders even when depressive neuroses (dysthymic disorders) were omitted.

Table 14.7 provides data about the associations of the various anxiety disorders with both suicide and nonfatal suicidal behaviors (Bliss, 1980; Coryell et al., 1982; Coryell, 1988; McDowall et al., 1968; Morrison, 1982; Putnam, Guroff, & Silverman, 1986; Ross, Norton, & Wozney, 1989; Solomon & Solomon, 1982; Weissman, Klerman, Markowitz, & Ouellette, 1989; Woodruff, Clayton, & Guze, 1972). The unanimous finding (six of six studies) that suicide is rare in obsessive–compulsive disorder is especially notable (Coryell, Noyes, & House, 1986; Gittleson, 1966; Hollingsworth, Tanguay, Grossman, & Pabst, 1980; Kopp, Felsovaly, Skrabski, & Tringer, 1977; Rosenberg, 1968; Woodruff et al., 1972).

Personality Disorders

As a general rule, personality disorders are linked to nonfatal suicidal behaviors rather than to suicide. Several sources suggest that the nature of self-destructive behavior in personality disorders is less serious than in depression (McHugh & Goodell, 1971), and it has been characterized as

TABLE 14.7. Anxiety Disorders and the Frequency of Suicidal Behavior

Disorder	Nonfatal suicidal behaviors	Suicide
Panic	20%; o/e, 2.62[a] (1)	5% (1)
Obsessive–compulsive	No increase (4)	No increase (2)
Somatoform	Increase (2)	No increase (2)
Dissociative (multiple personality)[b]	71–91%	2.1% (1)

Note. Numbers of studies are in parentheses.
[a]o/e, ratio of observed to expected deaths; remains elevated even when coexisting major depression and substance abuse are controlled for.
[b]Many co-occurring diagnoses.

"common, repetitive and usually not serious" and "often engaged in . . . without lethal intent" (Frances, Fyer, & Clarkin, 1986, p. 292). Personality disorders are said to aggravate the possibility of suicidal behaviors, and this may be due either to additive severity of the psychopathology or to specific comorbidity relationships. In four of six studies of borderline personality disorder (BPD), suicidal behaviors were more frequent and more serious if comorbidity with affective or substance abuse disorders was also present (Friedman, Aronoff, Clarkin, Corn, & Hurt, 1983; Fyer, Frances, Sullivan, Hurt, & Clarkin, 1988; Kullgren, 1988; Paris, Nowlis, & Brown, 1989; Shearer, Peters, Quaytman, & Wadman, 1988; Stone, Stone, & Hurt, 1987).

Because personality disorders do not appear as the principal diagnosis in most patients, it is possible that their frequency in those exhibiting suicidal behaviors may have been underestimated in the majority of studies, which assigned only one diagnosis per patient or used a hierarchy of diagnoses. This classification bias does not, however, explain two recent studies in which the frequency of personality disorders was underrepresented in samples of inpatient suicides. Modestin (1989) found that only 10.7% of suicides had personality disorder diagnoses, whereas 29.5% of a control group of nonsuicide inpatients had such diagnoses. Kullgren (1988) found that BPD was not overrepresented among completed suicides in an inpatient sample (12%), relative to the percentage of patients diagnosed as borderline on the unit (14–20%).

Although Friedman et al. (1983) reported that patients with 6 of 10 "other personality disorders" reported a suicide attempt history on the lifetime Schedule for Affective Disorders and Schizophrenia, the most important associations with suicidal behavior have been noted for antisocial personality disorder (ASPD), BPD, hysterical personality disorder (somatization disorder), and homosexuality. Frances et al. (1986) offer an excellent summary. Miles (1977) concluded that 5% of those with ASPD eventually complete suicide. A similar median figure of 6.5% has been calculated from eight follow-up studies of BPD patients (Akiskal et al., 1985; Friedman et al., 1983; Kroll, Carey, & Sines, 1985; Kullgren et al., 1986; McGlashan, 1986; Paris, Brown, & Nowlis, 1987; Pope, Jonas, Hudson, Cohen, & Tohen, 1983; Stone et al., 1987). In both ASPD and BPD, the lifetime history of suicide attempts is much higher than expected, ranging from 11% to 72% in ASPD (Garvey & Spoden, 1980) and from 75% to 92% in BPD (Fyer et al., 1988). An earlier report (Woodruff et al., 1972) mentions a suicide attempt history in 50% of homosexuals. Harry's (1989) review of this topic cites three further references to suicidal behavior in gay and lesbian youths. This data base is too thin and the studies too overinterpreted to allow meaningful conclusions at present.

Assessed Suicide Risk of the Five Clinical Cases, Based Only on Mental Disorder Diagnoses

Heather B: *Low* for suicide, *High* for nonfatal suicidal behavior.

Ralph F: *High.* Psychotic features and accompanying substance abuse add to the risk already associated with major depressive disorder. Chronic and debilitating physical disease further increases the risk, as does the maladaptive coping reflected by the asthma. Sexually transmitted disease could indicate increased risk taking in regard to personal health and safety.

John Z: *High.* Risk in major depressive disorder is greater with increasing severity.

Faye C: If atypical psychosis in schizotypal personality (principal diagnosis) with obsessional traits, *low*. Principal diagnosis and personality traits are not associated with suicide. Atypical psychosis is usually transient. There are many different views about suicide in atypical psychosis, however, with recent evidence that risk is moderate to high.

If paranoid schizophrenia with temporal lobe epilepsy, *moderate*. Well-compensated subchronic course with long-standing depressive adaptation suggests low risk. This is modified to next greater level of risk by the temporal lobe epilepsy, with its known increased suicide risk.

If schizoaffective disorder, *high*. This is a combination of affective disorder with psychosis, and both are known high-risk parameters.

José G: *High.* Risk in major depressive disorder increases with accompanying substance dependence disorder. Chronic physical diseases with little hope of improvement further increase the risk.

If organic mental syndrome, *low.*

THE RELATIONSHIPS BETWEEN MENTAL DISORDERS AND SUICIDAL BEHAVIORS

An Artifact of Definition?

If suicide is defined as a life-ending event occurring only during a state of mental disorder ("all suicides are insane"), any appraisal of the contribution of mental disorders to assessing and predicting suicide becomes frivolous. Several sources, including the psychological autopsy data, provide information about the mental state near the time of their death of those who kill themselves. Beskow (1979) reported that 93% of suicides were mentally disorganized at the time of death. Beisser and Blanchette (1961) and Achté et al. (1966) stated that 83% and 65%, respectively, of their suicides were depressed. The finding that persons about to commit suicide have disturbed and disturbing feelings and thoughts in the face of such an irreversible decision should not be surprising or unexpected. Their mental disturbance may truly reflect the distress of making this weighty decision. This is not mental disorder as it has been understood and defined for purposes of present-day study and treatment. It is also *not necessarily* the consequence of some pre-existing mental disorder. It would be pointless and circular to argue that the psychological turmoil generated in deciding about suicide is mental disorder, and that this mental disorder is itself one of the factors that at some earlier time led to the very consideration of the suicide option. It is even less appropriate to use the observation of mental disorganization near the time of suicide to infer that mental disorder has contributed to the decision for death, and to conclude that its presence in others increases their likelihood of suicide. Much of this confusion might be resolved by recalling the distinctions between signs/symptoms and disorders elaborated earlier. (To review, signs and symptoms of behavioral, cognitive, and/or affective disturbance are necessary but not sufficient to define a state of mental disorder.)

The introduction of observed behaviors as part of the criteria to operationally define mental disorders, (e.g., in DSM-III) has furthered the explanation of the relationship between suicide and mental disorders as an artifact of definition. Two DSM-III-R disorders, major depression and BPD, include suicidal behaviors among the criteria that can be used to define the disorders. In major depression, five behaviors from a list of nine possibilities, one of which is suicidal behaviors, must be present. For BPD, five of eight behaviors must be present; again, suicidal behaviors are among these possibilities. Because both disorders *may* be defined by the presence of suicidal behaviors, any association between these diagnoses and suicidal behaviors represents circular logic and as a result must be discounted. Predicting the likelihood of suicide from the presence of these two mental disorders may thus have no value. Because the criteria for dysthymic disorder and histrionic personality disorder as defined in DSM-III also include suicidal behaviors as one of the behavioral items to consider in making those diagnoses, the invalidating argument must be extended to include them.

This is a very real dilemma. In the studies reviewed here and elsewhere, each of these disorders is noted to have a significant association with suicidal behaviors. Although no resolution is offered here, two additional points can be considered:

1. It is likely that those who constructed the categories of mental disorder and their criteria accepted the relationship as an evident and observable fact. Derived from the wisdom of clinical observation over the course of time, the association was enshrined as part of the definition. As an assumption concerning specific mental disorders, any effort to demonstrate or to question it is irrelevant. This may seem arbitrary, but the theory of science incorporates such assumptions in order to further the progress of knowledge development within a specific paradigm. This explanation is uncomfortable, both because it blocks the process of further scientific inquiry and because there is sparse evidence that the issue of linkage between mental disorder and suicide received serious scientific scrutiny in the North American behavioral sciences literature before 1950.

2. Friedman et al. (1983) approached this issue more pragmatically by diagnosing their sample of BPD patients with and without the self-harm criterion. Of 36 patients, 31 still qualified for the diagnosis when the self-harm criterion was excluded from consideration as part of the defining list of behaviors. Of more importance, this included all 28 patients who had a history of nonfatal suicidal behaviors, and both of the 2 patients who completed suicide. The association of BPD with suicide remained strong even when the possibility of definitional artifact was excluded. Sims (1984) pursued the same logic in showing that the linkage of anxiety disorders (neuroses) to suicidal behavior remained even when the subgroup of depressive neuroses (equivalent to dysthymic disorder) whose definition included suicidal behaviors was segregated in the analysis. For the examples of persons at risk considered in this text, all three persons with major depres-

sive disorder (Ralph, John, and José) would have retained that diagnosis even if suicidal ideation had been excluded from consideration in evaluating the presence of disorder.

The possibility that the association between mental disorders and suicidal behaviors is a definitional artifact cannot be totally discarded, but this argument should not be valued as strongly as it has been.

An Artifact of Observation?

If mental disorder is inferred from and sometimes even defined by the presence of suicide, it is equally possible that suicide may be determined as the cause of death, on the basis of data that the deceased person had a prior history of mental disorder. This may occur most often when the circumstances of death are uncertain and an open or undetermined verdict is unavoidable unless the background of the person is considered. Based on a possibly unwarranted linking of the disorder and the cause of death, the finding of death by suicide in such cases artificially inflates the strength of the relationship between mental disorders and suicide. This becomes even more problematic when this verdict is later used by others as part of an argument to illustrate the association of mental disorder to suicide.

The issues of timing and directionality must also be considered in evaluating epidemiological studies that report an increased frequency of suicidal behavior over a lifetime in association with specific mental disorders. Although both behavioral disorders have occurred in the same person during his or her life, the suicidal behavior may have taken place before the mental disorder and in fact may be entirely unrelated to it. Studies observing such an association are useful pointers for further exploration, but cannot be used alone to predict any relationship between mental disorders and suicide.

The Effect of Treatment?

Both Pokorny (1983; see Chapter 6, this volume) and Hawton (1987) have pointed out a restriction in our data base of information about the relationship between mental disorders and suicide. If a mental disorder is a strong predictor of suicide, and some treatment program is available, society and its helpers will use that treatment to prevent the suicide if at all possible. If treatment is successful and the suicide is prevented, the single datum representing that person, which would have contributed to the data base relating mental disorder and suicide, will never appear. The relationship of suicide outcome to the predictor variable of mental disorder will be weakened by effective treatments. From another viewpoint, Hawton (1987) commented that our knowledge of the relationship between suicide and mental disorders is based only on those persons who die anyway, in spite of treatment. Khuri and Akiskal (1983), Avery and Winokur (1978), Jamison (1986), Flood and Seager (1968), Morrison (1982), and Medlicott and Medlicott (1969) all subscribe to the view that our understanding of the relationships between specific diagnoses and completed suicide has, in fact, been influenced by the implementation of modern treatments for mental disorders. Specifically, they refer to the success of electroconvulsive therapy and psychopharmacological preparations in the treatment and prophylaxis of recurrent mood disorders.

Increases in suicide among psychiatric populations have been noted in Norway, The Netherlands, Sweden, Denmark, and Switzerland over the past three decades. Although there is much controversy, numerous authors (Barner-Rasmussen et al., 1986; Beskow, 1987; De Graaf, 1982; Hesso, 1977) speculate that newer treatment approaches, including community or holistic psychiatry and even psychopharmacology, may actually contribute to suicide in those with mental disorders.

Relationship Possibilities

This review reaffirms the findings of Miles (1977) and others who have previously investigated suicidal behaviors in persons with psychiatric disorders. A linkage or association does exist, and its varying strength for different disorders implies that the psychopathology or course of the disorder itself is an important consideration. An association does not, however, mean that mental disorders are a direct cause for suicide. A number of other explanations can be considered, and it is possible that one of these mechanisms might prove a better predictor for suicide outcome in mental disorders than the disorder(s) with which it is associated. With brief examples, these possibilities are presented in Table 14.8. Understanding these mechanisms and specifying the exact nature of the processes involved may be important for treatment and prevention activities. Even if incompletely understood, the association still aids in identifying persons with mental disorders as being at increased risk of suicide.

The last of the possible relationships in Table 14.8 deserves elaboration. Pattison and Kahan (1983), and more recently Favazza, DeRosear, and Conterio (1989), have proposed the inclusion of "deliberate self-harm" as a specific mental disorder in a future revision of the DSM classification system. Van Egmond and Diekstra (1990) have proposed an operational definition of "parasuicide" that could also be adapted for this purpose. Certainly their description lies within the boundaries of mental disorder as defined by the DSM classification. As a scientific strategy, the inclusion of

TABLE 14.8. Possible Relationships of Mental Disorders to Suicidal Behaviors

Mechanism	Examples
Cause or consequence	
Direct cause or consequence	
Vehicle	Psychotic thinking: command hallucinations, depressive delusions
Risk factor	Low concentrations of 5-hydroxyindoleacetic acid (5-HIAA) linked to violent, impulsive suicide
	Severity of disorder related to suicide
Indirect complication	
Iatrogenic	Emphasis on early discharge, community care
	Direct behavioral toxicity of antipsychotics(?), fluoxetine, phenobarbital
Illness (mal)adaptation	Hopelessness of chronic disorder (e.g., schizophrenia)
	Suicide orientation schema in nonverbal learning disorder
Interaction	
Additive, aggravating	Axis II personality disorders (e.g., borderline, antisocial) increase frequency of suicidal behaviors in other disorders
	Dual diagnoses (depression) have increased suicidal behaviors
	Alcohol or other substance abuse + depression → suicide as a result of psychological and pharmacological disinhibition
Predisposing (cofactor)	
Releasing	One phenotype of bipolar affective disorder releases some genetically based suicide factor
	Atypical psychosis in substance abuse
Suppressing	Obsessive–compulsive disorder
	Alcohol or other substance abuse replaces direct suicidal behavior
Co-occurrent/coexisting factor	
"Equivalent" form	Substance abuse as indirect suicide
	Suicidal behavior as a defining criterion of the disorder
Comorbid factor	
Common etiology	Genetic-spectrum concept with variable expression
	Isolation (Sainsbury, 1986) or loneliness (Gove & Hughes, 1980) leads both to suicide and to substance abuse/depression
Independent etiology	Chance occurrence
	"Deliberate self-harm" defined as a unique mental disorder

suicidal behaviors in the classification system would have definite advantages. Because DSM allows the specification of multiple diagnoses, the reporting of suicidal behaviors would be encouraged. In cases where this diagnosis was comorbid with another disorder, any linkage could then be investigated without inferring a pre-existing relationship. This suggestion will undoubtedly alarm many persons who are interested in and concerned about suicide. It is important to realize that such an undertaking would not imply or require that suicidal behavior be considered a manifestation of psychopathology, or that it necessarily be designated a form of psychopathology. Like several other disorders in DSM-III-R that are described as "proposed diagnostic categories needing further study," deliberate self-harm could be a convention adopted for just these purposes. Although it would be controversial, major benefits to our understanding of suicidal behavior might be realized.

CONCLUSIONS

Despite the diversity of methods and the various terminologies in the available studies, the box scores and graphic summaries presented in this chapter allow some conclusions to be set forth with reasonable confidence.

1. Persons with mental disorders engage in suicidal behaviors more often than the general population. This finding holds both for suicide and for nonfatal suicidal behaviors. The increased likelihood of suicide in persons with mental disorders is significant when all causes of death are considered and is estimated at approximately five times that of the general population in the several years after an episode of mental health contact. Although not as important in the magnitude of its predictive ability as prior suicidal behavior, a history of diagnosed mental disorder is a valuable predictor in assessing the likelihood of suicidal behavior.

2. The presence of a specific mental disorder diagnosis and any subtype of it is likely to be of even greater value in prediction (Table 14.9). This conclusion suggests that the association is more than an artifact of definition, a consequence of labeling, or a general linkage to patienthood.

3. When coexisting disorders are identified, the risk is even greater. The explanation for this is unresolved. It may represent an interaction between disorders that increases risk, or it may be an indication that more (or more severe) psychopathology is the important determinant.

4. The diagnosis of a mental disorder is not a sufficient explanation for suicidal behavior. Among the heterogeneity of causes, mental disorders can

TABLE 14.9. The Frequency of Suicidal Behaviors in Mental Disorders: A Summary

Mental disorder	Suicide	Nonfatal suicidal behaviors
Affective disorders	+++	++
Bipolar	++	
Major depression (unipolar)	+++	
Psychotic/melancholic	+++	
Reactive, neurotic	++	
Chronic, recurrent	++	
Secondary depression	++	
Adjustment disorder, depressed	++	++
Schizophrenias	++	
Paranoid schizophrenia	++	
Other psychoses	+	
Substance abuse	++	++
Personality disorders		
Antisocial	+	+++
Borderline	+	+++
Anxiety disorders		
Panic	+	+
Obsessive–compulsive	−	−
Dissociative	0	+
Eating disorders	+	++
Developmental disorders	0	+
Organic mental disorders	0	
Mental retardation	0	0

Note. In relation to the general population: −, less than; 0, equal to; +, ++, +++, increasingly greater than.

lay claim to a position in the first rank of the matrix of causation. But the issue is complex, and multiple explanations may be operating simultaneously. Along with many others, Cohen, Test, and Brown (1990) reaffirm the ultimate importance of listening to the person in distress. Any other conclusion would be most surprising, given our awareness of the multifactorial and multidetermined origins of suicidal behaviors.

REFERENCES

Achté, K. A., Stenback, A., & Teravainen, H. (1966). On suicides committed during treatment in psychiatric hospitals. *Acta Psychiatrica Scandinavica, 42*(3), 272–284.

Akiskal, H. S., Chen, S. E., Davis, G. C., Puzantian, V. R., Kashgarian, M., & Bolinger, J. M. (1985). Borderline: An adjective in search of a noun. *Journal of Clinical Psychiatry, 46*, 41–48.

American Psychiatric Association. (1987). *Diagnostic and statistical manual of mental disorders* (3rd ed., rev.). Washington, DC: Author.

Angst, J. (1980). Verlauf unipolar depressiver, bipolar manisch–depressiver and schizo-affectiver Erkrankungen and Psychosen: Ergebnisse einer prospekitven Studie. *Fortschrift für Neurologie und Psychiatrie, 48,* 3–30.

Avery, D., & Winokur, G. (1978). Suicide, attempted suicide, and relapse rates in depression. *Archives of General Psychiatry, 35,* 749–753.

Barner-Rasmussen, P. (1986). Suicide in psychiatric patients in Denmark, 1971–1981: II. Hospital utilization and risk groups. *Acta Psychiatrica Scandinavica, 73,* 449–455.

Barner-Rasmussen, P., Dupont, A., & Bille, H. (1986). Suicide in psychiatric patients in Denmark, 1971–1981: I. Demographic and diagnostic description. *Acta Psychiatrica Scandinavica, 73,* 441–448.

Barraclough, B. M. (1987). The suicide rate of epilepsy. *Acta Psychiatrica Scandinavica, 76*(4), 339–345.

Barraclough, B. M., & Pallis, D. J. (1975). Depression followed by suicide: A comparison of depressed suicides with living depressives. *Psychological Medicine, 5,* 55–61.

Beck, A. T., Davis, J. H., Frederick, C. J., Perlin, S., Pokorny, A. D., Schulman, R. E., Seiden, R. H., & Wittlin, B. J. (1973). Classification and nomenclature. In H. L. P. Resnik & B. Hathorne (Eds.), *Suicide prevention in the seventies* (pp. 7–12). Washington, DC: U.S. Government Printing Office.

Beisser, A. R., & Blanchette, J. E. (1961). A study of suicides in a mental hospital. *Diseases of the Nervous System, 22*(7), 365–369.

Berglund, M. (1984). Suicide in alcoholism. *Archives of General Psychiatry, 41,* 888–891.

Berglund, M., Krantz, G., Lundqvist, G., & Therup, L. (1987). Suicide in psychiatric patients. *Acta Psychiatrica Scandinavica, 76,* 431–437.

Berglund, M., & Nilsson, K. (1987). Mortality in severe depression. *Acta Psychiatrica Scandinavica, 76,* 372–380.

Berglund, M., & Smith, G. J. W. (1988). Post-diction of suicide in a group of depressive patients. *Acta Psychiatrica Scandinavica, 77,* 504–510.

Beskow, J. (1979). Suicide and mental disorder in Swedish men. *Acta Psychiatrica Scandinavica* (Suppl. 277), 1–138.

Beskow, J. (1987). The prevention of suicide while in psychiatric care. *Acta Psychiatrica Scandinavica, 76*(Suppl. 336), 66–75.

Bigler, E. D. (1989). On the neuropsychology of suicide. *Journal of Learning Disabilities, 22*(3), 180–185.

Birtchnell, J., & Alarcon, J. (1971). Depression and attempted suicide: A study of 91 cases seen in a casualty department. *British Journal of Psychiatry, 118,* 289–296.

Black, D. W., Warrack, G., & Winokur, G. (1985a). The Iowa record-linkage study. *Archives of General Psychiatry, 42,* 71–75.

Black, D. W., Warrack, G., & Winokur, G. (1985b). Excess mortality among psychiatric patients. *Journal of the American Medical Association, 253*(1), 58–61.

Black, D. W., Warrack, G. & Winokur, G. (1985c). The Iowa record-linkage study: II. Excess mortality among patients with organic mental disorders. *Archives of General Psychiatry, 42,* 78–81.

Black, D. W., & Winokur, G. (1986). Prospective studies of suicide and mortality in psychiatric patients. *Annals of the New York Academy of Sciences, 487,* 106–113.

Black, D. W., Winokur, G., & Nasrallah, A. (1987). Suicide in subtypes of major affective disorder: A comparison with general population suicide mortality. *Archives of General Psychiatry, 44*(10), 878–880.

Black, D. W., Winokur, G., & Nasrallah, A. (1988). Effect of psychosis on suicide risk in 1,593 patients with unipolar and bipolar affective disorders. *American Journal of Psychiatry, 145*(7), 849–852.

Black, D. W., Yates, W., Petty, F., Noyes, R., Jr., & Brown, K. (1986). Suicidal behaviour in alcoholic males. *Comprehensive Psychiatry, 27*(3), 227–233.

Bliss, E. L. (1980). Multiple personality: A report of fourteen cases with implications for schizophrenia and hysteria. *Archives of General Psychiatry, 37,* 1388–1397.

Bolin, R., Wright, R., Wilkinson, M., & Lindner, C. (1968). Survey of suicide among patients on home leave from a mental hospital. *Psychiatric Quarterly, 42*(1), 81–89.

Borg, S. E., & Stahl, M. (1982). Prediction of suicide: A prospective study of suicides and controls among psychiatric patients. *Acta Psychiatrica Scandinavica, 65,* 221–232.

Brent, D. A. (1986). Overrepresentation of epileptics in a consecutive series of suicide attempters seen at a children's hospital, 1978–1983. *Journal of the American Academy of Child Psychiatry, 25*(2) 242–246.

Brent, D. A., Kupfer, D. J., Bromet, E. J., & Dew, M. A. (1988). The assessment and treatment of patients at risk for suicide. In A. J. Frances & R. E. Hales (Eds.), *Review of psychiatry* (Vol. 7, pp. 353–385). Washington, DC: American Psychiatric Press.

Bryan, D. P., & Herjanic, B. (1980). Depression and suicide among adolescents and young adults with selective handicapping conditions. *Exceptional Education Quarterly, 1*(2), 57–65.

Buda, M., Tsuang, M. T., & Fleming, J. A. (1988). Causes of death in DSM-III schizophrenics and other psychotics (atypical group): A comparison with the general population. *Archives of General Psychiatry, 45*(3), 283–285.

Burke, A. W. (1983). The proportional distribution of suicide among mental hospital deaths and persons in the general population. In J. P. Soubrier & J. Vedrinne (Eds.), *Depression et suicide* (pp. 204–208). Paris: Pergamon Press.

Ciompi, L. (1976). Late suicide in former mental patients. *Psychiatria Clinica, 9,* 59–63.

Cohen, L. J., Test, M. A., & Brown, R. L. (1990). Suicide and schizophrenia: Data from a prospective community treatment study. *American Journal of Psychiatry, 147*(5), 602–607.

Commission on Professional and Hospital Activities. (1978). *The International Classification of Diseases, Ninth Revision, Clinical Modification.* Ann Arbor; MI: Author.

Copas, J. B., & Robin, A. (1982). Suicide in psychiatric in-patients. *British Journal of Psychiatry, 141,* 503–511.

Coryell, W. (1988). Panic disorder and mortality. *Psychiatric Clinics of North America, 11*(2), 433–440.

Coryell, W., Noyes, R., & Clancy, J. (1982). Excess mortality in panic disorder: A comparison with primary unipolar depression. *Archives of General Psychiatry, 39,* 701-703.

Coryell, W., Noyes, R., & House, D. (1986). Mortality among outpatients with anxiety disorders. *American Journal of Psychiatry, 143*(4), 508-510.

d'Elia, G., von Knorring, L., & Perris, C. (1974). Non-psychotic depressive disorders: A ten year follow-up. *Acta Psychiatrica Scandinavica* (Suppl. 255), 173-186.

Dassori, A. M., Mezzich, J. E., & Keshavan, M. (1990). Suicidal indicators in schizophrenia. *Acta Psychiatrica Scandinavica, 81,* 409-413.

De Graaf, A. C. (1982). Mededeling uit het centrale patientenregister. *Tijdschrift voor Psychiatrie, 24*(7-8), 507-512.

Dorpat, T. L., & Boswell, J. W. (1963). An evaluation of suicidal intent in suicide attempts. *Comprehensive Psychiatry, 4*(2), 117-125.

Drake, R. E., & Ehrlich, J. (1985). Suicide attempts associated with akathisia. *American Journal of Psychiatry, 142*(4), 499-501.

Durkheim, E. (1951). *Suicide: A study in sociology* (J. A. Spaulding & G. Simpson, Trans.). Glencoe, IL: Free Press. (Original work published 1897)

Dyck, R. J., Bland, R. C., Newman, S. C., & Orn, H. (1988). Suicide attempts and psychiatric disorders in Edmonton. *Acta Psychiatrica Scandinavica,* 77(Suppl. 338), 64-71.

Eastwood, M. R., Henderson, M. D., & Montgomery, I. M. (1972). Personality and parasuicide: Methodological problems. *Medical Journal of Australia, 1*(4), 170-175.

Eastwood, M. R., Stiasny, S., Meier, H. M., & Woogh, C. M. (1982). Mental illness and mortality. *Comprehensive Psychiatry, 23*(4), 377-385.

Egeland, J. A., & Sussex, J. N. (1985). Suicide and family loading for affective disorders. *Journal of the American Medical Association, 254*(7), 915-918.

Evenson, R. C., Wood, J. B., Nuttall, E. A., & Cho, D. W. (1982). Suicide rates among public mental health patients. *Acta Psychiatrica Scandinavica, 66,* 254-264.

Farberow, N. L. Ganzler, S., Cutter, F., & Reynolds, D. (1971). An eight-year survey of hospital suicides. *Suicide and Life-Threatening Behavior, 1*(3), 184-202.

Farberow, N. L., & McEvoy, T. L. (1966). Suicide among patients with diagnoses of anxiety reaction or depressive reaction in general medical and surgical hospitals. *Journal of Abnormal Psychology, 71*(4), 287-299.

Farberow, N. L., Shneidman, E. S., & Neuringer, C. (1966). Case history and hospitalization factors in suicides of neuropsychiatric hospital patients. *Journal of Nervous and Mental Disease, 142*(1), 32-44.

Favazza, A. R., DeRosear, L., & Conterio, K. (1989). Self-mutilation and eating disorders. *Suicide and Life-Threatening Behavior, 19*(4), 352-361.

Fawcett, J., Scheftner, W., Clark, D., Hedeker, D., Gibbons, R., & Coryell, W. (1987). Clinical predictors of suicide in patients with major affective disorders: A controlled prospective study. *American Journal of Psychiatry, 144*(1), 35-40.

Fernando, S., & Storm, V. (1984). Suicide among psychiatric patients of a district general hospital. *Psychological Medicine, 14,* 661-672.

Flood, R. A., & Seager, G. P. (1968). A retrospective examination of psychiatric case records of patients who subsequently committed suicide. *British Journal of Psychiatry, 114,* 443-450.

Forssman, H., & Jansson, B. (1960). Follow-up study of 849 men admitted for mental disorders to the psychiatric ward of a general hospital. *Acta Psychiatrica et Neurologica Scandinavica, 35*(5), 57–72.

Frances, A., Fyer, M., & Clarkin, J. (1986). Personality and suicide. *Annals of the New York Academy of Sciences, 487,* 281–293.

Friedman, R. C., Aronoff, M. S., Clarkin, J. F., Corn, R., & Hurt, S. W. (1983). History of suicidal behaviour in depressed borderline inpatients. *American Journal of Psychiatry, 140*(8), 1023–1026.

Fyer, M. R., Frances, A. J., Sullivan, T., Hurt, S. W., & Clarkin, J. (1988). Suicide attempts in patients with borderline personality disorder. *American Journal of Psychiatry, 145*(6), 737–739.

Gardner, A., & Rich, C. (1988). Eating disorders and suicide. In R. Yufit (Ed.), *Proceedings of the 21st Annual Meeting of the American Association of Suicidology* (pp. 171–172). Denver: American Association of Suicidology.

Garvey, M. J., & Spoden, F. (1980). Suicide attempts in antisocial personality disorder. *Comprehensive Psychiatry, 21*(2), 146–149.

Gittleson, N. L. (1966). The relationship between obsessions and suicidal attempts in depressive psychosis. *British Journal of Psychiatry, 112,* 889–890.

Goldney, R. D., Positano, S., Spence, N. D., & Rosenman, S. J. (1985). Suicide in association with psychiatric hopsitalization. *Australian and New Zealand Journal of Psychiatry, 19,* 177–183.

Gordon, R. G. (1929). Certain personality problems in relation to mental health illness with special reference to suicide and homicide. *British Journal of Medical Psychology, 9*(60).

Gove, W. R., & Hughes, M. (1980). Reexamining the ecological fallacy: A study in which aggregate data are critical in investigating the pathological effect of living alone. *Social Forces, 58*(4), 1157–1177.

Guze, S. B., & Robins, E. (1970). Suicide and primary affective disorders. *British Journal of Psychiatry, 117,* 437–438.

Hagnell, O., & Rorsman, B. (1979). Suicide in the Lundby study: A comparative investigation of clinical aspects. *Neuropsychobiology, 5,* 61–73.

Hagnell, O., Lanke, J., & Rorsman, B. (1981). Suicide rates in the Lundby Study: Mental illness as a risk factor for suicide. *Neuropsychobiology, 7,* 248–253.

Harris, A. (1938). The prognosis of anxiety state. *British Medical Journal, ii,* 649.

Harry, J. (1989). Sexual identity issues. In L. Davidson & M. Linnoila (Eds.), *Report of the Secretary's Task Force on Youth Suicide: Vol. 2. Risk factors for youth suicide* (DHHS Publication No. 89-1622, pp. 131–142). Washington, DC: U.S. Government Printing Office.

Hasin, D., Grant, B., & Endicott, J. (1988). Treated and untreated suicide attempts in substance abuse patients. *Journal of Nervous and Mental Disease, 176*(5), 289–294.

Hatsukami, D., Eckert, E., Mitchell, J. E., & Pyle, R. (1984). Affective disorder and substance abuse in women with bulimia. *Psychological Medicine, 14,* 701–704.

Haugland, G., Craig, T. J., Goodman, A. B., & Siegel, C. (1983). Mortality in the era of deinstitutionalization. *American Journal of Psychiatry, 40*(7), 848–852.

Hawton, K. (1987). Assessment of suicide risk. *British Journal of Psychiatry, 150,* 145–153.

Hayes, M. L., & Sloat, R. S. (1988). Learning disability and suicide. *Academic Therapy, 23*(5), 469–475.

Helzer, J. E., & Przybeck, T. R. (1988). The co-occurence of alcoholism and other psychiatric disorders in the general population and its impact on treatment. *Journal of Studies on Alcohol, 49*, 219–224.

Hesso, R. (1977). Suicide in Norwegian, Finnish, and Swedish psychiatric hospitals. *Archiv für Psychiatrie und Nervenkrankheiten, 224*, 119–127.

Hillard, J. R., Ramm, D., Zung, W. W. K., & Holland, J. M. (1983). Suicide in a psychiatric emergency room population. *American Journal of Psychiatry, 140*(4), 459–462.

Hirschfeld, R., & Davidson, L. (1988). Risk factors for suicide. In A. J. Frances & R. E. Hales (Eds.), *Review of psychiatry* (Vol. 7, pp. 307–333). Washington, DC: American Psychiatric Press.

Hoberman, H. M., & Garfinkel, B. D. (1988). Completed suicide in children and adolescents. *Journal of the American Academy of Child and Adolescent Psychiatry, 27*(6), 689–695.

Hollingsworth, C. E., Tanguay, P. E., Grossman, L., & Pabst, P. (1980). Long-term outcome of obsessive–compulsive disorder in childhood. *Journal of the American Academy of Child Psychiatry, 19*(1), 134–144.

Innes, G., & Millar, W. M. (1970). Mortality among psychiatric patients. *Scottish Medical Journal, 15*, 143–148.

James, I. P., & Levin, S. (1964). Suicide following discharge from psychiatric hospital. *Archives of General Psychiatry, 10*, 67–71.

Jamison, K. R. (1986). Suicide and bipolar disorders. *Annals of the New York Academy of Sciences, 487*, 301–315.

Kerr, T. A., Schapira, K., & Roth, M. (1969). The relationship between premature death and affective disorders. *British Journal of Psychiatry, 115*, 1277–1282.

Khuri, R., & Akiskal, H. S. (1983). Suicide prevention: The necessity of treating contributory psychiatric disorders. *Psychiatric Clinics of North America, 6*(1), 193–207.

Kopp, M. S., Felsovaly, A., Skrabski, A., & Tringer, L. (1977). Clinical epidemiological study of mental disorders. *Activitas Nervosa Superior*(Praha), *19*(2, Suppl.), 385–387.

Kovacs, M., & Puig-Antich, J. (1989). "Major psychiatric disorders" as risk factors for suicide. In L. Davidson & M. Linnoila (Eds.), *Report of the Secretary's Task Force on Youth Suicide: Vol. 2. Risk factors for youth suicide* (DHHS Publication No. 89-1622, pp. 143–159). Washington, DC: U.S. Government Printing Office.

Kowalchuk, B., & King, J. D. (1989). Adult suicide versus coping with nonverbal learning disorder. *Journal of Learning Disabilities, 22*(3), 177–179.

Kraft, D. P., & Babigian, H. M. (1976) Suicide by persons with and without psychiatric contacts. *Archives of General Psychiatry, 33*, 209–215.

Kroll, J. L., Carey, K. S., & Sines, L. K. (1985). Twenty-year followup of borderline personality disorder: A pilot study. In C. Shagass (Ed.), *Biological psychiatry 1985: Proceedings of the IVth World Congress of Biological Psychiatry*. New York: Elsevier.

Kullgren, G. (1988). Factors associated with completed suicide in borderline personality disorder. *Journal of Nervous and Mental Disease, 176*(1), 40–44.

Kullgren, G., Renberg, E., & Jacobsson, L. (1986). An empirical study of borderline personality disorder and psychiatric suicides. *Journal of Nervous and Mental Disease, 174*(6), 328–331.

Lester, D., & Beck, A. T. (1975). Attempted suicide in alcoholics and drug addicts. *Journal of Studies on Alcohol, 36*(1), 162–164.

Lester, D., & Beck, A. T. (1976). Suicidal behavior in neurotics and psychotics. *Psychological Reports, 39*, 549–550.

Levy, S., & Southcombe, R. H. (1953). Suicide in a state hospital for the mentally ill. *Journal of Nervous and Mental Disease, 117*, 504–514.

Lipschutz, L. S. (1942). Some administrative aspects of suicide in the mental hospital. *American Journal of Psychiatry, 99*, 181–187.

MacDonald, M. (1977). The inner side of wisdom: Suicide in early modern England. *Psychological Medicine, 7*, 565–582.

Martin, R. L., Cloninger, C. R., Guze, S. B., & Clayton, P. J. (1985). Mortality in a follow-up of 500 psychiatric outpatients. *Archives of General Psychiatry, 42*, 58–66.

Matthews, W. S., & Barabas, G. (1982). Suicide and epilepsy: A review of the literature. *Psychosomatics, 22*(6), 515–524.

McDowall, A. W. T., Brooke, E. M., Freeman-Browne, D. L., & Robin, A. A. (1968). Subsequent suicide in depressed in-patients. *British Journal of Psychiatry, 114*, 749–754.

McGlashan, T. H. (1986). The Chestnut Lodge follow-up study: III. Long-term outcome of borderline personalities. *Archives of General Psychiatry, 43*, 2–30.

McHugh, P. R., & Goodell, H. (1971). Suicidal behavior: A distinction in patients with sedative poisoning seen in a general hospital. *Archives of General Psychiatry, 25*, 456–464.

Medlicott, R. W., & Medlicott, P. A. W. (1969). Suicide in and after discharge from a private psychiatric hospital over a period of eighty-six years. *Australian and New Zealand Journal of Psychiatry, 3*, 137–144.

Miles, C. P. (1977). Conditions predisposing to suicide: A review. *Journal of Nervous and Mental Disease, 164*, 231–247.

Modestin, J. (1989). Completed suicide in personality disordered inpatients. *Journal of Personality Disorders, 3*(2), 113–121.

Modestin, J., & Hoffmann, H. (1989). Completed suicide in psychiatric inpatients and former inpatients. *Acta Psychiatrica Scandinavica, 79*, 229–234.

Modestin, J., & Kopp, W. (1988). Study on suicide in depressed inpatients. *Journal of Affective Disorders, 15*, 157–162.

Morgan, H. G., Burns-Cox, C. J., Pocock, H., & Pottle, S. (1975). Deliberate self-harm: Clinical and socio-economic characteristics of 368 patients. *British Journal of Psychiatry, 127*, 564–574.

Morrison, J. R. (1982). Suicide in a psychiatric practice population. *Journal of Clinical Psychiatry, 43*(9), 348–352.

Mościcki, E., O'Carroll, P., Rae, D., Locke, B., Roy, A., & Regier, D. (1988). Suicide attempts in the Epidemiologic Catchment Area study. *Yale Journal of Biology and Medicine, 61*, 259–268.

Murphy, S. L., Rounsaville, B. J., Eyre, S., & Kleber, H. D. (1983). Suicide attempts in treated opiate addicts. *Comprehensive Psychiatry, 24*, 79–87.

Murphy, G. E., & Wetzel, R. D. (1990). The lifetime risk of suicide in alcoholism. *Archives of General Psychiatry, 47*, 383–392.

Myers, D. H., & Neal, C. D. (1978). Suicide in psychiatric patients. *British Journal of Psychiatry, 133*, 38–44.

Newson-Smith, J. G. B., & Hirsch, S. R. (1979). Psychiatric symptoms in self-poisoning patients. *Psychological Medicine, 9*, 493–500.

Niskanen, P., Lonnqvist, K. A., & Rinta-Manty, R. (1974). Suicides in Helsinki psychiatric hospitals in 1964–1972. *Psychiatrica Fennica*, 275–280.

Noyes, R., Clancy, J., Hoenk, C. R., & Slymen, D. J. (1978). Anxiety neurosis and physical illness. *Comprehensive Psychiatry, 19*, 407–413.

Nuttall, E. A., Evenson, R. C., & Cho, D. W. (1980). Patients of a public state mental health system who commit suicide. *Journal of Nervous and Mental Disease, 168*(7), 424–427.

Odegard, O. (1967). Mortality in Norwegian psychiatric hospitals, 1950–1962. *Acta Genetica et Statistica Medica, 17*, 137–153.

Paris, J., Brown, R., & Nowlis, D. (1987). Long-term follow-up of borderline patients in a general hospital. *Comprehensive Psychiatry, 28*(6), 530–535.

Paris, J., Nowlis, D., & Brown, R. (1989). Predictors of suicide in borderline personality disorder. *Canadian Journal of Psychiatry, 34*, 8–9.

Pattison, E. M., & Kahan, J. (1983). The deliberate self-harm syndrome. *American Journal of Psychiatry, 140*(7), 867–872.

Perris, C., Beskow, J., & Jacobsson, L. (1980). Some remarks on the incidence of successful suicide in psychiatric care. *Social Psychiatry, 15*, 161–166.

Pokorny, A. D. (1960). Characteristics of forty-four patients who subsequently committed suicide. *Archives of General Psychiatry, 2*, 315–323.

Pokorny, A. D. (1964). Suicide rates in various psychiatric disorders. *Journal of Nervous and Mental Disease, 139*(6), 499–506.

Pokorny, A. D. (1983). Prediction of suicide in psychiatric patients: Report of a prospective study. *Archives of General Psychiatry, 40*, 249–257.

Pope, H. G., Jonas, J. M., Hudson, J. I., Cohen, B. M., & Tohen, M. (1983). The validity of DSM-III borderline personality disorder. *Archives of General Psychiatry, 40*, 23–30.

Prasad, A., & Kumar, N. (1988). Suicidal behavior in hospitalized schizophrenics. *Suicide and Life-Threatening Behavior, 18*(3), 265–269.

Putnam, F. W., Guroff, J. J., & Silberman, E. K. (1986). The clinical phenomenology of multiple personality disorder: A review of 100 recent cases. *Journal of Clinical Psychiatry, 47*(6), 285–293.

Retterstol, N., Hesso, R., & Ekeland, H. (1985). *Suicide in young people—the development in Scandinavia: A seven year series for Oslo*. Paper presented at the 13th International Congress for Suicide Prevention and Crisis Intervention, Vienna.

Rich, C. L., Fowler, R. C., & Young, D. (1986). Suicide and psychosis: Changing patterns. In S. R. Sandler (Ed.), *Proceedings of the 19th Annual Meeting of the American Association of Suicidology* (pp. 94–95). Denver: American Association of Suicidology.

Rich, C. L., Fowler, R. C., & Young, D. (1989). Substance abuse and suicide: The San Diego study. *Annals of Clinical Psychiatry, 1,* 79-85.

Robin, A. A., Brooke, E., & Freeman-Browne, D. (1968). Some aspects of suicide in psychiatric patients in Southend. *British Journal of Psychiatry, 114,* 739-747.

Roose, S. P., Glassman, A. H., Walsh, B. T., Woodring, S., & Vital-Herne, J. (1983). Depression, delusions, and suicide. *American Journal of Psychiatry, 140*(9), 1159-1162.

Rorsman, B., Hagnell, O., & Lanke, J. (1985). *Death from suicide and accident and mental disorder in the Lundby Study.* Paper presented at the 13th International Congress for Suicide Prevention and Crisis Intervention, Vienna.

Rosenberg, C. M. (1968). Complications of obsessional neurosis. *British Journal of Psychiatry, 114,* 477-478.

Ross, C. A., Norton, G. R., & Wozney, K. (1989). Multiple personality disorder: An analysis of 236 cases. *Canadian Journal of Psychiatry, 34,* 413-418.

Rourke, B., Young, G. C., & Leenaars, A. A. (1987). A childhood learning disability that predisposes those afflicted to adolescent and adult depression and suicide risk. *Journal of Learning Disabilities, 22*(3), 169-175.

Roy, A. (1982). Risk factors for suicide in psychiatric patients. *Archives of General Psychiatry, 39,* 1089-1095.

Roy, A. (1986). Suicide in schizophrenia. In A. Roy (Ed.), *Suicide* (pp. 97-112). Baltimore: Williams & Wilkins.

Sainsbury, P. (1986). Depression, suicide and suicide prevention. In A. Roy (Ed.), *Suicide* (pp. 73-88). Baltimore: Williams & Wilkins.

Scheftner, W. A., Young, M. A., Endicott, W. C., Fogg, L., Clark, D. C., & Fawcett, J. (1988). Family history and five-year suicide risk. *British Journal of Psychiatry, 153,* 805-809.

Schuckit, M. A. (1985). The clinical implications of primary diagnostic groups among alcoholics. *Archives of General Psychiatry, 42*(11), 1043-1049.

Shearer, S. L., Peters, C. P., Quaytman, M. S., & Wadman, B. E. (1988). Intent and lethality of suicide attempts among female borderline inpatients. *American Journal of Psychiatry, 145*(11), 1424-1427.

Shneidman, E. S., Farberow, N. L., & Leonard, C. V. (1962, February 1). *Suicide-evaluation and treatment of suicidal risk among schizophrenic patients in psychiatric hospitals* (Medical Bulletin, Department of Medicine and Surgery). Washington, DC.: Veterans Administration.

Silver, M. A., Bohnert, M., Bect, A. T., & Marcus, D. (1971). Relation of depression to attempted suicide and seriousness of intent. *Archives of General Psychiatry, 25,* 573-576.

Sims, A. (1984). Neurosis and mortality. *Journal of Psychosomatic Research, 28,* 353-362.

Sims, A., & Prior, P. (1978). The pattern of mortality in severe neuroses. *British Journal of Psychiatry, 133,* 299-305.

Sletten, I. W., Brown, M. L., Evenson, R. C., & Altman, H. (1972). Suicide in mental hospital patients. *Diseases of the Nervous System, 33*(5), 328-334.

Solomon, R. S., & Solomon, V. (1982). Differential diagnosis of the multiple personality. *Psychological Reports, 51,* 1187-1194.

Sternlicht, M., Pustel, G., & Deutsch, M. R. (1970). Suicidal tendencies among institutionalized retardates. *Journal of Mental Subnormality*, *16*(31, Pt. 2), 93–102.

Stone, M. H., Stone, D. K., & Hurt, S. (1987). The natural history of borderline patients treated by intensive hospitalization. *Psychiatric Clinics of North America, 10*(2), 185–206.

Temoche, A., Pugh, T., & MacMahon, B. (1964). Suicide rates among current and former mental institution patients. *Journal of Nervous and Mental Disease, 138*, 124–130.

Tsuang, M. T., Dempsey, G. M., & Fleming, J. A. (1979). Can ECT prevent premature death and suicide in 'schizoaffective' patients? *Journal of Affective Disorders, 1*, 167–171.

Tyrer, P., Remington, M., & Alexander, J. (1987). The outcome of neurotic disorders after out-patient and day hospital care. *British Journal of Psychiatry, 151*, 57–62.

Urwin, P., & Gibbons, J. L. (1979). Psychiatric diagnosis in self-poisoning patients. *Psychological Medicine, 9*, 501–507.

van Egmond, M., & Diekstra, R. F. W. (1990). The predictability of suicidal behavior: The results of a meta-analysis of published studies. *Crisis, 11*(2), 57–84.

Viesselman, J. O., & Roig, M. (1985). Depression and suicidality in eating disorders. *Journal of Clinical Psychiatry, 46*, 118–124.

Vinoda, K. S. (1966). Personality characteristics of attempted suicides. *British Journal of Psychiatry, 112*, 1143–1150.

Virkkunen, M. (1974). Suicides in schizophrenia and paranoid psychoses. *Acta Psychiatrica Scandinavica* (Suppl. 250).

Weeke, A., Vaeth, M., & Juel, K. (1985). *Suicides among manic-depressives.* Paper presented at the 21st Nordic Congress on Psychiatry, Odense, Denmark.

Weissman, A. N., Beck, A. T., & Kovacs, M. (1979). Drug abuse, hopelessness, and suicidal behaviour. *International Journal of the Addictions, 14*(4), 451–464.

Weissman, M. M. (1974). The epidemiology of suicide attempts, 1960 to 1971. *Archives of General Psychiatry, 30*, 737–746.

Weissman, M. M., Klerman, G., Markowitz, J., & Ouellette, R. (1989). Suicidal ideation and suicide attempts in panic disorder and attacks. *New England Journal of Medicine, 321*(18), 1209–1214.

Westermeyer, J. F., & Harrow, M. (1989). Early phases of schizophrenia and depression: Prediction of suicide. In R. Williams & J. T. Dalby (Eds.), *Depression in schizophrenics* (pp. 153–169). New York: Plenum Press.

Wheeler, E. O., White, P. D., Reed, W. E., & Cohen, M. E. (1950). Neurocirculatory asthenia (anxiety neurosis, effort syndrome, neuroasthenia): A 20-year follow-up study of 173 patients. *Journal of the American Medical Association, 142*, 878–888.

Whitters, A. C., Cadoret, R. J., & Widmer, R. B. (1985). Factors associated with suicide attempts in alcohol abusers. *Journal of Affective Disorders, 9*, 19–23.

Williams, R., & Dalby, J. T. (Eds.). (1989). *Depression in schizophrenics.* New York: Plenum Press.

Wilson, G. C., Jr. (1968). Suicide in psychiatric patients who have received hospital treatment. *American Journal of Psychiatry, 125*(6), 752–757.

Winokur, G., & Tsuang, M. (1975). The Iowa 500: Suicide in mania, depression and schizophrenia. *American Journal of Psychiatry, 132*(6), 650–651.

Woodruff, R. A., Clayton, P. J., & Guze, S. B. (1972). Suicide attempts and psychiatric diagnosis. *Diseases of the Nervous System, 33*, 617–621.

World Health Organization. (1978). *Mental disorders: Glossary and guide to their classification in accordance with the ninth revision of the International Classification of Diseases.* Geneva: Author.

Zilber, N., Schufman, N., & Lerner, Y. (1989). Mortality among psychiatric patients—the groups at risk. *Acta Psychiatrica Scandinavica, 79*, 248–256.

Zilboorg, G. (1936). Differential diagnostic types of suicide. *Archives of Neurology and Psychiatry, 35*, 270–291.

CHAPTER 15

Alcoholism and Drug Abuse

David Lester, Ph.D.
Center for Studies of Suicide, Blackwood, New Jersey

Substance abuse is sometimes viewed as a self-destructive behavior. For example, Menninger (1938) included substance abuse in his category of "chronic suicide," since he felt that substance abuse may be motivated in part, consciously or unconsciously, by suicidal impulses. Alternatively, perhaps, suicide and substance abuse may be expressions of the same underlying variable, such as social disorganization or an oral personality.

Substance abusers appear to have a higher incidence of suicidal behavior than nonabusers. It may be that substance abuse disrupts the social relationships of people and impairs their work performance, leading to social isolation and social decline; that it increases their impulsivity and lowers their restraints; or that it increases their self-deprecation and depression, tendencies that may increase the probability of suicidal behavior (Kendall, 1983).

Alcoholism may also make the self-destructive medications (e.g., antidepressant drugs) often used for suicide more lethal to the body, and alcohol itself may be used in conjunction with medications to provide a more lethal concoction. Furthermore, the substances that can be abused are also those that can be used to commit suicide. Thus, people have committed suicide by overdosing on such drugs as heroin and cocaine. It should also be noted that in the planning and the execution of a suicidal action, individuals often use alcohol and other drugs to achieve a state of mind in which it is easier to carry out their suicidal plan.

The present chapter addresses two issues: (1) Can substance abuse be a predictor of suicidal behavior? (2) Will the useful predictors of suicidal behavior differ in substance abusers and nonabusers? Let us first turn to the incidence of suicide in substance abusers.

SUICIDAL BEHAVIOR IN SUBSTANCE ABUSERS
Alcohol Abusers

Many recent studies have reported an excess of alcoholics among completed suicides. For example, Wihelmsen, Elmfeldt, and Wedel (1983) found an excess of alcoholics among Swedish completed suicides; Knop and Fischer (1981) found an excess of of alcoholics among duodenal ulcer patients who completed suicide; and Fawcett et al. (1987) found an excess of alcohol abusers among patients with affective disorder who completed suicide. Similarly, many recent studies have reported an excess of completed suicides among alcoholics (Agren & Jakobsson, 1987; Barr, Antes, Ottenberg, & Rosen, 1984; Babigan, Lehman, & Reed, 1985; Berglund & Tunving, 1985; Lindberg & Agren, 1988; Ohara et al., 1989). Indeed, Beck and Steer (1989) found that alcoholism was the strongest single predictor of subsequent completed suicide in a sample of attempted suicides.

In a community survey, Weissman, Myers, and Harding (1980) found that 24% of alcoholics had attempted suicide, as compared to 5% of those with other diagnoses. A similar excess of attempted suicides has been reported by Gomberg (1989) and by Vaglum and Vaglum (1987) in alcoholic female psychiatric patients. Nace, Saxon, and Shore (1983) found an excess of attempted suicides only among those alcoholics who also were diagnosed concomitantly as having borderline personality disorder. Bascue and Epstein (1980) also discovered a high incidence of suicide attempts in alcoholics. Smith (1986), however, found no association between alcohol use and suicidal involvement in a sample of young adults.

Garvey, Tuason, Hoffman, and Chastek (1983) found a higher incidence of alcohol abuse in patients with affective disorders who attempted suicide than in those who did not. Robinson and Duffy (1989) found a higher incidence of alcohol abuse in attempted suicides who used cutting than in those who used overdoses. Gaines and Richmond (1980), however, found no association between suicidal gestures and alcohol abuse in military trainees. It seems that the evidence for an association between alcohol abuse and attempted suicide is not as consistent as the evidence for an association between alcohol abuse and completed suicide.

In a recent review of the literature, Roy and Linnoila (1986) estimated that on average about 18% of alcoholics subsequently complete suicide and that 21% of suicides are alcoholics. Thus, not only is the suicide rate substantially elevated among alcoholics, but suicide is a cause of death for a substantial percentage of alcoholics.

Drug Abusers

An increased suicide rate has been found in narcotic addicts (O'Donnell, 1969) and opioid addicts (Watterson, Simpson, & Sells, 1975). However,

Barner-Rasmussen, Dupont, and Bille (1986) found an average rate of suicide for psychiatric patients diagnosed as substance abusers. Bagley (1989) reported a higher rate of substance abuse in adolescents who completed suicide, and Allebeck, Allgulander, and Fisher (1988) found a higher rate of both narcotic and alcohol abuse in conscripts who completed suicide.

Tardiff, Gross, Wu, Stajic, and Millman (1989) found that 7% of the deaths of in a sample of cocaine abusers were suicides. Wetli (1983) reported that 11% of deaths in persons taking methaqualone were suicides. Tunving (1988) found that 31% of the deaths in a group of young drug addicts were suicides. Beck and Steer (1989), however, claimed that drug abuse did not predict subsequent completed suicide in a sample of attempted suicides.

Drug abusers have been found to have high rates of attempted suicide (Frederick, Resnick, & Wittlin, 1973; Hatsukami, Mitchell, Eckert, & Pyle, 1986; Janofsky, Spear, & Neubauer, 1988; Kosten & Rounsaville, 1988; McKenry, Tishler, & Kelley, 1983; Murphy, Rounsaville, Eyre & Kleber, 1983; Saxon, Kuncel, & Aldrich, 1978; Saxon, Kuncel, & Kaufman, 1980). Gaines and Richmond (1980) found more drug abuse in military trainees who made mild suicidal gestures than in those who did not. Moise, Kovach Reed, and Bellows (1982), however, found an excess of suicide attempts among female drug abusers only in whites. There is no evidence yet to indicate that some drugs are more strongly associated with suicidal behavior than others, and almost all drugs have been implicated in the association.

Both Farberow, Litman, and Nelson (1988) and Kirkpatrick-Smith, Rich, Bonner, and Jans (1989) found that suicidal ideation was associated with alcohol and drug abuse in adolescents in the community, and that substance abuse added significantly to the ability to predict suicidal ideation in a multiple-regression analysis. Smith (1986) found that marijuana, cocaine and tobacco (cigarette) use were each weakly associated with more suicidal involvement in a sample of young adults. Weissman, Klerman, Markowitz, and Ouellette (1989) reported that drug and alcohol abuse predicted attempted suicide in people who had suffered from panic disorders at some point in their lives. However, Levy and Deykin (1989) found that substance abuse was associated with suicidal ideation and attempts only in male college students. Simonds and Kashani (1979) found a higher incidence of attempted suicide in delinquents who had abused phencyclidine than in those who had not. Haycock (1989) reported that prisoners who made serious attempts at suicide were more likely to have opiate dependence than those who made suicidal gestures.

Discussion

It is clear that substance abuse appears to be associated with suicidal behavior—both with completed suicides and suicide attempts. Several questions need to be addressed in future research. First, how does the increased risk of suicidal behavior in substance abusers compare with the increased risk when other psychiatric symptoms or syndromes are present? For example, is the risk of suicidal behavior greater if the individual has already attempted suicide or if the individual has a major affective disorder? How should these symptoms/ syndromes be rated in relation to one another? In the classic suicide prediction scale devised by the Los Angeles Suicide Prevention Center (Whittemore, 1970), affective disorder is given a higher rating than alcoholism.

Other questions that must be addressed include the following: Are different abused substances associated with different risks for subsequent suicidal behavior? Is substance abuse a better predictor by itself or in combination with other factors (such as an affective disorder or borderline personality disorder)? Finally, is the increased risk of suicide identified in the research to date found for all groups (by gender, race, psychiatric status, etc.), or only for some of these groups?

PREDICTING SUICIDAL BEHAVIOR IN SUBSTANCE ABUSERS

Many studies have compared substance abusers with a history of attempted suicide and those with no such history. The identifying characteristics are shown in Table 15.1 for alcohol abusers and in Table 15.3 for drug abusers. It should be noted that all of these studies have focused on *previous* attempts at suicide. Similarly, many studies have compared substance abusers who have completed suicide with those who have not, and the results of these studies are summarized in Tables 15.2 and 15.4 for alcohol and drug abusers, respectively.

Several features of this information are noteworthy. First, many of the variables identified as predictive of suicide are similar to those identified for nonabusers. For example, psychiatric disturbance is predictive of subsequent suicide in all individuals, not simply substance abusers. Second, many of the variables that may differentiate suicidal abusers from nonsuicidal abusers have been identified by only one or two groups of investigators. The usefulness of these variables as predictors must therefore be considered suspect until this research can be replicated by others. Third, the major lacuna in the information is for variables that might predict completed suicide in drug abusers; only one study was located that addressed this question. Fourth, the most fruitful predictor variables may turn out to be those related specifically to the substance abuse, since these variables are unique to the substance abuser. Thus, they may add to the predictive power of variables common to all of those for whom we wish to predict subsequent suicidal behavior.

So far, no research has explored the usefulness of these variables in predicting subsequent suicidal behavior; perhaps this chapter may stimu-

TABLE 15.1. Predictors of Attempted Suicide in Alcohol Abusers

Alcohol abuse symptoms
  Delirium tremens absent (Kockott & Feuerlein, 1968)
  Delirium tremens present (Hasin, Grant, & Endicott, 1988)
  Began drinking earlier in life (Black, Yates, Potty, Noyes, & Brown, 1986; Buydens-Branchey, Branchey, & Nourair, 1989; Hesselbrock, Hesselbrock, Szymanski, & Weidenman, 1988; Koller & Castanos, 1968)
  Severer alcoholism (Black et al., 1986; Hasin et al., 1988; Hesselbrock et al., 1988; Schuckit, 1986; Whitters, Cadoret, Troughton, & Widmer, 1987)
  More often gamma (rather than delta) alcoholics (Lesch, Walter, Mader, Musalek, & Zeiler, 1988)
  More often members of Alcoholics Anonymous (Palola, Dorpat, & Larson, 1962)
  Less often on skid row (Palola et al., 1962)
  At least one alcoholic parent (Gomberg, 1989; Hesselbrock et al., 1988)
Psychiatric symptoms
  More psychiatrically disturbed (Hagnell, Nyman, & Tunving, 1973; Hesselbrock et al., 1988; Lesch et al., 1988; Schuckit, 1986)
  Any psychiatric diagnosis (Weissman, Myers, & Harding, 1980)
  More neurosis (Hagnell et al., 1973; Hesselbrock et al., 1988)
  More anxiety/panic attacks or disorders (Gomberg, 1989; Hagnell et al., 1973; Hasin et al., 1988; Hesselbrock et al., 1988)
  More paranoia and aggression (Hagnell et al., 1973)
  More socially withdrawn (Lesch et al., 1988)
  More antisocial behavior when young and adult (Hasin et al., 1988; Hesselbrock et al., 1988; Schuckit, 1986)
  Major depression/depressed (Black et al., 1986; Hesselbrock et al., 1988, for men only; Lesch et al., 1988; Whitters, Cadoret, & Widmer, 1985)
  Drug abuse (Bissell & Skorina, 1987; Gomberg, 1989; Hasin et al., 1988; Hesselbrock et al., 1988; Schuckit, 1986; Whitters et al., 1985)
  Used psychotropic drugs in past (Blankfield, 1989)
  Multiple diagnoses (Whitters et al., 1985)
  More psychiatrically disturbed relatives (Schuckit, 1986)
  If antisocial personality disorder, more violence (Whitters et al., 1987)
Demographic characteristics
  Less often married (Hesselbrock et al., 1988)
  More often separated/divorced (Schuckit, 1986)
  More deteriorating social status (Lesch et al., 1988)
  Younger (Hasin et al., 1988; Hesselbrock et al., 1988)

late such a study. Motto (1980), however, has addressed the problem of predicting suicide in alcohol abusers. He interviewed 3,006 depressed or suicidal individuals admitted to a hospital and coded the responses to 186 questions. Of this sample, 978 individuals met the criteria for alcohol abuse and could be followed up for 2 years. The alcohol abusers were divided into two groups: one for identifying the variables that predicted completed suicide, and another for cross-validating the variables. Motto identified 11 variables: more than two prior attempts; ambivalence in present suicide at-

TABLE 15.2. Predictors of Completed Suicide in Alcohol Abusers

---

Alcohol abuse symptoms
  Late stages of alcoholism (Robins & Murphy, 1965)
Psychiatric symptoms
  More depressed/hopeless (Beck, Steer, & McElroy, 1982)
  More prior suicidal behavior (Kapamadzija, Souljanski, & Skendzic, 1979; Ritson, 1968)
  Higher neuroticism scores (Koller & Castanos, 1968)
  More affective disorder (Haberman, 1979)
  Less psychosis (Kapamadzija et al., 1978)
  If prior suicide attempt, more precautions taken (Beck, Steer, & Trexler, 1989)
Demographic and social characteristics
  Older (Zmuc, 1968)
  Younger and active alcoholics (Thorarinsson, 1979)
  Male (Kapamadzija et al., 1979)
  Married (Haberman, 1979; Kapamadzija et al., 1979; Zmuc 1968)
  White (Haberman, 1979)
  Employed (Haberman, 1979)
  Worse financial and marital situation (Kapamadzija et al., 1979)
  Last-born (Ritson, 1968)
  More often from broken homes (Kapamadzija et al., 1979)
  More self-critical (Ritson, 1968)
  More attached to mothers (Ritson, 1968)
  Better physical health (Kapamadzija et al., 1978)
  More often raised by nonparent (Koller & Castanos, 1968)

---

tempt; negative/mixed attitude toward the interviewer; over $1,000 in financial resources; living in hotel/apartment or unstable living arrangements; high intelligence; opposite-sex parent emotionally disturbed; poor health; health getting worse; no moves in the past year; and recent changes in job stability. In the cross-validation study, this risk scale identified 60% of the suicides and 36% of the nonsuicides as being at high risk. Motto noted that the degree of differentiation was not as precise as he would wish. It is also noteworthy that none of the 11 variables identified by Motto included information about the alcohol abuse. Future investigators need to apply the methodology described by Motto to validate the usefulness of the variables identified in Tables 15.2 and 15.4 for predicting completed suicide in substance abusers.

DIFFERENTIAL PREDICTION

Many years ago, in discussing the problem of predicting suicide in general, Lettieri (1974) suggested that it would be useful to devise scales specifically tailored for different sociodemographic groups. He presented separate scales for young and old men and for young and old women. Lettieri's work

TABLE 15.3. Predictors of Attempted Suicide in Drug Abusers

Drug Abuse Symptoms
    Oral abuse (rather than intravenous) (Gossop, Cobb, & Connell, 1975)
    If heroin addict, glue sniffer (D'Amanda, Plumb, & Taintor, 1977)
    Used LSD and cocaine (Harris, Linn, & Hunter, 1979)
    More blackouts from drug use (Harris, et al., 1979)
    Used alcohol (Davidson, 1979; Harris et al., 1979)
    Used hashish and heroin less (Davidson, 1979)
    Experienced withdrawal from barbiturates (Ward & Schuckit, 1980)
    More often drug-dependent (Davidson, 1979)
    Polydrug users (Davidson, 1979; Ward & Schuckit, 1980)
    In opiate abusers, heavy use of amphetamines/barbiturates and sedatives/inhal-
        ants (Murphy, Rounsaville, Eyre, & Kleber, 1983)
    In opiate abusers, less use of marijuana (Murphy et al., 1983)
    In opiate abusers, more severely addicted (Murphy et al., 1983)
Psychiatric symptoms
    More psychiatrically disturbed (Cavaiola, 1988; Davidson, 1979; Harris et al., 1979;
        Murphy et al., 1983; Ward & Schuckit, 1980)
    Psychiatric disturbance in mother (Ward & Schuckit, 1980)
    Sociopathy (Ward & Schuckit, 1980)
    History of hyperactivity (Ward & Schuckit, 1980)
    More learning disabilities/temper tantrums/accident proneness (Berman &
        Schwartz, 1989)
    In opiate abusers, sibling alcoholic/depressed (Murphy et al., 1983)
    In opiate abusers, father psychiatrically disturbed (Murphy et al., 1983)
    More neuroticism and introversion (Murphy et al., 1983)
    Higher depression score (Murphy et al., 1983)
Demographic and social characteristics
    More often from broken homes (Davidson, 1979)
    More parental conflict (Berman & Schwartz, 1989)
    More asthma and other illnesses (Berman & Schwartz, 1989)
    White (Kosten & Rounsaville, 1988; Ward & Schuckit, 1980)
    Female (Kosten & Rounsaville, 1988; Ward & Schuckit, 1980)
    More often raised in foster homes/orphanages (Murphy et al., 1983)
    Parental physical abuse (Murphy et al., 1983)

suggests that in the present endeavor, for example, a scale could be developed to predict suicide in male alcoholics that would differ from a scale designed to predict suicide in female alcoholics. Different scales might be designed for substance abusers of different ages, for individuals with different psychiatric diagnoses, and for individuals abusing different drugs.

Data supporting these possibilities exist. For example, male alcoholics appear to have much higher suicide rates than female alcholics. It has been argued that alcoholism in women is less disturbing to their lives, since they are less likely to hold jobs, and since their alcoholism is probably less disruptive of their families' lives than the alcoholism of men (Rushing, 1969). Thus, perhaps female alcholics experience less stress than male alco-

TABLE 15.4. Predictors of Completed Suicide in Drug Abusers

More psychiatric disturbance in relatives (Tunving, 1988)
More alcohol abuse (Tunving, 1988)
Less intravenous drug use (Tunving, 1988)
More prison sentences (Tunvung, 1988)

holics, and so are less likely to commit suicide. Male and female alcoholics also differ quite considerably in social-psychological characteristics, such as family history of psychiatric disorder, developmental experiences, and drinking behavior (Linnoila, Erwin, Ramm, Cleveland, & Brindle, 1980). There are many more cases diagnosed of sociopathy among male alcoholics and of affective disorder among female alcoholics. Persons of these psychiatric subtypes have very different reasons for suicide. For example, the sociopathic individual who commits suicide is more likely to have experienced a disruptive childhood and recent social disruptions than the affectively disordered individual who commits suicide (Robins & O'Neal, 1958), and these differences may account for the differences in the backgrounds of male and female alcoholic suicides. Therefore, it may prove quite useful to have separate predictive scales for suicide for male and female alcoholics.

It has also been noted that alcoholic suicides are quite old. Barraclough, Bunch, Nelson, and Sainsbury (1974) found that their alcoholic suicides had been abusing alcohol for about 25 years and had an average age of 51. Suicide may be more common in these middle-aged alcoholics because of the higher mortality of elderly alcoholics from physical diseases resulting from their alcoholism (Goodwin, 1973). It may be also that middle age is the period of most stress for alcoholics. This may be the time when their marriages break up and during which they experience severe job difficulties. It is found, for example, that alcoholics who complete suicide are less likely to be married than other suicides and than nonsuicidal alcoholics. Again, then, different predictive scales may be in order for young, middle-aged, and elderly alcoholics.

WHY ARE ALCOHOLISM AND SUICIDE ASSOCIATED?

Roy and Linnoila (1986) suggested four reasons why alcoholism and suicide may be associated. First, evidence from animal studies indicates that alcohol causes changes in the turnover of several neurotransmitters in the brain. A recent review of physiological research into suicide (Lester, 1988) concluded that serotonin is the neurotransmitter most likely to be involved in suicidal and depressive behavior, and that alcoholism may have an impact on suicidal behavior through its impact on the serotonergic system.

Second, Roy and Linnoila noted that depression and depressive disorder are common in alcoholics as well as in their relatives. Alcoholism itself also produces depressive symptoms. Thus, it may be that concomitant depression is the mediating factor in producing the high suicide rate in alcoholics. Two other mediating variables may be the experience of a personality disorder (commonly noted in substance abusers who are suicidal) and the experience of recent stressful life events (see Yufit & Bongar, Chapter 27, this volume).

The association between depression and alcoholism is especially important. Depression is a powerful associate of (and predictor of) suicide, and if the association between alcoholism and suicide is simply a result of the mediation of depression, than alcoholism will never be as powerful a predictor of suicide as depression. Alcoholism is associated with depression, depression is common in the relatives of alcoholics, and alcoholism is common in the relatives of depressive patients (Goodwin, 1973). In addition, alcoholism itself produces depression. Thus, future research must compare and contrast the relative power of depression and alcoholism in predicting suicide.

BIOCHEMICAL PREDICTORS OF SUICIDE IN ALCOHOLICS

There has been a tremendous growth in studies of the biochemistry of suicide in recent years, and there have been many claims that biochemical predictors of suicide will soon be discovered. Since, as I have noted above, there is also much research into the biochemistry of alcoholism, there is the possibility of identifying biochemical predictors of suicide in alcoholics. It must be borne in mind that the biochemical research on suicides is primarily carried out because many suicides are depressed, and so study of the suicidal person promises to provide further knowledge about the biochemistry of depression. Such knowledge will be welcome, because there is no one sound biochemical theory of depression at the present time.

Elsewhere (Lester, 1988), I recently reviewed the biochemical research on suicides and identified only four replicable results: Suicide was associated with abnormal responding on the dexamethasone suppression test, lower levels of 5-hydroxyindoleacetic acid in the cerebrospinal fluid, a lower epinephrine–norepinephrine ratio in the urine, and lower levels of serotonin in the central nervous system. Three of these findings implicate the serotonergic system in suicide. I noted that other suggestions had been made for the role of serotonin, but without good supporting empirical evidence. It has been suggested, for example, that the serotonergic system is implicated in assaultive aggression (van Praag, 1986) and in aggressive/impulsive behavior (Brown & Goodwin, 1986).

Roy and Linnoila (1989) have recently reviewed some of the biochemical research on alcoholism. They concluded that the serotonergic system may be involved in Type II alcohol abuse (alcoholism associated with an early onset, a genetic predisposition, antisocial personality traits, and the seeking of alcohol for its euphoric effects). Thus, Roy and Linnoila infer an association between the serotonergic system and impulsive behavior.

The conclusions to be drawn from this research would seem to be that we are a long way from having a clear idea of the biochemical causes of depression, suicide, impulsive behavior, or assaultive behavior. It is unlikely that a specific biochemical predictor of suicide will soon be discovered, since the potential predictors appear to be associated with a wide variety of other pathological behaviors.

DISCUSSION OF THE APPLICABLE CASE STUDIES

Ralph F, the 16-year-old white male, was an alcohol abuser, though the interviewer felt that the severity of the abuse was exaggerated by Ralph. As well as obvious risk factors in other areas of functioning, the alcohol abuse itself enables us to evaluate Ralph's suicide potential on the basis of the risk factors identified above.

Ralph, though young, was beginning to abuse other drugs as well as alcohol. Though at the time of his interview he had used only cigarettes and marijuana, both of these have been implicated in predicting suicidal behavior in alcohol abusers (McKenry et al., 1983; Smith, 1986). Furthermore, Ralph was young, and so his pattern of drug use was developing and changing. He might eventually abuse other drugs. Ralph's alcohol abuse, as he reported it, would appear to be severe; withdrawal was associated with hallucinations. Ralph was also depressed, and there was a history of depression, suicide, and psychiatric disturbance among his relatives. Thus, there is the suggestion of an inherited and biochemical basis for his depression and alcohol abuse. Finally, Ralph had experienced recent stressful life events, severe enough to precipitate asthma attacks.

If the interviewer was correct in assuming that Ralph exaggerated his alcohol abuse, then the risk factors for suicide based on the substance abuse would be moderate. But if we take Ralph at his word, and if we remember that Ralph was still young and developing patterns of behavior, then the long-term risk factors for suicide based on his substance abuse would be fairly high.

The other case with substance abuse was José G, the 64-year-old Hispanic male. José had a history of alcohol abuse combined with recent stress from his injury and permanent disability. José's increased alcohol use at the time of the interview seemed to be directly related to, and secondary to, his depression, although the alcohol abuse may have made his depression worse. Furthermore, though José had a history of alcohol abuse, it had never been severe enough to impair his work record, which was evidently a source of pride and self-identity for him. The interviewer would seem to be correct in referring to the alcohol use as "heavy use" rather than as "abuse." In José's case, then, the substance abuse would not markedly increase the estimate of his suicide potential, with one caveat: If José were to be given medication, thought would have to be given to the lethality of the medication in overdose when combined with alcohol, as well as to the question of whether José might make a suicide attempt when intoxicated.

DISCUSSION AND CONCLUSIONS

This review of the literature has clearly indicated that substance abuse is associated with an increased likelihood of suicide—a conclusion that makes sense if we agree with Menninger's (1938) view that substance abuse itself is a self-destructive (and suicidal) behavior. Thus, substance abuse may be considered to be a predictive sign for suicide. Despite this, many previously devised scales for predicting suicide do not include substance abuse as a predictive sign. For example, Lettieri (1974) included alcoholism only on his scale for older females. Thus, much research needs to be done to pinpoint the groups for which substance abuse is a useful predictive sign.

This review has also indicated a large number of possible variables that might predict completed suicide in alcoholics and in drug abusers. Far more research has been conducted on alcoholics than on drug abusers. For alcoholics, one alcohol abuse symptom, six psychiatric symptoms, and 13 demographic and social variables have been identified as potential predictors of completed suicide in at least one study (see Table 15.2). In contrast, only one study has been conducted on completed suicide in drug abusers, and only four variables have been identified (see Table 15.4). Thus, much research is needed to identify potential predictive signs of completed suicide in drug abusers. In addition, these potential predictive signs for completed suicide must be validated (and cross-validated) in future research. Despite the enthusiastic reports in the biochemical literature about the potential of biochemical variables to predict suicide, the present review has found little evidence for any reliable predictors. If biochemical predictors are ever identified, it will not be for many years.

In conclusion, this review has established a program for future research, rather than revealing already validated predictive scales for suicide in substance abusers. I hope that it will stimulate scholars to pursue this interesting and important topic in the prediction of suicide.

REFERENCES

Agren, G., & Jakobsson, S. W. (1987). Validation of diagnosis on death certificates for male alcoholics in Stockholm. *Forensic Science International, 33*, 231-241.

Allebeck, P., Allgulander, C., & Fisher, L. D. (1988). Predictors of completed suicide in a cohort of 50,465 young men. *British Medical Journal, 297*, 176-178.

Babigan, H. M., Lehman, A. F., & Reed, S. K. (1985). Suicide epidemiology and psychiatric care. In R. Cohen-Sandler (Ed.), *Proceedings of the 18th Annual Meeting of the American Association of Suicidology* (pp. 73-74). Denver: American Association of Suicidology.

Bagley, C. (1989). Profiles of youthful suicide. *Psychological Reports, 65*, 234.

Barner-Rasmussen, P., Dupont, A., & Bille, H. (1986). Suicide in psychiatric patients in Denmark 1971-1981. *Acta Psychiatrica Scandinavica, 73*, 449-455.

Barr, H. L., Antes, D., Ottenberg, D. J., & Rosen, A. (1984). Mortality of treated alcoholics and drug addicts. *Journal of Studies on Alcohol, 45*, 440-452.

Barraclough, B. M., Bunch, J., Nelson, B., & Sainsbury, P. (1974). A hundred cases of suicide. *British Journal of Psychiatry, 125*, 355-373.

Bascue, L., & Epstein, L. (1980). Suicide attempts and experiences of hospitalized alcoholics. *Psychological Reports, 47*, 1233-1234.

Beck, A. T., & Steer, R. A. (1989). Clinical predictors of eventual suicide. *Journal of Affective Disorders, 17*, 203-209.

Beck, A. T., Steer, R. A., & McElroy, M. (1982). Relationships of hopelessness, depression and previous suicide attempts to suicidal ideation in alcoholics. *Journal of Studies on Alcohol, 43*, 1042-1046.

Beck, A. T., Steer, R. A., & Trexler, L. D. (1989). Alcohol abuse and eventual suicide. *Journal of Studies on Alcohol, 50*, 202-209.

Berglund, M., & Tunving, K. (1985). Assaultive alcoholics 20 years later. *Acta Psychiatrica Scandinavica, 71*, 141-147.

Berman, A. L., & Schwartz, R. (1989). Suicide attempts among adolescent drug users. In D. Lester (Ed.), *Suicide '89* (pp. 64-66). Denver: American Association of Suicidology.

Bissell, L., & Skorina, J. K. (1987). One hundred alcoholic women in medicine. *Journal of the American Medical Association, 257*, 2939-2944.

Black, D. W., Yates, W., Potty, F., Noyes, R., & Brown, K. (1986). Suicidal behavior in alcoholic males. *Comprehensive Psychiatry, 27*, 227-233.

Blankfield, A. (1989). Female alcoholics. *Acta Psychiatrica Scandinavica, 79*, 355-362.

Brown, G., & Goodwin, F. (1986). Human aggression and suicide. *Suicide and Life-Threatening Behavior, 16*, 223-243.

Buydens-Branchey, L., Branchey, M. H., & Noumair, D. (1989). Age of alcoholism onset. *Archives of General Psychiatry, 46*, 225-230.

Cavaiola, A. A. (1988). Chemical dependency and adolescent suicide. In D. Lester (Ed.), *Suicide '88* (pp. 167-168). Denver: American Association of Suicidology.

D'Amanda, C., Plumb, M., & Taintor, Z. (1977). Heroin addicts with a history of glue sniffing. *International Journal of the Addictions, 12*, 255-270.

Davidson, F. (1978). Suicide and the abuse of drugs. In H. Z. Winnick & L. Miller

(Eds.) *Aspects of suicide in modern civilization* (pp. 220-227). Jerusalem: Academic Press.

Farberow, N. L., Litman, R. E., & Nelson, F. L. (1988). A survey of youth suicide in California. In R. Yufit (Ed.), *Proceedings of the 21st Annual Meeting of the American Association of Suicidology* (pp. 298-300). Denver: American Association of Suicidology.

Fawcett, J., Scheftner, W., Clark, D., Hedeker, D., Gibbons, R., & Coryell, W. (1987). Clinical predictors of suicide in patients with major affective disorders. *American Journal of Psychiatry, 144*, 35-40.

Frederick, C., Resnick, H., & Wittlin, B. (1973). Self-destructive aspects of hard core addiction. *Archives of General Psychiatry, 28*, 579-585.

Gaines, T., & Richmond, L. (1980). Assessing suicidal behavior in basic military trainees. *Military Medicine, 145*, 263-266.

Garvey, M. J., Tuason, V., Hoffman, N., & Chastek, J. (1983). Suicide attempters, nonattempters and neurotransmitters. *Comprehensive Psychiatry, 24*, 332-336.

Gomberg, E. S. (1989). Suicide risk among women with alcohol problems. *American Journal of Public Health, 79*, 1363-1365.

Goodwin, D. (1973). Alcohol in suicide and homicide. *Quarterly Journal of Studies on Alcohol, 34*, 144-156.

Gossop, M., Cobb, J., & Connell, P. (1975). Self-destructive behavior in oral and intravenous drug-dependent groups. *British Journal of Psychiatry, 126*, 266-269.

Haberman, P. (1979). Cause of death in alcoholics. In *Proceedings of the 10th International Congress for Suicide Prevention* (pp. 108-115). Vienna: International Association for Suicide Prevention.

Hagnell, O., Nyman, E., & Tunving, K. (1973). Dangerous alcoholics. *Scandinavian Journal of Social Medicine, 1*, 125-131.

Harris, R., Linn, M. W., & Hunter, K. (1979). Suicide attempts among drug abusers. *Suicide and Life-Threatening Behavior, 9*, 25-32.

Hasin, D., Grant, B., & Endicott, J. (1988). Treated and untreated suicide attempts in substance abuse patients. *Journal of Nervous and Mental Disease, 176*, 289-294.

Hatsukami, D., Mitchell, J. E., Eckert, E. D., & Pyle, R. (1986). Characteristics of patients with bulimia only, bulimia with affective disorder and bulimia with substance abuse. *Addictive Behaviors, 11*, 399-406.

Haycock, J. (1989). Manipulation and suicide attempts in jails and prisons. *Psychiatric Quarterly, 60*, 85-98.

Hesselbrock, M., Hesselbrock, V., Szymanski, K., & Weidenman, M. (1988). Suicide attempts and alcoholism. *Journal of Studies on Alcohol, 49*, 436-442.

Janofsky, J. S., Spear, S., & Neubauer, D. N. (1988). Psychiatrists' accuracy in predicting violent behavior on an inpatient ward. *Hospital and Community Psychiatry, 39*, 1090-1094.

Kapamadzija, B., Souljanski, M., & Skendzic, S. (1978). Alcoholics and non-alcoholics in committed suicides. In V. Aalberg (Ed.), *Proceedings of the 9th International Congress for Suicide Prevention* (pp. 311-315). Helsinki: Finnish Association for Mental Health.

Kendall, R. E. (1983). Alcohol and suicide. *Substance and Alcohol Actions/Misuse, 4,* 121-127.

Kirkpatrick-Smith, K., Rich, A., Bonner, R., & Jans, F. (1989). Substance abuse and suicidal ideation among adolescents. In D. Lester (Ed.), *Suicide '89* (pp. 90-91). Denver: American Association of Suicidology.

Knop, J., & Fischer, A. (1981). Duodenal ulcer, suicide, psychopathology and alcoholism. *Acta Psychiatrica Scandinavica, 63,* 346-355.

Kockott, G., & Feuerlein, W. (1968). The relationship between suicide attempts and delirium tremens. In N. L. Farberow (Ed.), *Proceedings of the 4th International Congress for Suicide Prevention* (pp. 71-74). Los Angeles: Delmar.

Koller, K. M., & Castanos, J. N. (1968). Attempted suicide and alcoholism. *Medical Journal of Australia, 2,* 835-837.

Kosten, T. R., & Rounsaville, B. J. (1988). Suicidality among opioid addicts. *American Journal of Drug Abuse, 14,* 357-369.

Lesch, O. M., Walter, H., Mader, R., Musalek, M., & Zeiler, K. (1988). Chronic alcoholism in relation to attempted or effected suicide. *Psychiatrie et Psychobiologie, 3,* 181-188.

Lester, D. (1988). *The biochemical basis of suicide.* Springfield, IL: Charles C Thomas.

Lettieri, D. J. (1974). Suicidal death prediction scales. In A. T. Beck, H. L. P. Resnik, & D. J. Lettieri (Eds.), *The prediction of suicide* (pp. 163-192). Bowie, MD: Charles Press.

Levy, J. C., & Deykin, E. Y. (1989). Suicidality, depression and substance abuse in adolescence. *American Journal of Psychiatry, 146,* 1462-1467.

Lindberg, S., & Agren, G. (1988). Mortality among male and female hospitalized alcoholics in Stockholm 1962-1983. *British Journal of Addiction, 83,* 1193-1200.

Linnoila, M., Erwin, C., Ramm, D., Cleveland, P., & Brendle, A. (1980). Effects of alcohol on psychomotor performance of women. *Alcoholism, 4,* 302-305.

McKenry, P., Tishler, C., & Kelley, C. (1983). The role of drugs in adolescent suicide attempts. *Suicide and Life-Threatening Behavior, 13,* 166-175.

Menninger, K. (1938). *Man against himself.* New York: Harcourt, Brace & World.

Moise, R., Kovach, J., Reed, B. G., & Bellows, N. (1982). A comparison of black and white women entering drug abuse treatment programs. *International Journal of the Addictions, 17,* 35-49.

Motto, J. A. (1980). Suicide risk factors in alcohol abuse. *Suicide and Life-Threatening Behavior, 10,* 230-238.

Murphy, S. L., Rounsaville, B., Eyre, S., & Kleber, H. (1983). Suicide attempts in treated opiate addicts. *Comprehensive Psychiatry, 24,* 79-89.

Nace, E. P., Saxon, J. J., & Shore, N. (1983). A comparison of borderline and nonborderline alcoholic patients. *Archives of General Psychiatry, 40,* 54-56.

O'Donnell, J. A. (1969). *Narcotic addicts in Kentucky.* Chevy Chase, MD: National Institute of Mental Health.

Ohara, K., Suzuki, Y., Sugita, T., Kobayashi, K., Tamefusa, K., Hattori, S., & Ohara, K. (1989). Mortality among alcoholics discharged from a Japanese hospital. *British Journal of Addiction, 84,* 287-291.

Palola, E., Dorpat, T., & Larson, W. (1962). Alcoholism and suicidal behavior. In

D. Pittman & C. Snyder (Eds.), *Society, culture and drinking patterns* (pp. 511-534). New York: Wiley.

Ritson, E. B. (1968). Suicide among alcoholics. *British Journal of Medical Psychology, 41*, 235-242.

Robins, E., & Murphy, G. E. (1965). The physician's role in the prevention of suicide. In L. Yochelson (Ed.), *Symposium on suicide* (pp. 84-91). Washington, DC: George Washington University Press.

Robins, E., & O'Neal, P. (1958). Culture and mental disorder. *Human Organization, 16*(4), 7-11.

Robinson, A. D., & Duffy, J. C. (1989). A comparison of self-injury and self-poisoning from the Regional Treatment Center, Edinburgh. *Acta Psychiatrica Scandinavica, 80*, 272-279.

Roy, A., & Linnoila, M. (1986). Alcoholism and suicide. *Suicide and Life-Threatening Behavior, 16*, 244-273.

Roy, A., & Linnoila, M. (1989). CSF studies of alcoholism and related behaviors. *Progress in Neuro-Psychopharmacology and Biological Psychiatry, 13*, 505-511.

Rushing, W. (1969). Suicide and the interaction of alcoholism (liver cirrhosis) with the social situation. *Quarterly Journal of Studies on Alcohol, 30*, 93-103.

Saxon, S., Kuncel, E., & Aldrich, S. (1978). Drug abuse and suicide. *American Journal of Drug and Alcohol Abuse, 5*, 485-495.

Saxon, S., Kuncel, E., & Kaufman, E. (1980). Self-destructive behavior patterns in male and female drug abusers. *American Journal of Drug Abuse, 7*(1), 19-29.

Schuckit, M. A. (1986). Primary men alcoholics with histories of suicide attempts. *Journal of Studies on Alcohol, 47*, 78-81.

Simonds, J., & Kashani, J. (1979). Phencyclidine use in delinquent males committed to a training school. *Adolescence, 14*, 721-725.

Smith, G. M. (1986). Interrelations among measures of depressive symptomatology, other measures of psychological distress, and young adult substance use. In G. L. Klerman (Ed.), *Suicide and depression among adolescents and young adults* (pp. 301-315). Washington, DC: American Psychiatric Press.

Tardiff, K., Gross, E., Wu, J., Stajic, M., & Millman, R. (1989). Analysis of cocaine-related fatalities. *Journal of Forensic Sciences, 34*, 53-63.

Thorarinsson, A. A. (1979). Mortality among men alcoholics in Iceland. *Journal of Studies on Alcohol, 40*, 704-718.

Tunving, K. (1988). Fatal outcome in drug addiction. *Acta Psychiatrica Scandinavica, 77*, 551-566.

Vaglum, S., & Vaglum, P. (1987). Differences between alcoholic and nonalcoholic female psychiatric patients. *Acta Psychiatrica Scandinavica, 76*, 309-316.

van Praag, H. (1986). Affective disorders and aggressive disorders. *Suicide and Life-Threatening Behavior, 16*, 102-132.

Ward, N., & Schuckit, M. (1980). Factors associated with suicidal behavior in poly-drug abusers. *Journal of Clinical Psychiatry, 41*, 379-385.

Watterson, O., Simpson, D., & Sells, S. (1975). Death rates and causes of death among opioid addicts in community drug treatment programs during 1970-1973. *American Journal of Drug and Alcohol Abuse, 2*(1), 99-111.

Weissman, M. M., Klerman, G. L., Markowitz, J. S., & Ouellette, R. (1989). Suicidal ideation and suicide attempts in panic disorder and attacks. *New England Journal of Medicine, 321,* 1209–1214.

Weissman, M. M., Myers, J. K., & Harding, P. S. (1980). Prevalence and psychaitric heterogeneity of alcoholism in a U.S. urban community. *Journal of Studies on Alcohol, 41,* 672–681.

Wetli, C. V. (1983). Changing patterns of methaqualone abuse. *Journal of the American Medical Association, 249,* 621–626.

Whittemore, K. (1970). *Ten centers.* Atlanta: Lullwater Press.

Whitters, A. C., Cadoret, R. J., Troughton, E., & Widmer, R. B. (1987). Suicide attempts in antisocial alcoholics. *Journal of Nervous and Mental Disease, 175,* 624–626.

Whitters, A. C., Cadoret, R. J., & Widmer, R. B. (1985). Factors associated with suicide attempt in alcohol abusers. *Journal of Affective Disorders, 9,* 19–23.

Wihelmsen, L., Elmfeldt, D., & Wedel, H. (1983). Causes of death in relation to social and alcohol problems among Swedish men aged 35–44 years. *Acta Medica Scandinavica, 213,* 263–268.

Zmuc, M. (1968). Alcohol and suicide. *Alcoholism, 4,* 38–44.

Suicide Notes, Communication, and Ideation

Antoon A. Leenaars, Ph.D., C.Psych.
Private Practice, Windsor, Ontario, Canada

To be seriously concerned with understanding suicide leads one to a most challenging task, the prediction of suicide. The problem of predicting those who will eventually kill themselves is one that has plagued suicidology since the origins of the field. Traditional sources for efforts at suicide prediction include interviews with those who have made nonfatal suicide attempts, general statistics, and interviews with third parties (survivors). Each of these sources has brought clinicians closer to predicting the event. Yet there is at least one other source that I believe can be rewarding in our quest—namely, personal documents (Allport, 1942).

Although there is considerable controversy surrounding the usefulness of personal documents and other introspective communications (Runyan, 1982; Windelband, 1904), Allport (1942) contended that personal documents have a significant place in social science. Allport made a clear case for their use, citing the following as goals: learning about the person (such as his or her ideation); advancing nomothetic and idiographic understanding; and aiding in the aims of science in general—understanding, prediction, and control. These are the very aims of sound assessment and prediction of suicide.

Perhaps the most personal document of all is the suicide note. It is the unsolicited communication of a suicidal person, usually written minutes before the suicidal death. It is an invaluable starting point for comprehending the suicidal act and for predicting such events.

THE RELATIONSHIP BETWEEN
COMMUNICATION AND IDEATION

Suicide notes are without question communications—written communications (Hayakawa, 1957). Often such a note is a final communication, a last desperate act of saying something to someone. To comprehend the communication, we must understand the relation of the note to ideation, which itself may well be hidden from direct observation.

The problem of the relation between communication (including written forms such as notes) and thought (or ideation) is a historical one. Some thinkers, such as Muller (1887), have suggested that the two are simply identical. A few, such as Berkeley (see Bolton, 1972), have seen no relation at all. Numerous schools of thought (e.g., association psychology, Gestalt psychology, the Wurzburg school) have expanded on the relation, all with different points of view. Today the relation between communication and ideation is acknowledged to exist, but it remains complex and controversial (e.g., Bolton, 1972; Piaget, 1968, 1972; Vygotsky, 1962). The relation is seen as not merely associational or static, but rather as dynamic. To present a comprehensive discussion of such a relationship is well beyond the scope of this chapter; let it suffice to say that the relation is not a thing but a process.

Ideation is for oneself, whereas communication is usually for others (Vygotsky, 1962). This difference in function reflects real differences in process. Often our thoughts are more abstract than our specific words. Judgments need to be made regarding whether a specific written or oral communication is a reflection of a thought. Yet we have to study words, talk, notes, diaries, and the like to infer ideation. We typically communicate in words, although, as Furth (1966) has shown, thinking is possible without language (e.g., in the deaf). We cannot directly study a person's ideation. We infer it, given the relation of thought to words.

In line with the subject of this volume, it is important to note that ideation is engendered by our needs, pain, interests, and so forth. As I have said, the relationship between word and thought is dynamic. Vygotsky (1962) stated, "The relation between thought and word is a living process" (p. 153). Freud (1901/1960, 1916–1917/1963) proposed that needs, wishes, and so on, although often repressed in the unconscious, are expressed in dreams and everyday life (e.g., verbal expressions, writings). Freud (1916–1917/1963) further suggested that conscious and unconscious ideation can be assessed in communication. As Vygotsky (1962) noted on the dynamic relation, "A word is a microcosm of human consciousness" (p. 153). This is the main tenet of the thematic tradition that is espoused here.

It is my belief that this is why the study of suicide notes has been so fruitful. Suicide notes are windows to the mind of the deceased. In the same way, other communications (e.g., talk, diaries) of a suicidal person offer us a living link to his or her ideation.

CONSIDERATIONS PRELIMINARY TO PREDICTION

Interpretation of clinical material usually includes or implies prediction of the client's future behavior, as well as a description of the client's present ideation. We can go so far as to say that prediction from clinical material (communications, notes, diaries, etc.) is one of the primary purposes of interpretation in a clinical setting. The interpretation "This client is suicidal" is certainly a prediction that the client is in danger of attempting and/or completing suicide. How do we make such a prediction? If we are to answer this question, we should not see prediction as separate from understanding.

During this century, applied psychology has been involved with the use of tests to study intelligence, memory, anxiety, depression, and many other constructs. One of the major movements has been the projective one. Henry Murray (1943), following the earlier pioneer, Herman Rorschach, saw the projective procedures as "useful in any comprehensive study of personality" (p. 1). These procedures are based on the premise that people, when they speak or write, "draw on the fund of their experiences and express their sentiments and needs, whether conscious or unconscious" (1943, p. 1). Murray's description of how the process operates was, in part, derived from Freud's description of defensive operation, but Murray stressed that the process is natural and that defensiveness may or may not play a role (see Exner, 1986). As simply put by John Exner, "any stimulus situation that is not structured to elicit a specific class of response, as are arithmetic tests, true–false inventories, and the like, may evoke the projective process" (1986, p. 16). Murray's Thematic Apperception Test (TAT) is a prime example within this tradition. Through an error in printing, one of the cards in the TAT (Card 16) was a blank card; it was retained, however, in the TAT itself. Elsewhere, I (Leenaars, 1988a) have argued that a suicide note can be seen, as it were, as a response to this blank card of the TAT. Suicide notes can thus be seen as similar to the communications in the TAT and other thematic tests. Both types of communications are windows to a person's ideation and can be analyzed for "thematic meaningfulness" (Shneidman, 1949, 1951).

It is likely that a layperson, without the benefit of any constructs or templates to understand suicide, may make valid and important interpretations (with some beginner's luck). However, no true clinician would engage in such action, especially in terms of predicting life and death. Pertinent and sound understanding is needed in suicide prediction. What is required, as I see it, is a theoretical context for suicide and personality functioning in general, which will enable us to understand the communication (and, by implication, the ideation) of a potential suicidal individual and its potential implications for prediction. The templates (or constructs or frames) proposed here not only provide such a view, but have at least some empirical support. As a word of caution, Murray (1943) has noted that some interpretations may "do more harm than good, since the apparent plausibility of clever interpretations creates convictions which merely serve to confirm the interpreter in the error of his ways" (p. 6).

REVIEW OF THE LITERATURE

One reason, if not *the* reason, why it is so difficult to predict suicide is that usually we deal only with the end result. In other mental health areas, we are not faced with this obstacle. For example, if we wish to predict a learning disability, we can make some interpretations, check them out, try again, and so forth. In suicide, obviously, we cannot do this. As Joseph Zubin (1974) has argued, given this situation, "unraveling the causes after the fact is well, highly impossible" (p. 4). I contend that, to a certain extent, it *is* possible. We are, however, restricted *at this time* by a fact noted by James Diggory (1974): "The belief that suicidal behaviors are predictable can be valid only as a belief *in principle*, not *in fact*" (italics in original; p. 59).

Over the last few decades, despite these and similar critical observations, numerous attempts at constructing tests for suicide prediction and related phenomena have been made. Probably one of the best tests is Shneidman's (1973) simple measure (or, more accurately, question): "During the last 24 hours, I felt my chances of actually killing myself (committing suicide and ending my life) were: absent, very low, low medium, fifty-fifty, high medium, very high, extra high (came very close to actually killing myself)" (p. 384). Clinical experience has shown that many patients can predict their own suicide potential (and are often relieved to find someone willing to talk about their own ominous prediction).

Aaron Beck and his colleagues (e.g., Beck, 1967; Beck & Beamesderfer, 1974; Beck, Beck, & Kovacs, 1975; Beck, Kovacs, & Weissman, 1979; Beck, Schuyler, & Herman, 1974; Beck, Weissman, Lester, & Trexler, 1974) are probably most noteworthy in their endeavors to construct scales for prediction related to suicide. Their tests include the Beck Depression Inventory, the Hopelessness Scale, the Suicide Intent Scale, and the Scale for Suicide Ideation. The research on these scales, including very critical reviews and research, is too vast to be discussed here (see Weishaar & Beck, Chapter 22, this volume, for more details). Many other possible scales presented to assess and predict suicide; this volume outlines many of these (see especially Eyman & Eyman, Chapter 9, and Rothberg & Geer-Williams, Chapter 10).

One critical observation is in order here, however: I believe that our search for *the* test of predicting a behavior as complicated as suicide is a wishful fancy. There is no such test. Clinicians wishing to understand and predict any behavior have long since abandoned the notion of using one instrument. To use just one test is, in effect, to regress to the days of phrenology, when it was believed that if we could find the right bump on a person's head we would know his or her personality, IQ, and the like—and, I assume, his or her suicidal tendencies. Even the earliest use of standardized tests in psychology (e.g., Galton's questionnaire methods, Cattell's mental tests, Binet's test) was criticized as needing to address this problem (Anastasi, 1982). In response to the recognition of such simplification, clinicians developed the battery approach and acknowledged the need to use their clinical judgment to understand the results. To predict suicide, I believe that we must adopt such a comprehensive approach, or we will be forever searching for the "bump" that will tell all.

Instruments of prediction equally call for reflection. Motto (1985) has provided us with some important insights into problems about prediction, which are worthy of review here. He cites the following: a suitable criterion measure (predictive validity); the extent to which the scale agrees with other measures (concurrent validity); applicability of the scale to various populations; the willingness of crisis workers, physicians, and other clinicians to use a scale that is not consistent with their own intuition; and the use of a rater who knows what the scale measures (criterion contamination). There is at least one additional concern that is fundamental to prediction and the development of a test—namely, the base rate problem, or the frequency of a given condition in a population to which the test is applied (Meehl & Rosen, 1955). All of these problems remain challenges in our efforts to predict and, if I may add, to control suicide.

SUICIDE NOTES

Suicide notes are ultrapersonal documents (Leenaars, 1988a; Shneidman, 1980). They are the unsolicited productions of suicidal persons, usually written minutes before death. They are an invaluable starting point for comprehending the suicidal act, and for understanding how people who actually commit suicide both resemble and differ from the rest of us who have only imagined it (Leenaars, 1988a; Leenaars & Balance, 1984a; Shneidman, 1980, 1985; Shneidman & Farberow, 1957a).

It should be noted at the beginning, however, that the study of suicide notes has a number of limitations. Only about 12–15% of suicides leave notes (Leenaars, 1988a; Shneidman, 1985; Shneidman & Farberow, 1957a). Thus, any conclusions about the psychology of suicide (and implications for test construction) based on the study of notes probably contain some bias.

However, since the first systematic study of suicide notes, few differences have been reported between individuals who leave notes and those who have not. Erwin Stengel (1964) noted:

> Whether the writers of suicide notes differ in their attitudes from those who leave no notes behind it is impossible to say. Possibly, they differ from the majority only in being good correspondents. At any rate, the results of the analysis of suicide notes are in keeping with the observation[s] . . . common to most suicidal acts. (pp. 44-45)

Sampling differences exist, given the nature of some suicides. Fishbain, D'Achille, Barsky, and Aldrich (1984) reported that those who make suicide pacts more frequently leave notes. Fishbain, Fletcher, Aldrich, and Davis (1987) noted that subintentional suicides (e.g., those who die as a result of Russian roulette) are significantly less likely to leave notes. Researchers have reported differences in various aspects of samples. Michel (1988) reported that young people are more likely to leave suicide notes, whereas Posener, LaHaye, and Cheifetz (1989) found no such higher rate. Samples may vary; we (Leenaars & Lester, 1988-1989) have pointed out that caution is in order when conclusions are being drawn from small samples. Elsewhere (Leenaars, 1988a) I have attempted to address this problem by creating a large archive of notes. Generally, in regard to psychological characteristics that may be relevant to assessment of suicidal risk, no differences have been reported between those who do and those who do not write notes.

This is not to say that my current position is without controversy. It is often asserted that any behavior engaged in by only 12-15% of suicides is quite likely to reflect differences from the 85-88% who do not. However, a review of the literature, including the proceedings of the recent conferences of the American Association of Suicidology, has produced no studies supporting this view. Studies that included suicide notes as a variable found no empirical differences. There may be phenotypic differences (e.g., writing a note itself), but no genotypic ones have been found. At this time, we can only conclude that we *do not know* whether there are differences (or what such differences are, if they exist) between those who write suicide notes and those who do not.

Other questions about the usefulness of suicide notes are as follows: Can an acutely suicidal individual provide a clear account of the suicide? Can such an individual give a relatively complete account of the suicide? And are the notes in a sample representative? Such problems, however, should be placed in perspective by the observation that other sources (suicide attempters, statistics, third parties) have their own limitations (Maris, 1981). Furthermore, it strikes me that these questions are ubiquitous for any evaluation of an individual, regardless of the data being used, and will call into play the skill of the evaluator in interpreting the validity of the data he or she collects.

Early research (e.g., Wolff, 1931) on suicide notes largely utilized an anecdotal approach that incorporated descriptive information. Subsequent methods of study have primarily included classification analysis and content analysis. Currently, there are over 70 published articles on suicide notes; an extensive review with an annotated bibliography has been presented elsewhere (Leenaars, 1988a). Some of this research is very relevant in showing the predictive power of notes. Shneidman and Farberow's early studies (Shneidman & Farberow, 1957a, 1957b; Farberow & Shneidman, 1957) indicated that suicidal individuals are prone to fallacies in their ideational processes; that the wish to kill, the wish to be killed, and the wish to die are evident; and that the suicidal person departs with hate and self-blame. Subsequent studies have isolated the following clinically relevant factors in notes:

Psychic tension (Wagner, 1960)

Depression (Capstick, 1960)

Mental confusion (Spiegel & Neuringer, 1963)

Unfulfillable desires, high perturbation, intolerable inner tension, unrealistic expectations of others, personal devaluation, and feelings of worthlessness (Bjerg, 1967)

Hostility (Tuckman & Ziegler, 1968)

Positive affect (e.g., "love"; Oglivie, Stone, & Shneidman, 1969)

Heightened dependency needs, problems in maintaining relationships, and veiled aggression (Darbonne, 1969)

A view of the act as justified, and a need to be forgiven for it (Jacobs, 1971)

Involvement with fantasy (Lester, 1971)

Inability to distinguish the subjective from the objective, oversimplification, thinking that everything is obvious, rigidity, fatalism, projection, and inability to distinguish between feelings and the outside world (Tripodes, 1976)

Constriction (Henken, 1976)

Ambivalence (i.e., simultaneous presence of love and hate), shame, and disgrace (Shneidman, 1980)

Idiosyncrasies in ideation (Shneidman, 1981)

Cognitive impairment in positive evaluation (Schwilbe & Rader, 1982)

Negating specific people, places, and things, while seeing generalized others as more positive (Edelman & Renshaw, 1982)

A fatalistic attitude (Peck, 1983)

Ambivalent attachment to a person (Posener et al., 1989)

Only a very few of the above-cited studies on suicide notes have utilized a theoretical–conceptual analysis, despite the belief since the first formal study of suicide notes that such contributions are rich in potential (Shneid-

344   SPECIFIC PREDICTORS OF SUICIDE

man & Farberow, 1957a). In a series of studies spanning well over a decade (e.g., Leenaars, 1979, 1985, 1986, 1987, 1988a, 1988b, 1989a, 1989b, 1990; Leenaars & Balance, 1981, 1984a, 1984b, 1984c; Leenaars, Balance, Wenckstern, & Rudzinski, 1985), my colleagues and I have introduced a logical, empirical approach to suicide notes—one that not only includes a method for the theoretical analysis of suicide notes, but is also calculated to augment the effectiveness of previous controls. Essentially, this method, which has been outlined in detail elsewhere (Leenaars, 1988a; Leenaars & Balance, 1984a), calls for the notes to be treated as an archival source and subjected to the scrutiny of control hypotheses, following an *ex post facto* research design (Kerlinger, 1964). Suicide notes are recast in different theoretical contexts (hypotheses, theories, models, etc.); lines of evidence for each of these positions can then be pursued in the data, utilizing Carnap's (1931/ 1959) logical and empirical procedure for such investigations. These positivistic procedures call for translating of theoretical formulations into observable (specific) "protocol sentences" in order to test the formulations. The protocol sentences constitute the meaning of the theory as they are matched empirically, by independent judges, with the actual data. Next, conclusions are developed from the verified protocol sentences to facilitate model building and test construction.

To date, the theories of 10 suicidologists have been investigated in this way (Leenaars, 1988a). Specifically, studies of Alfred Adler, Ludwig Binswanger, Sigmund Freud, Carl Jung, Karl Menninger, George Kelly, Henry Murray, Edwin Shneidman, Harry Stack Sullivan, and Gregory Zilboorg were undertaken. (Certainly the views of these thinkers do not present all of the psychological variables that might prompt someone to commit suicide; however, these individuals are generally recognized as having given us a rich history of theory about suicide.) These investigations produced 23 protocol sentences that highly predicted (described) the content of suicide notes (i.e., one standard deviation above the mean of all observations), as well as 18 protocol sentences that significantly discriminated genuine suicide notes from simulated (control) suicide notes (i.e., they were generally observed infrequently in genuine notes, compared to the former 23). Both sources of information have utility in understanding suicide and, by implication, in predicting suicide. The protocol sentences (each with an indication whether it is a predictive clue [P], or a discriminative clue [D], or both) can be found in Appendix 16. Subsequently, these same 36 protocol sentences (since 5 sentences both predicted and discriminated the content in suicide notes) were reduced to a meaningful empirical nosology, by means of a cluster analysis (Leenaars, 1989a). The method itself called for a new sample of suicide notes, with controls for age (young, middle and late adulthood) and sex, to be analyzed by independent judges. The 35 sentences (1 sentence was eliminated because it was not observed) were grouped into eight discrete clusters, which accounted for 56% of the variance.

The eight groupings, with a few descriptive statements, are as follows:

I. *Unbearable Psychological Pain.* The common stimulus in suicide is unendurable psychological pain (Shneidman, 1985). Although, as Menninger (1938) noted, other motives (elements, wishes) are evident, the suicidal person primarily perceives that he or she wants to flee from a trauma or catastrophe. The person feels boxed in, rejected, deprived, forlorn, distressed, and especially hopeless and helpless. The situation is unbearable, and the person desperately wants a way out of it. The suicide, as Murray (1967) noted, is functional because it abolishes painful tension for the individual; it provides relief from intolerable suffering.

II. *Interpersonal Relations.* The suicidal person has problems in establishing or maintaining relationships. The suicide is often related to unsatisfied or frustrated affiliation (attachment) needs, although other needs may also be evident (e.g., achievement, autonomy, dominance).

III. *Rejection-Aggression.* The rejection-aggression hypothesis was documented by Stekel in a famous 1910 meeting of the Psychoanalytic Society in Freud's home in Vienna (see Friedman, 1910/1967). Suicide may be a turning back upon oneself of murderous impulses (wishes, needs) that have been directed against a traumatic event, most frequently rejection by another person. Suicide may be veiled aggression—that is, "murder in the 180th degree" (Menninger, 1938).

IV. *Inability to Adjust.* Depressed people are not the only ones who kill themselves. Although the majority of suicides may not fit best into any specific nosological classification, manic-depressive disorders, obsessive-compulsive disorders, schizophrenic disorders, psychopathic disorders, and others have been related to some suicides (Leenaars, 1988a; Sullivan, 1962a, 1962b). All these disorders can be seen to reflect an inability to adjust.

V. *Indirect Expressions.* Complications, ambivalence, redirected aggression, unconscious implications, and other indirect expressions (or behavior) are often evident in suicide.

VI. *Identification-Egression.* Freud (1917/1957, 1920/1955) hypothesized that an intense identification (or bond) to a lost or rejecting person is critical in understanding the suicidal person; Zilboorg (1936) showed that this is also true of an identification with any ideal (e.g., health, young age, employment, freedom). If this emotional need is not met, the suicidal person experiences a deep discomfort (pain) and wants to be gone, to be elsewhere, to exit—to egress.

VII. *Ego.* The person himself or herself is a critical aspect of the suicidal act. Often, a relative weakness in the person's capacity to develop constructive tendencies and to overcome his or her personal difficulties is evident.

VIII. *Cognitive Constriction.* The common cognitive state in suicide is constriction (Shneidman, 1985). Constriction (i.e., rigidity in thinking, narrowing of focus, tunnel vision, concreteness, etc.) is the major component of the cognitive state in suicide. The suicidal person perceives only permutations and combinations of a trauma (e.g., poor health, rejection by the spouse).

Appendix 16.1 presents the protocol sentences in these eight groupings. Research on these protocol sentences has indicated that there are no differences between the following: males and females (Leenaars, 1988a, 1988c, 1989a); individuals who use different methods (Leenaars, 1990); and individuals who kill themselves at symbolic ages (e.g., 40, 60) and other ages (Phillips & Leenaars, 1990). Notes that research subjects judge to be obviously genuine do not differ from notes that they do not perceive as real (Leenaars & Lester, 1990). Recent research (Leenaars, Lester, Wenckstern, Rudzinski, & Brevard, 1992) also indicates that there are no differences on these protocol sentences between suicide notes and parasuicide notes. Parasuicide notes are communications written by individuals who attempted but did not complete suicide (or engaged in some other form of parasuicidal behavior, including ideation).

The last-mentioned study (Leenaars et al., 1992) is pertinent here because it suggests that the protocols have applicability to both suicide and parasuicide. In this study, a comparison of suicide notes written by individuals who killed themselves and notes by individuals who attempted but did not complete suicide, we undertook the comparison of the eight patterns (and individual protocol sentences) as possible predictors of the communications of completers and attempters. The attempts of the parasuicides were of moderate to high lethality. No difference on the eight clusters was found, and only one difference on a protocol sentence was noted—namely, that attempters saw themselves more often as too weak to cope with life's difficulties, although their notes were not more frequently judged to be indicative of pathology. Although there are differences between attempters and completers (see Leenaars et al., 1992; Shneidman, 1985), it may well be that the psychological characteristics outlined here are as applicable to attempters as to completers. It is likely that there is a continuum of suicidal behavior, not merely a dichotomy of attempters and completers. If so, the suicidal profile identified elsewhere (e.g., Leenaars 1988a, 1989a) may be clinically useful in understanding not only suicide but also parasuicidal behavior. The profile may well thus be clinically useful in assessing and predicting both suicide and parasuicide.

It is important to note about the profile, however, that it reveals age differences (Leenaars, 1988a, 1989a) as well as age × sex differences (Leenaars, 1989a, 1989b). In particular, young adults (chronological age = 18–25) differ most from other adults in their suicide notes and, by implication, their suicides. These differences occur in several essential patterns; however, they are differences of degree, not of presence or absence, since the eight clusters occur across the adult lifespan.

Still further research is needed. For example, we are currently research-ing the notes of adolescents and the terminally ill. However, the line of research completed to date would suggest that this profile may be useful in understanding not only notes but other suicidal communications, and, by implication, ideation.

THEMATIC GUIDE FOR SUICIDE PREDICTION

From this research, the Thematic Guide for Suicide Prediction (TGSP) has been developed (Leenaars, 1988d). The structure of the TGSP is thus based on many years of research on suicide notes, in which suicide has been recognized as a human malaise with considerable psychological variability. The TGSP is a 35-item measure that can be applied to an individual's communication, whether written or spoken, following the long tradition of thematic measurement. It provides an inferential guide to suicidal ideation. The guide consists of eight separate subscales (which correspond to the clusters identified above), with predictive and differentiating items: Unbear-able Psychological Pain, Interpersonal Relations, Rejection–Aggression, Inability to Adjust, Indirect Expressions, Identification–Egression, Ego, and Cognitive Constriction. It is critical to understand that the TGSP is not a test like the TAT or other projective tests; it is an analysis and interpreta-tion of actual archival materials. It is a guide or outline for assessment or evaluation of the spoken or written words of an individual. It also allows one to assess and qualitatively predict a person's suicidal ideation, follow-ing the premise that prediction is based on understanding. It provides the templates, much like the views on interpretation presented on the TAT in Shneidman's (1951) book *Thematic Test Analysis*. The TGSP is presented in Appendix 16., with specific instructions (derived from the research), identifying data, and so on.

At this point, it may be prudent to describe a clinical observation and some limitations of this thematic analysis tool, noted in its development. The guide should be approached with at least two constructs in mind: perturbation and lethality. "Perturbation" refers to how upset (disturbed, agitated, sane-insane) the individual is; it can be rated as low, medium, or high (or, alterna-tively, on a 1–9 scale). Lethality is roughly synonymous with "likelihood of death" (and is an important dimension in understanding any potentially suicidal individual). Like perturbation, lethality can be rated as low, medium, or high (or, alternatively, on a 1–9 scale). Both are covered in the TGSP and are probably not independent of any prediction of suicide. Of critical impor-tance in suicide is that it is lethality, not perturbation, that kills. All sorts of people are highly perturbed, but not all are suicidal by any means.

Our research experience with independent judges, outlined in detail elsewhere (Leenaars, 1988a), has raised a number of concerns having to do with raters. First, one can probably only use professionally trained raters. Attempts to utilize, for example, undergraduate psychology students have produced very unreliable results, suggesting the problem of clinical prediction. Second, raters can be, in the terminology of Exner (1986), "overincorporaters" or "underincorporaters." The former are slow, excessive, and overly perfectionistic; the latter are *very* quick, which results in poor ratings and excessive blunders. Third, motivational issues may affect the judgments. My colleagues and I have also noted that the more frequently a client's protocols are matched (or verified) with the items of the TGSP, the more ominous the predictive value of those items becomes. However, it should be remembered that some items have a differentiating value despite their infrequent occurrence. As one uses the guide with an individual's communications (whether written or oral), an infrequently observed item on the TGSP may well be important in understanding that individual.

One possible critical response to the TGSP is the following: It seems to generate numbers, but what these numbers tell us about suicide prediction is not clear. Such a comment, I believe, is based largely on a statistical approach to prediction—the quantitative approach. This is only one avenue in assessment, and in its rigid form is discrepant from the projective movement. The use of only the statistical view is a "cognitively simple" (as George Kelly used the term) construal of assessment. I believe that to predict suicide, we need the statistical approach, the projective approach, and other approaches as well. It should be borne in mind that the TGSP should not be used alone or in a vacuum. Rather, it should be utilized within a context that includes other tests, judgments, and forms of assessment. There is no *single* test for suicidality.

It should also be noted that the TGSP is only at a proposal stage; it needs to meet further requirements for development. It is, as noted previously, a *guide* for assessment or evaluation of available communication. Research is currently underway with the TGSP. Problems such as reliability, validity, and norms, need to be addressed; also data need to be gathered for different groups (attempters, contemplators, psychiatric inpatients, etc.). However, even at this stage, the TGSP should at least provide the clinician with constructs (or templates) to understand the suicidal person.

APPLICATION OF THE METHOD
TO THE FIVE CLINICAL CASES

In the cases provided for this text (see Chapter 12), only the description of Heather B provides enough clinical material for an application of the TGSP that would have any utility. However, even here, there are problems: Some of the data were furnished by Heather's mother, not Heather; some of the data were indirect (results of the Rorschach, TAT, etc.); and our research on adolescents with the protocol sentences is incomplete at this time. Yet an attempt is made here to provide an analysis of this case, although caution is in order. TGSP items scored "yes" for all five cases are also provided, albeit reluctantly. The problem is not that the scoring is not valid; rather, the case material available to us is clinically sparse. The TGSP should be based on actual archival material, not narrow case summaries, if it is to allow us to understand and thus to predict suicide.

Interpretation of Heather's case

I. *Unbearable Psychological Pain.* Heather appeared to be in pain, wanting to flee. Distress and grief were clearly evident, especially in the following journal entry: "I'm sorry . . . When you told me he was dead, I didn't believe you. How could I? My dad was always there. For seven years and what do I get? A grave and a photo? What else? . . . I should have cried. But I didn't. I'm sorry, Daddy. I miss you." The death of her father was probably a painful trauma, which she was unable years later to accept.

II. *Interpersonal Relations.* Heather's note about her father suggested defeat, something that she could not overcome. There was a similar theme in her response to Card 1 of the TAT: "He can't learn it right now." Her needs, notably attachment, were probably frustrated and unsatisfied. Her note to her former friend, Robin, also expressed this message. It would seem accurate to conclude that Heather's problems were both current and historical. Her interpersonal relations were disturbed, and these (especially her relations to her dead father), I suspect, were keeping her under a constant strain.

III. *Rejection–Aggression.* Heather's personality was not adequately developed. Even at a manifest level, she called herself "stupid." The story in Card 1 of the TAT also suggested this theme. Her journal entry about her father clearly suggested a deep hurt. Themes of rejection and ideas of aggression toward self and, more indirectly, toward others (e.g., father, mother), were evident. Direct anger toward her stepfather, her school, and her peers was clearly evident in her written material and her mother's report.

IV. *Inability to Adjust.* Heather's inability to adjust was evident in her note about her father. She saw herself as too weak. Her TAT stories suggested themes of hopelessness and futility. Although more data than those provided in Chapter 12 would be needed to make a diagnosis of a mental disorder (Leenaars, 1991), the available material does suggest that a serious disorder might well be present.

V. *Indirect Expressions.* Themes of aggression turned inward were evident. The mother's report about Heather's self-destruction would seem to verify this. Unconscious implications, especially in her note about her father, appeared to be present; however, further data would be needed to ascertain the nature of these processes.

VI. *Identification-Egression.* Heather both directly and indirectly communicated an identification with her lost father. She wanted to egress. She wrote, "I want to run away, not come back. . . . I need some air." She even communicated that she was "suicidal"—itself an egressive thought.

VII. *Ego.* Unresolved ego problems were evident in both Heather's writings and her mother's report. Heather suggested that she deserved to be punished ("Leave me alone to inflict self pain"). Indeed, there were at least three clear messages about antagonistic, unassimilated obstacles in her ego. She lacked constructive tendencies (e.g., attachment, love).

VIII. *Cognitive Constriction.* Heather appeared to be intoxicated by her overpowering emotions and perceptions. She wrote, "My mentality is so severely corrupted, distorted, and disturbed." In her journal entry about her father, she wrote about being overwhelmed with his death ("My dad was always there") Her last statement is, I believe, most important in understanding Heather: "I'm sorry, Daddy. I miss you."

Scoring for the Five Cases

TGSP scoring for each of the five clinical cases is summarized below. The numbers refer to the protocol sentences for which a "yes" response was deemed appropriate.

> *Heather B*: 1, 2, 4, 5, 7, 8, 9, 10, 11, 12, 13, 15, 17, 19, 20, 21, 22, 23, 25, 26, 27, 28, 29, 30, 31, 32, 33, 34
> *Ralph F*: 15, 17, 23 (e?), 33
> *John Z*: 2, 4, 15, 17, 23 (e?), 32, 33
> *Faye C*: 2, 4, 7, 8, 9, 11, 13, 15, 21, 23 (a?), 27, 29, 30, 33, 34
> *José G*: 2, 4, 7, 8, 11, 15, 19, 20, 21, 25, 30, 32, 33, 34, 35

The fact that Heather's case material resulted in the highest number of items with "yes" responses does *not* mean that she was the most suicidal. Heather's case material was simply the most extensive and clinically rich (although I do believe that Heather's development would need to be monitored as she moved into adulthood). This is a problem with the data: They are not qualitatively and quantitatively equivalent. No clinician would base a prediction *only* on any of the case material provided for this book. Furthermore, as noted above, the TGSP can only be useful as part of a battery approach.

CONCLUDING REMARKS

Although this point of view is not without controversy, I believe that suicide notes (and other personal communications) constitute a microcosm of human ideation. They are an invaluable starting point not only for understanding what Herman Melville called the "damp, drizzly November of my soul" (see Murray, 1967), but also for assessing and predicting suicide and parasuicidal behavior. Indeed, in my school of thought, understanding and prediction are intertwined. Although much more research is needed, suicide notes as a form of communication—and the TGSP, which was developed from the research on notes—constitute a neglected source for understanding and prediction. Suicide notes have predictive power.

It is likely that no communication of any person (e.g., a suicide note) will provide all of the information needed to assess and predict suicide. Such a communication—and, by implication, ideation—will have to be placed in the context of that person's life. It is likely that a number of tests, interviews, and scales will be needed to predict such a complex human behavior as suicide. No one test or guide may be the answer. There is no one "bump on the head" that will tell us *whether* a patient is suicidal or not, much less *how* suicidal that person is. The TGSP is only one tool. Furthermore, all instruments of prediction ultimately depend on the skill of the clinician. In that sense, suicide prediction is a task like many others that a sound clinician faces—a problem of understanding a number of evaluations of the same person.

REFERENCES

Allport, A. (1942). *The use of personal documents in psychological science.* New York: Social Science Research Council.

Anastasi, A. (1982). *Psychological testing,* (5th ed.). New York: Macmillan.

Beck, A. T. (1967). *Depression: Clinical, experimental and theoretical aspects.* New York: Hoeber.

Beck, A. T., & Beamesderfer, M. (1974). Assessment of depression: The depression inventory. In P. Pichot (Ed.), *Modern problems in pharmacopsychiatry: Vol. 7. Physiological measures of psychopharmacology.* Basel: Karger.

Beck, A. T., Beck, R., & Kovacs, M. (1975). Classification of suicidal behaviors: I. Quantifying intent and medical lethality. *American Journal of Psychiatry, 132,* 285-288.

Beck, A. T., Kovacs, M., & Weissman, A. (1979). Assessment of suicidal intent: The Scale for Suicide Ideation. *Journal of Consulting and Clinical Psychology, 47,* 343-352.

Beck, A. T., Schuyler, D., & Herman, I. (1974). Development of suicidal intent scales. In A. T. Beck, H. L. P. Resnik, & D. J. Lettieri (Eds.), *The prediction of suicide.* Bowie, MD: Charles Press.

Beck, A. T., Weissman, A., Lester, D., & Trexler, L. (1974). The measurement of pessimism: The Hopelessness Scale. *Journal of Consulting and Clinical Psychology, 42,* 861-865.

Bjerg, K. (1967). The suicidal life space: Attempts at reconstruction from suicide notes. In E. Shneidman (Ed.), *Essays in self-destruction*. New York: Science House.

Bolton, N. (1972). *The psychology of thinking*. Edinburgh: Constable.

Capstick, A. (1960). Recognition of emotional disturbance and the prevention of suicide. *British Medical Journal, i,* 1179–1182.

Carnap, R. (1959). Psychology in physical language. In A. Ayer (Ed.), *Logical positivism*. New York: Free Press. (Original work published 1931)

Darbonne, A. (1969). Study of psychological content in the communications of suicidal individuals. *Journal of Consulting and Clinical Psychology, 33,* 590–596.

Diggory, J. (1974). Predicting suicide: Will-o-the-wisp or reasonable challenge? In A. T. Beck, H. L. P. Resnik, & D. J. Lettieri (Eds.), *The prediction of suicide*. Bowie, MD: Charles Press.

Edelman, A., & Renshaw, S. (1982). Genuine versus simulated suicide notes. An issue revisited through discourse analysis. *Suicide and Life-Threatening Behavior, 12,* 103–113.

Exner, J. (1986). *The Rorschach: A comprehensive system. Vol. 1. Basic foundation,* (2nd ed.). New York: Wiley.

Farberow, N., & Shneidman, E. (1957). Suicide and age. In E. Shneidman & N. Farberow (Eds.), *Clues to suicide*. New York: McGraw-Hill.

Fishbain, D., D'Achille, L., Barsky, S., & Aldrich, T. (1984). A controlled study of suicide pacts. *Journal of Clinical Psychiatry, 45,* 154–157.

Fishbain, D., Fletcher, J., Aldrich, T., & Davis, J. (1987). Relationship between Russian roulette deaths and risk-taking behavior: A controlled study. *American Journal of Psychiatry, 144,* 564–567.

Freud, S. (1955). The psychogenesis of a case of homosexuality in a woman. In J. Strachey (Ed. and Trans.), *The standard edition of the complete psychological works of Sigmund Freud,* (Vol. 18). London: Hogarth Press. (Original work published 1920)

Freud, S. (1957). Mourning and melancholia. In J. Strachey (Ed. and Trans.), *The standard edition of the complete psychological works of Sigmund Freud,* (Vol. 14). London: Hogarth Press. (Original work published 1917)

Freud, S. (1960). The psychopathology of everyday life. In J. Strachey (Ed. and Trans.), *The standard edition of the complete psychological works of Sigmund Freud* (Vol. 6). London: Hogarth Press. (Original work published 1901)

Freud, S. (1963). Introductory lectures on psycho-analysis. In J. Strachey (Ed. and Trans.), *The standard edition of the complete psychological works of Sigmund Freud* (Vols. 15 and 16). London: Hogarth Press. (Original work published 1916–1917)

Friedman, P. (Ed.) (1967). *On suicide*. New York: International Universities Press. (Original work published 1910)

Furth, H. (1966). *Thinking without language*. New York: Free Press.

Hayakawa, S. (1957). Suicide as a communicative act. *ETC., 15,* 46–51.

Henken, V. (1976). Banality reinvestigated: A computer-based content analysis of suicidal and forced death documents. *Suicide and Life-Threatening Behavior, 6,* 36–43.

Jacobs, J. (1971). A phenomenological study of suicide notes. In A. Geddens (Ed.), *The sociology of suicide*. London: Cass.

Kerlinger, F. (1964). *Foundations of behavioral research*. New York: Holt, Rinehart & Winston.

Leenaars, A. A. (1979). *A study of the manifest content of suicide notes from three different theoretical perspectives: L. Binswanger, S. Freud, and G. Kelly*. Unpublished doctoral dissertation, Windsor, Ontario, Canada.

Leenaars, A. A. (1985). Freud's and Shneidman's formulations of suicide investigated through suicide notes. In E. S. Shneidman (Chair), *Suicide notes and other personal documents in psychological science*. Symposium conducted at the meeting of the American Psychological Association, Los Angeles.

Leenaars, A. A. (1986). A brief note on the latent content in suicide notes. *Psychological Reports, 59*, 640–642.

Leenaars, A. A. (1987). An empirical investigation of Shneidman's formulations regarding suicide: Age and sex. *Suicide and Life-Threatening Behavior, 17*, 233–250.

Leenaars, A. A. (1988a). *Suicide notes*. New York: Human Sciences Press.

Leenaars, A. A. (1988b). Are women's suicides really different from men's? *Women and Health, 18*, 17–33.

Leenaars, A. A. (1988c). The suicide notes of women. In D. Lester (Ed.), *Why women kill themselves*. Springfield, IL: Charles C Thomas.

Leenaars, A. A. (1988d). *A Thematic Guide for Suicide Prediction: A proposal*. Paper presented at the 21st Annual Meeting of the American Association of Suicidology, Washington, DC.

Leenaars, A. A. (1989a). Suicide across the adult life span: An archival study. *Crisis, 10*, 132–151.

Leenaars, A. A. (1989b). Are young adults' suicides psychologically different from those of other adults? (The Shneidman Lecture). *Suicide and Life-Threatening Behavior, 19*, 249–263.

Leenaars, A. A. (1990). Do the psychological characteristics of the suicidal individual make a difference in the method chosen for suicide? *Canadian Journal of Behavioural Science, 22*, 385–392.

Leenaars, A. A. (1991). *Suicide notes in the courtroom*. Manuscript submitted for publication.

Leenaars, A. A., & Balance, W. (1981). A predictive approach to the study of manifest content in suicide notes. *Journal of Clinical Psychology, 37*, 50–52.

Leenaars, A. A., & Balance, W. (1984a). A logical empirical approach to the study of the manifest content in suicide notes. *Canadian Journal of Behavioural Science, 16*, 248–256.

Leenaars, A. A., & Balance, W. (1984b). A predictive approach to Freud's formulations regarding suicide. *Suicide and Life-Threatening Behavior, 14*, 275–283.

Leenaars, A. A., & Balance, W. (1984c). A predictive approach to suicide notes of young and old people from Freud's formulations regarding suicide. *Journal of Clinical Psychology, 40*, 1362–1364.

Leenaars, A. A., Balance, W., Wenckstern, S. & Rudzinski, D. (1985). An empirical investigation of Shneidman's formulations regarding suicide. *Suicide and Life-Threatening Behavior, 15*, 184–195.

Leenaars, A. A., & Lester, D. (1988-1989). The significance of the method chosen for suicide in understanding the psychodynamics of the suicidal individual. *Omega, 19*, 311-314.

Leenaars, A. A., & Lester, D. (1990). What characteristics of suicide notes are salient for people to allow perception of a suicide note as genuine? *Death Studies, 14*, 25-30.

Leenaars, A. A., Lester, D., Wenckstern, S., Rudzinski, D., & Brevard, A. (1992). A comparison of suicide notes and parasuicide notes. *Death Studies, 16*.

Lester, D. (1971). Choice of method for suicide and personality: A study of suicide notes. *Omega, 2*, 76-80.

Maris, R. (1981). *Pathways to suicide: A survey of self-destructive behaviors*. Baltimore: John Hopkins University Press.

Meehl, P., & Rosen, A. (1955). Antecedent probability and the efficiency of psychometric signs, patterns, or cutting scores. *Psychological Bulletin, 52*, 194-216.

Menninger, K. (1938). *Man against himself*. New York: Harcourt, Brace & World.

Michel, K. (1988). Suicide in young people is different. *Crisis, 9*, 135-145.

Motto, J. (1985). Preliminary field testing of a risk estimator for suicide. *Suicide and Life-Threatening Behavior, 15*, 139-150.

Muller, M. (1887). *The science of thought* (2 Vols). New York.

Murray, H. (1943). *Thematic Apperception Test manual*. Cambridge, MA: Harvard University Press.

Murray, H. (1967). Death to the world: The passions of Herman Melville. In E. S. Shneidman (Ed.), *Essays in self-destruction*. New York: Science House.

Oglivie, D., Stone, P., & Shneidman, E. S. (1969, March). Some characteristics of genuine versus simulated suicide notes. *Bulletin of Suicidology*, pp. 19-26.

Peck, D. (1983). The last moments of life: Learning to cope. *Deviant Behavior, 4*, 313-332.

Piaget, J. (1968). *Structuralism* (C. Maschler, Trans.). New York: Harper & Row.

Piaget, J. (1972). Language and thought from the genetic point of view. In P. Adams (Ed.), *Language in thinking*, Harmondsworth, England: Penguin.

Phillips, D. & Leenaars, A. A. (1990). [Suicide notes at symbolic ages]. Unpublished raw data.

Posener, J., LaHaye, A., & Cheifetz, P. (1989). Suicide notes in adolescence. *Canadian Journal of Psychiatry, 34*, 171-176.

Runyan, W. (1982). In defense of the case study method. *American Journal of Orthopsychiatry, 52*, 440-446.

Schwilbe, M., & Rader, K. (1982). Content analytic studies of emotionality in suicide letters and other texts written near death. *Zeitschrift für Klinische Psychologie Forschung und Praxis, 11*, 280-291.

Shneidman, E. S. (1949). Some comparison among Four Picture Test, Thematic Apperception Test, and Make a Picture Test. *Rorschach Research Exchange and Journal of Projective Techniques., 13*, 150-154.

Shneidman, E. S. (1951). *Thematic test analysis*. New York: Grune and Stratton.

Shneidman, E. S. (1973). Suicide. In *Encyclopedia Britannica*, 21st ed., Vol. 14 (pp. 383-385). Chicago: William Benton.

Shneidman, E. S. (1980). *Voices of death*. New York: Harper & Row.

Shneidman, E. S. (1981). Logical content analysis. In E. S. Shneidman, *Suicide thoughts and reflections, 1960–1980*. New York: Human Sciences Press.

Shneidman, E. S. (1985). *Definition of suicide*. New York: Wiley.

Shneidman, E. S., & Farberow, N. (Eds.). (1957a). *Clues to suicide*. New York: McGraw-Hill.

Shneidman, E., S., & Farberow, N. (1957b). The logic of suicide. In E. S. Shneidman & N. Farberow (Eds.), *Clues to suicide*. New York: McGraw-Hill.

Spiegel, D., & Neuringer, C. (1963). Role of dread in suicidal behavior. *Journal of Abnormal and Social Psychology, 66*, 507–511.

Stengel, E. (1964). *Suicide and attempted suicide*. Harmondsworth, England: Penguin.

Sullivan, H. S. (1962a). Schizophrenia as a human process. In H. Perry, N. Gorvell, & M. Gibbens (Eds.), *The collected works of Harry Stack Sullivan*, (Vol. 2). New York: Norton.

Sullivan, H. S. (1962b). The fusion of psychiatry and social sciences. In H. Perry, N. Gorvell, & M. Gibbens (Eds.), *The collected works of Harry Stack Sullivan*, (Vol. 2). New York: Norton.

Tripodes, P. (1976). Reasoning patterns in suicide notes. In E. Shneidman (Ed.), *Suicidology: Contemporary developments*. New York: Grune & Stratton.

Tuckman, J., & Ziegler, R. (1968). A comparison of single and multiple note writers among suicides. *Journal of Clinical Psychology, 24*, 179–180.

Vygotsky, L. (1962). *Thought and language* (E. Hanfmann & G. Vakar Eds. and Trans.). Cambridge, MA: The MIT Press.

Wagner, F. (1960). Suicide notes. *Danish Medical Journal, 7*, 62–64.

Windelband, W. (1904). *Geschichte und Naturwissenschaft*. Strassburg, Germany: Hertz.

Wolff, H. (1931). Suicide notes. *American Mercury, 24*, 264–272.

Zilboorg, G. (1936). Suicide among civilized and primitive races. *American Journal of Psychiatry, 92*, 1347–1369.

Zubin, J. (1974). Observations on nosological issues in the classification of suicidal behavior. In A. T. Beck, H. L. P. Resnik, & D. J. Lettieri (Eds.), *The prediction of suicide*. Bowie, MD: Charles Press.

APPENDIX 16.1
THEMATIC GUIDE FOR SUICIDE PREDICTION

I. Client Data

Date _____

Name _____ Age _____ Sex _____

Date of Birth _____ Marital Status _____

Education Status _____ _____
(years)   (degrees)

Current Employment _____

II. Suicidal Experience

1. Has the client ever seriously contemplated suicide? (If yes, note particulars)
_____

2. Has the client ever attempted suicide? (If yes, note particulars)
_____

3. Does the client know anyone who attempted suicide? (If yes, indicate family, acquaintance, etc.) _____

4. Does the client know anyone who committed suicide? (If yes, indicate family, acquaintance, etc.) _____

III. Referral Data

1. Purpose _____

2. What is the referral question? _____
_____

3. What is the presenting problem? _____
_____

IV. Interview Situation

1. Observations _____
_____
_____

2. Other procedures (e.g., tests, interviews) _____
_____

V. Interpretations

1. Perturbation rating: Low   Medium   High
   Scale equivalent   1 2 3   4 5 6   7 8 9
2. Lethality rating: Low   Medium   High
   Scale equivalent   1 2 3   4 5 6   7 8 9
3. Guide summary:
   Scores 1: 1, 2, 3, 4, 5, 6;   II: 7, 8, 9, 10, 11, 12;   III: 13, 14, 15, 16, 17, 18, 20;
   IV: 21, 22, 23 (, other:);   V: 24, 25, 26;   VI: 27, 28, 29;   VII: 30, 31,
   32;   VIII: 33, 34, 35.
   Conclusions: _____

   _____
   _____
   _____
   _____
   _____

VI. Remarks

   _____
   _____
   _____
   _____
   _____

INSTRUCTIONS

Your task will be to verify whether the statements provided below correspond or compare to the contents of the client's protocols (e.g., interview, written reports). The statements provided below are classifications of the possible content. You are to determine whether the client's protocols provide a particular or specific instance of each classification or not. Your comparison should be based on one or more observable examples; however, the classification may be more abstract than the specific instances. Thus, you will have to make judgments about whether the particular content of a protocol should be included in a given classification or not. Your task is to conclude "yes" or "no."

I. Unberable Psychological Pain   *Circle One*

1. The person communicates flight from one of the following: pain, incurable disease, the threat of helpless senility, a violent death; anticipated rejection or fear of becoming dependent; or self-depreciation, feelings of sexual or general inadequacy, humiliation, unknown danger. *However*, the solution of suicide

does not appear to be caused only by such a single thing; other
motives (elements, wishes) appear to be evident. (P & D)[1]   Yes   No

2. The following emotional states are evident: pitiful forlornness,
deprivation, distress, and/or grief. (P & D)   Yes   No

3. The person, who appears to have arrived at the end of his/her
limited social interest, sees his/her suicide as a solution for an
urgent problem and/or the injustices of life. (P)   Yes   No

4. A clash is evident between a demand of adaptation and the individual's constitutional inability to meet the challenge. (P)   Yes   No

5. It appears that although suicide does not have adaptive (survival) value, suicide does have adjustive value for the individual. suicide is functional because it abolishes painful tension
for the individual; it provides relief from intolerable suffering.
(P)   Yes   No

6. The person is in a state of heightened disturbance (perturbation); that is, he/she feels boxed in, rejected, harassed, unsuccessful, and especially hopeless and helpless. (P)   Yes   No

II. Interpersonal Relations

7. Unresolved problems in the individual are evident; he/she has
suffered defeat, at least for the time being, and there is something he/she cannot evade or overcome. His/her weak spots in
every sense of the word are evident. (P)   Yes   No

8. The stressor appears to be unsatisfied or frustrated needs (e.g.,
achievement, affiliation, autonomy, dominance, etc.), although
it may be difficult to determine precisely which needs are operating. (P)   Yes   No

9. The communications allow one to conclude that the solution
of suicide appears to be determined by the individual's history
and the present interpersonal situation. (P)   Yes   No

10. The person appears to be under stress from a situational factor,
which changes a relatively unvarying disturbance in interpersonal relations to one that is increasing to a traumatic degree.
(P)   Yes   No

11. The person's communications indicate that his/her field of interpersonal relations is disturbed. A positive development in
those some disturbed relations is held as the only possible way
to go on living, but such a development is seen as not forthcoming. (P)   Yes   No

12. There is direct or indirect evidence or inference of too great an
attachment and too intimate (and primitive) a relationship, no
matter how conventionally correct, of the individual to any

---

1. The letter P refers to a specific highly predictive variable, whereas the letter D refers to a specific differentiating variable.

other person (e.g., family member), keeping him/her under the constant strain of having wishes (e.g., closeness, incestuous desires) stimulated and inhibited at one and the same time. (D)   Yes   No

III. Rejection–Aggression

13. The communications suggest that the person's personality (ego) organization is not adequately developed ("primitive," "weak") and narcissistic. (P & D)   Yes   No

14. It appears that the unconscious has created a situation in which death is desired, partly in order to hurt/attack someone else, or as an act of revenge toward someone who has slighted him/her. One can conclude that the person, by attacking himself/herself, is likely attacking another person. (P)   Yes   No

15. The person communicates the existence of a traumatic event (e.g., an unmet love, a failing marriage, disgust with one's work) that results in a deep hurt, desperation, and ultimately suicide itself. (P)   Yes   No

16. Although the person may not state this directly, there is evidence that a particular, significant other person (or persons), who was a destructive influence in the individual's past, is the target of the self-destruction. Self-destruction may not be the only goal of the individual; the individual may well calculate that the act would have a prolonged evil effect on this other person (or persons). (P)   Yes   No

17. The person communicates that he/she is preoccupied with a person that he/she has lost or who has rejected him/her. (D)   Yes   No

18. The person communicates that he/she is feeling quite ambivalent (i.e., affectionate and hostile toward a lost or rejecting person). (D)   Yes   No

19. The person communicates feelings and/or ideas of vengefulness and aggression toward himself/herself; however, he/she appears to be angry toward someone else. (D)   Yes   No

20. the person communicates that he/she is turning back upon himself/herself murderous impulses that have been directed against someone else. (D)   Yes   No

IV. Inability to Adjust

21. The individual considers himself/herself too weak to overcome his/her personal difficulties, and therefore (in revenge) rejects everything at one fell swoop in order to escape the feeling of inferiority, and/or to act intelligent according to his/her goal of coping with the difficulties of life (with disregard to the community—a beloved person, a teacher, society, or the world at large). (P)   Yes   No

22. The person points out, with passionate eloquence and with flawless logic (from his/her perspective), that life is hard, bitter, futile, and hopeless; that it entails more pain than pleasures; that there is no profit or purpose in it for him/her and no conceivable justification fr living on. (P)   Yes   No

23. There is evidence of *one* of the following serious disorders of social behavior: Yes   No

Other disorder:

a. There is evidence consistent with the "down phase" of a manic-depressive disorder. For example, there is a sort of all-embracing (grandiose) negative self-appraisal—he/she is no good, has never been any good, and has caused everyone else a great deal of trouble, which can only be ended by destroying himself/herself.

b. There is evidence consistent with a diagnosis of schizophrenia. For example, the schizophrenic wants to end his/her life quite incidentally to some fantastic procedure for the remedy of his/her distress: to be reborn, to protect others from some delusional contamination, to save the world, to demonstrate omnipotence, and the like.

c. There is evidence consistent with the diagnosis of obsessive-compulsive disorder. For example, the individual exhibits obsessional characteristics such as overwhelming suicidal thoughts with unlimited attention to the detail of such an act.

d. There is evidence consistent with a diagnosis of psychopathic disorder. For example, the individual's communications are a tool for ensuring attention of others, but the act itself will likely be an accidental misjudgment—too great a dose of poison, too long a delay in calling for help, and so forth.

e. There is evidence consistent with a diagnosis of depressive disorder. For example, the person exhibits a "reverie" of self-depreciating statements and appears to be very restrictive in thoughts and actions.

f. There is no evidence of a serious specific disorder, but the protocols appear to be expressed by an individual who is so baffled in his/her attempt to subjugate his/her interests that a paralysis of interest in others and in future possibilities of self has progressed to the point at which life has become colorless and completely wholly unattractive. (P)

V. Indirect Expressions

24. The person communicates ambivalence (e.g., complications, concomitant contradictory feelings, attitudes, and/or thrusts). (P & D)   Yes   No

25. The individual's aggression appears to have been turned inward. Themes of humility, submission and devotion, subordination, flagellation, or masochism are evident. (P)   Yes   No

26. The person's communications appear to have unconscious psychodynamic implications. (D)   Yes   No

VI. Identification–Egression

27. There is evidence for egression (defined as a person's intended departure from a region of distress, chiefly with the aim of terminating the pain he/she has been suffering and achieving relief) and desertion (e.g., from the suicide's closest bonded person). (P)   Yes   No

28. The person communicates that he/she is in some direct or indirect fashion identifying with a rejecting or lost person. (D)   Yes   No

29. An unwillingness to accept sickness, old age, or too many painful emotions not only makes it possible for the individual to accept death willingly, even to seek it; it also generally leads him/her to project his/her ideal beyond life (e.g., the hereafter), where life is eternal and forever devoid of any discomfort. (D)   Yes   No

VII. Ego

30. A "complex" is evident; that is, something discordant, unassimilated, and antagonistic exists (e.g., symptoms, ideas), perhaps as an obstacle, pointing to unresolved problems in the individual. (P)   Yes   No

31. The person communicates that his/her suicide is a fulfillment of punishment (i.e., self-punishment). (D)   Yes   No

32. The communications indicate that the person wishes to die; that is, suicide is accomplished because of some relative weakness in the capacity for developing constructive tendencies (e.g., attachment, love). (D)   Yes   No

VIII. Cognitive Constriction

33. The person communicates evidence of adult trauma (e.g., poor health, rejection by the spouse, being married to a competing spouse). (P & D)   Yes   No

34. The person appears to be figuratively intoxicated or drugged by his/her overpowering emotions and constricted logic and perception. (D)   Yes   No

35. There is a poverty of thought, exhibited by the individual's expressing only permutations and combinations of grief-provoking content. (D)   Yes   No

CHAPTER 17

The Relationship of Nonfatal Suicide Attempts to Completed Suicides

Ronald W. Maris, Ph.D.
University of South Carolina

In 1981 I wrote: "It is tempting to assume that the key to prediction and control of suicide is buried somewhere in the deceptively transparent observation that in order to kill yourself, you must first make an attempt" (p. 264). On average, over their lifetimes about 10–15% of individuals making nonfatal suicide attempts eventually go on to kill themselves (see Figure 17.1; Roy & Linnoila, 1990; cf. Retterstol, 1974). Of course, it is also true that 85–90% of nonfatal suicide attempters never kill themselves. Depending on their age and sex, nonfatal suicide attempters outnumber suicides completers by at least 8 or 10 to 1. Although it is a little confusing, one could describe Figure 17.1 by saying *either* that "only" 10–15% of suicide attempters ever complete suicide *or* that "fully" 30–40% of suicide completers have made at least one prior nonfatal suicide attempt (depending on which set area A + B is taken as a proportion of). Prior suicide attempters are at a relatively high risk of completing suicide. The suicide rate in the United States is about 12 per 100,000 per year, but 15,000 per 100,000 (i.e., 15 per 100) for prior suicide attempters over their lifetimes.

One commonly held belief about the psychosocial development of suicides is that some lifelong precursors (e.g., a family history of suicide; loss of a parent at an early age; isolation and/or inability to get along with other people; work, marital, or sexual problems; recurring episodes of depressive illness; alcohol and/or drug abuse; etc.) interact with acute stressors to "trigger" initial nonfatal suicide attempts (Clark, Gibbons, Fawcett, & Scheftner, 1989). The initial suicide attempt can be seen as having both benefits and costs to the attempter. On the positive side, nonfatal suicide attempts almost always get attention from family members, friends, and professionals. The attempter is usually allowed to assume a "sick role," and ordinary responsibilities are often temporarily suspended. Suicide attempts may even be cathartic or purging, with a short-term elevation of affect.

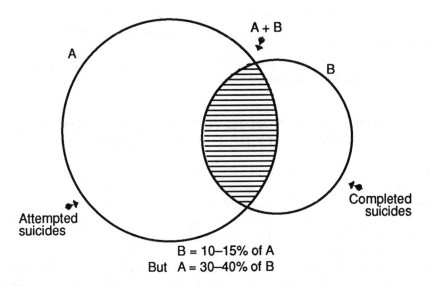

FIGURE 17.1. Relationship of attempted suicide to completed suicide. From *Pathways to Suicide: A Survey of Self-Destructive Behaviors* (p. 266), by R. W. Maris, 1981, Baltimore: Johns Hopkins University Press. Copyright 1981 by The Johns Hopkins University Press. Reprinted by permission.

On the negative side, the attention resulting from a suicide attempt is sometimes stigmatizing and may make it more difficult for the individual to maintain a healthy identity. People may be sympathetic with suicide attempters, but they are also likely to be angry. Suicide attempts inconvenience and manipulate others. Many people believe that, unlike physical illnesses, suicide attempts are intentional and to a degree are unnecessary. After a period of recuperation, the attempter is expected to give up the "sick role" and to resume more normal, preattempt behavior and responsibilities. In short, suicide attempters incur costs. The problems that were associated with the first suicide attempt tend to recur, in part because of the suicide attempt itself.

Attempting suicide may become a conditioned reaction. The suicide attempter may learn to adapt to stress and life events by repeated self-destructive behaviors. However, subsequent suicide attempts may be made with more lethal methods. In part, this may be the case because the attempter is older and more hopeless. Furthermore, to get a positive response from significant others, the attempter may have to appear more dramatic and serious in his or her subsequent efforts. Of course, more lethal attempts may also provoke elevated anger and frustration from those individuals who are affected. Hospitalization may now be unavoidable. Community resources may begin to dry up, and supportive individuals may become increasingly impatient with the suicide attempter. Finally, perhaps after a few more nonfatal attempts, there may appear to be no way out of this progressively intolerable life situation except to complete suicide. The major problem with the stereotypic suicidal career just outlined is that a large part of it is simply not true for the usual suicide completer (e.g., for older males).

NONFATAL ATTEMPTS VERSUS COMPLETIONS: COMPLEXITY OF THE RELATIONSHIP

The relationship between nonfatal suicide attempts and eventual suicide completion is complex. First, there is considerable comorbidity and inter-action in the etiology of suicide. Table 1.1 in Chapter 1 of this book reminds us of other major factors predicting completed suicide. In addition to prior nonfatal suicide attempts, they include the following (which are by now well known): depressive illness; alcoholism and drug abuse; suicide idea-tion; use of lethal methods to attempt suicide; social isolation; hopelessness; being an older, white male; a family history of suicide and/or mental disorder; work problems; marital and relational problems; stress, anger, and irritability; serotonergic disturbances; physical illness; and *repetition* and *interaction* of all of these factors (usually over "suicidal careers" of 20–30 years).

A second problem is that most suicide completers make a relatively small number of attempts before completing suicide. Tables 17.1 and 17.2 reveal that in my Chicago survey (Maris, 1981), 70–75% of all suicide com-pleters made only one fatal attempt. If we focus on older (over age 45) white males (who are "typical" suicides in many respects), then fully *88% made a single, fatal suicide attempt.* Thus, although nonfatal suicide attempts predict some suicides, they obviously do not predict about 75–90% of all completed suicides (depending on the age and sex of the attempters). Note in Table 17.2 that among suicide completers in the Chicago sample, only females made a significant number of multiple suicide attempts before completing suicide. This is particularly true for younger females; 16% of completers in this group made five or more nonfatal suicide attempts before completing suicide.

Third, a clear reason why there are relatively few suicide attempts before completion (especially among men) is that lethal methods, particu-larly guns and hanging, tend to be used. Table 17.3 (from a now somewhat dated Chicago survey) shows the preponderance of firearms used to attempt suicide (among completers). Turning to contemporary data (National Cen-ter for Health Statistics, 1990) in Table 17.4, we see that firearms now constitute the method of first choice for *both* men and women (64% and 39.8%, respectively). Thus, in the United States suicide prevention is highly related to gun control. Hanging is the preferred second method for men,

TABLE 17.1. Number of Suicide Attempts
by Suicide Completers, Chicago ($n = 246$)

Number of attempts	%[a]
1	70.0
2	13.8
3	4.8
4	3.9
5	3.5
6	0.0
7	1.1
8 or more	0.7
DK[b]	2.2
Total	100.0

Note. Data from *Pathways to Suicide: A Survey of Self-Destructive Behaviors* by R. W. Maris, 1981, Baltimore: Johns Hopkins University Press. Copyright 1981 by The Johns Hopkins University Press. Adapted by permission.
[a]Percentages slightly different from "total" column in Table 17.2 due to different number of cases.
[b] In this and subsequent tables, DK means "don't know."

especially in jails, prisons, and hospitals. Women are still much more likely than men to overdose on drugs and medications (25% of all female suicides) and to utilize a broader panorama of methods.

Fourth, it is well known that while males outnumber females 3 or 4 to 1 in their suicide completion rates (McIntosh & Jewell, 1986), females tend to exceed males in nonfatal suicide attempt rates and in rates of depressive illness (an important precursor of suicide). This suggests that the social and

TABLE 17.2. Number of Suicide Attempts; by Suicide Completers, by Sex and Age (%), Chicago ($n = 266$)

Number of attempts	Male		Female		Total
	≤ 45	>45	≤ 45	>45	
1	79	88	50	71	75
2–4	19	10	34	26	20
5+	0	0	16	3	3
DK	2	2	—	—	2
Total	100	100	100	100	100
(n)	(55)	(90)	(44)	(77)	(266)

Note. From *Pathways to Suicide: A Survey of Self-Destructive Behaviors* (p. 268) by R. W. Maris, 1981, Baltimore: Johns Hopkins University Press. Copyright 1981 by The Johns Hopkins University Press. Reprinted by permission.

TABLE 17.3. Methods Used to Attempt Suicide for Suicide Completers, Chicago (*n* = 246)

Method	%
Firearms, explosives	27.4
Hanging	17.1
Gases (esp. carbon monoxide)	10.5
Poisons, medications	19.3
Cutting, piercing	7.7
Jumping from heights	6.1
Drowning	1.1
Other	6.1
DK	4.9
Total	100.0

Note. From *Pathways to Suicide: A Survey of Self-Destructive Behaviors* (p. 268) by R. W. Maris, 1981, Baltimore: Johns Hopkins University Press. Copyright 1981 by The Johns Hopkins University Press. Reprinted by permission.

TABLE 17.4. Percentage of Completed U.S. Suicides (1987) by Method and Gender

	Gender	
Method	Male (%)	Female (%)
Firearms (E955.0–955.4)	64.0	39.8
Drugs/medications (E950.0–950.5)	5.2	25.0
Hanging (E953.0)	13.5	9.4
Carbon monoxide (E952.0–952.1)	9.6	12.6
Jumping from a high place (E957)	1.8	3.0
Drowning (E954)	1.1	2.8
Suffocation by plastic bag (E953.1)	0.4	1.8
Cutting/piercing instruments (E956)	1.3	1.4
Poisons (E950.6–950.9)	0.6	1.0
Other[a]	2.5	3.2

Note. The data are from National Center for Health Statistics (1990).
[a]Includes gases in domestic use (E951), other specified and unspecified gases and vapors (E952.8–952.9), explosives (E955.5), unspecified firearms and explosives (E955.9), and other specified or unspecified means of hanging, strangulation, or suffocation (E953.8–953.9).

psychiatric dynamics of at least some types of female suicides are different from those of male suicides. The suicide attempts of younger females more often involve changes in interpersonal relationships and family responsibilities, as well as motivations of revenge and perhaps of anger (Kaplan & Klein, 1989).

Fifth, in the Chicago survey (Maris, 1981), my colleagues and I also inquired how long the time interval was between a suicide attempt and death, as well as who found a suicide. Table 17.5 indicates, as expected that 50–75% (depending on how the "don't know" responses would be distributed) of all suicide completers died within an hour after attempting suicide. Table 17.6 reveals that suicide completers were much more likely than nonfatal suicide attempters to be responded to (the actual question was "Who was primarily involved in trying to save the suicide attempter's life?") by no one, police officers, or firefighters, and much less likely to be responded to by family members or friends. These factors clearly contributed to their suicide attempts' being fatal. One is reminded here of Weisman and Worden's (1974) "risk–rescue rating scale," in which suicide outcome is conceived of as a joint product of the lethality of the attempt and the probability of effective intervention. It is interesting to note that virtually no interventions were reported by psychotherapists, crisis workers, or suicide prevention center workers for either attempters or completers.

TABLE 17.5. Time Interval between Suicide Attempt and Completion (%), Chicago

Time interval between attempt and death	Percentage of completed suicides
1 week or more	7
4–6 days	3
2–3 days	2
4–24 hours	3
2–3 hours	6
1 hour or less	15
Instantaneous death	34
DK	30
Total	100
(n)	(266)

Note. From *Pathways to Suicide: A Survey of Self-Destructive Behaviors* (p. 284) by R. W. Maris, 1981, Baltimore: Johns Hopkins University Press. Copyright 1981 by The Johns Hopkins University Press. Reprinted by permission.

TABLE 17.6. Types of Interveners in Suicide Attempts; by Nonfatal Attempters and Completers (%), Chicago

Type of intervener	Suicide attempts by attempters	Suicide attempts by completers
Family member	48	26
Friends	19	6
Police/fireman	5	21
Physician	6	6
Psychotherapist	0	0
Suicide prevention or crisis center worker	0	0
Other	3	2
None	11	33
Don't know	8	5
Total	100	100
(*n*)	(64)	(266)

Note. From *Pathways to Suicide: A Survey of Self-Destructive Behaviors* (p. 283) by R. W. Maris, 1981, Baltimore: Johns Hopkins University Press. Copyright 1981 by The Johns Hopkins University Press. Reprinted by permission.

PERCEIVED CAUSES AND PRECURSORS OF NONFATAL ATTEMPTS VERSUS COMPLETIONS

What actually predicts fatal suicide attempts may be any one of a number of antecedents acting singly or in concert, over a lifetime or just one hour. Of course, an important theoretical assumption we make is that most suicides occur in the context of a whole life history ("suicidal careers") and typically display a multicausal network. Table 17.7 reveals that the primary reported causes (reports were primarily from spouses) of suicide attempts among suicide completers in the Chicago survey (now somewhat dated [Maris, 1981]) were depression, hopelessness, anger, and other mental problems, especially for female completers (a difference-of-proportions test between males and females produced a z score of 3.1, which was significant at the .001 level). Although it may appear self-evident that very few happy people kill themselves, there is considerable evidence that the relationship between depression and suicide is much more complex than is usually realized. It can also be seen that with increasing age physical problems understandably play a larger role in suicide attempts, particularly for men (z for male completers $= 2.75$, $p = .01$). Fourteen percent of male suicides under age 45 were reported as having primarily physical problems. For males over 45, physical problems were seen as the major cause of the suicide attempts in 36% of the cases. Work problems were also more important among older males, as was the death of a significant other for both older men and women (data not presented in Table 17.7). All emotional problems seemed somewhat less central for older suicides.

Finally, divorce or separation was mentioned as a cause of suicide attempts primarily for male suicide completers and younger female nonfatal attempters. Male suicides were more highly associated with divorce than were female suicides. Although the sample was small and somewhat unreliable when divided by cause, general interpersonal problems were the second most frequently mentioned cause of suicide attempts for nonfatal suicide attempters. Feelings of anger, and divorce and separation, were important attempt causes for female nonfatal suicide attempters. Hopelessness and depression were moderately strong causes for both men and women, although these variables appeared to be less powerful causes for female nonfatal attempters than they were for female completers. When first and last suicide attempts were compared by cause, there were no significant variations. This finding is in part an artifact, since for completers "first" and

TABLE 17.7. Perceived Cause of Last Suicide Attempt by Nonfatal Suicide Attempters and Suicide Completers by Sex and Age (%), Chicago

| | Suicide attempters | | | | Suicide completers | | | |
| | Male | | Female | | Male | | Female | |
Cause	≤45	>45	≤45	>45	≤45	>45	≤45	>45
Mental problems (including hopelessness, depression, and anger)	56	—	46	50	56	40	74	65
Physical problems (including hospitalization)	—	—	3	17	14	36	16	21
Alcoholism, drug abuse	—	—	7[a]	—	4[b]	3[b]	5[b]	—
Loss (including job, divorce, separation, children, death)	—	—	17	—	22	15	—	7
General interpersonal problems (including sexual problems)	44	—	21	33	2	5	5	3
Other (including arrest, being jailed)	—	—	—	—	2	1	—	2
Total	100	—	100	100	100	100	100	100
(n)	(9)		(29)	(6)	(49)	(88)	(40)	(73)

Note. Cause of last attempt is missing for 19 attempters and 15 completers. From *Pathways to Suicide: A Survey of Self-Destructive Behaviors* (p. 273) by R. W. Maris, 1981, Baltimore: Johns Hopkins University Press. Copyright 1981 by The Johns Hopkins University Press. Reprinted by permission.
[a]All drug abuse.
[b]Predominantly alcoholism.

"last" suicide attempts tended to be the same. However, even when multiple suicide attempts were made, there did not seem to be much change in major causes of the attempts.

It remains for a comparison to be made between the more remote causes of suicide and the immediate situational precursors or "trigger" factors. In the Chicago survey (Maris, 1981), each informant for each subject was asked to describe in detail what happened the week immediately preceding the suicide attempt or natural death. It was thought that such a question might provide insight into the factors that could be "triggering" or precipitating the attempts. In the question on causes of attempts, an effort was made to single out the events that were more remote from the suicide attempt. Thus, causes were more likely to be long-term life problems, whereas the precursor question was "Why did the suicide attempt or death occur in *this week* rather than in some other?"

Table 17.8 does reveal some differences between long-term causes and immediate precursors of suicide attempts. Depression and hopelessness were still the most important precursors of completed suicide, but physical problems, general interpersonal problems, and work problems all seemed to be slightly more important as situational precursors than as long-term causes. For the nonfatal suicide attempters, depression and hopelessness were also

TABLE 17.8. Immediate (Week Before) Precursor Symptoms for Nonfatal Suicide Attempters, Suicide Completers, and Natural Deaths (%), Chicago

Immediate situational precursor symptoms[a]	Natural deaths	Suicide attempters	Suicide completers
Mental problems (depression, hopelessness, anger)[b]	31	88	83
Physical problems	75	13	40
Alcoholism	14	14	18
Drug abuse	1	30	6
Loss (including job, divorce, separation, death)	6	14	18
General interpersonal problems	17	78	54
Hospitalization	69	3	7
Financial problems	3	14	17
(n)	(71)	(64)	(266)

Note. Because respondents could check more than one precursor, solumns do not total 100%. From *Pathways to Suicide: A Survey of Self-Destructive Behaviors* (p. 274) by R. W. Maris, 1981, Baltimore: Johns Hopkins University Press. Copyright 1981 by The Johns Hopkins University Press. Reprint by permission.
[a]Precursor symptoms could be checked more than once. Interviewers did not ask for the one most common symptom, as they did with causes.
[b]For mental problems, $z = -8.7$, $p > .001$ (natural deaths vs. completers).

the most important situational precursors, with general interpersonal problems a close second. Loneliness, anger, drug abuse, and sexual problems followed roughly in order of mention (data not presented in Table 17.8). For the sample of natural deaths, of course, physical problems and hospitalization were cited most often.

When major situational differences were contrasted for natural deaths, nonfatal attempters, and suicide completers (not all data are presented in Table 17.8), suicide completers and nonfatal attempters scored high on depression and hopelessness, whereas natural deaths scored low; drug abuse was a situational problem primarily for nonfatal suicide attempters; work problems were most prevalent among suicide completers; interpersonal problems were most often mentioned by nonfatal suicide attempters; physical problems were salient among natural deaths and to a lesser degree among suicide completers; feelings of anger and sexual problems distinguished the nonfatal attempters; and, finally, problems with arrest and imprisonment were mentioned only for the suicide completers.

The evidence in Tables 17.7 and 17.8 indicates that suicide attempts are not "triggered"; that is, the immediate precursors of suicide attempts are not very different from their long-term causes. For the most part, the same factors seem to be operating in the week before the suicide attempt or death as are present as long-term causes of suicide attempts. One key to predicting suicide is that lifelong repetition of similar problems breaches an adaptive threshold in some individuals but not in others (and we need to know why this happens). Apparently, almost anyone can (and routinely does) weather single, acute crises. Suicidal hopelessness is made up of very different stuff: repeated loss, repeated depression and hospitalization, progressive loss of social support, repeated failures, recurring physical illnesses, and the like.

FACTORS THAT PREDICT COMPLETED SUICIDES

Most of the rest of this chapter is concerned with identifying factors that predict which suicide attempters will eventually go on to complete suicide (cf. Table 1.1 of this book). Table 17.9 is an early effort by Tuckman and Youngman (1968) to differentiate categories of high and low suicide risk for 3,800 attempted suicides. "High-risk" factors were defined as those factors associated with statistically significant higher completed suicide rates among attempters. They included the following: being male, white, and 45 years of age or older; being separated, widowed, or divorced; living alone; being unemployed or retired; being in poor physical health; having a mental disorder; being alcoholic; having had medical care within 6 months of the suicide attempt; using methods of firearms, hanging, jumping, or drowning; attempting in warm months; making the attempt at home; being discovered immediately; not reporting suicidal intent to others; leaving a

TABLE 17.9. Suicide Rate per 100,000 Population among 3,800 Attempted Suicides, by High- and Low-Risk Categories of Risk-Related Factors

Factor	High-risk category	Suicide rate	Low-risk category	Suicide rate	Odds ratio of suicide rates (high vs. low risk)
Age	45 years of age and older	24.0	Under 45 years of age	9.4	2.5
Sex	Male	19.9	Female	9.2	2.2
Race	White	14.3	Nonwhite	8.7	1.6
Marital status	Separated, divorced, widowed	12.5	Single, married	8.6	1.5
Living arrangements	Alone	48.4	With others	10.1	4.8
Employment status[a]	Unemployed, retired	16.8	Employed	14.3	1.2
Physical health	Poor (acute or chronic condition in the 6-month period preceding the attempt)	14.0	Good	12.4	1.1
Mental condition	Nervous or mental disorder, mood or behavioral symptoms including alcoholism	19.1	Presumably normal, including brief situational reaction[b]	7.2	2.7
Medical care (within 6 months)	Yes	16.4	No	10.8	1.5

Method	Hanging, firearms, jumping, drowning	28.4	Cutting or piercing, gas or carbon monoxide, poison, combination of other methods, other	12.0	2.4
Season	Warm months (April–September)	14.2	Cold months (October–March)	10.9	1.3
Time of day	6:00 A.M.–5:59 P.M.	15.1	6:00 P.M.–5:59 A.M.	10.5	1.4
Where attempt was made	Own or someone else's home	14.3	Other type of premises, out of doors	11.9	1.2
Time interval between attempt and discovery	Almost immediately reported by person making attempt	10.9	Later	7.2	1.5
Intent to kill (self-report)	No[b]	14.5	Yes	8.5	1.7
Suicide note	Yes	16.7	No[b]	12.3	1.4
Previous attempt or threat	Yes	25.2	No[b]	11.0	2.3

Note. From "Assessment of Suicide Risk in Attempted Suicides" (p. 196) by J. Tuckman and W. F. Youngman, 1968, In H. L. P. Resnik (Ed.), *Suicidal Behaviors: Diagnosis and Management* (pp. 190–197), Boston: Little, Brown. Copyright 1968 by Little, Brown & Company, Inc. Reprinted by permission.
[a]Does not include housewives and students.
[b]Includes cases for which information on this factor was not given in the police report.

suicide note; and making prior suicide attempts. Eventual suicide was particularly likely (see odds ratios) when an attempter lived alone, had some mental disorder, and/or had symptoms of alcoholism. Interaction effects of individual predictors were not calculated. Although these data are by now somewhat dated, the sample was large and the predictor variables identified compare well with more recently identified predictors (such as those listed in Table 1.1).

Tables 17.10 and 17.11 summarize several other relevant studies from 1965 to 1989 concerning suicide attempters who later went on to complete suicide (cf. Lönnqvist, Niskanen, Achte, & Ginman, 1975). Some overall generalizations can be made for these studies:

1. Prior suicide attempters have an average suicide completion rate of about 1% per year.
2. The probability of completing suicide is especially high in the first year or two after the initial nonfatal suicide attempt.
3. At least two studies found that older males were more likely to go on to complete suicide than were other age and sex groups.
4. Isolation (lack of contact with a psychiatric facility, as well as living alone), alcoholism and other substance abuse, and having a history of self-poisoning were more common among suicide completers (cf. Greer & Lee, 1967).
5. Other factors related to suicide completion mentioned include insomnia (especially terminal insomnia), depressive illness, and prior suicide attempts. In addition, Beck, Steer, Kovacs, and Garrison (1985), in their longitudinal study, found that a score of 10 or more on their Hopelessness Scale correctly identified 91% of all eventual suicides.

TABLE 17.10. Results of a Follow-Up Examination of Suicide Attempters after an Observation Period of 31–42 Years

	Absolute figures			Percent		
	M	W	M + W	M	W	M + W
Alive	33	66	99	35.5	48.5	43.2
Dead by suicide	13	12	25	14.0	8.8	10.9
Dead from other causes	44	52	96	47.3	38.2	41.9
Unknown	3	6	9	3.2	4.4	3.9
Total	93	136	229	100.0	99.9	99.9

Note. M, men; W, women. From "Attempted Suicides—35 Years Afterwards" (p. 77) by K. G. Dahlgren, 1977, *Suicide and Life-Threatening Behavior*, 7(2), 75–79. Copyright 1977 by the American Association of Suicidology. Reprinted by permission.

TABLE 17.11. Percentage of Completed Suicides among Prior Nonfatal Suicide Attempters by Time to Completion and Major Factors in Completion

Study	% completed suicides	Time to completion (years)	Greatest risk of repeat attempt	Major factor in completion
Motto (1965)	8	5	—	Lack of contact with psychiatric facility
Pokorny (1965)	3.4	4.6	First 2 years	—
Rosen (1970)	1	1	—	Depression, insomnia, being older, living alone
Paerregaard (1975)	11	10	First year	Being older, being male, prior suicide attempts
Dahlgren (1977)	10.9	35	—	Being male
Beck, Steer, Kovacs, & Garrison (1985)	7	5–10	—	Hopelessness
Wang, Nielsen, Bille-Brahe, Hansen, & Kolmos (1985)	10	3	First year	—
Cullberg, Wasserman, & Stefensson (1988)	3.7	8–10	—	Substance abuse, alcoholism
Hasseanyeh, O'Brien, Holton, Hurren, & Watt (1989)	3	1.5	—	History of self-poisoning

It should be noted that several related issues have not been thoroughly addressed in this chapter. For example, not much has been said about why some initial nonfatal suicide attempters make repeated or multiple suicide attempts (Barnes, 1986; Favazza, 1989), or about why some initial suicide attempters never repeat suicidal behaviors (aside from the fact that many first attempts are fatal).

DISCUSSION

It is necessary for us to speculate as to why some nonfatal suicide attempters go on to complete suicide—in other words, for us to go theoretically beyond the available data. First, in a sense, the only permanent resolution to many life problems is to be dead. Under certain limited circumstances (one has to be very careful here), suicide can be eminently rational (Maris, 1982). Second, many suicides are less a matter of choice than they are a product of a compulsion or of behavioral bankruptcy. Individuals with long histories of recurrent depressive illness, alcoholism, failed interpersonal relationships, and so forth tend to have limited adaptive repertoires. Third, alcoholism tends to protect one against suicide early on, but after 20–25 years (if not earlier) it exacerbates suicide potential. It has been hypothesized that alcohol transiently raises both serotonin and 5-hydroxindoleacetic acid (5-HIAA, a metabolite of serotonin), but depletes it in the long run (Ballenger, Goodwin, Major, & Brown, 1979). As Asberg, Traskman, & Thoren (1976) have demonstrated, lower levels of 5-HIAA are positively associated with (violent) suicide outcomes (cf. Arango et al., 1990).

Fourth, loss of social support is often critical to suicide outcome. Suicide completers often are socially isolated and/or rejected (as reflected in the concepts of "driving the other person to suicide" and negative interaction). Many times, the individual's psychotherapist or physician is the last person meaningfully involved with the would-be suicide. Numerous traits of suicide completers (e.g., alcoholism, living alone, divorce, unemployment, aggression and irritability, depression, etc.) separate them from crucial social supports that could have prevented their suicide. Finally, suicide completers usually have chronic suicidal careers, with accumulated developmental debits and stagnation. This can include many indirect self-destructive behaviors that interact with and potentiate one another (Farberow, 1980): for example, chronic alcohol and other substance abuse (including abuse of cigarettes and other forms of tobacco); failed interpersonal relationships; sexual promiscuity; malignant masochistic rituals; repeated stress; anorexia, bulimia, or obesity; early sexual and other physical abuse; overwork and/or too heavy an investment in one's work; lack of sleep and exercise; failure to treat medical problems; and recurring mental disorders. Obviously, the list could go on and on.

APPLICATION TO THE FIVE CLINICAL CASES

I have tried to apply what this chapter has revealed about the relationship of nonfatal suicide attempts and completed suicide to the five clinical cases discussed throughout this book (see Table 17.12). Problems immediately arise with such an attempt, however. Most obviously, none of the cases (with the possible exception of John Z) made explicit suicide attempts. Four of the cases did have suicidal ideation, but then so does about 24% of the general population at some time in their lives (Linehan & Laffaw, 1982). The suicide methods planned by the individual cases are more useful. We know that Ralph F contemplated jumping, that John considered hanging, and that José G had a gun and was formerly a hunter. Of course, all of these methods are highly lethal. We also know that Ralph and John both had

TABLE 17.12. Application of Suicide Attempt Data to the Five Clinical Cases

Suicide attempt and related data	Heather B	Ralph F	John Z	Faye C	José G
1. Suicide attempt	?	No	Yes	No	No
2. Number of attempts	—	—	2?	—	—
3. Method/plan	Cutting	JUMPING	Plastic bag, HANGING	—	Had gun
4. Suicide note	—	—	—	—	—
5. Suicide or attempt in family	—	YES	Yes (sister)	—	—
6. Suicide ideas	YES	YES	Yes	Yes	—
7. Time after attempt	—	—	—	—	—
8. Sex	Female	Male	Male	Female	Male
9. Age	13	16	39	49	64
10. Race	White	White	White	White	Hispanic
11. Marital status	Single	Single	Married	SINGLE	Married
12. Employment	Student	Student	LAID OFF	Public health	OUT OF WORK
13. Physical illness	—	Yes	—	Yes	YES
14. Medical care	—	Yes	—	—	Yes
15. Mental disorder (esp. depression)	Yes	Yes	YES (depression)	YES (psychosis)	Yes (depression)
16. Psychiatric or psychological care	Yes	Yes	Yes	Yes	Yes
17. Angry, irritable	Yes	Yes	—	—	Yes
18. Hopelessness	—	Yes	—	—	Yes
19. Insomnia	No	Yes	Yes	Yes	Yes
20. Alcoholism	—	YES	—	—	Yes
21. Drug abuse	No?	Yes	—	—	Yes
22. Social isolation (living arrangement)	Yes (but family present)	No	No	Yes	Yes
23. Season	—	—	—	—	—

Note. Items in capital letters indicate particularly salient factors in each case.

histories of suicide or suicide attempts in their families. Heather B's suicide ideation was less lethal, since she claimed only to have "cut her arm." So, on the basis of explicit suicide attempts and related data (items 1 to 7 in Table 17.12), I would be most concerned that Ralph, John, and José might eventually commit suicide. Notice, too, how many cells in Table 17.12 are either blank or uncertain. Much of the information we need to predict suicide simply is not available. Often it is not even collected or considered by clinicians.

In our five cases, suicide attempt data by themselves are not very helpful in trying to predict who the eventual suicides might be. What if we were to add consideration of other predictor variables (viz., 8 to 23 in Table 17.12), crude as they may be? It has been argued throughout this volume that suicide prediction and assessment are issues of comorbidity and interaction; they should be based on single-variable predictors. On the basis of factors 8 to 23, Ralph and José would continue to appear very suicidal. In both cases, numerous other variables known to be associated with completed suicide were involved. Although Ralph was young, he had a major problem with alcohol abuse. As for José, not only was he an older male, but he had also lost a long-time job with little hope of recovering it or even the ability to work again; furthermore, he had several nagging physical illnesses.

The cases of John and Faye also show some cause for concern of eventual suicide. John had been laid off and was unable to keep his home or support his family; he was very depressed as well. On the basis of the suicide attempt data alone, Faye would not appear to be very suicidal. However, she also had psychotic-like symptoms (including feelings of depersonalization) and was single and lived alone. Although she was a female, Faye was in the maximum age range for female suicides. In contrast to the other cases, Heather would continue to have low apparent suicide lethality, when we examine other factors. For example, she was a young female; she had few if any vegetative depressive symptoms (e.g., she was sleeping and eating well); she had a supportive and concerned family; and even though she was quite agitated, most of her complaints seemed to derive from rather routine adolescent life transition situational reactions. Furthermore, none of Heather's clinical symptoms seemed to be florid or extreme. On the basis of the data examined in this chapter, I would rank the suicide potential of the five cases (from high to low) as follows: (1) José, (2) Ralph, (3) John, (4) Faye, and (5) Heather. All of the cases except Heather could easily be eventual completed suicides.

REFERENCES

Arango, V., Ernsberger, P., Marzuk, P. M., Chen, J.-S., Tierney, H., Stanley, M., Reis, D. J., & Mann, J. J. (1990). Autoradiographic demonstration of increased serotonin 5-HT$_2$ and beta-adrenergic receptor binding sites in the brain of suicide victims. *Archives of General Psychiatry, 47*(11), 1038-1048.

Asberg, M., Traskman, L., & Thoren, P. (1976). 5-HIAA in the cerebrospinal fluid: A biochemical suicide predictor? *Archives of General Psychiatry, 33*, 1193-1197.

Ballenger, J., Goodwin, F., Major, L., & Brown, G. (1979). Alcohol and central serotonin metabolism in man. *Archives of General Psychiatry, 36*, 224-227.

Barnes, R. A. (1986). The recurrent self-harm patient. *Suicide and Life-Threatening Behavior, 16*(4), 399-408.

Beck, A. T., Steer, R. A., Kovacs, M., & Garrison, B. (1985). Hopelessness and eventual suicide: A 10 year prospective study of patients hospitalized with suicidal ideation. *American Journal of Psychiatry, 142*(5), 559-563.

Clark, D. C., Gibbons, R. D., Fawcett, J., & Sheftner, W. A. (1989). What is the mechanism by which suicide attempts predispose to later suicide attempts? *Journal of Abnormal Psychology, 98*(1), 42-49.

Cullberg, J., Wasserman, D., & Stefansson, C. G. (1988). Who commits suicide after a suicide attempt? *Acta Psychiatrica Scandinavica, 77*, 598-603.

Dahlgren, K. G. (1977). Attempted suicides: 35 years afterwards. *Suicide and Life-Threatening Behavior, 7*(2), 75-79.

Farberow, N. L. (Ed.). (1980). *The many faces of suicide: Indirect self-destructive behavior.* New York: McGraw-Hill.

Favazza, A. R. (1989). Why patients mutilate themselves. *Hospital and Community Psychiatry, 40*(2), 137-145.

Greer, S., & Lee, H. A. (1967). Subsequent progress of potentially lethal suicide attempts. *Acta Psychiatrica Scandinavica, 43*, 361-371.

Hassanyeh, F., O'Brien, G., Holton, A. R., Hurren, K., & Watt, L. (1989). Repeat self-harm: An 18 month follow-up. *Acta Psychiatrica Scandinavica, 79*, 265-267.

Kaplan, A. G., & Klein, R. B. (1989). Women and suicide. In D. Jacobs & H. N. Brown (Eds.), *Suicide: Understanding and responding* (pp. 257-284). Madison, CT: International Universities Press.

Linehan, M. M., & Laffaw, J. A. (1982). Suicidal behaviors among clients of an outpatient psychology clinic versus the general population. *Suicide and Life-Threatening Behavior, 12*(4), 234-239.

Lönnqvist, J., Niskanen, P., Achte, K. A., & Ginman, L. (1975). Self-poisoning with follow-up considerations. *Suicide and Life-Threatening Behavior, 5*(1), 39-46.

Maris, R. W. (1981). *Pathways to suicide: A survey of self-destructive behaviors.* Baltimore: Johns Hopkins University Press.

Maris, R. W. (1982). Rational suicide. *Suicide and Life-Threatening Behavior, 12*(1), 3-16.

McIntosh, J. L., & Jewell, B. L. (1986). Sex difference trends in completed suicide. *Suicide and Life-Threatening Behavior, 16*(1), 16-27.

Motto, J. A. (1965). Suicide attempts: A longitudinal view. *Archives of General Psychiatry, 13*, 516-520.

National Center for Health Statistics. (1990). *Vital statistics of the United States, 1987: Vol. 2. Mortality* (Part A). Washington, DC.: U.S. Government Printing Office.

Paarregaard, G. (1975). Suicide among attempted suicides: A 10 year follow-up. *Suicide and Life-Threatening Behavior, 5*(3), 140-144.

Pokorny, A. D. (1965, May). *A follow-up study of 618 suicidal patients.* Paper presented at the annual meeting of the American Psychiatric Association, New York.

Retterstol, N. (1974). The future fate of suicide attempters. *Suicide and Life-Threatening Behavior, 4*(4), 203–211.

Roy, A., & Linnoila, M. (1986). Alcoholism and suicide. In R. Maris (Ed.), *Biology of suicide* (pp. 162–191). New York: Guilford Press.

Roy, A., & Linnoila, M. (1990). Monoamines and suicidal behavior. In H. M. Van Praag, R. Plutchik, & A. Apter (Eds.), *Violence and suicidology: Perspectives in clinical and psychological research* (pp. 141–183). New York: Brunner/ Mazel.

Rosen, D. H. (1970). The serious suicide attempt. *American Journal of Psychiatry, 127*(6), 764–770.

Tuckman, J., & Youngman, W. F. (1968). Assessment of suicide risk in attempted suicides. In H. L. P. Resnik (Ed.), *Suicidal behaviors: Diagnosis and management* (pp. 190–197). Boston: Little, Brown.

Wang, A. G. (1985). Attempted suicide in Denmark: Assessment of repeated suicidal behavior. *Acta Psychiatrica Scandinavica, 72,* 389–394.

Weisman, A., & Worden, W. J. (1974). Risk–rescue rating in suicide assessment. In A. T. Beck, H. L. P. Resnik, & D. J. Lettieri (Eds.), *The prediction of suicide* (pp. 193–213). Bowie, MD: Charles Press.

CHAPTER 18

Methods of Suicide

John L. McIntosh, Ph.D.
Indiana University at South Bend

The method that an individual chooses for suicide is influenced by a number of factors and has a major impact on the likelihood of a fatal outcome. Demographic characteristics of those who perform suicidal actions have also been observed to be associated with the choice of specific methods of suicide. This chapter reviews the literature on suicide methods and their lethality, and also presents current U.S. demographic data on the subject.

LETHALITY

Methods employed in suicide vary widely in their dangerousness and likelihood of resulting in death—that is, in their lethality. "Lethality" may refer either to the present risk of death by the method chosen or to the future risk of death by suicide conveyed by a present action. In this chapter, the term "lethality" is most often used to refer to the probability or likelihood of death. This reflects the prevalent use of the word in the suicide literature as well (e.g., Smith, Conroy, & Ehler, 1984). However, it should be noted that methods chosen in nonfatal suicide acts may have clinical implications for future risk of death by suicide (e.g., Card, 1974; Pallis & Barraclough, 1977–1978), and this literature is briefly discussed here as well.

Card (1974) studied completed suicides in a Pennsylvania county during a 5-year period, as well as attempts in the same county during 2 years. He calculated the probability of death for each method by dividing the number of deaths in which the method was employed by the total number of "incidents" (attempts and completions) using the method. This resulted in the following order of methods by lethality (from most to least lethal): gunshot, carbon monoxide, hanging, drowning, plastic bag over head, impact, fire, poison, drugs, gas, cutting. Card emphasized, however, "that this ordering does not mean that the less lethal methods . . . cannot or do not kill or seriously injure.

All we can conclude from our lethality rankings of the methods is that, statistically speaking, the less lethal methods do not result in as many deaths, proportionately speaking, as the more lethal methods" (p. 41).

Card also obtained a measure of the probability of death by suicide in the future among attempted suicides. He termed this the "risk" of suicide and determined this risk for each method listed above. The likelihood of attempters' committing suicide in the future varied from most to least in the following order of their original attempt methods: plastic bag over head, carbon monoxide, drowning, gas, poison, gunshot, impact, cutting, drugs, hanging, and fire. The different rank orderings and other data analyses led Card to argue that "lethality" and "risk" are two distinct concepts. Others have scrutinized and questioned these data, but agree that a suicide attempt of serious lethality is generally associated with increased future suicide likelihood (for a general discussion of this issue, see Maris, Chapter 17, this volume). The description of the case of John Z (see Berman, Chapter 12) contains reports of two separate attempts (by placing a plastic bag over his head and later by hanging). Although the authenticity of these reports could not be verified, the first attempt would be associated with a high suicide risk rating, according to Card's findings.

Smith et al. (1984) constructed a Lethality of Suicide Attempt Rating Scale. This scale was developed to provide a reliable measure of the seriousness of a suicide attempt (either past or present), as well as a measure that could be administered by a wide range of mental health and other personnel. This scale may be useful to clinicians in more accurately determining the event in a treatment context. The excellent discussion of this instrument includes tables of drugs and their lethal range; definitions of the 11 rating scale points are also provided, with examples of methods potentially seen at each point. These examples include cutting and ingestion at each of the 11 points and clearly show that lethality is not exclusively determined by a general category of method (e.g., drugs) alone. At the same time, the methods suggested as most likely to end in death by Card (1974) occur predominantly above the "equivocal" level of 5.0, where death becomes probable to almost certain.

At least two general factors contribute to the likelihood of death by a particular method. Suicide methods for which the time between the initiation of a suicidal act and death is greater will probably be lower in lethality. These methods, especially drugs and poisons, allow for the possibility of detection and intervention, as well as of changing one's mind and seeking help (Weisman & Worden, 1986). Another related factor in lethality is the potential for and availability of medical intervention related to that method. The possibility that medical professionals can save the life of a suicide attempter is generally far greater if the attempter has taken drugs or lost blood through cutting than if the individual has used a firearm, jumped from a height, suffocated, hanged, or drowned.

In brief, therefore, it would seem that the lethality of suicide methods, from a probability-of-death perspective, can be determined. In the case of nonfatal suicide attempts, this information, when coupled with other clinical information, may have immediate implications for treatment and assessment; it may also have useful implications for future suicide risk.

FACTORS AFFECTING METHOD CHOICE

A number of factors may influence an individual's decision regarding method in a suicidal act. The availability of a method is among such factors. Ready access to a method (e.g., drugs, poisons, firearms, etc.) and/or familiarity with it may increase the likelihood that it will be chosen in suicide. One aspect of familiarity with a method is one's expectations regarding the method. Lester (1988b) asked college students which method of suicide they would choose. Factors such as painlessness, availability, and nondisfigurement appealed to those choosing drug overdose, whereas the students selecting guns cited the quickness of this method.

The intent and motivation of the suicidal individual may also determine the method selected. For example, Fox and Weissman (1975) studied 258 suicide attempters and compared those who had used pill ingestion to those who had used violent methods (shooting, jumping, wrist cutting). Among those ingesting pills, the suicide attempt was found to be more impulsive, the attempters' intention of actually killing themselves was low, and the act was more often motivated so as to obtain attention from others. On the other hand, the actions of the violent attempters were more carefully planned, their intent to die was higher, and their motivation centered upon self-directed hostility. Thus, the methods chosen by these individuals appeared to depend at least partially on the level of their intention to die and on the effect they desired.

Sites associated with suicides may also enter into the choice of method. For example, Seiden and Spence (1983-1984) discuss the suggestion and psychological/symbolic elements associated with the Golden Gate Bridge in San Francisco. Other landmarks or publicized sites may likewise influence local decisions regarding suicide methods.

Gender has been found to be a major demographic factor in the choice of suicide methods (e.g., Evans & Farberow, 1988, p. 200). As will be shown below with current demographic data, females have traditionally utilized less lethal methods (especially solid and liquid poisons) in their suicides and nonfatal attempts in much higher proportions than have males. Males have employed more lethal methods (especially firearms) as their major methods of suicide and in substantially higher proportions than have women. In recent times, however, there has been an increase in the use of firearms among both sexes (and nearly all demographic groups; see, e.g.,

McIntosh & Santos, 1982, 1985–1986; see also Boor, 1981; Boyd, 1983; Markush & Bartolucci, 1984). Even when the increases in firearms are taken into account, however, both the greater use of solid and liquid poisons among women and the more frequent choice of firearms among men remain.

The sex differences in suicide method choice have been attributed to several differential aspects of socialization. Lester (1972, 1988b) has observed that women choose less lethal methods of suicide, especially drugs, to avoid disfigurement. In other words, society has taught women to have a greater concern for bodily appearance, and this may even prevail in their consideration of how they will look in death. The less violent, less lethal methods are generally associated with less disfigurement, whereas firearms and hanging in particular are not.

Seiden (1977) suggested that women in general have a weaker intent to die than do men and that the "upbringing and differing cultural expectations" for the sexes are factors. Marks (1977) argues that the sociocultural perspective best explains sex differences in method choice. Marks, as Lester (1988b) did, asked college students about the acceptability of nine methods of suicide. Students were also asked which method was most often used by members of their own sex and why. Marks found that drugs/poison were most "acceptable" to both sexes (more so to females than to males); firearms were acceptable to a lesser degree to more than half the males, but only about one-third of females. Females associated drugs/poison with their gender, citing their painlessness, ease of use, accessibility, availability, familiarity, and lack of messiness. Males associated masculinity with firearms as a means of destruction, and in choosing firearms mentioned their quickness, ease of use, efficiency, accessibility, availability, and familiarity.

Age is another demographic variable that has been associated with suicide method differences. It has been suggested that older adults use more lethal methods of suicide (e.g., Jarvis & Boldt, 1980). We (McIntosh & Santos, 1985–1986) compiled U.S. suicide data by age for 1960–1978 and found that among completed suicides there was confirming evidence for the use of more lethal methods (firearms and hanging) among white males and blacks of both sexes, but not among white females. Firearm use increased for all groups over the time of study, but among white females the young clearly utilized lethal methods most often, whereas the old used the two methods comparably. The major difference was attributable to the use of firearms. White females under 30 utilized firearms at levels comparable to poisons, whereas a lower proportion of those under 55 used firearms and only a small proportion did so at age 65 and above (hanging was low for all age groups). It may be speculated that the variation in white females' firearm use by age is due to a cohort difference. Older adult females were socialized to view firearm use as masculine and poisons as feminine, to perhaps a greater degree than middle-aged females and a much greater degree than young females. The increases in female firearm use, therefore, have been observed in the young groups and not among the elderly. As this cohort of elderly women is "replaced" by these now younger cohorts of women with different socialization backgrounds, we might expect the choice in methods to resemble the pattern found overall for the young and for white males and blacks of both sexes. It should be noted that elderly black females, like males of both races, used lethal methods (predominantly firearms) at high and increasing levels throughout the time period of study.

Even for less lethal methods such as poisoning, however, there are significant age differences. A recent study (Woolf, Fish, Azzara, & Dean, 1990) of older adults who died from serious poisoning in Massachusetts (suicide/intentional poisonings represented 82 of 152 deaths) found that older adults were more likely than the young to die from poisoning-related deaths. Higher and increased rates for poisoning suicides among the old were also observed by Sims (1974) for Canada from 1950 to 1969.

Explanations for age-related differences in suicide methods include (1) greater intent to die among the old as compared to the young, which is reflected in the choice of more lethal methods (e.g., McIntosh, Hubbard, & Santos, 1981); (2) ready availability of large quantities of drugs to be used in overdose by older adults, because of increased physical health problems and depression (e.g., Woolf et al., 1990); and (3) socialization and historically produced experiences, among the current cohort of elderly men at least (e.g., military and rural backgrounds in larger proportions), that would increase familiarity with firearms. Furthermore, the old seem more likely to die than the young following suicide attempts by any methods, because of general physical decline, poorer recuperative powers (McIntosh et al., 1981), greater vulnerability to the toxic effects of drugs (Woolf et al., 1990), and greater social isolation and living alone (which decreases the likelihood of detection and potential intervention with methods where this is applicable).

Few studies have focused on racial or ethnic differences in suicide methods. In addition to the study (McIntosh & Santos, 1985–1986) noted above, we (McIntosh & Santos, 1982) presented U.S. national data from 1923 to 1978 for specific ethnic groups. For all ethnic groups, it was generally observed that firearm use increased whereas poisons declined. Among all ethnic groups with the exception of Chinese- and Japanese-Americans (i.e., among whites, blacks, and Native Americans), firearms were the method most often employed by the late 1970s by those of both sexes. The use of hanging was generally low, and solid and liquid poisons were utilized in higher proportions among females than males. Among both Japanese- and Chinese-American males and females, hanging was the method most often utilized in suicide, although it declined over time while firearm use increased.

A final factor to be considered in the choice of suicide methods is the geographic and sociocultural environment of the individual. Marks and colleagues (Marks & Abernathy, 1974; Marks & Stokes, 1976) have suggested that, like socialization with respect to sex (as discussed above), geographic region of residence/origin may also predispose individuals toward certain suicide method choices via transmitted values and practices. This argument is applied more specifically to the choice of firearms in suicide. Investigating U.S. regional differences from 1940 to 1965, Marks and colleagues found that in all regions males preferred firearms, and with the exception of Southern women all women preferred poisoning. Southern women, like Southern men, preferred firearms. They concluded that a part of the "Southern" experience includes the acceptability, familiarity, and availability of firearms. Peterson, Peterson, O'Shanick, and Swann (1985) applied similar reasoning with respect to native Texan self-inflicted gunshot wounds treated at a trauma center. Consistent with this reasoning, my colleagues and I (Osgood, McIntosh, & Covey, 1989) found higher proportionate use of firearms among both elderly males and females in Virginia, compared to the elderly in the nation as a whole. Taylor and Wicks (1980) contend that the location of an individual within his or her social structure is relevant for the selection of suicide methods, and that a simple regional socialization explanation such as Marks and colleagues suggest is inadequate.

In a related note, Doerner (1983) has suggested that the high homicide rate in the South may not be interpretable as a "regional culture of violence," but as a lack of medical resources. In other words, it may not be "Southernness" that produces high homicide rates with gunshot wounds, but rather the fact that Southern states generally have less access to and less adequate medical resources, which are "a critical intervening factor in the production of homicide rates" (p. 1). By the same reasoning, if this is a factor in firearm homicides in the South, it is quite likely a partial explanation for the firearm suicide rates as well.

Farmer and Rohde (1980) suggest that the low utilization of hanging in many cultures seems to have at least two possible components: Either the rates are low for all methods, or hanging is found repulsive by the populace because of its association with capital punishment within that culture. Hanging then is seen as a dishonorable death in such cultures (e.g., England) and therefore is not as often considered acceptable for suicide. On the other hand, in cultures or subcultures where social customs and socialization differ in this regard, the use of hanging as a method may be high. For example, as noted above, hanging is common as a method of suicide among Asian-Americans and in several Asian cultures (e.g., McIntosh & Santos, 1982).

DEMOGRAPHY OF METHODS OF SUICIDE

Attempted Suicide/Parasuicide

The literature on attempted suicide is extremely consistent in its observation that poisoning accounts for as much as 90% of all nonfatal suicide attempts. Among other methods, self-cutting usually ranks after poisoning and is most often characteristic of younger individuals. The potentially more lethal methods, such as shooting, drowning attempts, and jumping from heights, are generally employed by older adults (e.g., Hawton & Catalan, 1982; Kreitman, 1977; Weissman, 1974; Wexler, Weissman, & Kasl, 1978).

Completed Suicide

The National Center for Health Statistics compiles (in annual volumes of *Vital Statistics of the United States*) official mortality data for the United States. Included in these figures are data for suicide deaths by method. To provide current data for suicide methods, the 3-year average figures for 1985–1987 (National Center for Health Statistics, 1988a, 1988b, 1988c, 1988d, 1989, 1990) are presented here. Official data have frequently been criticized as biased (e.g., Lester, 1972, Chapter 1), but the bias may not be as great as suggested (e.g., Sainsbury & Jenkins, 1982). Farmer and Rohde (1980, especially pp. 442-443) discuss difficulties with respect to specific suicide methods. These problems make it likely that certification of death by methods such as poisoning or drowning may be less reliable and more often misclassified than suicides by firearms or hanging. Therefore, official mortality data may be considered the most conservative estimate of actual figures (e.g., Allen, 1984).

As can be seen in Table 18.1, the utilization of suicide methods in the United States by sex is generally as reported earlier in the literature (e.g., McIntosh & Santos, 1982, 1985-1986). Firearms accounted for more than half of all suicide deaths for 1985-1987. Hanging, strangulation, and suffocation ranked a distant second, with solid and liquid poisons and gas poisoning close behind. These four categories accounted for all but 7% of suicides in this time period. For males compared to the nation as a whole, firearms were utilized in even higher proportions and hanging was again a distant second, while gas poisoning and solid and liquid poisoning each accounted for fewer than 10% of suicides. Although firearms ranked first for females as well, the gap between firearms and solid and liquid poisons was small by comparison with the male first-to-second gap. Gas poisoning and hanging each accounted for 12% of female suicides.

With respect to age, the 1985-1987 data (see Table 18.2) showed higher use of firearms by the old than by other groups, especially among males (see Table 18.3), as reported elsewhere (McIntosh & Santos, 1985-1986). The utilization of firearms decreased in proportion for females, as has also been noted in the literature. However, even among females in older adulthood, the higher choice of firearms in suicide is readily apparent—a striking change from earlier reports.

The available information regarding race/ethnicity also provides support for earlier data compilations (McIntosh & Santos, 1982), with few exceptions (see Table 18.4). All groups, with the exception of Japanese- and

TABLE 18.1. Methods of Suicide in the United States by Sex, 1985–1987

Method	Both sexes combined			Males			Females		
	No. of suicides	% of total	Mean rate	No. of suicides	% of total	Mean rate	No. of suicides	% of total	Mean rate
All methods	91,153	100.00	12.6	71,643	100.00	20.3	19,510	100.00	5.3
Firearms[a]	53,652	58.86	7.4	45,866	64.02	13.0	7,786	39.91	2.1
Hanging[b]	13,105	14.38	1.8	10,771	15.03	3.1	2,334	11.96	0.6
Solid and liquid poisons	9,113	10.00	1.3	4,087	5.70	1.2	5,026	25.76	1.4
Gas poisoning	8,948	9.82	1.2	6,538	9.13	1.9	2,410	12.35	0.6
All other methods	6,335	6.95	0.9	4,381	6.12	1.2	1,954	10.02	0.5

Note. Mean suicide rates for the 3-year period 1985–1987 employed population estimates for the midpoint year 1986, published in U.S. Bureau of the Census (1988). The other suicide data are from National Center for Health Statistics (1988a, 1988b, 1988c, 1988d, 1989, 1990). Some advance data for 1987 were provided by the National Center for Health Statistics prior to their appearance in *Vital Statistics of the United States, 1987.*
[a]"Firearms" refers to the category "Firearms and explosives" in all tables.
[b]"Hanging" refers to the category "Hanging, strangulation, and suffocation" in all tables.

TABLE 18.2. Methods of Suicide in the United States by Age Groupings, 1985–1987

Method	15–24			25–44			45–64			65+		
	No. of suicides	% of total	Mean rate	No. of suicides	% of total	Mean rate	No. of suicides	% of total	Mean rate	No. of suicides	% of total	Mean rate
All methods	15,165	100.00	13.0	34,513	100.00	15.2	22,132	100.00	16.4	18,527	100.00	21.2
Firearms	9,100	60.00	7.8	18,671	54.10	8.2	13,190	59.60	9.8	12,250	66.10	14.0
Hanging	2,878	18.98	2.5	5,157	14.94	2.3	2,457	11.10	1.8	2,332	12.59	2.0
Solid and liquid poisons	973	6.42	0.8	4,194	12.15	1.8	2,578	11.65	1.9	1,318	7.11	1.5
Gas poisoning	1,398	9.22	1.2	4,032	11.68	1.8	2,317	10.47	1.7	1,186	6.40	1.0
All other methods	816	5.38	0.7	2,459	7.12	1.1	1,590	7.18	1.2	1,441	7.78	1.6

Note. The data are from U.S. Bureau of the Census (1988) and National Center for Health Statistics (1988a, 1988b, 1988c, 1988d, 1989, 1990) (see Table 18.1 footnote for details).

TABLE 18.3. Methods of Suicide in the United States by Age and Sex Groupings, 1985–1987

Method	15–24		25–44		45–64		65+	
	No. of suicides	% of total	No. of suicides	% of total	No. of suicides	% of total	No. of suicides	% of total
Males								
All methods	12,652	100.00	27,054	100.00	16,332	100.00	14,973	100.00
Firearms	7,856	62.09	15,562	57.52	10,987	67.27	11,104	74.16
Hanging	2,567	20.29	4,443	16.42	1,856	11.36	1,669	11.15
Solid and liquid poisons	491	3.88	2,158	7.98	963	5.90	460	3.07
Gas poisoning	1,092	8.63	3,064	11.33	1,545	9.46	831	5.55
All other methods	646	5.11	1,827	6.75	981	6.00	909	6.07
Females								
All methods	2,513	100.00	7,459	100,00	5,800	100.00	3,554	100.00
Firearms	1,244	49.50	3,109	41.68	2,203	37.98	1,146	32.25
Hanging	311	12.38	714	9.57	601	10.36	663	18.66
Solid and liquid poisons	482	19.18	2,036	27.30	1,615	27.84	858	24.14
Gas poisoning	306	12.18	968	12.98	772	13.31	355	9.99
All other methods	170	6.76	632	8.47	609	10.50	532	14.97

Note. The data are from National Center for Health Statistics (1988a, 1988b, 1988c, 1988d, 1989, 1990).

TABLE 18.4. Methods of Suicide in the United States by Ethnicity and Sex, 1985–1987

Method	Both sexes		Males		Females	
	No. of suicides	% of total	No. of suicides	% of total	No. of suicides	% of total
Whites						
All methods	83,741	100.00	65,714	100.00	18,027	100.00
Firearms	49,709	59.36	42,487	64.65	7,222	40.06
Hanging	11,438	13.66	9,385	14.28	2,053	11.39
Solid and liquid poisons	8,465	10.11	3,783	5.76	4,682	25.97
Gas poisoning	8,726	10.42	6,363	9.68	2,363	13.11
All other methods	5,403	6.45	3,696	5.62	1,707	9.47
Blacks						
All methods	5,650	100.00	4,653	100.00	997	100.00
Firearms	3,256	57.63	2,802	60.22	454	45.54
Hanging	1,034	18.30	935	20.09	99	9.93
Solid and liquid poisons	474	8.39	229	4.92	245	24.57
Gas poisoning	164	2.90	137	2.94	27	2.71
All other methods	722	12.78	550	11.82	172	17.25
Native Americans ("Indian")						
All methods	653	100.00	539	100.00	114	100.00
Firearms	346	52.99	300	55.66	46	40.35
Hanging	203	31.09	184	34.14	19	16.67
Solid and liquid poisons	55	8.42	18	3.34	37	32.46
Gas poisoning	14	2.14	11	2.04	3	2.63
All other methods	35	5.36	26	4.82	9	7.89
Chinese-Americans						
All methods	213	100.00	116	100.00	97	100.00
Firearms	43	20.19	30	25.86	13	13.40
Hanging	96	45.07	40	34.48	56	57.73
Solid and liquid poisons	22	10.33	12	10.34	10	10.31
Gas poisoning	7	3.29	5	4.31	2	2.06
All other methods	45	21.13	29	25.00	16	16.49
Japanese-Americans						
All methods	216	100.00	131	100.00	85	100.00
Firearms	64	29.63	51	38.93	13	15.29
Hanging	88	40.74	47	35.88	41	48.24
Solid and liquid poisons	28	12.96	14	10.69	14	16.47
Gas poisoning	12	5.56	6	4.58	6	7.06
All other methods	24	11.11	13	9.92	11	12.94

Note. The data are from National Center for Health Statistics (1988a, 1988b, 1988c, 1988d, 1989, 1990).

Chinese-Americans employed firearms most frequently in their suicides (including white females). Among Japanese- and Chinese-Americans, the utilization of hanging as the most prominent method of suicide is a marked difference from all other ethnic groups for which there are data (national data are currently unavailable for Hispanics). The only exception to earlier national figures in this regard is the use of firearms and hanging in essentially equal proportions (but a slightly higher figure for firearms) among Japanese-American males.

EXPLANATIONS FOR TRENDS IN METHOD USE

The decline in deaths by poisons has been addressed by several authors. These explanations usually focus on females, who have traditionally employed poisons in their suicides and continue to utilize them in much higher proportions than do males. We (McIntosh & Santos, 1982) suggested that advances in medical technology over time have probably improved rescue effectiveness to such an extent that potentially fatal suicidal acts more often result in nonfatal attempts. The existence of trauma centers in most major urban areas probably also benefits those using methods such as poisoning most, because a greater possibility for survival generally exists. Hassan and Tan (1989) make the same suggestion with respect to overall declines in nonviolent suicide attempts in Australia (and rates among women) from 1901 to 1985. Similar statements are made by Becker et al. (1987) for self-poisoning individuals in Heidelberg, Germany.

Another explanation regarding declines in the utilization of less lethal methods of suicide has centered on the alternative choice of lethal methods. The reasoning is that individuals are committing suicide with highly lethal methods in greater numbers, rather than employing less lethal methods. That is, there is a displacement of method choice, rather than (or in addition to any) lessening in the deaths by less lethal methods (e.g., Clarke & Mayhew, 1989; Farmer & Rohde, 1980; Rich, Young, Fowler, Wagner, & Black, 1990). Although inadequate data have been presented to test this contention fully, there is some evidence that this does not entirely explain the declines for less lethal methods. Those who are rescued, are successfully treated, are prevented from committing suicide, or survive their attempt by one method do not inevitably or necessarily attempt or commit suicide by another method or in another location (e.g., Clarke & Mayhew, 1989; Lester, Fong, & D'Angelo, 1989; Peterson et al., 1985; Seiden, 1978). Interestingly, Card (1974) found that those who received *no* treatment following their suicidal acts had the highest subsequent suicide rate, whereas those who were treated in intensive care units had a relatively low suicide rate. The likelihood of referral for mental health treatment in these two instances may have influenced subsequent actions.

The decreased use of gas and carbon monoxide in suicide has also been discussed in the literature. The decrease in suicide in general and suicide by toxic domestic gas in particular since World War II in Britain has been well documented (e.g., Brown, 1979; Clarke & Mayhew, 1989; Farmer, 1979; Kreitman, 1976) and has been attributed to the detoxification of domestic gas. Similarly, declines in suicide by auto exhaust have been related to its detoxification (Clarke & Lester, 1987; Hays & Bornstein, 1984; Lester, 1989). Lester (1988b) has also suggested that in addition to the fact that auto exhaust now contains less carbon monoxide, suicide by auto exhaust requires "more technical skills (disconnection of the auto-emission control system) or a longer period of isolation so that the minute quantities of carbon monoxide can eventually cause death (which makes intervention by others more likely)" (p. 314).

The factors of medical technological advances and availability of medical resources have also been credited with saving the lives of more individuals who employ firearms than in the past (e.g., Peterson et al., 1985). More often, however, the increases associated with firearms—as has been discussed, and as trends demonstrate—have greatly overwhelmed any lessening effect produced by technological advances with respect to this method. Increases in American firearm use in general (Farmer & Rohde, 1980), by women (Frierson, 1989), and by children (Fingerhut & Kleinman, 1989) have been attributed to the nonrestrictive firearm legislation in the United States compared to most other Western nations, and the resultant wide availability of and increased familiarity with firearms.

From the viewpoint of prevention, the implication of nearly all these explanations is that we need to lessen the lethality of methods of suicide or to lessen the availability of highly lethal methods. This translates into measures such as careful prescribing of medications and coordination of prescriptions among physicians in the case of poisons, and erecting barriers for bridges or high places associated with suicide (e.g., Seiden, 1978). A large and growing literature in recent years recommends the restriction of firearms, the most commonly employed and lethal of suicide methods (e.g., Boor & Bair, 1990; Boyd, 1983; Clarke & Jones, 1989; Lester, 1988a; Lester & Murrell, 1982; Medoff & Magaddino, 1983; Sloan, Rivara, Reay, Ferris, & Kellermann, 1990).

In summary, methods of suicide vary greatly in their lethality. The use of firearms in U.S. suicides has increased, while the use of less lethal methods has generally decreased. The choice of methods is influenced by many personal and social factors that change with time. The differential lethality of suicide methods calls for attention to this aspect in present treatment, as well as in the assessment of future suicide risk. Additional research is needed to determine more precisely the effectiveness of restriction of methods in suicide prevention, as well as the role of suicide methods in the prediction of suicidal behavior.

REFERENCES

Allen, N. (1984). Suicide statistics. In C. L. Hatton & S. M. Valente (Eds.), *Suicide: Assessment and intervention* (2nd ed., pp. 17–31). Norwalk, CT: Appleton-Century-Crofts.

Becker, U., Bohme, K., Breitmaier, J., Drisch, D., Schaefer, D. O., Kulessa, C. H. E., & Wahl, P. (1987). Self-poisoning in Heidelberg, 1974–1980. *Crisis, 8*, 103–111.

Boor, M. (1981). Methods of suicide and implications for suicide prevention. *Journal of Clinical Psychology, 37*, 70–75.

Boor, M., & Bair, J. H. (1990). Suicide rates, handgun control laws, and sociodemographic variables. *Psychological Reports, 66*, 923–930.

Boyd, J. H. (1983). The increasing rate of suicide by firearms. *New England Journal of Medicine, 308*, 872–874.

Brown, J. H. (1979). Suicide in Britain: More attempts, fewer deaths, lessons for public policy. *Archives of General Psychiatry, 36*, 1119–1124.

Card, J. J. (1974). Lethality of suicidal methods and suicide risk: Two distinct concepts. *Omega, 5*, 37–45.

Clarke, R. V., & Jones, P. R. (1989). Suicide and increased availability of handguns in the United States. *Social Science and Medicine, 28*, 805–809.

Clarke, R. V., & Lester, D. (1987). Toxicity of car exhausts and opportunity for suicide. *Journal of Epidemiology and Community Health, 41*, 114–120.

Clarke, R. V., & Mayhew, P. (1989). Crime as opportunity: A note on domestic gas suicide in Britain and The Netherlands. *British Journal of Criminology, 29*, 35–46.

Doerner, W. G. (1983). Why does Johnny Reb die when shot? The impact of medical resources upon lethality. *Sociological Inquiry, 53*, 1–15.

Evans, G., & Farberow, N. L. (1988). *The encyclopedia of suicide.* New York: Facts on File.

Farmer, R., & Rohde, J. (1980). Effect of availability and acceptability of lethal instruments on suicide mortality. *Acta Psychiatrica Scandinavica, 62*, 436–446.

Farmer, R. D. T. (1979). Suicide by different methods. *Postgraduate Medical Journal, 55*, 775–779.

Fingerhut, L. A., & Kleinman, J. C. (1989). Firearm mortality among children and youth. *Advance Data from Vital and Health Statistics of the National Center for Health Statistics*, No. 178 (whole issue).

Fox, K., & Weissman, M. (1975). Suicide attempts and drugs: Contradiction between method and intent. *Social Psychiatry, 10*, 31–38.

Frierson, R. L. (1989). Women who shoot themselves. *Hospital and Community Psychiatry, 40*, 841–843.

Hassan, R., & Tan, G. (1989). Suicide trends in Australia, 1901–1985: An analysis of sex differentials. *Suicide and Life-Threatening Behavior, 19*, 362–380.

Hawton, K., & Catalan, J. (1982). *Attempted suicide: A practical guide to its nature and management.* New York: Oxford University Press.

Hays, P., & Bornstein, R. A. (1984). Failed suicide attempt by emission gas poisoning. *American Journal of Psychiatry, 141*, 592–593.

Jarvis, G. K., & Boldt, M. (1980). Suicide in later years. *Essence, 4*, 145–158.

Kreitman, N. (1976). The coal gas story: United Kingdom suicide rates, 1960–71. *British Journal of Preventative and Social Medicine, 30,* 86–93.

Kreitman, N. (1977). *Parasuicide.* New York: Wiley.

Lester, D. (1972). *Why do people kill themselves?: A summary of research findings on suicidal behavior.* Springfield, IL: Charles C Thomas.

Lester, D. (1988a). Research note: Gun control, gun ownership, and suicide prevention. *Suicide and Life-Threatening Behavior, 18,* 176–180.

Lester, D. (1988b). Why do people choose particular methods for suicide? *Activas Nervosa Superior, 30,* 312–314.

Lester, D. (1989). Changing rates of suicide by car exhaust in men and women in the United States after car exhaust was detoxified. *Crisis, 10,* 164–168.

Lester, D., Fong, C. A., & D'Angelo, A. A. (1989). Chronic suicide attempters who switch methods and those who do not. *Perceptual and Motor Skills, 69,* 1390.

Lester, D., & Murrell, M. E. (1982). The preventive effect of strict gun control laws on suicide and homicide. *Suicide and Life-Threatening Behavior, 12,* 131–140.

Marks, A. (1977). Sex differences and their effect upon cultural evaluations of methods of self-destruction. *Omega, 8,* 65–70.

Marks, A., & Abernathy, T. (1974). Toward a sociocultural perspective on means of self-destruction. *Life-Threatening Behavior, 4,* 3–17.

Marks, A., & Stokes, C. S. (1976). Socialization, firearms, and suicide. *Social Problems, 23,* 622–629.

Markush, R. E., & Bartolucci, A. A. (1984). Firearms and suicide in the United States. *American Journal of Public Health, 74,* 123–127.

McIntosh, J. L., Hubbard, R. W., & Santos, J. F. (1981). Suicide among the elderly: A review of issues with case examples. *Journal of Gerontological Social Work, 4,* 63–74.

McIntosh, J. L., & Santos, J. F. (1982). Changing patterns in methods of suicide by race and sex. *Suicide and Life-Threatening Behavior, 12,* 221–233.

McIntosh, J. L., & Santos, J. F. (1985–1986). Methods of suicide by age: Sex and race differences among the young and old. *International Journal of Aging and Human Development, 22,* 123–139.

Medoff, M. H., & Magaddino, J. P. (1983). Suicides and firearm control laws. *Evaluation Review, 7,* 357–372.

National Center for Health Statistics. (1988a). *Vital statistics of the United States, 1985: Vol. 2. Mortality* (DHHS Publication No. 88-1101, Part A). Washington, DC: U.S. Government Printing Office.

National Center for Health Statistics. (1988b). *Vital statistics of the United States, 1985: Vol. 2. Mortality* (DHHS Publication No. 88-1102, Part B). Washington, DC: U.S. Government Printing Office.

National Center for Health Statistics. (1988c). *Vital statistics of the United States, 1986: Vol. 2. Mortality* (DHHS Publication No. 88-1122, Part A). Washington, DC: U.S. Government Printing Office.

National Center for Health Statistics. (1988d). *Vital statistics of the United States, 1986: Vol. 2. Mortality* (DHHS Publication No. 88-1114, Part B). Washington, DC: U.S. Government Printing Office.

National Center for Health Statistics. (1989). *Vital statistics of the United States, 1987: Vol. 2. Mortality* (DHHS Publication No. 89-1102, Part B). Washington, DC: U.S. Government Printing Office.

National Center for Health Statistics. (1990). *Vital statistics of the United States, 1987: Vol. 2. Mortality* (DHHS Publication No. 90-1101, Part A). Washington, DC: U.S. Government Printing Office.

Osgood, N. J., McIntosh, J. L., & Covey, N. R. (1989). *A study of suicide among the elderly of Virginia* (Final report to the Virginia Department for the Aging). Richmond: Virginia Department for the Aging. (Summary of the report appears as House Document No. 32, *The problems of suicide and substance abuse by the elderly and the impact of family care giving on employee work performance.* Richmond: Commonwealth of Virginia.)

Pallis, D. J., & Barraclough, B. M. (1977-1978). Seriousness of suicide attempt and future risk of suicide: A comment on Card's paper. *Omega, 8,* 141-149.

Peterson, L. G., Peterson, M., O'Shanick, G. J., & Swann, A. (1985). Self-inflicted gunshot wounds: Lethality of method versus intent. *American Journal of Psychiatry, 142,* 228-231.

Rich, C. L., Young, J. G., Fowler, R. C., Wagner, J., & Black, N. A. (1990). Guns and suicide: Possible effects of some specific legislation. *American Journal of Psychiatry, 147,* 342-346.

Sainsbury, P., & Jenkins, J. S. (1982). The accuracy of officially reported suicide statistics for the purposes of epidemiological research. *Journal of Epidemiology and Community Health, 36,* 43-48.

Seiden, R. H. (1977). Suicide prevention: A public health/public policy approach. *Omega, 8,* 267-276.

Seiden, R. H. (1978). Where are they now? A follow-up study of suicide attempters from the Golden Gate Bridge. *Suicide and Life-Threatening Behavior, 8,* 203-216.

Seiden, R. H., & Spence, M. (1983-1984). A tale of two bridges: Comparative suicide incidence on the Golden Gate and San Francisco-Oakland Bay Bridges. *Omega, 14,* 201-209.

Sims, M. (1974). Sex and age differences in suicide rates in a Canadian province: With particular reference to suicides by means of poison. *Suicide and Life-Threatening Behavior, 4,* 139-159.

Sloan, J. H., Rivara, F. P., Reay, D. T., Ferris, J. A. J., & Kellermann, A. L. (1990). Firearm regulations and rates of suicide: A comparison of two metropolitan areas. *New England Journal of Medicine, 322,* 369-373.

Smith, K., Conroy, R. W., & Ehler, B. D. (1984). Lethality of suicide attempt rating scale. *Suicide and Life-Threatening Behavior, 14,* 215-242.

Taylor, M. C., & Wicks, J. W. (1980). The choice of weapons: A study of methods of suicide by sex, race, and region. *Suicide and Life-Threatening Behavior, 10,* 142-149.

U.S. Bureau of the Census. (1988). United States population estimates, by age, sex, and race: 1980 to 1987. *Current Population Reports,* Series P-25, No. 1022.

Weisman, M. D., & Worden, J. W. (1986). Risk-rescue rating in suicide assessment. In A. T. Beck, H. L. P. Resnik, & D. J. Lettieri (Eds.), *The prediction of suicide* (2nd ed., pp. 193-213). Philadelphia: Charles Press.

Weissman, M. M. (1974). The epidemiology of suicide attempts, 1960 to 1971. *Archives of General Psychiatry, 30,* 737–746.

Wexler, L., Weissman, M. M., & Kasl, S. V. (1978). Suicide attempts 1970–1975: Updating a United States study and comparisons with international trends. *British Journal of Psychiatry, 132,* 180–185.

Woolf, A., Fish, S., Azzara, C., & Dean, D. (1990). Serious poisonings among older adults: A study of hospitalization and mortality rates in Massachusetts 1983–85. *American Journal of Public Health, 80,* 867–869.

Isolation, Seclusion, and Psychosocial Vulnerability as Risk Factors for Suicide Behind Bars

Ronald L. Bonner, Psy.D.
Federal Correctional Institution, Schuylkill, Pennsylvania
Private Practice, Harrisburg/Selinsgrove, Pennsylvania

You asked me what my reasons for living were, Doc. I ain't got none. My old lady is shacked up with my partner. Never gonna see my kids again. I got 30 more years to do in this fuckin' hole. And I'm tired of all the bullshit. That's all it is, bullshit! Fuck it, who would care if I hung up anyway? (Therapy transcript with "Mickey," a suicidal inmate)

Over the past 20 years, the problem of suicide behind bars has been given increasing attention (e.g., Bonner & Rich, 1990a, 1990b; Danto, 1973; Irwin, 1970; Ogloff & Otto, 1989; Salive, Smith, & Brewer, 1989; Schimmel, Sullivan, & Mrad, 1988). Suicide is the leading cause of death of inmates in jail facilities (National Sheriffs' Association, 1985), and the suicide rate in jails has been estimated to be approximately nine times higher than that of the general population (Hayes & Rowan, 1988). Suicide in prisons has also been recognized as a major cause of death of inmates, and the prison suicide rate has been identified as several times higher than that of the general population (Salive et al., 1989). Prevalence rates of mental illness have long been recognized as disproportionately high among inmates, with estimates ranging from 16% to 66%, depending upon the type of facility (Gibbs, 1982; Ogloff & Otto, 1989; Teplin, 1983). The increasing attention has resulted in recent developments in risk identification research, correctional mental

The views expressed in this chapter represent those of the author and do not necessarily reflect the Federal Bureau of Prisons or the U.S. Department of Justice.

health care standards, and suicide prevention programs (Cox, Landsberg, & Pravati, 1989; O'Leary, 1989; Rowan & Hayes, 1988; Sovronsky & Shapiro, 1989). Significant progress has been made programmatically, and there is preliminary evidence of its impact on suicide rates (e.g., Cox et al., 1989; Schimmel et al., 1988).

The key to continued progress in suicide prevention behind bars is an empirical understanding of the *process* by which certain inmates become suicidal while incarcerated. The present chapter first presents a selected review of major research on suicide behind bars. Second, it is argued that a process-based, stress–vulnerability model of suicide, as advocated in the general suicidology literature, would provide increased understanding and added utility in theory, risk assessment, and prevention programming for corrections. Within this paradigm, the role of select risk factors is considered, including isolation, seclusion, and absence of psychosocial coping resources. Finally, with these considerations in mind, liability issues and health care standards are reviewed, together with implications for future research and clinical efforts in suicide prevention behind bars.

REVIEW OF MAJOR RESEARCH

Typically, the study of suicide behind bars has taken a retrospective, descriptive approach to the problem. Utilizing sociodemographic analysis and historical autopsy methodology, researchers have studied various sociodemographic, historical, and incidental characteristics associated with inmate populations of suicide victims. Through these efforts, investigators have attempted to construct "typical" profiles of common characteristics of suicide victims within correctional facilities.

Perhaps the most comprehensive examination within this research to date is the research conducted by the National Center for Institutions and Alternatives. In 1979, Lindsay Hayes and Barbara Kajdin, funded by the National Institute of Corrections, conducted a national survey of suicides in this country's jails and police lockups. Utilizing an in-depth questionnaire assessing various sociodemographic and historical factors associated with an inmate's suicide, they identified approximately 419 jail suicides in 1979 (Hayes & Kajdin, 1981). A number of key characteristics were identified in this population of victims. The majority of victims were white (67%) and under the age of 32 (75%); almost all were male (97%). The majority of victims were isolated in marital status (54% single, 15% separated/divorced). Most of the victims had been incarcerated for nonviolent offenses (over 73%), with a significant number arrested for drug or alcohol offenses. According to the jail administrators surveyed, approximately 60% of the suicide victims had been under the influence of drugs or alcohol at the time of their incarceration.

In addition, Hayes and Kajdin identified some significant characteristics about the suicide event itself. First, approximately 50% of the suicides occurred during the 9 P.M.–6 A.M. shift, when less staff supervision was available. Almost all (96%) of the victims completed suicide by hanging, usually with material from beds or clothing. A shocking finding was that over 50% of the victims completed suicide within the first 24 hours of incarceration; furthermore, two out of every three suicides (68%) occurred while the victims were held in isolation or seclusion (frequently known as "segregation," the "hole," the "drunk tank," or the "bullpen"). Paradoxically, the research team discovered that many of the victims had been placed in isolation or seclusion because they were considered abnormal, intoxicated, or in some cases suicidal upon booking.

On the basis of this research, Hayes and Kajdin (1981) constructed a hypothetical profile of the "typical" suicide victim in this country's jails:

> An inmate committing suicide in jail was most likely to be a 22 year old, white, single male. He would have been arrested for public intoxication, the only offense leading to his arrest, and would presumably be under the influence of alcohol and/or drugs upon incarceration. Further, the victim would not have a significant history of prior arrests. He would have been taken to an urban county jail and immediately placed in isolation for his own protection and/or surveillance. However, [after] less than three hours of incarceration, the victim would be dead. He would have hanged himself from material from his bed (such as a sheet or pillowcase). The incident would have taken place on a Saturday night in September, between the hours of midnight and 5 A.M.. Jail staff would have found the victim, they say, within 15 minutes of the hanging. Later, jail records would indicate [that] the victim did not have a history of mental illness or previous suicide attempt. (p. 58)

In 1985–1986, Hayes and Joseph Rowan replicated this national study to determine the stability and generalizability of these results. They found 453 jail suicides in 1985 and 401 such suicides in 1986 (Hayes & Rowan, 1988). Through statistical projection, these investigators estimated the annual suicide rate in U.S. jails to be approximately 107 inmates per 100,000— that is, approximately nine times higher than the rate in the general population. Most interesting, despite the 6- to 7-year gap between the original research and the replication, the various sociodemographics of the suicide victims remained relatively constant, as outlined in Table 19.1. Again, the majority of victims were white, male, young, and single or divorced. The victims were generally arrested for nonviolent offenses and were intoxicated at the time of their arrest. Most of the suicides again took place by hanging within the first 24 hours of incarceration. Once again, the majority of the victims were housed in isolation or segregation at the time of their suicide. Again, the jail administrators surveyed suggested that many of the victims were placed in isolation for abnormal behavior; yet approximately 89% of

TABLE 19.1. Common Characteristics of Suicide Victims in U.S. Jails between 1985 and 1986

Characteristics	Jail suicide victims (%)
Sex	
Male	94.4
Female	5.6
Race	
White	71.6
Black	15.7
Other	12.7
Age	
17 or younger	3.6
18–22	16.2
23–27	26.5
28–32	21.0
33–37	15.0
38–42	8.7
43–47	3.3
48–53	3.3
54–older	2.4
Marital status	
Single	51.6
Married	27.6
Separated/divorced	16.9
Widowed	1.4
Common-law	2.5
Offense	
Property	19.9
Alcohol/drug	26.8
Minor other	28.6
Violent	24.7
Intoxication upon arrest	
Alcohol	43.8
Drugs	6.8
Alcohol/drugs	9.7
Neither	39.7
Length of incarceration before suicide	
0–3 hours	28.5
4–6 hours	9.3
7–9 hours	4.5
10–12 hours	2.1
13–18 hours	1.8
19–24 hours	5.2
25–48 hours	6.6
2–14 days	15.0
After 14 days	27.0
Prior suicide attempts	
Yes	15.9
No	84.1

(continued)

TABLE 19.1. (continued)

Characteristics	Jail suicide victims (%)
Prior mental illness	
Yes	19.3
No	80.7
Housed in isolation/segregation	
Yes	66.9
No	33.1

Note. Data from *National Study of Jail Suicides: Seven Years Later* by L. M. Hayes and J. R. Rowan, 1988, Alexandria, VA: National Center for Institutions and Alternatives. Copyright 1988 by the National Center for Institutions and alternatives. Adapted by permission.

the victims had not been specifically screened for suicide intention upon booking!

Several studies of local jail populations have reported relatively similar findings for suicide victims within jails. In an evaluation of jail suicides in Ohio, Hardyman (1983) found that most of the victims were white, young, and single. They had generally been arrested for nonviolent offenses, often drug- or alcohol-related. Most of the victims had died by hanging within the first 24 hours of incarceration. A study of police lockups in Massachusetts reported much the same results, with 74% of the victims having been intoxicated upon arrest and most of the suicides having occurred within the first 4 hours of incarceration (Special Commission to Investigate Suicide in Municipal Detention Centers, 1984). A recent study of Detroit's Wayne County Jail reported 36 suicides over a 20-year span (Burtka, DuRand, & Smith, 1988). Again, similar victim characteristics were found: All died by hanging, two-thirds of the suicides occurred during the night shift, most of the victims were either single or divorced, and approximately 90% of the victims were alone in isolated cells at the time of the suicide act.

In addition to these common characteristics for suicide victims within jails, some local studies have identified other potentially significant risk factors for suicide. Interestingly, many of these factors have also been identified in the general suicidology literature. Psychiatric disorder and a history of previous suicide attempts have been linked with certain jail suicide victims (Danto, 1973; Fawcett & Marrs, 1973). A study of suicides in New York State indicated that approximately 55% of the suicide victims had been hospitalized for psychiatric illness or emotional problems on at least one occasion (New York State Commission of Corrections, 1982). A recent literature review by Ivanoff (1989) noted that a significant number of studies found mood disturbances of depression, hopelessness, and anger in the histories of jail suicide victims. He also noted the prevalence of common suicide verbalization and gestures prior to the suicides, as well as common triggers of life stress and interpersonal loss. Diagnoses of mood disorder (including major depression and bipolar disorder) and schizophrenia have been cited in the histories of many suicide victims behind bars (Sherman & Morschauser, 1989).

Although research on nonfatal suicide attempts behind bars has unfortunately been scarce, two recent studies have shed light on risk factors in this area. LeBrun (1990), in studying the characteristics of male suicide attempters in the Sacramento County (California) jail, discovered that over 75% of the attempters had a psychiatric treatment history. Common diagnoses were major depression, bipolar disorder, and schizophrenia. Approximately 70% of the attempters had made suicide threats or verbalizations before their attempts, and they often had a history of previous suicidal behavior. Finally, it was determined that the suicide attempts were often precipitated by negative life events, such as relationship loss or legal conflicts. A study by Hopes (1986), utilizing a control group, found significant differences between inmate attempters and nonattempters on several variables. Attempters had significantly more histories of alcohol/drug abuse, suicidal ideation, hopelessness, previous suicide attempts, and intoxication upon booking than did nonattempter inmates.

Although research on suicide in jails has been given increasing attention, research on suicide in prisons has lagged behind. Whereas "jails" are generally short-term holding or presentencing facilities, "prisons" are long-term detention facilities where inmates who have been convicted serve out their sentences. Until recently, it has been assumed that suicide, although a problem for inmates in jails as they face the initial crisis of incarceration, is not a significant problem for inmates who advance to prison to serve out their time. This assumption, however, has not been supported. Suicides in prisons are disproportionately high (e.g., Salive et al., 1989), although they remain somewhat different from suicides in jails and are often triggered for different reasons.

In what is probably the most comprehensive suicide study of prisons to date, the Federal Bureau of Prisons conducted a retrospective analysis of suicides in federal prisons from 1983 to 1987, inclusive (Schimmel et al., 1988). Table 19.2 outlines some of the common characteristics of suicide victims in this study. In this 5-year period, 43 documented suicides were identified; this figure was extrapolated to an approximate annual rate of 24 suicides per 100,000 inmates. All of the victims were male, and most were older (i.e., 25 years or over). Race was generally distributed evenly: 16 suicides were committed by whites, 12 by blacks, and 15 by Hispanics (10 of the Hispanics were Mariel Cuban detainees). In contrast to the jail data, these victims represented three significant sentence clusters: 28% were serving sentences longer than 20 years, usually for a violent offense; 19% of the victims were Cuban detainees; and 19% of the victims were in the presentenc-

TABLE 19.2. Common Characteristics of Suicide Victims in U.S. Federal Prisons between 1983 and 1987

Characteristics	Prison suicide victims (%)
Sex	
Male	100
Female	0
Race	
White	37
Black	28
Hispanic	35
Age	
19–24	9
25–34	33
34–44	47
45–54	11
55–older	0
Sentence length	
Presentence	19
20 years +	28
Cuban detainees	19
Prior suicide attempts	
Yes	49
No	51
Prior mental illness	
Yes	45
No	55
Housed in isolation/segregation	
Yes	63
No	37

Note. Data from *Suicide Prevention Workgroup Report: A 1983–1987 Analysis* by D. Schimmel, J. Sullivan, and D. Mrad, 1988, Washington, DC: U.S. Department of Justice, Federal Bureau of Prisons.

ing cluster. Generally, the long-term offenders committed suicide after serving approximately 5 years of their sentence.

In regard to precipitant factors, these investigators were able to identify specific negative life events or stressors for each cluster of victims. In the group serving lengthy sentences, the victims generally had encountered severe problems within the institution, such as interpersonal conflict or being labeled a "snitch." For the presentencing group, both legal and family problems appeared to precipitate the suicides. Presumably for the Cuban detainees, the uncertain and seemingly hopeless future regarding deportation contributed to their desperation and suicidality. Approximately 45% of the suicide victims had documented histories of mental illness, including diagnoses of depression and psychosis. Approximately half (49%) of the victims had documented histories of previous suicide attempts. Similarities to the jail data were found in the circumstances of the suicides: The most popular method of suicide in federal prisons was by hanging (79%); a high percentage (48%) of the suicides occurred between midnight and 5 A.M., presumably when less staff supervision was available; and finally, once again, many of the victims (63%) were held in isolation or segregation at the time of the suicide act.

A more recent study in the Maryland state prison system (Salive et al., 1989) reported similar results. Through retrospective analysis of prison records, the investigators found that 37 male suicides occurred between the years of 1979 and 1987. Extrapolation generated an estimated annual suicide rate of 40 suicides per 100,000 inmates—a rate approximately three times higher than that of the general population. The following common characteristics of the suicide victims were identified: The majority of the victims were white, were between the ages of 25 and 34, were serving a life sentence in a maximum-security institution, and had committed suicide after serving approximately 4 years of the sentence by hanging. Unfortunately, data on psychiatric history, precipitant factors, and place of suicides were not reported.

To summarize the selected research, the following generalizations and distinctions can be made. First, suicide behind bars, in both jails and prisons, is a major problem. It is the leading cause of death of inmates in jails. The rates are significantly higher than that of the general population: The rate in jails is approximately nine times higher, and that in prisons is approximately two to three times higher. Second, it appears from sociodemogrpahic and historical retrospective analyses that suicides behind bars share a number of common characteristics, but that several distinctions can be made between jail and prison facilities. In jails, suicide victims are generally young, first-time offenders who have been arrested for minor offenses (often drug- or alcohol-related). Generally, these jail victims are single, separated, or divorced, and are usually intoxicated at the time of their arrest. They usually commit suicide within the first 24 hours of incarceration. In prisons, suicide victims are generally older, are serving long-term sentences for major offenses, and have histories of psychiatric illness and suicidal behavior. These prison victims generally commit suicide after several years of incarceration, and their actions are frequently precipitated by severe problems within the institution. Both jail and prison victims usually commit suicide by hanging between the hours of midnight and 5 A.M. Most significantly, most of the suicides in jail and prisons occur while the victims are held in isolation or seclusion (segregation). Furthermore, it is alarming to note that the jail research implies that many of the victims are placed in isolation for suspected abnormal behavior; yet they often are not screened specifically for suicidal intentions.

Given the current state of suicide research in corrections, it is possible to construct "typical" profiles of suicide victims. Common characteristics, including age, sex, marital status, criminal offense, psychiatric history, drug/alcohol abuse, method of suicide, and place of suicide, can be utilized to generate such a profile. This information obviously has been extremely important in identifying the problem of suicide behind bars, as well as in sensitizing correctional administrators and staff to inmates at risk. Such research has also provided useful information for suicide prevention efforts in corrections (Cox et al., 1989) and has had an impact on mental health care standards for jails and prisons (O'Leary, 1989).

In spite of these advancements, suicide research in corrections has been limited on several counts. First, the research has generally been retrospective and descriptive. The descriptors have been gathered after the fact (of suicide), and therefore their etiological and/or developmental role in the process of suicide is unclear. In addition, with very few exceptions, suicide research in corrections has not utilized a control group, so that it remains unclear whether the sociodemographic/historical descriptors actually differentiate inmates who do from inmates who do not commit suicide. The base rates for many of these descriptor characteristics are probably high for the inmate population in general; such variables, therefore, may be of limited utility in risk assessment and prediction (i.e., the statistical problem of false positives may be a factor). Finally, and perhaps most importantly, this research to date has narrowly conceptualized suicide as a static, isolated event and has associated it with other static factors (e.g., sociodemographics). Such an approach cannot explain or account for the *process* by which certain inmates, while incarcerated, eventually decide to end their lives at a given point in time within a particular life condition. To put the problem simply, the process by which certain inmates become suicidal within the context of a life condition behind bars has not been addressed. Such data would appear to be crucial for advancements in risk assessment technology and prevention programming efforts.

SUICIDE AS A PROCESS: A STRESS-VULNERABILITY MODEL

To turn to the general suicidology literature, a growing body of theory and research over the past decade suggests that suicide is best defined as a complex, biopsychosocial process that evolves over time and across life conditions (e.g., Beck, Kovacs, & Weissman, 1975, 1979; Bonner, 1990; Bonner & Rich, 1987, 1988a, 1988b, 1991; Braucht, 1979; Maris, 1981, 1986; Mikawa, 1973; Rich & Bonner, 1987a, 1991; Shneidman, 1985). In this view, suicide is not viewed simply as the act of self-inflicted death, but as a process by which certain maladaptive processes of an individual (transpiring at any or all system levels of biological, psychological, and sociocultural vulnerability), interacting with particular demands of environmental life conditions (e.g., negative life stress) over time, result in varying degrees of suicidal intention (i.e., ideation, contemplation, attempts, and completion), which ultimately may culminate in suicide. This process is generally viewed within a stress–coping paradigm: Certain individuals, as a result of varying vulnerabilities (or risk factors), are thought to be ill equipped to handle certain stressful life events, and over time may reach a psychological breaking point. At this breaking point, such vulnerable individuals are thought to be unable to see, generate, and/or effect viable coping responses, and therefore come to see suicide as perhaps the only viable option for dealing with intolerable life circumstances. Although varying vulnerabilities and stressful life conditions may affect suicide intention differently for each individual, the common psychological theme in the suicide process is a "hopeless" state of mind (Beck, Steer, Kovacs, & Garrison, 1985; Beck et al., 1975; Bonner & Rich, 1988b, 1991; Fawcett et al., 1987; Kashani, Reid, & Rosenberg, 1989; Minkoff, Bergman, & Beck, 1973). At this state, an individual loses all options for coping and resolving stressful life circumstances, and comes to view his or her future as only worsening. Suicide thus comes to be seen as the only way out of a desperate, hopeless condition.

To apply this process-based view to suicide behind bars, it becomes quite clear that incarceration is a very negative life condition that may overwhelm or exhaust one's coping repertoire (e.g., Bonner, 1987; Bonner & Rich, 1990, 1992; Hayes & Kajdin, 1981; Hayes & Rowan, 1988; Rowan & Hayes, 1988). Initially, incarceration may represent loss of freedom, loss of familial and social support, fear of the unknown, fear for one's safety, uncertainty and fear about one's future, embarrassment and guilt, and poor environmental conditions. In time, incarceration may bring about added stressors, such as loss of outside relationships, conflicts within the institution, victimization, further legal frustration, physical and emotional breakdown, and a wide variety of other problems in living. Coupled with such negative life stress, individuals with psychosocially vulnerabilities (including psychiatric illness, drug/alcohol intoxication, marital/social isolation, suicidal coping history, and deficiencies in problem-solving ability) may be unable to cope effectively and in time may become hopeless (e.g., Bonner & Rich, 1990; Schotte & Clum, 1982, 1987). Risk assessment and prevention programming in corrections, therefore, must be process-oriented, coping-focused, and systematically and methodically targeted toward an inmate's mental state, affective state, and psychosocial context (Bonner, 1990).

A plethora of research has implicated the powerful role of social isolation, loneliness, and interpersonal loss in negative stress reactions, psychological breakdown, and major depressive illness (e.g., Brown, 1979; Cohen & Willis, 1985; Henderson et al., 1978; Holahan & Moos, 1981; Lin, Ensel, Simeone, & Kuo, 1979; Rich & Bonner, 1987b, 1989; Swindle, Cronkite, &

Moos, 1989). Braucht (1979) has suggested that suicidal individuals lack important social supports and resources for effective coping with life stress and problems of living. By holding life stress constant, Braucht found that alienated and isolated individuals were at a significantly higher risk for suicide than were individuals with close family ties and strong social supports. Demographic/sociological research (e.g., Cazzuli, Invernizzi, & Vitalie, 1974/1977; Dublin, 1967; Maris, 1969; McCulloch & Phillip, 1973) has consistently found that people who lead isolated lives, devoid of contact with family, friends, and community, are most at risk for suicide. Moreover, significant interpersonal loss, loneliness, and isolation have been shown to exacerbate the effects of negative life stress and to heighten the risk for suicidal behavior (e.g., Bonner & Rich, 1988a, 1988b, 1991; Braucht, 1979; Giddens, 1971; Kreitman, 1977). Trout (1980). in an extensive review of the literature on loneliness and the social environment of suicidal individuals, concluded that "social isolation has a primary and direct role in suicide" (p. 19).

The function of social support in adaptive, coping behavior or the lack thereof has been viewed from several perspectives. Most recently, social support has been viewed as a form of protection or "buffering" from the negative effects of life stress. According to Lazarus and Folkman (1984), social support prevents negative stress reactions by making harmful or threatening life experiences seem less consequential. Furthermore, social support provides important resources for adaptive coping and problem solving when stress occurs (Cassel, 1976). Resources such as emotional support, social information and feedback, and tangible support have all been shown to help individuals solve and cope more effectively with life's problems and stressors (Schaefer, Coyne, & Lazarus, 1982). Consequently, lonely and isolated people appear to be at a heightened risk for maladaptive coping and negative stress reactions. In time, with repeated stress, lonely and isolated individuals may be apt to reach a psychological breaking point, to become hopeless, and ultimately to become suicidal (see also Yufit & Bongar, Chapter 27, this volume).

It has also been suggested that the absence of social support and the presence of isolation and loneliness affect suicide vulnerability by creating intense psychological pain and the "cry for help" impulse. Suicidal behavior has been viewed as a unique response of communication in which the suicidal individual is making a desperate "cry for help" to the social environment (e.g., Breed, 1972; Giddens, 1971; Kreitman, 1977; Shneidman, 1985). According to Breed (1972), "Isolation represents the beginning of a climax of self-destruction, because the human being is a social being, and without communication he loses his humanity" (p. 16). Lonely and isolated individuals have been shown to experience intense emotional discomfort and feelings of depression (Brown & Harris, 1978; Peplau & Perlman, 1982). Such feelings are thought to interfere with an individual's ability to establish stable and satisfying relationships, causing him or her to withdraw from the social environment (Rich & Bonner, 1989). Consequently, the isolated individual is hypothesized to be unable to elicit support and feedback in his or her emotional distress and crisis, and thus to come to perceive himself or herself as helpless and hopeless. The suicidal individual, experiencing a chronic sense of human social isolation, emotional pain, and hopelessness, is seen as resorting to suicidal behavior as the ultimate plea for help to those around him or her (Shneidman, 1985).

Finally, not only has the role of isolation and loneliness been linked with the development of suicide intention, but learning theorists have suggested that it also becomes a key variable in the maintenance of suicidal behavior. According to Zich (1984), the manner in which suicidal behavior (including threats, gestures, and attempts) is received by the social environment will determine whether such behavior will become a generalized coping response for future stress and emotional crises. Individuals who threaten or attempt suicide are often viewed as attention seekers who are trying to manipulate others for social attention and reinforcement, with little intention of actually killing themselves (Freeman, Wilson, Thigpen, & McGee, 1974; Zich, 1984). Consequently, the response given by the social environment is often avoidant, negative, and/or ambivalent. With this social reaction, the suicidal individual is thought to be likely to increase the frequency of his or her suicidal behavior in a further attempt to secure social support, only in turn to alienate those around him or her further (Frederick & Resnik, 1971; Zich, 1984). With repeated failure, the individual may plunge into complete alienation and despair, and perhaps may take his or her life to exit a most painful and distressing existence. Given the potent social/interpersonal conditioning of this vicious cycle, the nature of suicide as a process becomes apparent, as do the reasons why frequent ideation and a past history of gestures and attempts are often the best risk predictors for ultimate suicide (Beck, Resnik, & Lettieri, 1974; Patsiokas & Clum, 1977; Shneidman, 1985; Shneidman & Farberow, 1961).

APPLICATION OF THE MODEL
TO SUICIDE BEHIND BARS

With these considerations in mind, it is possible to return to the topic of suicide behind bars with a sensitivity to the potent role of social isolation and negative life stress. First, as the available demographic data have indicated repeatedly, suicide behind bars tends to be committed by inmates who are isolated in marital status—that is, single, divorced, or separated (e.g., Hardyman, 1983; Hayes & Kajdin, 1981; Hayes & Rowan, 1988). This finding is perhaps best understood functionally as creating a certain coping vulnerability for these inmates in handling the stress of incarceration, in addition to representing the absence or loss of important psychosocial resources for effective coping. Second, similar to suicides in the general population, inmate suicides have been shown to be precipitated or triggered by significant interpersonal losses, including relationship breakup, family problems, and conflict with peers (in this case, fellow inmates) (e.g., Ivanoff, 1989; LeBrun, 1990; Rowan & Hayes, 1988; Schimmel et al., 1988). All of these precipitants are negative life events that bring about alienation, isolation, and in some cases fear of violent attack. The inmate who has been labeled a "snitch," for example, not only is ostracized and alienated from the inmate community, but is often placed at significant risk for violent attack or homicide. Isolated inmates who encounter negative life stress and problems of living are apt to be ill equipped and unprepared to cope with their circumstances. Because they lack important emotional and social resources, their feelings of loneliness may become crippling. In time, these inmates are likely to experience emotional breakdown, to withdraw further, to become hopeless, and perhaps to see suicide as the only viable option for coping with a desperate, intolerable life condition.

In order to test out these clinical contentions, my mentor and I recently conducted some preliminary research in a jail population (Bonner & Rich, 1990, 1992). Volunteer inmates completed self-report measures of loneliness, psychosocial resources, perceived stress of incarceration, hopelessness, depression, and suicidal ideation. Table 19.3 reveals moderately high correlations between the various vulnerability factors and suicidal ideation. Furthermore, a hierarchical-regression analysis demonstrated that loneliness and absence of psychosocial resources interacted with jail stress to predict suicidal intention, independently of depressed mood. In other words, inmates who were psychosocially vulnerable (i.e., alienated, lonely, and without social resources and support), and who also experienced incarceration as a very threatening and stressful life event, were most at risk for becoming hopeless and considering suicide as a viable option to deal with their circumstances. Although these results are obviously preliminary and in need of extension and cross-validation, they underscore the importance of understanding suicide behind bars as a stress–vulnerability process—one in which isolation and lack of psychosocial supports and resources operate as potent mediators in suicidal intention.

IMPLICATIONS FOR RESEARCH, TREATMENT, AND CORRECTIONS PROCEDURES

The understanding that certain inmates become vulnerable to the effects of negative life stress (brought about at least in part by incarceration) through a variety of biopsychosocial paths (including isolation and loneliness) makes the placement, observation, and evaluation of these inmates critical issues. The recognition that most suicide victims behind bars are placed in

TABLE 19.3. Psychosocial Correlates of Suicide Intent in a Jail Population

	2	3	4	5	6	7
1. Suicide ideation	.41*	.44*	−.42*	−.54*	.61*	.76*
2. Jail stress		.30*	−.36*	−.09	.42*	.36*
3. Loneliness			−.31*	−.32*	.50*	.43*
4. Irrational beliefs				.08	−.48*	−.32*
5. Reasons for living					−.40*	−.63*
6. Depression						.67*
7. Hopelessness						

Note. From "Psychosocial Vulnerability, Life Stress, and Suicide Ideation in a Jail Population: A Cross-Validation Study" (p. 218) by R. L. Bonner and A. R. Rich, 1990, *Suicide and Life-Threatening Behavior, 20*(3), 213–224. Copyright 1990 by the American Association of Suicidology. Reprinted by permission.
*$p < .05$.

isolation or segregation becomes most disturbing. Moreover, paradoxically, many of these inmates are placed in isolation for seemingly abnormal behavior or intoxication, but often are not screened specifically for suicide intention. One can only imagine the devastating impact of social isolation on vulnerable inmates, who are experiencing severe stress and alienation and are perhaps considering suicide. The mental state of such individuals may well place them at a heightened risk for plunging into total despair and hopelessness. Whether an inmate is going through the frightening experience of initial incarceration, or is in an agitated state of drug/alcohol withdrawal, or has just been told by his girlfriend (perhaps his only reason for living) that she is leaving him, or has come to be labeled a "snitch" and fears a violent death, or is paranoid and fearful because of an underlying psychotic reaction—in any of these situations, placement in isolation may only serve to intensify emotional breakdown and psychological despair, and perhaps may be the final loss to push a person to suicide.

Although none of the five clinical cases discussed in this volume was a jail or prison inmate, it is instructive to consider what might become of each one if he or she were to be incarcerated. Each individual's psychosocial vulnerability and life stress conditions were unique, but their common psychological themes were emotional pain and hopelessness. One can only imagine the devastating additional impact of incarceration, social isolation, and abandonment on these individuals. In the case of John Z, for example, what would the circumstances of incarceration and being housed in isolation add to his psychological picture? This individual had experienced a major life loss (that of profession); felt embarrassed, worthless, and hopeless as a person and provider; and was tortured by feelings of agitation and depression. Should he find himself arrested, one would only expect the stress to increase his feelings of depression and humiliation. If he were to be left alone in isolation with no access to social support or contact, John could easily plunge into complete emotional despair, and perhaps commit suicide to exit this most painful existence. Likewise, would not isolation or segregation of Faye C intensify her emotional fear and despair? Seemingly under the control of a psychotic illness, Faye was fearful, confused, and unable to make sense of her world. While no doubt feeling a sense of loss of connection to others, Faye was also tormented by thoughts that people were against her and wanted to harm her. If she found herself incarcerated in an 8 × 8 cell, alone, might not her fear, paranoia, and fragile state of mind deteriorate into hopelessness and suicidal despair?

According to correctional suicidology expert Joseph Rowan (1989), the most important element in suicide prevention behind bars is the *presence of human interaction*. Vulnerable, potentially suicidal inmates need close observation, access to meaningful support networks, and appropriate therapeutic intervention. Whereas isolation and loneliness exacerbate life stress and contribute to hopelessness and suicide intent, the presence of social support and the availability of psychosocial resources buffer or protect a person from the negative effects of life stress, and provide vital resources to enhance successful coping. In this light, Rowan has noted that, in fact, the mere placement of inmates in dormitories or in cells with other inmates significantly decreases the risk of suicide, simply through the social presence of and interaction with the other inmates.

Other important social interventions are evolving for suicidal inmates. The "buddy system" is a program in which select inmates are trained to observe and provide peer counseling for inmates who are having a difficult time adjusting to incarceration (e.g., Manning, 1989). Often, suicidal inmates are housed and placed through such a "buddy system" to facilitate coping via positive support networks. The Federal Bureau of Prisons utilizes a "suicide companion" program, in which select inmates are trained to monitor suicidal inmates and to provide interpersonal communication and support for inmates in crisis (Schimmel et al., 1988). In some circumstance, a formal suicide watch will be carried out, in which a suicidal inmate is placed under constant observation by staff and/or inmates until he or she emerges from the crisis. These programs richly illustrate the vital role of social support in suicide prevention behind bars.

As an aside, it is interesting to note that segregation or isolation has been primarily designed in penology for inmates who break the rules of the institution, who cannot function in the population, who "act out," who are "disruptive," or who are "manipulative." In this function, isolation has also been used to control inmates who exhibit abnormal behavior and in some cases suicidal intent. Frequently, for example, inmates who exhibit suicidal gestures or who make actual attempts are viewed as "manipulative" and "attention-seeking"—as trying to manipulate the environment in order to obtain a more favorable outcome. Consequently, such cases are often not taken seriously, with the attitude that corrections personnel should not "give in" to the behaivor. Hence, such cases are generally approached with inattention as well as continuance of isolation. Although there is certainly no question that in an inmate population, often characterized by severe sociopathic personality disturbance, acting out and manipulative behavior (including self-injurious behavior) will occur, control tactics of isolation and inattention are not solutions.

Haycock (1989) has recently demonstrated that manipulative or suicidal intention may actually have little influence in the severity or potential lethality of self-injurious behavior. Whether they are manipulative behaviors or not, self-injurious gestures or suicide attempts can result in death. To return to the learning literature on the learning and maintenance of suicidal behavior, researchers have suggested that inattention and avoidance by the social enviroment typically result in an increase of suicidal behavior, in an effort to secure the social support and attention the person needs. The bottom line is that inmates who exhibit suicidal behaivor or self-injurious behavior are in need of social intervention, not social isolation. For suicidal inmates, programs that foster close supervision, social support, and access to or development of psychosocial resources are crucial. For acting-out, potentially self-injurious inmates, programs with close supervision and behavioral management strategies will be crucial in protecting and modifying such behavior. Not only is isolation inappropriate, but a plethora of research suggests that ultimately it can be deadly.

Although theoretical and empirical efforts in understanding suicide behind bars have lagged behind the process-based research of general clinical suicidology, it is fortunate that programmatic efforts, increasing litigation, and evolving correctional mental health care standards have implicated suicide as a stress–vulnerability process that can be identified and prevented. Courts generally have viewed suicide prevention in correctional facilities as as right of humane treatment afforded by the U.S. Constitution. According to the National Sheriffs' Association (1985), under the Eighth Amendment of the Constitution, inmates are protected from cruel and unusual punishment. The neglect of an inmate's medical needs has been viewed as a violation of this amendment. Suicidal intention has been primarily viewed as the outcome of mental health needs that are in need of identification, treatment, and appropriate social monitoring.

O'Leary (1989), in a recent excellent review of the legal literature on correctional suicide, notes that courts have held facilities responsible for detecting suicide risk, as well as for protecting inmates against the occurrence of suicide. Liability has consistently been found in cases where facilities have failed to identify inmates obviously at risk, including inmates with major mental illness, intoxication, specific suicide intention, and psychiatric or suicidal history. Courts have also made judgments of liability against institutions that have failed to provide adequate supervision of suicidal inmates or training for correctional staff members in suicide prevention, as well as against institutions with poor structural conditions that inhibit monitoring and close supervision of inmates. O'Leary (1989) further notes that judgments of liability have ensued when staff members have been deliberately indifferent to inmates exbititing suicidal intention or mental illness, including failure to provide mental health treatment services, failure to provide consistent visual monitoring, and failure to remove housing items that might be used to carry out a suicide. Finally, courts have strongly recognized the nature of suicide as a process and the impact that physical isolation and seclusion have on suicide behind bars. According to O'Leary (1989), placement of suicidal inmates in isolation has been recognized by the courts as leading to a "morbid state of mind" in which liability for wrongful deaths has been demonstrated.

With growing litigation and increasing recognition of the problem, national standards for suicide prevention in correctional facilities have been developed, in the pursuit of promoting humane conditions of confinement and reducing liability in lawsuits. Hayes (1989) recently conducted a review of a number of national standards for suicide prevention in correctional facilities. According to the standards of the American Correctional Association (cited in Hayes, 1989), policy and procedure should require that all suicidal inmates be under constant observation by staff, and that all inmates who are incarcerated receive visual observation at least every 30 minutes. In addition, the standards dictate that policy and procedure require all inmates to be screened for mental illness and suicide risk upon arrival at an institution. Finally, the standards require that a written suicide prevention program be developed and approved by qualified mental health professionals at each institution. All staff members are required to be trained in the implementation of the program, including screening, identification, and supervision of suicidal inmates.

In the most comprehensive standards to date, the National Commission of Correctional Health Care (cited in Hayes, 1989) dictates the following. Correctional facilities are required to have a written plan for identifying and responding to suicidal inmates. The institution's plan must include the following elements: First, the institution is responsible for the identification of inmates at risk for suicide upon arrival at the facility. Second, all staff members must be trained to recognize and understand various verbal and behavioral cues that indicate suicide risk. Third, staff members must be trained in interpersonal communication and ways of responding to inmates in emotional crises. Fourth, institutions must have available mental health services for further evaluation and treatment. Fifth, facilities must also have written procedures for monitoring suicidal inmates, as well as for documenting consistent visual checks. Finally, the standards specifically state that suicidal inmates should *not* be placed in isolation or segregation, but instead should be continually monitored by the staff. It is also recommended that inmates, when possible, should be housed with other inmates in a dormitory setting and checked at least every 10–15 minutes.

SUMMARY AND CONCLUSIONS

In summary, the problem of suicide behind bars has been given growing attention. It is now recognized that incarceration can be a strong risk factor for self-inflicted death, particularly for inmates who are psychosocially vulnerable and ill equipped to handle this stressful life condition. Correctional researchers have discovered common population characteristics of suicide victims, including drug/alcohol intoxication, mental illness, verbal and behavioral indications of suicidal intention, past history of suicidal behavior, mood disturbances (especially depression), isolated marital status, and specific precipitants or negative life events (interpersonal loss, family problems, peer conflict, and a variety of other negative life stressors). One of the most dramatic findings from this research has been that most suicide victims behind bars are placed in isolation or segregation before they commit suicide.

An in-depth review of the general suicidology literature suggests that suicide is best understood as a stress–vulnerability process, whereby certain individuals are unprepared, ill equipped, and/or at a loss for resources to cope effectively with incarceration. Specific risk factors, such as loneliness, isolation, and alienation, appear to be particularly potent in coping breakdown and leave individuals vulnerable and exposed to the impact of negative life events; the interaction of these factors and events can lead to emotional breakdown, and in time, under certain conditions, to suicidal action. The use of physical isolation or seclusion for such individuals no doubt only further intensifies this process. Although research has not specifically addressed the processual nature of suicide behind bars, court decisions and developing national standards have strongly echoed the view that suicide is a process, with typically observable physical signs of maladaptive coping and suicide intention, which in most cases can be reversed or prevented. Encouraging work is now being done on the programmatic level, and there is evidence for the positive impact of this work in preventing suicide behind bars. Researchers likewise will need to become proactive and process-oriented in the study of suicide behind bars.

After all has been said and done, we must remember that suicide behind bars, like suicide in general, is a very personal process that stems fundamentally from problems in living. To the suicidal individual, these problems seem too overwhelming, feel too painful, and appear too hopeless to go on living with. In spite of personal prejudices, punitive attitudes, and the paramilitary structure of our correctional systems, the success of suicide prevention programs will necessarily depend on our willingness and ability to understand suicide from the point of view of the vulnerable inmate. Ultimately, our efforts will be measured by our responsiveness to "Mickey's" poignant question, quoted at the beginning of this chapter: "Who would care if I hung up anyway?"

REFERENCES

Beck, A. T., Kovacs, M., & Weissman, A. (1975). Hopelessness and suicidal behavior: An overview. *Journal of the American Medical Association, 234*(11), 1146-1149.

Beck, A. T., Kovacs, M., & Weissman, A. (1979). Assessment of suicidal intent: The Scale for Suicide Ideation. *Journal of Consulting and Clinical Psychology, 47*, 343-352.

Beck, A. T., Resnik, H. L. P., & Lettieri, D. J. (Eds.). (1974). *The prediction of suicide.* Bowie, MD: Charles Press.

Beck, A. T., Steer, R. A., Kovacs, M., & Garrison, B. (1985). Hopelessness and eventual suicide: A 10 year prospective study of patients hospitalized with suicidal ideation. *American Journal of Psychiatry, 142*, 559-563.

Bonner, R. L. (1987). *Suicide and its prevention: A training program for correctional officers.* Palm Beach, FL: Palm Beach County Sheriff's Department.

Bonner, R. L. (1990). A "M.A.P." to the clinical assessment of suicide risk. *Journal of Mental Health Counseling, 12*(2), 231-236.

Bonner, R. L., & Rich, A. R. (1987). Toward a predictive model of suicidal behavior: Some preliminary data in college students. *Suicide and Life-Threatening Behavior, 17*(1), 50-63.

Bonner, R. L., & Rich, A. R. (1988a). A prospective investigation of suicidal ideation: A test of a model. *Suicide and Life-Threatening Behavior, 18*(3), 245-258.

Bonner, R. L., & Rich, A. R. (1988b). Negative life stress, social problem solving appraisal, and hopelessness: Implications for suicide research. *Cognitive Therapy and Research, 12*(6), 849-856.

Bonner, R. L., & Rich, A. R. (1990). Psychosocial vulnerability, life stress, and suicidal ideation in a jail population: A cross-validation study. *Suicide and Life-Threatening Behavior, 20*(3), 213-224.

Bonner, R. L., & Rich, A. R. (1991). Predicting vulnerability to hopelessness under conditions of negative life stress: A longitudinal analysis. *Journal of Nervous and Mental Disease, 179*(1), 29-32.

Bonner, R. L., & Rich, A. R. (1992). Dysfunctional cognitions and hopelessness in a correctional population. *Journal of Offender Rehabilitation, 17*(3-4), 71-79.

Braucht, G. (1979). Interactional analysis of suicidal behavior. *Journal of Consulting and Clinical Psychology, 47*, 653-669.

Brown, G. W. (1979). The social etiology of the London depression studies. In R. A. Pepue (Ed.), *The psychobiology of the depressive disorders: Implications for the effects of stress* (pp. 263-289). New York: Academic Press.

Brown, G. W., & Harris, T. (1978). *Social origins of depression.* London: Tavistock.

Breed, W. (1972). Five basic components of a basic suicidal syndrome. *Suicide and Life-Threatening Behavior, 2*, 3-18.

Burtka, G. J., DuRand, C. J., & Smith, J. W. (1988). *Completed suicides in Detroit's Wayne County Jail*. Paper presented at the 21st Annual Meeting of the American Association of Suicidology, Washington, DC.

Cassel, J. (1976). The contribution of the social environment to host resistance. *American Journal of Epidemiology, 104*, 107-123.

Cassuli, C. L., Invernizzi, G., & Vitalie, A. (1974). Suicide, attempted suicide, and the community. *Socijalna Psihijatrija, 2*, 267-291. (From *Psychological Abstracts*, 1977, *57*, Abstract No. 6050).

Cohen, S., & Wills, R. (1985). Stress, social support, and the buffering hypothesis. *Psychological Bulletin, 98*, 310-357.

Cox, J. F., Landsberg, G., & Pravati, M. (1989). The essential components of a crisis intervention program for local jails: The New York Local Forensic Suicide Prevention Crisis Service Model. *Psychiatric Quarterly, 60*(2), 103-118.

Danto, B. J. (Ed.). (1973). *Jail house blues*. Orchard Lake, MI: Epic.

Dublin, L. I. (1967). Suicide: An overview of a health and social problem. *Bulletin of Suicidology*, pp. 25-30.

Fawcett, J., & Maris, B. (1973). Suicide at the county jail. In B. Danto (Ed.), *Jail house blues*. Orchard Lake, MI: Epic.

Fawcett, J., Scheftner, W., Clark, D., Hedeker, D., Gibbens, R., & Coryell, W. (1987). Clinical predictors of suicide in patients with major affective disorder: A controlled prospective study. *American Journal of Psychiatry, 144*(1), 35-40.

Frederick, C. J., & Resnik, H. L. P. (1971). How suicidal behaviors are learned. *American Journal of Psychotherapy, 25*, 37-55.

Freeman, D. J., Wilson, K., Thigpen, J., & McGee, R. K. (1974). Assessing intention to die in self-injury behavior. In C. Neuringer (Ed.), *Psychological assessment of suicidal risk*. Springfield, IL: Charles C Thomas.

Gibbs, J. J. (1982). Problems and priorities: Perceptions of jail custodians and social service providers. *Journal of Criminal Justice, 11*, 327-338.

Giddens, A. (1971). A typology of suicide. In A. Giddens (Ed.), *The sociology of suicide*. London: Cass.

Hardyman, P. L. (1983). *The ultimate escape: Suicide in Ohio's jails and temporary detention facilities, 1980-1981*. Columbus: Ohio Bureau of Adult Detention Facilities and Services.

Hayes, L. M. (1989). National standards of jail suicide prevention. *Jail Suicide Update, 2*(2), 1-6.

Hayes, L. M., & Kajdin, B. (1981). *And darkness closes in . . . : National study of jail suicides*. Washington, DC.: National Center for Institutions and Alternatives.

Hayes, L. M., & Rowan, J. R. (1988). *National study of jail suicides: Seven years later*. Alexandria, VA: National Center for Institutions and Alternatives.

Haycock, J. (1989). Manipulation and suicide attempts in jails and prisons. *Psychiatric Quarterly, 60*(1), 85-98.

Henderson, S., Byrne, D. G., Duncan-Jones, P., Adecik, S., Scott, R., & Steele, G. P. (1978). Social bonds in the epidemiology of neurosis: A preliminary investigation. *British Journal of Psychiatry, 132*, 463-466.

Holahan, C. J., & Moos, R. H. (1981). Social support and psychological distress: A longitudinal analysis. *Journal of Abnormal Psychology, 90*, 365-370.

Hopes, B. G. (1986). *Jail suicides: Prevention through prediction.* Cincinnati, OH: Hamilton County Justice Center.

Irwin, J. (1970). *The felon.* Englewood Cliffs, NJ: Prentice-Hall.

Ivanoff, A. (1989). Identifying psychological correlates of suicidal behavior in jail and detention facilities. *Psychiatric Quarterly, 60*(1), 73-84.

Kashani, J. H., Reid, J. C., & Rosenberg, T. (1989). Levels of hopelessness in children and adolescents: A developmental perspective. *Journal of Consulting and Clinical Psychology, 57*(4), 496-499.

Kreitman, N. (Ed.). (1977). *Parasuicide.* Chichester, England: Wiley.

Lazarus, R. S., & Folkman, S. (1984). *Stress, appraisal, and coping.* New York: Springer.

LeBrun, L. D. (1990). Characteristics of male suicide attempts in the Sacramento County jail, 1985-1987. *Jail Suicide Update, 2*(4), 1-4.

Lin, L., Ensel, W. M., Simeone, R. S., & Kuo, W. (1979). Social support, stressful life events, and illness: A model and an empirical test. *Journal of Health and Social Behavior, 20,* 108-119.

Manning, R. (1989). A suicide prevention program that really works. *American Jails, 3*(1), 18-24.

Maris, R. W. (1969). *Social forces in urban suicide.* Homewood, IL: Dorsey Press.

Maris, R. W. (1981). *Pathways to suicide: A survey of self-destructive behaviors.* Baltimore: Johns Hopkins University Press.

Maris, R. W. (Ed.). (1986). *Biology of suicide.* New York: Guilford Press.

McCulloch, J. W., & Phillip, A. S. (1973). *Suicidal Behavior.* Elmsford, NY: Pergamon Press.

Mikawa, J. K. (1973). An alternative to current analysis of suicidal behavior. *Psychological Reports, 32,* 323-330.

Minkoff, K., Bergman, E., & Beck, A. T. (1973). Hopelessness, depression, and attempted suicide. *American Journal of Psychiatry, 130,* 455-459.

National Sheriffs' Association. (1985). *Suicide: The silent signals* [Videotape]. Alexandria, VA: Author.

New York State Commission of Corrections, Medical Review Board. (1982). *Suicide in state and local correctional facilities: A three year study.* Albany: New York State Commission of Corrections.

Ogloff, J. R., & Otto, R. K. (1989). Mental health intervention in jails. In P. Keller & S. Heyman (Eds.), *Innovations in clinical practice: A source book* (Vol. 8) (pp. 357-370). Sarasota, FL: Professional Resource Exchange.

O'Leary, W. D. (1989). Custodial suicide: Evolving liability considerations. *Psychiatric Quarterly, 60*(1), 31-71.

Patsiokas, A., & Clum, G. A. (1977). *Parasuicide: Implications of prediction research for etiology and treatment.* Unpublished manuscript, Virginia Polytechnic Institute and State University.

Peplau, L. A., & Perlman, D. (1982). *Loneliness: A sourcebook of current theory, research, and therapy.* New York: Wiley.

Rich, A. R., & Bonner, R. L. (1987a). Concurrent validity of a stress-vulnerability model of suicidal ideation and behavior: A follow-up study. *Suicide and Life-Threatening Behavior, 17*(4), 265-270.

Rich, A. R., & Bonner, R. L. (1987b). Interpersonal moderators of depression in college students. *Journal of College Student Personnel, 26,* 337–342.

Rich, A. R., & Bonner, R. L. (1989). Support for a pluralistic approach to the treatment of depression. *Journal of College Student Development, 30,* 426–431.

Rich, A. R., & Bonner, R. L. (1991). *A process model of suicidal behavior.* Manuscript submitted for publication.

Rowan, J. R. (1989). Jail/correctional officers with "street attitudes" incur lawsuits. *American Jails, 3*(1), 13–17.

Rowan, J. R., & Hayes, L. M. (1988). *Training curriculum on suicide detection and prevention in jails and lock-ups.* Alexandria, VA: National Center for Institutions and Alternatives.

Salive, M. E., Smith, G. S., & Brewer, T. F. (1989). Suicide mortality in the Maryland state prison system, 1979–1987. *Journal of the American Medical Association, 262*(3), 365–369.

Schaefer, C., Coyne, J. C., & Lazarus, R. S. (1982). The health related functions of social support. *Journal of Behavioral Medicine, 4,* 381–406.

Schimmel, D., Sullivan, J., & Mrad, D. (1988). *Suicide Prevention Workgroup report: A 1983–1987 analysis.* Washington, DC.: U.S. Department of Justice, Federal Bureau of Prisons.

Schotte, D. E., & Clum, G. A. (1982). Suicidal ideation in a college population: A test of a model. *Journal of Consulting and Clinical Psychology, 50,* 690–696.

Schotte, D. E., & Clum, G. A. (1987). Problem solving skills in suicidal psychiatric patients. *Journal of Consulting and Clinical Psychology, 55*(1), 49–54.

Sherman, L. G., & Morschauser, P. C. (1989). Screening for suicide risk in inmates. *Psychiatric Quarterly, 60*(2), 119–138.

Shneidman, E. S. (1985). *Definition of suicide.* New York: Wiley.

Shneidman, E. S., & Farberow, N. L. (1961). Statistical comparisons between attempted and committed suicide. In N. L. Farberow & E. S. Shneidman (Eds.), *The cry for help.* New York: McGraw-Hill.

Sovronsky, H. R., & Shapiro, I. (1989). The New York State Model Suicide Prevention Training Program for Local Correctional Officers. *Psychiatric Quarterly, 60*(2), 139–150.

Special Commission to Investigate Suicide in Municipal Detention Centers. (1984). *Final report: Suicide in Massachusetts lock-ups, 1973–1984.* Boston.

Swindle, R. W., Cronkite, R. C., & Moos, R. H. (1989). Life stressors, social resources, coping, and the 4-year course of unipolar depression. *Journal of Abnormal Psychology, 98*(4), 468–477.

Teplin, L. A. (1983). The criminalization of the mentally ill: Speculation in search of data. *Psychological Bulletin, 94,* 54–67.

Trout, D. L. (1980). The role of social isolation in suicide. *Suicide and Life-Threatening Behavior, 10,* 10–23.

Zich, J. M. (1984). A reciprocal control approach to the treatment of repeated parasuicide. *Suicide and Life-Threatening Behavior, 14,* 36–51.

C H A P T E R   2 0

Risk Assessment and Prevention of Youth Suicide in Schools and Educational Contexts

Robert D. Felner, Ph.D.
Angela M. Adan, Ph.D.
University of Illinois
Morton M. Silverman, M.D.
University of Chicago

Over the past three decades, youth suicide has become a mental and public health problem of epidemic proportions. Currently, documented cases make suicide the second leading killer of all youths aged 15-24 in the United States, and there are similarly heightened rates among children and young adolescents. The startling rise in these rates has brought with it a national call for more intensive and effective actions to reduce the terrible human and economic toll. In the search for such solutions, the recognition that epidemics are not ever eradicated or even significantly reduced solely through the treatment of afflicted individuals has been a guiding focus (Albee, 1982). With this understanding has come a major emphasis on the development of effective risk assessment, prediction, and prevention strategies for youth suicide.

In this chapter, we consider a number of the issues that need to be addressed in the pursuit of more effective means for predicting and preventing youth suicide. These two processes are linked, with the latter built on the former. That is, the identification of prediction variables should clarify those factors that contribute to the onset of disorder, and thus should define the factors that prevention strategies should attempt to change. Furthermore, the salience of the prediction variables identified as etiological contributors to youth suicide can be assessed by observing changes in the incidence of youth suicide accompanying changes in levels of predictor variables that derive from prevention efforts. In this case we can see that prediction variables, if clearly and accurately identified, will also be the first-order targets of change in prevention efforts. Our discussion attempts to place the issues in the context of relevant literature—not only literature pertaining directly to suicide, but relevant research and theory on the prediction and enhancement of youth mental health outcomes more generally.

CENTRAL ISSUES IN YOUTH SUICIDE PREDICTION AND PREVENTION

The impetus for prevention programming, including youth suicide initiatives, stems from the recognition of a number of significant obstacles to service delivery confronted by more traditional "clinical" strategies. Clinical studies have consistently shown that individuals in need of services often fail to seek them out or do so only after problems have become severe or reached crisis proportions. In the case of children and youths these difficulties are magnified, as this population is even less likely to be self-referred to clinical services. Moreover, the adequacy of procedures for identifying those youths "at risk" or in serious need of mental health services is often questionable, as is the relevance of these assessment and prediction efforts for intervention (Felner, DuBois, & Adan, 1991). Too often there are few clear links between the assessments conducted and the interventions carried out. In the case of youth suicide prevention, the full set of these issues is well illustrated by recent findings that many youths who are at risk for youth suicide cannot be effectively identified; that those who are correctly identified as at risk are unlikely to go to traditional settings for service; and that even if the first two factors are overcome, there may be a lack of access to the necessary professionals or of economic resources (Alcohol, Drug Abuse and Mental Health Administration, 1989).

This last finding underscores another issue that must be addressed in the design of all mental health programs. That is, both human and economic resources to address mental health problems are limited and relatively scarce (Albee, 1959; Sarason & Lorentz, 1979); local, state, or national efforts that do not attend to this scarcity in their design will be doomed to implementation failure, no matter how potentially effective the program. Still another question about a reliance on traditional services pertains to the issue of the efficacy of the procedures. As long ago as the early 1960s (Joint Commission on Mental Health and Mental Disabilities, 1961), the efficacy of traditional clinical models of intervention for all populations, but especially for children and youths, was seriously questioned. Muehrer (1990) raises more specific questions about the efficacy of such interventions, in a recent review of the literature on the treatment of individuals who have made prior suicide attempts. He notes that the results obtained through this avenue have been disappointing at best, with only a relatively small proportion of these clients attaining outcomes that may be termed "successful."

Although this finding may make clinicians feel initially defensive, it should not do so—at least if considered in the full context of the development of disorders. Clearly, treatment is a tertiary care strategy for individuals. That is, most individuals who have already made suicide attempts may safely be labeled as having serious disorders and adjustment problems, many of which may have been present or developing for an extended period. Given this state of affairs, it should not be surprising that tertiary interventions are less than optimally effective. Rather, it is the reverse that should surprise us: That is, given how long many of the problems seen in tertiary care strategies have been developing or have been "in place," and how severe they typically are by the time such help is sought, we should be surprised that treatment efforts often do produce at least some lasting positive results.

Recognition of the unmanageable and sometimes unnecessary difficulties and expense of a delivery system that depends on "reactive" treatment strategies, as well as of the predictably poor success attained with those who have had enduring disorders, has led to an emphasis on early intervention and prevention strategies as critical parts of the continuum of care in mental health. This is not to say that effective treatments will not be required for those who still develop serious disorders, as seems to be inevitable (at least at present). Rather, these strategies must be combined in a complementary fashion, with prevention and intervention efforts cutting the flow of those in need of tertiary care to a level that can be handled with available resources. Such strategies may also encourage those in need to come in earlier for services, thereby increasing the potential efficacy of treatment efforts. Such strategies are also far more humane. Even in cases where all levels of intervention might ultimately result in positive outcomes, the personal costs to the clients and their families will be far less if we can decrease the often painful processes and life disruptions that lead to or accompany suicide attempts. Finally, we must recognize that a strategy focusing on the treatment of those who have made attempts or are very close to committing such acts is unacceptable, in that before help is provided to many of these individuals tragic actions may have already occurred, including the loss of many lives. Having discussed the benefits of prevention and the problems associated with tertiary approaches more generally, we now discuss these benefits and problems as they relate more specifically to school-based prediction and prevention efforts.

ISSUES IN THE DESIGN OF SCHOOL-BASED PREDICTION AND PREVENTION EFFORTS

Approaches to youth suicide that focus on early intervention and prevention have attempted to address many of the concerns described above. That is, they have sought to develop care delivery systems for youth suicide that are proactive, that seek out youths in natural settings, and that are resource-efficient. Although numerous early intervention and prevention models have been put forth, few have attained the scope of, or been surrounded by as much controversy as, school-based programming prevention efforts. But to talk about "school-based" suicide prevention programs is to give the appearance of homogeneity to a highly diverse set of efforts—many of which may not even be appropriately labeled "prevention" programs. Often these programs have little more in common than their focal goals and the fact that they are associated with educational settings.

What is required for the further development and refinement of our programmatic efforts in this area, as well as of identification/prediction models that should accompany them, is an integrating framework that will allow us to examine these programs in a systematic fashion and thus to illuminate key areas of divergence. We hope that in the near future the research focus on such programs will shift from a consideration of some general classes of programs to a set of questions much closer to that used in well-designed therapy studies (Lambert, Shapiro, & Bergin, 1986). That is, what program level, with what elements, under what conditions, for which goals, and with what implementation characteristics (e.g., dosage, intensity, fidelity) is best for a particular population of youths?

To arrive at a framework that enables us to organize our thinking about prediction and preventive efforts in educational settings, perhaps the best way to start is by asking what appear to be some very innocent questions: (1) What do we mean by the concept of "prevention" when applied to youth suicide? (2) Whom does the program target? (3) What are the goals of suicide prevention programs? (4) What and where is the focus of intervention? (Felner & Felner, 1988). Let us now turn to each of these issues, and follow the paths they lead us on in the search for our unifying framework and implications for the prediction and prevention of youth suicide.

The Nature and Targeting of Prevention and Assessment for Prevention

The discussion of the prediction and prevention of youth suicide must start with clarity about just what we mean by "prevention." Although this is seemingly a straightforward question, there are actually several possible answers with quite different implications for programming. Here, two sets of conditions play key roles in shaping the answer to this question. The first set derives from the public health model of prevention. The second set of issues derives from the lack of precision that results from the use of this model in discussions of what it means to "prevent" youth suicide in terms of timing and targeting.

The Public Health Model and Multilevel Categorizations of "Prevention"

Most current "prevention" efforts can trace their roots back to the tripartite public health model. According to this model, there are three distinct "levels" of prevention—primary, secondary, and tertiary—that, combined, encompass the full range of traditional medical and human service interventions. "Tertiary prevention" refers to interventions with specific individuals who have an existing (often serious or severe) disorder. The word "prevention" is used here not in the sense of prevention of the disorder, but, instead, prevention of the residual and radiating effects that the persons' serious disorder may have on their lives and the lives of those around them. Prediction efforts at this level are concerned primarily with relapse and prognosis under different types of treatment.

"Secondary prevention" also focuses on identifying specific individuals, who in this case are showing early but clear signs of the focal disorder(s). The goals of "prevention" in this sense is the reduction of the intensity, severity, and duration of the disorder; again, this does not include prevention of its onset or reduction of its incidence in a population. In terms of risk assessment and prediction, such interventions are generally characterized by efforts to screen and identify specific individuals who are experiencing "preclinical" manifestations of the focal or associated disorder(s) (Lorion, Price, & Eaton, 1989).

It is only when we get to the level of "primary prevention" in the public health model that we are dealing with efforts focused on reduction of the incidence of new cases of the disorder in the overall population or subpopulation, rather than reduction of the effects of existing disorder. That is, primary prevention is by definition targeted to those individuals who do not yet "have" the disorder. Assessment and prediction efforts here have as their focus conditions that may place entire groups or populations at risk and are not dependent on the assessment of specific individuals.

Conceptual Problems with the Model

Recognition of the differential goals of the three levels of prevention brings into focus another critical dimension on which the three levels can and should be distinguished. This dimension is the level of analysis of the target of our efforts. That is, the level of prevention that is selected answers our second question: "Whom does the program target?" Primary prevention efforts are by definition population-focused. For prediction and assessment, the implication is that prescreening of specific individuals for the presence of preclinical states in order to define target groups—as is true for early intervention or tertiary care (Lorion et al., 1989)—is not justified under the rubric of primary prevention.

For the purposes of assessments to guide primary prevention, the concept of risk is defined epidemiologically, at the population level. Such risk statements must be recognized as conditional statements about the probability that any member of the given population or subpopulation will develop the focal disorder(s) later. What is often overlooked in many types of mental health studies is that the designation of being a member of the "at-risk" group conveys no information about specific members of that group, other than that they have been exposed to the condition of risk under consideration; "risk" designation is an actuarial statement. That is, if the conditional probabilities of disorder in a population are X, it is not the case that all members of that group possess X levels of predisposition or "riskiness" for disorder (Richters & Weintraub, 1990). Instead, assessment and prediction (risk statements) for program targeting are based on knowledge of probabilistic ways in which developmentally hazardous elements of the social context or biological characteristics of a population may disrupt positive developmental processes in the ecological framework of the lives of all persons in the cohort, even if we do not know the extent to which these processes have been disrupted for specific individuals. Thus, when considering these variables it is better to speak of "conditions of risk" rather than "at-risk individuals."

This brief discussion should make it clear that the public health model's grouping of three intervention levels under the construct of 'prevention' serves to perpetuate problematic conceptual confusions. If we are to develop the precision necessary for programmatic excellence, a fundamental shift must occur in the language of prevention (Felner & Felner, 1988). As we and others (e.g., Seidman, 1987) see it, a useful reformulation of the model is as follows: "Tertiary prevention" becomes "treatment"; "secondary prevention" becomes "early intervention"; and "primary prevention" alone assumes the mantle of "prevention."

These changes are more than semantic. If we adopt this point of view, we can now answer our first two questions: "What do we mean by the concept of 'prevention' when applied to youth suicide?" and "Whom does the program target?" In our reformulated framework, all prevention programs are targeted at populations and attempt the reduction of incidence of disorder. At other program levels, the goal may be to predict and reduce the prevalence of the *act* of youth suicide. But assessment and intervention efforts are still built around the existence of early stages of individual-level disorder. This view "makes explicit that *the phenomena of interest in prevention, our ways of understanding and conceptualizing them, and the delivery system approaches required, are all different from and in many ways unique from other levels of intervention*" (Felner, Silverman, & Felner, 1992; italics added).

The difficulties that may arise if we fail to attend to this critical distinction is well illustrated if we consider a review of the prevention of teenage suicide by Shaffer, Garland, Gould, Fisher, and Trautman (1988). Under the rubric of a review of "primary prevention" programs, these authors include such interventions as direct one-to-one psychiatric services, policy efforts, and school-based curricula. They also include what they call "secondary and tertiary interventions" in their discussion before attempting to come to some general conclusions about the efficacy of prevention efforts. Mixing these apples and oranges is simply inappropriate and leads to conclusions such as the following: "We believe that no matter how easy it is to rationalize a suicide, the act is almost always a sign of severe psychopathology and is therefore most appropriately an activity for the mental health professional" (Shaffer et al., 1988, p. 25). This may be true in early intervention and treatment, when individual disorder may be present. But in primary prevention we are still dealing with healthy (or at most vulnerable) individuals, and perhaps disordered or damaging contexts; in this case, educators or others (e.g., urban planners, housing professionals, recreation workers) may be as appropriately involved in change efforts as mental health professionals, if not more so.

To return to our reformulated model of intervention levels and its more carefully articulated distinctions among types of interventions, we can also see that while it is a useful starting point for developing a systematic approach to assessment and intervention in school-based youth suicide prevention efforts, it raises as many questions as it answers. Although it helps us understand what we mean by "prevention" and whom to target, it does not tell us how to do these things. Our next step is to address our third and fourth questions: "What are the goals of suicide prevention programs?" and "What and where is the focus of intervention?" Although these questions too appear to have been answered by our agreeing that prevention's targets should be population-level reduction of the incidence of disorder, this is a necessary but not sufficient element of the answer required, as we shall see.

Intervention Goals and Pathways to Disorder

Outcome Specificity

There are three dimensions on which the goals of any prevention or intervention activity can be organized. Thus far, we have considered two of these: (1) the timing of the intervention; and (2) the targets of the program. The third critical defining factor, not yet addressed, is whether the targeting is highly specific to a particular disorder or is focused on multiple problem outcomes.

A critical step in the design of youth suicide prediction and prevention efforts is clarification of the implicit or explicit models of "pathways" to disorder and adaptation that have guided the selection of the strategies employed (Felner & Felner, 1988). The strategies selected and their goals should follow directly from underlying understandings of etiological pathways (Felner et al., 1992). That is, a critical question we must be able to answer is this: "How are our assessment and intervention activities guided by our understanding of how our targeted outcomes emerge?"

Specific and relatively "generic" approaches to prevention programming reflect two quite different perspectives on pathways to youth suicide, which can be assessed against available theory and data. To oversimplify, a careful examination of youth suicide prevention programs reveals that a major dimension on which we can distinguish them (and prevention programs more generally) is that of the *degree of outcome specificity* that is sought. Some programs are very specific to youth suicide; others seek to build general competencies, to reduce stressors, and otherwise to influence that set of antecedent conditions that may relate both to youth suicide and to a broad array of potentially associated disorders.

Specific outcome approaches are exemplified by those school-based prevention programs that are most often labeled as "youth suicide prevention programs." These programs, for example, may provide information about suicide and associated symptomatology, means of early identification and referral, and other practices or data specific to suicide. They reflect a "specific disease prevention" model that rests heavily on classic medical and public health paradigms. This perspective holds that dysfunction is caused by *specific conditions* that interact with individual vulnerabilities, which are likewise *specifiable*. In this approach, prediction and prevention efforts are geared, respectively, to the identification of those unique "germs" or causal factors that maximize the prediction of youth suicide, and the subsequent removal of these conditions.

The "antecedent condition" perspective is reflected in programs that target the reduction of youth suicide through the modification of a broad set of conditions that may predispose individuals to or protect them against suicide and associated dysfunction. Although they have the prediction and prevention of youth suicide as central goals, these programs may make no mention of youth suicide in their titles. Instead, they carry such labels as "comprehensive health curricula," "life skills programs," "stress reduction and management programs," and "social competency development programming," to name but a few of these efforts. By contrast to the "specific disease" approach, this perspective (see, e.g., Felner & Felner, 1988; Felner, DuBois & Adam, 1991), holds that for a wide range of developmental outcomes, efforts to identify unique and/or specific etiological agents are neither appropriate nor supported by data (Sameroff & Fiese, 1989).

Although the two program types share certain elements, there are fundamental differences in assumptions about both the degree of outcome uniqueness and the specificity of risk pathways (for more extended discussions of these models, see Felner & Felner, 1988; Felner et al., 1992). To guide our decisions about which approach is more suited to the prediction and prevention of youth suicide in educational settings, let us briefly consider a selected review of empirical findings.

Pathways to Adaptation and Disorder in Youth Suicide

Two strands of research evidence appear most relevant to our questions. The first focuses on factors that predict, precede, or otherwise appear to be etiologically significant in the course of youth suicide. The second focuses on the co-morbidity of youth suicide and other disorders. Although these two stands are discussed separately, there is a high degree of overlap in the nature of the findings.

Predictors of Youth Suicide, Risk Assessment, and the Need for Theory. When we examine the literature on the prediction of suicide and the construction of assessment procedures or instruments that may be helpful in such prediction, we find an almost bewildering array of conditions that have been cited as contributing to suicide risk. Everything from the stresses and strains of everyday life to severe psychopathology and trauma has been cited. Indeed, it would be difficult to find some life experience, adaptive demand, or psychological difficulty that has not been shown to relate to suicide in one way or another. For example, Maris (1981) notes that "under the best of conditions life is often short, periodically painful, fickle, often lonely and anxiety generating. . . . only if the human condition were dramatically altered would suicide change much" (p. 6).

Studies of life stresses, social resources, and coping skills provide further support for the common antecedents to youth suicide and other mental health problems of children and youths (see Felner, Farber, & Primavera, 1983; Johnson, 1986). In this work, severe, prolonged, or unmanageable stress, the experience of major life transitions, and powerlessness are but a few of the conditions that appear to be associated with increased risk for an extraordinary variety of mental and physical disorders (Felner et al., 1983; Felner & Rowlison, 1986; Rappaport, 1987). By contrast, strong social support, a sense of self-efficacy, and well-developed coping skills or social competencies may all reduce the likelihood of a range of mental and physical disorders in the face of these and other conditions of risk or vulnerability (Felner, DuBois, & Adan, 1991).

Intervention research provides further evidence supportive of common early risk factors' relation to a broad array of later adaptive problems. Schweikert and Weikhart (1988) reported that disadvantaged youths who participated in early childhood education programs showed fewer negative outcomes (ranging from life-threatening behaviors and deliquency, to school failure, to the use of welfare services and unemployment) at a 15-year follow-up. Similarly, in discussing a major stressor that may be linked to youth suicide, Felner and Adan (1988) reported that a program that reduced the stressfulness and hazardous nature of a school context during a school transition reduced not only school failures and dropout rates, but also the development of psychological distress and symptomatology that may be related to suicide, delinquency, and other behavioral problems.

When we move from those experiences, resources, and capabilities that characterize daily life to less frequent, more pathological, and/or more severe conditions, we again find that a large number and broad range of such conditions have been cited as predictive of youth suicide. Mental illness or substance abuse of a parent (Pfeffer, 1989); a history of past or current sexual or physical abuse (Hawton, 1986); parental substance abuse, personal substance abuse, or personal mental health problems (Christie et al., 1988; Deykin, Levy, & Wells, 1987; Regier et al., 1990); family disorganization and other disruptions parent–child relationships (Pfeffer, 1989); negative social interactions and feelings of helplessness or hopelessness (Huffine, 1989); and academic and other life failures (Felner & Silverman, 1988) are but a few of the many factors that have been shown to relate, at least in the majority of studies in which they have been considered, to an increased risk for youth suicide attempts.

What should be clear is that in countless studies most if not all of these variables—both the factors pertaining to daily life and the more severe or pathological conditions—have also been shown to have high levels of associations with a broad array of other disorders, which are themselves often employed as predictors of youth suicide. For instance, Silverman (1989), in a review of the roots and co-occurrence of multiple disorders, notes that the antecedents of many problem behaviors are highly intercorrelated and that there may be a constellation of precursors or antecedents common to a broad range of clinical forms of dysfunction, including youth suicide. In a related vein, other authors (Felner & Felner, 1988; Felner et al., 1992; Sameroff & Fiese, 1989) note that data on developmental psychopathology provide additional substantiation for the existence of common antecedents to youth suicide and a number of the other disorders (e.g., substance abuse, depression) as well. These data also reveal the multicausal nature of these etiological pathways: Highly similar outcomes can result from very different combinations of risk factors, and very different outcomes can result from the same risk factors (Sameroff, Seifer, Barocas, Zax, & Greenspan, 1987). This understanding brings into focus the need to consider a second set of data that is relevant to our concerns—data pertaining to the comorbidity of disorders.

Comorbidity of Youth Suicide and Associated Disorders. The extent to which there are clear linkages in the emergence and nature of multiple forms of disorder, especially in childhood and adolescence, has only recently begun to receive attention. Previously, such associations and "mixed" diagnoses were often seen as "noise" deriving from imprecision in our ability to deal with diagnostic specificity—or, as in the studies described above, were seen as risk factors that may lead to the emergence of other disorders. But there is increasing recognition that disorders may in fact co-occur and/or evolve from one type to another, and that we need to attend to the phenomena of diagnostic instability and comorbidity as important in their own right. These phenomena may be potentially critical means of clarifying common mechanisms that contribute to the emergence of multiple disorders, as well as of increasing our understanding of how discrete conditions may emerge from such common mechanisms.

In highlighting the importance of comorbidity as a research focus for child psychiatric epidemiology, Rutter (1989) states, "Perhaps the most striking finding to emerge from all epidemiological studies undertaken up to now has been the extremely high levels of comorbidity" (p. 645). He goes on to note that until recently research findings have generally not been analyzed in ways that take comorbidity into account, leading perhaps to erroneous views of the specificity of the etiology of many disorders. When we apply the lens of comorbidity to viewing the question of the appropriate specificity of prediction and program design in youth suicide prevention, we find a number of features that may be useful.

Studies that focus on the nature of comorbidity in youth suicide also provide data convergent with those on the antecedents common to youth suicide and other disorders. Such studies provide compelling evidence that suggests the interrelatedness of youth suicide and a broad range of dysfunctions. High levels of substance abuse, depressive and other psychiatric symptoms, social and behavioral problems, and significant disruption in other spheres of socioemotional functioning have all been tied to suicide attempts in youths and young adults (Department of Health and Human Services, 1989). For example, some studies have found that a majority of youth suicide attempters in their samples show signs of significant abuse of alcohol or other drugs (Berman, 1990; Schuckit & Schuckit, 1989). In summarizing the data pertaining to the appropriateness of specifically focused versus more broadly based prevention efforts, Sameroff and Fiese (1989) argue that although "clear linkages have been found between some 'germs' and specific biological disorders, this has not been true for behavioral disorders . . . behavioral disturbances in the vast majority of cases are the result of factors more strongly associated with the psychological and social environment than any intrinsic characteristics of the affected individuals" (p. 24).

If we accept that these data support prevention strategies focused on antecedent conditions, we must still also recognize that even if we employ such prevention strategies there will be a continuing need for effective interventions with those who, despite such efforts, still develop serious, quite specific disorders. Thus, we must be certain that the development of an integrative framework encompasses a multi-element prediction, prevention, and intervention strategy—one that addresses what may appear on the surface to be incompatibility between the two levels of intervention. To address these apparent difficulties requires that we first recognize that "prevention" as employed in our reformulated model applied to the *unfolding* of a diagnosable mental health or social problem. Thus, in prevention the most immediate goal for any intervention strategy is to change those processes that lead to disorder. The corollary of this view is that "prediction" efforts are based on and concerned with the identification of these processes. That is, such efforts are seen as predicting not only the incidence of end-stage disorder (i.e., actual serious suicide attempts), but also the emergence or presence of pathogenic processes that may lead to this outcome. By contrast, when we are dealing with early intervention and treatment we are concerned with factors related to prognosis, not incidence. A critical concept in helping us bridge between these levels of intervention focus is that of "developmental trajectories" to youth suicide. In the most simple terms, the developmental trajectory of a disorder is the evolutionary history of that disorder (Felner & Felner, 1988). Let us consider this issue in more detail.

Developmental Trajectories to Disorder and the Issue of Onset in Intervention Levels: Disentangling Vulnerability, Risk, and Onset

To clarify what we mean by developmental trajectories and their implications for intervention, a useful starting point may be a return to our medical analogy. If we were to consider any action that reduces the occurrence of youth suicide, including the specific treatment of existing disorder, as a type of "prevention," this stance would be akin to saying that heart bypass surgery can be considered as a form of primary prevention of death from heart disease. Clearly, although the specific "final form" of the target disorder has not occurred, the processes leading to it (whether youth suicide or heart disease) may have been unfolding for some time. If we are targeting these unfolding processes at the population level, we are engaged in prevention. But if we identify pathogenic processes that are specific to identifiable individuals, we are engaged in secondary prevention (or, in our reformulated model, early intervention). Implicit, then, in our categorization scheme for intervention and prediction levels is a developmental model of disorder in which the conditions targeted not only become progressively severe but also progressively specific—first to the individual and then to the disorder, as we move closer to full clinical manifestation.

The adoption of a developmental perspective is a necessary but not a sufficient element in the design of effective prevention efforts (Felner et al., 1992). Such a conceptualization is still too broad to provide a clear understanding of the mechanisms that shape vulnerabilities, resilience, and the emergence of one specific outcome over others. To move closer to attaining this specificity, let us consider these latter issues as they pertain to the development of mental health problems and adaptive outcomes.

Onset, Vulnerability, Risk, and Resilience in Interactional and Diathesis Stress Models of Disorder. Most current perspectives on the evolution and emergence of disorder start with a fundamental "diathesis–stress" perspective. Diathesis–stress models hold that individuals may have either genetically based or environmentally acquired trait-like, individual-level vulnerabilities to the onset of a disorder. These vulnerabilities constitute the "diathesis" side of the equation and set the person's threshold of susceptibility to developmentally hazardous environmental conditions. Here, environmental conditions have two quite distinct roles. First, as suggested above, they may be sources from which vulnerabilities may be acquired. That is, acting as *predisposing factors*, environmental conditions may increase the probability that those within a given population will develop first-order outcome problems or "vulnerabilities" that create susceptibility to later disorder. Environmental stresses or conditions of risk may also affect developmental trajectories to disorder in a second fashion. Depending on the levels of vulnerabilities that have been previously acquired, these environmental factors may act as *precipitants* to the onset of more serious dysfunction.

In considering developmental trajectories from lesser to greater specificity of disorder, we may consider environmental and other population risk factors as more developmentally distant or "distal" from the onset of diagnosable conditions; they predispose individuals to a vulnerability to the broadest level of difficulties. By contrast, once individuals "acquire" vulnerabilities, the *specific manifestation* of a disorder that emerges (in the present case, youth suicide) will depend on or be triggered by identifiable, quite specific "risk" conditions that describe the person's recent, proximal life experiences (Felner et al., 1983, 1992). Without this understanding of developmental trajectories to disorder, these late-stage conditions are often mistaken for specific *causal* factors. With this formulation, we can now see that both the early, "broad-band," antecedent, predisposing conditions (both early risk factors and acquired vulnerabilities) and the later, quite specific condition that "shape" and precipitate the manifestation of a condition are each necessary for, but not alone sufficient for, the emergence of the disorder.

There is one more set of key points that derives from this model. That is, it should now be clear (1) that person-level vulnerabilities are themselves early problematic developmental outcomes that can be targeted by and reduced by prevention; (2) that these vulnerabilities result from risk conditions; (3) that the acquisition of vulnerabilities is not synonymous with the onset of disorder; and (4) that programs that target not only the reduction of risk factors but also the reduction of these vulnerabilities or that seek to develop and provide compensatory, "inoculatory" strengths, can reduce the incidence of our focal problem (i.e., youth suicide).

A next step in the development of our framework guiding prediction and prevention/intervention efforts is a greater explication of the actual developmental processes that produce the reciprocal influences of risk factors, vulnerabilities, resources, and developmental outcomes. It is to a model of those processes that we now turn.

THE TRANSACTIONAL-ECOLOGICAL MODEL OF DEVELOPMENTAL AND DISORDER

The "transactional-ecological" model is a framework that we and others (Felner & Silverman, 1988; Seidman, 1987) have argued offers the requisite levels of both comprehensiveness and specificity for the tasks confronted by prevention in focusing on the modification of developmental trajectories to disorder. As its name suggests, this model is derived from a conceptual synthesis of two other highly complementary frameworks—the "transactional" (e.g., Sameroff & Fiese, 1989) and "ecological" (e.g., Bronfenbrenner, 1979) models of development. A full discussion of these approaches is well beyond the scope of this chapter, but let us briefly attempt to capture the key features of each that bear on the current issues.

The transactional model articulated by Sameroff and Chandler (1975) and further developed by a number of authors since (e.g., Lorion et al., 1989; Sameroff & Fiese, 1989) emphasizes the reciprocal effects of a youth on his or her environmental context and vice versa. The ecological perspective, as articulated by Bronfenbrenner (1979) and others (e.g., Kelly, 1979; Rappaport, 1987; Vincent & Trickett, 1983), also emphasizes the "progressive, mutual accommodation between an active, growing human being and the changing properties of the settings in which the developing person lives" (Bronfenbrenner, 1979, p. 21).

To this emphasis on reciprocal process, the ecological model adds a focus on the ways in which the interactions between the person and his or her environment are affected by the relations *between settings* that define the person's life, and the broader contexts in which they may be nested. Thus, the degree to which each of the settings in which a child develops influences the effects of other settings becomes a factor that is necessary to consider, both in the assessment and prediction of developmental outcomes and in the design of prevention efforts. A focus on those settings that the child may never be directly involved in, but that shape the more direct developmental circumstances, is also part of this perspective. For example, parents' levels of stress and of received support may have an impact on their interactions with the child, and as such may constitute a potential focus for intervention; if so, these stress and support levels will need to be assessed, in order to determine their exact role in such interactions. Finally, the influence of broader social and political systems (e.g., poverty, the changing structure of the workplace, and racial inequality or other inequalities in opportunities) on the systems that define a child's day-to-day experience is also of concern (Bronfenbrenner, 1979). For example, in a climate in which jobs and economic prospects for those who do not go to college are declining, being shifted from the "college track" to the "general track" in high school may be a source of significantly more stress than it once was. Without assessment procedures that consider each of the potential levels of analysis, we may incorrectly assign weights to factors at the more proximal level that, in fact, may themselves be affected by changing conditions at higher levels. Now we also see that adopting a transactional–ecological view increases our ability to identify either developmentally hazardous conditions or developmentally facilitating/optimizing conditions as critical parts of our prediction and prevention efforts.

If we recognize that in the model of developmental psychopathology embodied in our transactional–ecological framework, disorder results from deviations in normal developmental processes, then the primary goals of preventive interventions are to "rebend" and otherwise modify these deviations in ways that bring the developmental processes into alignment with more typical, appropriate pathways. Assessment efforts focus primarily on the identification of these deviations and the conditions that produce them. Now, our earlier comment about the focus of change in prevention efforts can be restated as follows: "The target of prevention activities is the modification of developmentally hazardous processes that influence whole populations or subpopulations—not end-stage conditions in specific individuals." This understanding also helps us to address the assertion by Shaffer et al. (1988) that those who attempt suicide are always pathological. It may well be that a pathological or pathogenic process may always be present. But it also needs to be understood that this process may be external to the organism, or that it may only be dysfunctional because of the unique confluence of characteristics of the setting and person, neither of which would be pathological in itself (as in the example of changing economic conditions, above).

Let us consider, for instance, a "typical" early adolescent, with *appropriately* not fully developed or fully mature coping skills. Now if the adolescent is exposed to serious environmental stress that a mature adult might well be able to cope with (such as the chronic family disorganization discussed in the case of Ralph F in Chapter 12), the adolescent may be easily overwhelmed, and a suicide attempt may ensue—especially if, for example, alcohol use is also present. The "pathology" is not the youth's. His or her coping skills are normative, and some alcohol involvement is also (unfortunately) all too typical at this age. What is pathogenic here is the exposure to environmental demands beyond those that are developmentally appropriate, or perhaps an insufficiency of necessary environmentally based resources (e.g., support from family and friends). From a preventive perspective these resources should be developmentally assessed for their adequacy, so that if a youth cannot cope (even though he or she has all the resources that would be sufficient for an adult), this is not necessarily seen as a sign of disorder. Many of the problems we seek to prevent may in fact be attempts to adapt to disordered or hazardous contexts.

Thus, our targeted "problems" may stem from normal, typical processes in disordered or developmentally inappropriate circumstances. This perspective reduces the degree to which we need to infer the presence of pathology in the person; it thus allows us to shift our target of analysis in prediction efforts and subsequent intervention from the person alone, and to include more fully (and even primarily) the environment or setting level. The identification of developmentally hazardous or risk-predisposing conditions is now the basis of predictive and preventive efforts.

AN ORGANIZING FRAMEWORK FOR ASSESSMENT, PREDICTION, AND PREVENTION IN SCHOOL-BASED YOUTH SUICIDE EFFORTS

Given the overall framework at which we have arrived, let us now explain its utility for organizing and guiding school-based youth suicide assessment and prevention efforts. A critical feature of this perspective is its implications for the relationship between assessment/prediction and prevention programming. From the perspective we have developed above for prevention, those variables that constitute the focus of assessment efforts are also the same variables that either are the direct targets of change efforts or serve to focus such efforts. That is, assessment and intervention are inextricably intertwined.

It will be recalled that in our framework, prevention efforts are targeted at the modification of processes and factors that contribute to the incidence of disorder or the development of vulnerabilities at the *population* level rather than the *individual* level. The development, design, and evaluation of prevention programs involve a minimum of five steps that tie these processes together (Felner et al., in press). First, those charged with the design of the program should carefully articulate their assumptions about those processes that are operative in the acquisition of vulnerabilities predisposing individuals to youth suicide and associated disorders, and/or that precipitate disorder in the presence of vulnerabilities. Second, assessment efforts should focus on the presence and levels of these predisposing or precipitating processes. Third, prevention programming should be implemented that is designed to shift these processes in the direction of reducing the unwanted outcomes and increasing levels of adaptive developmental functioning. Fourth, assessment efforts should be brought to bear on the degree to which programming has modified the levels of these processes and/or vulnerabilities in the general population. Finally, assessment efforts should consider the degree to which changes brought about in the levels of the target processes or vulnerabilities actually "map on" to reductions in the focal disorder (in this case, youth suicide and suicide attempts).

In this five-step process, assessment focuses on outcomes/impacts at two levels: first, the changes considered in step 4; second, the shifts in levels of adaptive functioning considered in step 5. The former may be immediate or intermediate outcomes, depending on whether they are changes that derive directly from the intervention (e.g., reduced stressfulness of an environment) or that radiate from these direct changes (e.g., improved self-esteem and coping skills). The latter are focal or final outcomes. It should also be noted that the conditions that constitute and are the focus of the immediate- and intermediate-outcome assessments are the same conditions that serve as the basis of predictive assessments in step 2.

The antecedent-condition-focused, transactional–ecological model for prevention also provides a basis for deciding what the content focus will be at each of these steps in program design and assessment. Clearly, in this model our assumptions about relevant processes and vulnerabilities are driven by consideration of theoretical and empirical data that relate not only to youth suicide attempts in particular, but also to the developmental course of related conditions. Furthermore, within this category of variables we are concerned with processes that affect entire subsets of the population—processes that may cause most individuals exposed to them to develop critical vulnerabilities, and/or that may trigger disorder among a population that may already have heightened levels of vulnerabilities. In the first case, we may, for example, focus on the reduction of school-based conditions that are known to be harsh and potentially pathogenic (e.g., a large school with a great deal of flux, and/or conditions that lead to low expectancies of and investments in students by teachers). In the second case, we may focus our attention on the assessment and modification of conditions interacting with vulnerabilities that may be present at a heightened level among an entire subset of the population, which has already been exposed to vulnerability-predisposing conditions. For instance, the condition of poverty often leads to the acquired vulnerabilities of low expectations and poor school readiness; the levels of "precipitating" versus "protective" conditions in the school may be especially critical in the course of disorder in the presence of these vulnerabilities.

We see from this discussion that the conditions assessed in step 2 of our assessment and prevention process derive directly from these assumptions. So, to continue with our example, we might focus on those conditions that lead to low teacher expectations or support and high levels of setting flux;

on the presence of such low expectations and support; and/or on the hypothesized associated poor self-esteem and low personal expectations. Now we see that in prevention the focus of our assessment, prediction, and change efforts is on the following: (1) those elements of the environment(s) to which an entire subsample of the population is exposed, which either predispose them to the acquisition of vulnerabilities or interact with existing ones to precipitate youth suicide attempts; and (2) the presence of heightened levels of certain specific vulnerabilities in the exposed population, which are thought to be associated with the environmental conditions. It should also be kept in mind that prevention efforts may also be aimed at the enhancement of conditions that "inoculate" the members of a population through facilitating the development of competencies that increase resistance to negative environmental conditions. Thus, our assessment efforts must also consider the nature and levels of these conditions. In the now classic Albee (1982) model pertaining to factors that predict the incidence of the development of disorder (Figure 20.1), and in our expansion of that model (see Figure 20.2), preventive interventions may either attempt to reduce the pathogenic elements of environments or seek to strengthen the "host" population, in ways that reduce the incidence of a broad array of disorders. Employing a categorization scheme for school-based prevention programs suggested by Felner and Felner (1988), Table 20.1 presents a brief summary of some of the program models and types that have been employed in attempts to address the various elements of the "numerator" and "denominator" of our prediction and prevention "equation" in Figures 20.1 and 20.2.

As is seen in these models, conditions influencing the probability that different developmental outcome will emerge may reside in the person (e.g., population-level genetic factors or person-level acquired vulnerabilities), in the environment (e.g., stressors), or in some interaction of the two (e.g., individuals with heightened physiological responsivity to stress who are placed in high-demand environments). Assessment of personal predispositions and vulnerabilities (diatheses), and assessment of environmental demands and hazards (stresses), are both critical for predicting the onset and course of disorder. Furthermore, the implication for intervention is that in most cases along the continuum from diathesis (person-centered) to stress

$$\frac{\text{Stress}}{\text{Social resources} \star \text{Social competence} \star \text{Resources}}$$

FIGURE 20.1. Albee's model of factors that determine probability of psychopathology. Adapted from "Preventing Psychopathology and Promoting Human Potential" (p. 1046) by G. W. Albee, 1982, *American Psychologist, 37*(9), 1043–1050. Copyright 1982 by the American Psychological Association. Adapted by permission.

Risk and vulnerability
Pathogenic (stressful)   ★   Population vulnerabilities
elements of the environment

Pathogenic elements of the environment are conditions that predispose to the acquisition of vulnerabilities or precipitation of disorder. They include developmentally hazardous conditions and demands; major stresses; chronic stresses; inadequate resources; environmental conditions that are not well matched to the capacities, abilities, and personal characteristics of the setting population; limited environmental opportunities for positive goal attainment; and factors that limit opportunities (e.g., racism, prejudice, changing economic conditions).

Population vulnerabilities are any systematic elevations in biological, social, or emotional vulnerabilities that occur more often in the population being considered than in the general population, and that have been demonstrated to interact with the factors in any of the other domains to shape the potential course of developmental outcomes.

Host strengthening conditions
Social resources ★ Social competence ★ Resources ★ Population
                                                    vulnerabilities

---

	Expanded, these include but are not limited to the following:
Social resources:	Support systems and developmentally enhancing elements of the environment (teacher expectancies, classroom and school social climate).
Social competencies:	Social skills, decision-making abilities, cognitive and academic skills and knowledge, affective coping abilities, motivational "sets."
Resources:	Material and structural environmental opportunities in developmental contexts (home, school) for growth, self-sufficiency, and reaching prosocial desirable goals.

FIGURE 20.2. Expanded model of factors contributing to developmental trajectories to disorder and youth suicide that may be the focus of assessment and prevention efforts.

(environment-centered), the modification of conditions on one side of the continuum may influence the individual's probability of developing disorder, whether or not the existing risk conditions of concern are on the same side of the model or the other side. For intervention and prevention efforts, this interactive nature of the diathesis–stress model is particularly important when the risk conditions of concern may not be amenable to direct modification (e.g., genetic risk).

In both of these instances, the goal of the assessment is to understand those factors at the person and environment level that set the "threshold of vulnerability" of persons in that population, and the goal of the inter-

TABLE 20.1. A Brief Summary of School-Based Prevention Programs

Program focus	Program type	Target of change in Risk and vulnerability
Person-centered	Risk behavior modification Information provision Behavioral or academic skill enhancement Social competence enhancement Motivational change and affective coping	Programs in this section are based on the assumption that persons have certain deficits in one or more domains of competence that make them more vulnerable to environmental demands, and that training efforts in these areas can serve inoculatory functions.
Transactional	Facilitation of coping with life events and transitions Peer interaction enhancement Setting-related competence enhancement	Programs in this area are based on the assumption that there is some specific deficit or competence in the person that requires bolstering in order for the person to deal with some quite specific environmental hazards or stresses.
Ecological (setting-centered)	Modification of school social climate, structures, and regularities Teacher expectancy messages Increasing ecological congruence and support Resource enhancement and opportunity structure modification	These programs seek either (1) to provide necessary resources or conditions that facilitate positive development and coping; and/or (2) to modify or remove conditions in the environment that are developmentally damaging and hazardous.

vention is to shift the individual's threshold along the diathesis–stress continuum to reduce the likelihood that existing risk will result in new or further disorder. Of course, in those instances where the risk condition is itself amenable to change (e.g., environmental stress, emerging behavioral deficits) the intervention may be directly targeted to that condition. This too can modify the threshold of vulnerability of individuals in the target population.

If we extend these understandings to actual practice—the assessment of risk and design of prevention efforts in a school setting—we can see that the assessment for prevention may be significantly broader than those for early intervention and treatment. In the latter two instances, assessments are conducted primarily at the individual level and attempt to identify specific youths who are showing specific vulnerabilities or symptoms that have been shown to be associated with a heightened probability of suicide attempts. These vulnerabilities and symptoms may include suicidal ideation, previous attempts (indeed, these are among the major "risk" markers used in these program designs), and major changes in habits or affect (Hawton, 1986). Although each of these conditions may tell us whom to target, they actually tell us little about what to do or change. Furthermore, they require the often ineffectual and inefficient as well as resource-expensive strategy of individual screenings (Lorion et al., 1989). By contrast, let us examine the assessment levels and foci in prevention.

Assessments for the design of prevention efforts and prediction of incidence, based on the model we have explicated above, should occur at multiple levels of analysis. At a minimum, the first level of analysis should focus on school-related conditions that have been previously shown to (1) relate to the acquisition of vulnerabilities for both youth suicide and a broad array of associated mental health and behavioral problems (e.g., substance abuse); and/or (2) create conditions of stress or developmental hazard that may interact with existing vulnerabilities to precipitate either suicide attempts or associated disorders that futher enhance the population's level of vulnerability to youth suicide.

What should be clear at this point is that in a preventive approach the assessment of environmental/setting-level conditions within the school becomes an integral part of the process, not something that a clinician may simply do in passing. Furthermore, at least some of the elements of the setting that constitute the focus of assessment should be conditions that are potentially targets of the intervention efforts. Finally, assessment should also focus on the availability of resources that have been shown to be helpful to coping efforts (e.g., social support) and that facilitate the development of inoculatory competencies (e.g., teaching styles or processes that enhance critical thinking and decision-making skills).

A comprehensive review of the environmental factors in school settings that is well beyond the scope of this chapter. But it is also the case that certain well-established risk-potentiating and resilience-influencing factors that exist in school settings can be used as a starting point. Schools in which teachers have low expectations of students, are afforded little opportunity to know them well (as in large schools with little student overlap among teacher groups), and are themselves experiencing high levels of stress are assuredly hazardous. So too are school settings that convey little respect for students by engaging in such dehumanizing practices as removing the doors from restroom stalls so that students may have little privacy, or those in which there are high levels of fear, violence, and anxiety. Similarly, the recent report of the Carnegie Commission on the education of young adolescents (Carnegie Council on Adolescent Development, 1990) has noted that keeping students and teachers together in "teams" where they can develop a sense of belonging and interconnectedness (as in good middle schools rather than traditional junior high schools) reduces the degree of flux and chaos the students must confront in entering the school environment and provides for increased formal support and counseling during the critical years of early adolescence; as a result, it may enhance academic outcome and reduce the development of psychosocial difficulties. In similar fashion, Felner and his colleagues (Felner, Ginter, & Primavera, 1982; Felner & Adan, 1988) have shown that the stresses generated by exposure to much older peers, heightened demands for maturity, increased flux, anonymity, and lack of necessary support, all of which are confronted by students making the transition into large high schools from multiple "feeder" schools, can be reduced by restructuring the high school environment during the transition year or by creating modified "schools within schools."

At a second level of analysis, prevention-focused assessments should attempt to ascertain whether there are significant and/or heightened levels of specific vulnerabilities among those youths who comprise the population of the setting under consideration. These may vary greatly by setting and, as we will see, may interact with the characteristics of that setting. For example, youths in schools in upper-middle-class communities may have high levels of performance anxiety and excessively high aspirations, which result in poor academic self-esteem even in the presence of what (objectively) are excellent performance levels. Likewise, in university settings we are all too familiar with the case where a freshman whose skills and performance place him or her in the top 10% of that age group in the nation is surrounded by students with similar skills and ends up in "the bottom half of the top 10%". Without a setting that provides corrective feedback and reassurance, students like this may feel inadequate compared to their classmates, instead of recognizing their own skills as still excellent.

On the other end of the socioeconomic spectrum, youths in schools that serve low-income communities may be at risk because they come to school with lower levels of academic preparation than are necessary or optimal. Instead of attributing their need for additional work to poor preparation or resources, students in these schools may make self-attributions of academic incompetence. In many such schools, the majority of the students have lower-than-adaptive aspirations and expectations for the future—conditions that either relate directly to heightened levels of substance abuse and other risk behaviors associated with youth suicide, or predispose the students to other associated disorders (e.g., depression). What is critical in both the upper-middle-class and the low-income cases is that the schools in question have populations with known characteristics that predispose them to risk for heightened levels of specific vulnerabilities. Knowledge of these heightened levels of vulnerabilities in the school population should result in two forms of intervention in each case. The first form should be the development of school-wide programs that seek to directly modify the levels of the vulnerabilities in those populations (e.g., stress management and relaxation or coping skill development techniques for the high-stress school, and the teaching of goal setting and provision of didactic materials aimed at increasing aspirations in the low-income school). The second form should be the modification of the school environment in ways that reduce these vulnerabilities.

This second form of intervention suggests that the assessment for preventive interventions in school settings involves yet a third level of analysis. It will be recalled that critical features of the overall model are the transactional nature of adaptive efforts and the ecological appraisal of the degree of risk and vulnerability. Thus, the final element of the assessment process involves the consideration of the match between the characteristics of the environment and the vulnerabilities and strengths of the population in that school setting. Here the environment is of concern not as a *contributor* to the acquisition of vulnerabilities, but rather as a precipitating versus a protective factor for these previously acquired vulnerabilities. Thus, for example, Felner and Adan (1988) have shown that the degree of flux and low levels of teacher support that frequently accompany entry into a large high school are not risk-predisposing for students who come in highly prepared academically and/or with high levels of social skills. But for those whose skills are more marginal, or just above threshold for handling the demands of their prior school settings, the dramatic elevation in developmental demands that accompanies such a transition moves them into the risk range. It is critical to understand here that if these students were simply to move from one small elementary school to one small high school, fed only by that prior school, they might not show any vulnerability.

In a similar fashion, part of the assessment, as noted previously, involves consideration of the nature of other domains of the youths' lives that may interact with school characteristics. For example, in recent work Felner and his colleagues (Felner, DuBois, Brand, Adan, & Evans, 1991) have found that for youths from families where there are low levels of support for academic and personal achievement, supportive elements of the school environment, such as small class sizes and high levels of teacher support, may play critical compensatory roles in reducing adaptive difficulties and enhancing overall adjustment. But, for those students with high levels of family support for academic and personal development, school environments have little influence; in fact, these students appear able to weather even more developmentally hazardous school environments with some ease.

In summary, in a comprehensive assessment of the population's risk in a school setting or district, we need to know the following: (1) the levels and types of developmentally hazardous conditions, stressors, and protective factors that may be present in the school context; (2) the degree to which the population is characterized by the presence of particular vulnerabilities and competencies; (3) the ways in which the particular combination of setting and population characteristics that define the particular school or district interact to affect the acquisition of vulnerabilities or the precipitation of disorder; and (4) the degree to which other settings in which many members of the focal population are involved may increase or decrease the adaptive salience of any of the first three sets of conditions. Clearly, what we need to move forward on these issues in the future are multilevel school risk and vulnerability procedures that screen for those school conditions that are most socioemotionally salient to students; that provide an epidemiological assessment of the level of specific vulnerabilities in the focal population; and that provide a brief assessment of risk and resource characteristics of the other key developmental settings (e.g., families, the local community) in which the students are growing and functioning.

PREVENTION AS AN EXPERIMENTAL APPROACH TO ESTABLISHING THE ETIOLOGY OF DISORDER

Before closing, we would be remiss not to mention a critical way in which careful evaluation efforts built on the interlocking assessment and preventive intervention model described above may contribute not only to our understanding of their own efficacy, but to the development of a more general knowledge base that includes the further elaboration of etiologically significant pathways and predictors to youth suicide. Several authors (Felner et al., 1992; Mednick, Griffith, & Mednick, 1981) have noted that the core of this argument is that there are only two possible alternative strategies in the experimental testing of hypotheses about the causes of disorder. One is to attempt to systematically manipulate conditions in the lives of children or adults in accordance with our hypotheses about etiological factors, so as to induce mental disorder. Clearly, this option is totally unacceptable on ethical and humane grounds. The other experimental option is to develop hypotheses about the causes of disorder, to locate those who are naturally exposed to them, and then to systematically change these conditions in order to show that when they are removed (or when we introduce conditions hypothesized to be "protective"), then disorder does not emerge, whereas it does in those groups for whom we have not changed these conditions. That is, to test this model we want to show that nothing happened that otherwise would have occurred. It is in this fashion that well-designed youth suicide prevention programs can also contribute to our understanding of etiological pathways to youth suicide.

SUMMARY AND CONCLUDING COMMENTS

Over the past two decades, school-based youth suicide efforts have become an important element of our strategy in attacking this critical public health problem. Many of the early efforts in this area yielded quite disappointing results and, as in the case of the programs evaluated in recent work by Shaffer et al. (1990), often brought new problems with them while they solved others. There were multiple reasons for these failures. Across all levels of intervention, a lack of experience and appreciation for such issues as program intensity, dosage levels and duration, and external threats to program fidelity plagued first- and second-generation efforts. For prevention in particular, faulty and overly narrow conceptual frameworks of the nature of the problems with which we are dealing also hindered growth.

The value of what we have already learned and can still learn from these "failures" should not be underestimated. Much that is of value was learned from these early attempts and informed the work that followed. Moreover, in related work, comprehensive prevention efforts with children and youths have shown themselves to have far greater promise (Felner & Felner, 1988; Felner et al., 1991, in press) than their critics (e.g., Lamb & Zusman, 1979) have argued. There are now well-documented instances in which prevention efforts have been shown to reduce rates of serious socioemotional disorder in children and youths and to be cost-effective. But such documentation has not yet been adequately developed for youth suicide prevention programs in educational contexts. Still, the lessons of broad-based prevention programs provide an important and sound foundation upon which to build youth suicide prevention and evaluation efforts. Furthermore, the arguments in this should not be taken to mean that prevention-level efforts are the complete answer to reducing youth suicide. Even if we develop programs that are highly effective, some youths will still require additional, more traditional therapeutic measures. Prevention programs are not competitors with these approaches. Rather, youth suicide prevention programs in schools may be critical links in the mental health service delivery chain—not only reducing suffering in their own right, but alleviating the burden on more traditional services, to allow them to be more effective in meeting the demands placed upon them.

REFERENCES

Albee, G. W. (1959). *Mental health manpower trends.* New York: Basic Books.
Albee, G. W. (1982). Preventing psychopathology and promoting human potential. *American Psychologist, 37*(9), 1043–1050.
Berman, A. L. (1990, April). *The relationship between suicide and substance abuse.* Paper presented at the State of Illinois Department of Alcoholism and Substance Abuse Suicide Prevention Symposium, Springfield.
Bronfenbrenner, U. (1979). *The ecology of human development: Experiments by nature and design.* Cambridge, MA: Harvard University Press.
Christie, K. A., Burke, J. D., Regier, D. A., Rae, S. S., Boyd, J. H., & Locke, B. Z. (1988). Epidemiologic evidence for early onset of mental disorders and higher risk of drug use in young adults. *American Journal of Psychiatry, 145*, 971–975.
Department of Health and Human Services. (Ed.). (1989). *Proceedings of the DHHS Secretary's Task Force on Youth Suicide: Vol. 1. Overview and recommendations* (DHHS Publication No. ADM 89-1622). Washington, DC: U.S. Government Printing Office.

Deykin, E. Y., Levy, J. C., & Wells, V. (1987). Adolescent depression, alcohol and drug abuse. *American Journal of Public Health, 77,* 178–182.

Felner, R. D., & Adan, A. M. (1988). The school transitional environment project: An ecological intervention and evaluation. In R. H. Price, E. L. Cowen, R. P. Lorion, & J. Ramos-McKay (Eds.), *Fourteen ounces of prevention: A casebook for practitioners* (pp. 111–122). Washington, DC: American Psychological Association.

Felner, R. D., DuBois, D. L., & Adan, A. M. (1991). Community-based intervention and prevention: Conceptual underpinnings and progress toward a science of community intervention and evaluation. In C. E. Walker (Ed.), *Clinical psychology: Historical and research foundations* (pp. 459–510). New York: Plenum Press.

Felner, R. D., DuBois, D., Brand, S., Adan, A., & Evans, E. (1991). *Children in poverty: Mediated effects of educational and economic disadvantage.* Unpublished manuscript, University of Illinois, Institute for Government and Public Affairs, Evanston.

Felner, R. D., Farber, S. S., & Primavera, J. (1983). Transitions and stressful life events: A model for primary prevention. In R. D. Felner, L. A. Jason, J. N. Moritsugu, & S. S. Farber (Eds.), *Preventive psychology: Theory, research, and prevention* (pp. 191–215). Elmsford, NY: Pergamon Press.

Felner, R. D., & Felner, T. Y. (1988). Prevention programs in the educational context: A transactional–ecological framework for program models. In L. Bond, & B. Compas (Eds.), *Primary prevention in the schools.* Beverly Hills, CA: Sage.

Felner, R. D., Ginter, M. A., & Primavera, J. (1982). Primary prevention during school transitions: Social support and environmental structure. *American Journal of Community Psychology, 10,* 277–290.

Felner, R. D., & Rowlison, R. T. (1986). Unraveling the Gordian Knot in life change events: A critical examination of crises, stress, and transitional frameworks for prevention. In S. W. Auerbach & A. L. Stolberg (Eds.), *Children's life crisis events: Preventive intervention strategies* (pp. 39–63). New York: Hemisphere/McGraw-Hill.

Felner, R. D., & Silverman, M. M. (1988). Primary prevention: A consideration of general principles and findings for the prevention of youth suicide. *Proceedings of the DHHS Secretary's Task Force on Youth Suicide: Vol. 3. Prevention and intervention in youth suicide* (DHHS Publication No. ADM 88-1623, pp. 18–30). Washington, DC: U.S. Government Printing Office.

Felner, R. D., Silverman, M. M. (1989). Primary prevention: A consideration of general principles and findings for the prevention of youth suicide. In Alcohol, Drug Abuse and Mental Health Administration (Ed.), *Report of the Secretary's Task Force on Youth Suicide: Vol. 3. Prevention and intervention in youth suicide* (DHHS Publication No. ADM 89-1623, pp. 28–30). Washington, DC: U.S. Government Printing Office.

Felner, R. D., Silverman, M. M., & Felner, T. Y. (1992). Primary prevention: Conceptual and methodological issues in the development of a science of prevention in mental health and social intervention. In J. Rappaport & E. Seidman (Eds.), *Handbook of Community Psychology.* New York: Plenum Press.

Hawton, K. (1986). *Suicide and attempted suicide among children and adolescents.* Beverly Hills, CA: Sage.

Huffine, C. (1989). Social and cultural risk factors for youth suicide. In L. Davidson & M. Linnoila (Eds.), *Report of the Secretary's Task Force on Youth Suicide:*

Vol. 2. Risk factors for youth suicide (DHHS Publication No. ADM 89-1622, pp. 56–70). Washington, DC: U.S. Government Printing Office.

Johnson, D. L. (1989). Primary prevention of behavior problems in young children: The Houston Parent-Child Development Center. In R. H. Price, E. L. Cowen, R. P. Lorion, & J. Ramos-McKay (Eds.), *Fourteen ounces of prevention* (pp. 44–52). Washington, DC: American Psychological Association Press.

Johnson, J. H. (1986). *Life events as stressors in childhood and adolescence.* Beverly Hills, CA: Sage.

Joint Commission on Mental Health and Mental Disabilities. (1961). *Action for mental health.* New York: Basic Books.

Kelly, J. G. (Ed.). (1979). *Adolescent boys in high school: A psychological study of coping and adaptation.* Hillsdale, NJ: Erlbaum.

Lamb, H. R., & Zusman, J. (1979). Primary prevention in perspective. *American Journal of Psychiatry, 136,* 12–17.

Lambert, M. J., Shapiro, D. A., & Bergin, A. E. (1986) The effectiveness of psychotherapy. In S. L. Garfield & A. E. Bergin (Eds.), *Handbook of psychotherapy and behavior change* (3rd ed.), pp. 157–212). New York: Wiley.

Lorion, R. P., Price, R. H., & Eaton, W. W. (1989). The prevention of child and adolescent disorders: From theory to research. In D. Schaffer, I. Phillips, N. B. Enzer, M. M. Silverman, & V. Anthony (Eds.), *Prevention of mental disorders, alcohol and other drug use in children and adolescents.* (DHHS Publications No. ADM 89-1646, OSAP Prevention Monograph No. 2, pp. 55–96). Washington, DC: U.S. Government Printing Office.

Maris, R. W. (1981). *Pathways to suicide: A survey of self-destructive behaviors.* Baltimore: Johns Hopkins University Press.

Mednick, S. A., Griffith, J. J., & Mednick, B. R. (1981). Problems with traditional strategies in mental health research. In F. Schulsinger, S. A. Mednick, & J. Knop (Eds.), *Longitudinal research: Methods and uses in behavior science* (pp. 3–15). Boston: Martinus Nijhoff.

Muehrer, P. (1990). *Conceptual research models for preventing mental disorders* (DHHS Publication No. ADM 90-1713). Rockville, MD: National Institute of Mental Health.

Pfeffer, C. (1989). Family characteristics and support systems as risk factors for youth suicide. In L. Davidson & M. Linnoila (Eds.), *Report of the Secretary's Task Force on Youth Suicide: Vol. 2. Risk factors for youth suicide* (DHHS Publication No. ADM 89-1622). Washington, DC: U.S. Government Printing Office.

Rappaport, J. (1987). Terms of empowerment/exemplars of prevention: Toward a theory for community psychology. *American Journal of Community Psychology, 15,* 121–148.

Regier, D. A., Farmer, M. E., Rae, D. S., Locke, B. Z., Keith, S. J., Tudd, L. L., & Goodwin, F. K. (1990). Comorbidity of mental disorders with alcohol and other drug abuse: Results from the Epidemiologic Catchment Area. (ECA) study. *Journal of the American Medical Association, 264,* 2511–2518.

Richters, J., & Weintraub, S. (1990). Beyond diatheses: Toward an understanding of high-risk environments. In J. Rolf, A. S. Masten, D. Cicchetti, K. H. Nuechterlein, & S. Weitraub (Eds.), *Risk and Protective factors in the development of psychopathology* (pp. 67–96). Cambridge, England: Cambridge University Press.

Rutter, M. (1989). Isle of Wight revisited: Twenty-five years of child psychiatric epidemiology. *Journal of the American Academy of Child and Adolescent Psychiatry, 28*, 633–653.

Sameroff, A. J., & Chandler, M. J. (1975). Reproductive risk and the continuum of caretaking casualty. In F. D. Horowitz E. M. Hetherington, S. Scarr-Salapatek, & G. Siegal (Eds.), *Review of child development research* (Vol. 4, pp. 187–244). Chicago: University of Chicago Press.

Sameroff, A. J., & Fiese, B. H. (1989). Conceptual issues in prevention. In D. Schaffer, I. Phillips, N. B. Enzer, M. M. Silverman, & V. Anthony (Eds.), *Prevention of mental disorders, alcohol and other drug use in children and adolescents* (DHHS Publication No. ADM 89-1646, OSAP Prevention Monograph No. 2, pp. 23–54). Washington, DC: U.S. Government Printing Office.

Sameroff, A. J., Seifer, R., Barocas, R., Zax, M., & Greenspan, S. (1987). I.Q. score of 4-year-old children: Social–environmental risk factors. *Pediatrics, 79*, 343–350.

Sarason, S. B., & Lorentz, E. (1979). *The challenge of the resource exchange network.* San Francisco: Jossey-Bass.

Schuckit, M. A., & Schuckit, J. J. (1989). Substance use and abuse: A risk factor in youth suicide. In L. Davidson & M. Linnoila (Eds.), *Report of the Secretary's Task Force on Youth suicide: Vol. 2. Risk factors for youth suicide* (DHHS Publication No. ADM 89-1622, pp. 172–183). Washington, DC: U.S. Government Printing Office.

Schweikhert, L. J., & Weikart, D. P. (1988). The High/Scope Perry Preschool Program. In R. H. Price, E. L. Cowen, R. P. Lorion, & J. Ramos-McKay (Eds.), *Fourteen ounces of prevention: A casebook for practitioners* (pp. 53–66). Washington, DC: American Psychological Association.

Seidman, E. (1987). Toward a framework for primary prevention research. In J. A. Steinberg & M. M. Silverman (Eds.), *Preventing mental disorders: A research perspective.* (DHHS Publication No. ADM 87-1492, pp. 2–19). Washington, DC: U.S. Government Printing Office.

Shaffer, D., Garland, A., Gould, M., Fisher, P., & Trautman, P. (1988). Preventing teenage suicide: A critical review. *Journal of the American Academy of Child and Adolescent Psychiatry, 27*, 675–687.

Shaffer, D., Vieland, V., Garland, A., Rojas, M., Underwood, M., & Busner, C. (1990). Adolescent suicide attempters: Response to suicide prevention programs. *Journal of the American Medical Association, 264*, 3151–3155.

Silverman, M. M. (1989). Commentary: The integration of problem and prevention perspectives: Mental disorders associated with alcohol and drug use. In D. Schaffer, I. Phillips, N. B. Enzer, M. M. Silverman, & V. Anthony (Eds.), *Prevention of mental disorders, alcohol and other drug use in children and adolescents* (DHHS Publication No. ADM 89-1646, OSAP Prevention Monograph No. 2, pp. 7–22). Washington, DC: U.S. Government Printing Office.

Vincent, T. A., & Trickett, E. J. (1983). Preventive intervention and the human context: Ecological approaches to environmental assessment and change. In R. D. Felner, L. A. Jason, J. N. Moritsugu, & S. S. Farber (Eds.), *Preventive psychology: Theory, research, and prevention* (pp. 67–86). Elmsford, NY: Pergamon Press.

CHAPTER 21

Predicting and Preventing Hospital and Clinic Suicides

Robert E. Litman, M.D.
University of California at Los Angeles
Cedars-Sinai Hospital

At various times in the assessment and treatment of suicidal patients in hospitals and clinics, key decisions must be made, both by the clinician in charge and by the mental health staff. Examples are hospitalization itself and the timing of discharge; the institution and discontinuation of special observation and precautions; choices among treatment modalities; and the role of policy and procedure guidelines. The goal of this chapter is to clarify and amplify the process of making and implementing such decisions in both their clinical and ethical–legal aspects.

By contrast, the goal of suicide prevention is an ideal. Ideally, treatment in psychiatric hospitals would prevent suicides. But in fact suicides occur, sometimes in the hospital itself, and often in the weeks and months immediately following discharge from the hospital. Part of the explanation, of course, is that we do not completely understand the psychology of suicidal people, nor do we completely understand our interventions (e.g., antidepressant drugs, lithium carbonate, electroshock, and psychotherapy). More importantly, mental illness (and its treatment) is only one of many elements in the complex causation and prevention of suicide. Nevertheless, proper diagnosis and treatment of acute psychiatric disorders can often dramatically alter the risk for suicides.

It is fair to say that each suicidal patient is different, and that what is helpful for one may be harmful for another. Therefore, community standards expect the doctor, assisted by the staff, to give careful consideration to each important decision—to weigh the expected benefits against the anticipated risks and costs, after a competent effort to gather a reasonable amount of information about the patient, and especially about the patient's potential to commit suicide. There is a difference, however, between an "ideal" or "optimal" performance by the doctor and staff, which all professionals should strive to attain (Berman & Cohen-Sandler, 1982), and what people actually do in real situations. What courts call the "standard of care" is what the average competent and prudent professional would do, rather than some ideal of perfection.

SUICIDAL PATIENTS

In the argument over which is needed more, research on assessment or research on treatment, my choice is for efforts to improve treatment. We are already able to identify large numbers of suicidal patients, and know of many treatment failures. For example, Rich, Young, and Fowler (1986) reported that approximately 25% of suicides in San Diego had been in treatment when they killed themselves. Approximately half of the patients admitted to a psychodynamically oriented psychiatric treatment ward in Los Angeles, during the 3 years I was in charge of that ward, came there because they had attempted suicide or communicated thoughts of attempting suicide.

We often identify patients as "suicidal" because of associated "risk factors," which make these "suicidal" patients resemble people who have committed suicide. I have tried to quantify the concept of "suicide risk" as a statement of probability of suicide death within 1 year (Litman, 1974). For example, follow-up research indicates that, on average, patients who are hospitalized on a psychiatric unit after a suicide attempt commit suicide after discharge at the rate of 1 or 2 per 100 in the next year (see Discharge Planning and Discharge: below). This type of risk assessment is based on solid research but is not of much help for the hospital clinician, since any prediction based on statistical factors will predict a 95% probability that even the most suicidal person will still be alive 1 year later. Moreover, the emergency consultant is usually primarily concerned with evaluating the suicide danger for the next 48 or 72 hours, and after that, for the next few weeks (Motto & Bostrom, 1990).

EMERGENCY CONSULTATION

Emergency consultations occur in the context of concern and apprehension by the patient and/or relatives and friends, often because the patient has attempted or threatened suicide, or because he or she has expressed severe panic or serious depression. The focus of the consultation is on the present problem, its onset, its course, and the most recent cause for concern. Ideally, the emergency consultant would also have a more complete history of the presenting problem, gathering information from informants whenever possible to supplement the report of the primary patient. The purpose is to arrive at a tentative diagnosis if possible, and especially to determine whether the present situation represents a true crisis in the life of the patient or whether this patient is chronically suicidal—what Maris (1981) has called living a "career" of suicide. In a true crisis, the patient has been getting along with a reasonably good adjustment until one of life's hazards (e.g., a loss or threat of loss, an injury, or some other trauma) upsets the patient's psychological balance, causing that person to become perturbed and to consider suicide. Persons in crisis should have a great deal of support and crisis therapy beginning with the emergency consultation, because usually they recover and regain their former psychological level. By contrast, hospitalization is much less effective as a form of suicide prevention for persons who suffer from chronic suicidal psychiatric disorders, such as dysthymia with recurrent major depression, schizophrenia with suicidal ideas, alcoholism or other substance abuse, or personality disorder (Litman, 1989a). The special areas for assessment are stress, support, vulnerability, and suicidality.

Stress

In true crisis situations, the stress is obvious. An example I encounter frequently is that of the rejected husband of a divorcing wife. Some men, especially those with a great deal of unadmitted dependency, react with angry, destructive threats of suicide or even homicide. There is enough statistical reality to such threats to justify taking them quite seriously. There is some resemblance here to a terrorist threat; at least some wives see it that way. The intelligent response to such a threat is to play for time, to let hot feelings cool, and to negotiate. The emergency consultant may find himself or herself cast as mediator. For example, he or she may suggest a deal to the parties: If the wife will concede some time and the possibility down the line of a reconciliation, the husband will agree to enter the hospital for a period of cooling off and treatment.

Support

The consultant evaluates the amount and quality of the support available through people and through living circumstances. For example, some friends with whom a journalist was visiting brought him to the emergency room; he had been found with his head in the gas oven, attempting to asphyxiate himself. He was depressed over allegations that he had libeled a friend in his writing. The patient felt that the allegation was untrue, but that it would take a great deal of time and effort to defend himself. Beyond that, he was not completely sure whose side his wife was on. There were, however, numerous friends who rallied to his defense. In addition, the people he was visiting said that he could stay with them and they would not let him out of their sight, so a tentative decision was reached to treat him as an outpatient. I saw him daily or talked with him on the telephone, and observed that the suicide risk receded rapidly. He was eventually treated as an outpatient.

On the other hand, living alone is a risk factor, and sometimes the hospital is necessary to shelter a suicidal person from a hostile and provocative environment.

Vulnerability

Vulnerability is especially associated with psychiatric pathology, and with symptoms such as fear, panic, depression, helplessness, and hopelessness. Panic associated with depression has been overlooked in the past as a suicide danger signal (Fawcett, 1988; Weissman, Klerman, Markovitz, & Ouellette, 1989). The single most sensitive indicator of suicide potential is hopelessness.

My preferred psychodynamic model for suicidal vulnerability is adapted from Menninger and Freud (Litman, 1989b). In this concept, the mind is organized in levels or hierarchies of adaptational complexity. At times, in some people's lives, the organization falters because of stress and/ or disease. The vital balance is upset or perturbed, and the person regresses to less complex, more primitive levels of adaptation. Suicide is thus a result of a threat of regression to deep levels of adaptational disintegration; or, more accurately, suicide is the choice of death rather than of suffering disintegration. Some people cannot or will not tolerate the loss of their sense of a coherent self. Beyond the loss of money, health, and love as motivation for suicide because of grief and pain, there is a sense that threatened identity will be regained and confirmed by suicide: "If my life can't be my way, then it will be no way." This model emphasizes the importance of psychological support in crisis treatment.

Suicidality

What may be neglected or omitted in the emergency consultation is a painstaking investigation of the patient's suicidality. Where did the idea of suicide originate and how did it develop? What does it mean to the person? Under what circumstances would suicide be considered an option? Under what conditions in the future would the patient actually carry it out? If the patient has already made a suicide attempt, what was its meaning? Was it an appeal? If it was an appeal, has the message been heard, and has there been a reaction? Has there been a change in the patient's circumstances? What is the patient's estimate of the chance of repeating the suicide attempt? Part of the emergency assessment is to attempt to get involved with the patient and the patient's own ideas about the meaning of his or her suicidal thoughts and actions, to give a supportive interpretation about them, and to offer hope.

The Case of José G

The case of José G (see chapter 12 for full details) is an example of an emergency consultation. The presenting problem was José's depression over his forced retirement because of injury. His condition was complicated by certain physical problems (diabetes, a diabetes-related visual disorder and emphysema). He had a positive history of resourcefulness and industry, as well as a supportive home and family members who were concerned about him. The most serious complication was alcoholism. Thus the doctor would need to give this patient and family a hopeful attitude with regard to rehabilitation; perhaps to suggest another type of job with the railroad; and to recommend that the patient and family should involve themselves with Alcoholics Anonymous and Al-Anon. The diabetes and visual problems would need medical attention.

The one glaring omission in the consultation (as presented in Chapter 12) was the failure to investigate the potentiality for suicide. To what extent had José thought about ending it all, or felt that he would be better off dead? (He spontaneously said that he wished "the rail should have hit me on the head and ended it," but the clinician should have followed this up.) Could there come a time when he felt that he might take his own life? If he had some fear that this might happen, it would be a good idea to get his guns out of the house. Sometimes with a patient like José we discover in the emergency consultation that the patient has indeed had suicide thoughts and even gone through a rehearsal, thinking about a way to kill himself or herself. If the issue of hospitalization is raised and then rejected by the patient and the family, or postponed by both the patient and the doctor, it is important that the patient and family be warned that there is a danger of suicide. In addition, somebody should be with that patient and keep an eye on the patient, and, again, guns or other possible means of suicide should be removed.

THE DECISION TO HOSPITALIZE
General Considerations

Once the decision has been made to hospitalize the patient, care should be taken to implement this as rapidly and safely as possible, since this is a time of great tension and often ambivalence on the part of the patient and family. In making this decision, the patient and the family have to be informed of their treatment options and the special reasons why hospitalization is indicated, and they must give informed consent.

The advantages of hospitalization are many. In the first place, the patient is often taken out of a toxic environment (especially if it involves drugs and alcohol), removed from stress (temporarily, at least), and given shelter. In the hospital there is time and relative safety to assess the situation, consider options, to recall past strengths, and to regain perspective. The hospital is also a place where many different treatment resources are concentrated. In addition to the supportive milieu, there are psychological testing and psychological therapy; group therapy and various other specialties, such as occupational and art therapy; counseling for family members; and overall observation by the nurses and other members of the staff, who can keep track of the patient from hour to hour or from minute to minute if need be. Consultation (through case conferences and discussions with other physicians) is also easily available, and there are opportunities for physical examinations, medical treatments, and laboratory studies.

At the same time, hospitalization incurs risks. Hospitals are not always safe. I have estimated that there are about 300 suicides a year in psychiatric hospitals (Litman & Farberow, 1966), and several times that number in the immediate postdischarge period. Psychiatric hospitals are stigmatizing. For most people they are frightening, at least at first. Many people also feel that psychiatric hospitalization is a blow to their self-esteem. Some people interpret hospitalization negatively, as a sign that they are considered to be hopeless mental cases. Hospitalization may also remove patients from their chief sources of psychological support—for example, from their families (Conroy & Smith, 1983) or their work. There may be problems in the patients' lives that have to be resolved sooner or later, and these may only get worse while the patients are in the hospital. Finally, hospitalization is extremely expensive, and this may increase a depressed person's sense of guilt. Brent, Kupfer, Bromet, and Dew (1988) state quite correctly that it is difficult to provide evidence that inpatient hospitalization is a necessary or even always helpful therapeutic intervention for acutely suicidal patients. However, community standards and expert opinions strongly support this route for the high-risk patient, and ethical considerations may make a careful study of the problem impossible.

The Case of Faye C

The case of Faye C (again, see Chapter 12 for details) illustrates the value of brief hospitalization for a person who is chronically depressed and recurrently psychotic. It is vital to bear in mind Faye's great fear of hospitals. She was apparently in desperate need of treatment with antipsychotic drugs. Balancing the benefits of hospitalization against the risks, I would recommend a brief hospitalization aimed at handling the episode of psychosis, followed shortly by discharge. At all times with a patient such as Faye, there is a mild, chronic suicide risk that must be accepted, since suicide is unlikely unless the patient feels totally helpless and totally exposed to his or her magical fears and paranoid projections. Faye would need to be treated with a great deal of tact and kindness and support during her hospitalization, with the assurance that she would soon be discharged. Prolonged hospitalization could be quite damaging for Faye, and it would not be effective as suicide prevention.

THE DECISION NOT TO HOSPITALIZE

Many suicidal crises do not require hospitalization and can be resolved successfully with varying amounts of professional assistance. However, if hospitalization has been considered and rejected or postponed, ideally the psychiatrist will stay in reasonably close touch with the patient, monitoring the progress of the patient and his or her suicidal feelings; the psychiatrist should be prepared to re-evaluate the situation if the patient is not improving, or if there is an obvious barrier to developing a therapeutic alliance.

In the long view, as I have noted earlier, psychiatric treatment in hospitals has little to offer *as a form of suicide prevention* for persons who are chronically suicidal as a result of certain chronic mental disorders (e.g., dysthymia with recurrent major depression, addiction, schizophrenia, and borderline personality disorder). For them there is no quick guaranteed antisuicide prophylaxis, either through interpretation or through medication, and new developments in psychiatry and in public health have not made a dramatic change in their suicide rates. Recognizing that the basic element in treatment is a continuing stable and dependable doctor–patient relationship, many hospital emergency rooms have a "difficult patient, do not admit unless referred by treating psychiatrist" list. However, even chronically suicidal patients deserve careful consideration with consultation before admission is denied, and complete documentation is essential.

INVOLUNTARY COMMITMENT TO A PSYCHIATRIC UNIT
General Considerations

The decision to commit a patient involuntarily is never an easy one since it involves a political judgment as much as clinical judgment. Laws vary among the states, but essentially permit a qualified mental health professional to certify a patient to be held for 2 to 4 days, with various provisions for review by judicial authorities. The requirement is that the patient be evaluated as mentally ill and an imminent danger to self or others, or so gravely disabled by mental illness as to be unable to care for his or her most basic needs. Obviously, to hold persons behind locked doors against their will is a serious matter calling for a great deal of consideration, in which the risks must be carefully weighed against the benefits. For some suicidal people who are delusional, confused, or extremely agitated, the benefits are obvious. For some suicide attempters, commitment delivers a message that they are being taken seriously, and this in itself may be therapeutically beneficial.

Gutheil, Burszt, and Brodsky (1986) have described a process of evaluating competence on one hand and dangerousness on the other, and recommend involuntary commitment for those subjects who are relatively incompetent (out of control) and highly dangerous. They note the evaluation of competence in the medical chart, and give the patient several opportunities to understand what is happening—for example, by explaining, "I can only evaluate you on the basis of what you tell me." A great disadvantage of involuntary commitment is that it often interferes with the patient–doctor relationship. If there is a threat of incarceration, will the patient be open and trusting with the interviewer in describing his or her suicidal state of mind? Voluntary admission and the least restrictive alternative are preferable options. Often the resistance of a patient to entering the hospital can be dealt with by a sensitive interpretation of the patient's fear of the hospital. It must be kept in mind that for paranoid people it is obvious (to them) that the hospital is a front for their enemies. Many people are afraid that in the hospital they will be abused, so hospitalization is interpreted as a threat. Before such a patient is certified, the full extent of the possible negative side should be explored. Then the decision is a matter of clinical judgment.

The Case of John Z

The case of John Z (again, see Chapter 12) is an illustration of an emergency case that may well require involuntary hospitalization because the patient is a danger to self and others. John was exhibiting a high degree of suicide danger, involving a combination of depression and panic in a man who was in a crisis and was not responding to standard treatment as an outpatient. There had been almost 5 months of unsuccessful treatment complicated by suicidal thoughts and a couple of (reported) suicide attempts, and there had also been unsuccessful efforts to have the patient hospitalized. As the emergency consultant on this case I would call Dr. Smith (the patient's current psychiatrist), and with his cooperation (or not) I would move forcefully toward hospitalization, including involuntary commitment if needed. In the interim, I would advise John's wife not to let her husband out of her sight. Because there were financial problems, I would recommend taking him immediately to the local Veterans Affairs hospital (John was a Veitnam veteran). There he should be on suicide observation for the first 48 or 72 hours.

The actual level of suicide precautions would be determined by talking with John and observing him at the admission examination. He might be very relieved to be in the hospital, in which case only a low level of observation would be necessary. Or he might be extremely resistant and panicked in the hospital, in which case a high level of observation would be needed. In the hospital he will be placed on antidepressant medication and observed, and the staff should make efforts to be supportive and help him develop confidence in himself. If antidepressants did not work to relieve depression, electroshock treatment might have to be considered. John would have a reasonably good support system to return to when he left the hospital, but he would definitely need job counseling in order eventually to go back to work.

INITIAL AND ONGOING ASSESSMENT
Initial Considerations

The initial assessment takes place over the first 72 hours of hospitalization. This is the time when the patient is under the special stress of adjusting to the hospital, and the staff is getting acquainted with the patient; accordingly this is the time for special observation. It is important to be alert to the possibility of an unfortunate "weekend absentee" syndrome, when the patient comes in Friday night and is not assessed until Monday morning. Many hospitals have a routine assessment form that calls for a description of the patient's presenting problems and a history of their development, plus a special section for evaluation of suicide risk. Also included are a personal history, a family history, and a description of the patient's current mental status. The initial assessment includes a provisional diagnosis and a provisional treatment plan, plus the doctor's orders for the particular care that this patient will be given. All of this information is necessary for the information of the staff; it also provides a baseline set of observations against which the patient's progress can be measured.

Many hospitals provide for additional documentation by the hospital staff (e.g., a nursing plan and a psychosocial history) which is developed in association with the patient and the patient's family, looking forward to the time when the patient will be discharged.

The Interdisciplinary Team

Often the initial assessment includes opportunities for psychological testing and therapeutic interactions with psychologists, social workers, nurse therapists, and other staff members. All of these people together with the psychiatrist form an interdisciplinary team. I strongly recommend maximum use of the team approach in the hospital treatment of suicidal patients. This provides an opportunity for many different people to observe the patient from different points of view and to report back to their colleagues. In modern hospital practice, usually the psychiatrist is the leader of the team and takes the principal role in planning and especially in ordering and monitoring medications; however the psychological therapy may be administered principally by others on the team. To use a sports metaphor, the psychiatrist can be compared to the playing manager of a baseball team, who has a participating role as well as a managing role, but is definitely part of a team.

It is important to have harmony and agreement among the members of the team. They need to work out any differences they have in conferences and in discussion. They should communicate freely with one another and make written notes to one another in the chart as a basic method of keeping track of what is going on. Hospitals can facilitate communication among the members of the team by providing specific forms designed for the various team members (e.g., nurses' progress notes, social workers' progress notes, etc.), as well as the doctors' progress notes and order sheets. Sometimes patients are asked to fill in certain forms, such as self-descriptions, family histories, and descriptions of their plans and hopes for the future. Interdisciplinary staff conferences are generally held at regular intervals, and the patient is reassessed. Ideally, at these conferences the diagnosis is reviewed, the treatment plan is brought up to date, and there are modifications in the expectations and attitudes of the entire staff.

The Case of Ralph F

The case of Ralph F (again, see Chapter 12) illustrates ongoing assessment in the hospital. Ralph, age 16, was referred for a consultation focusing on suicide risk assessment. A number of risk factors were noted: Ralph did have a suicide plan; there was a history of alcohol abuse; and at times the suicide risk was especially high because Ralph felt helpless and hopeless. I would recommend immediate placement in a youth-oriented Twelve-Step program, but in addition he should have a full dose of an antidepressant drug. The suicide risk was high and probably chronic, and there would still be a suicide risk when he returned home, so there should be an effort to eliminate guns or other means of suicide from the home. It might possibly be helpful to consider some sort of school placement outside the home. In summary, a patient such as Ralph represents a serious, long-range, chronic suicidal problem calling for prolonged outpatient case management and therapy, with always a definite suicide risk. It is hard to assess what Ralph's auditory hallucinations might mean. They might not be important, or they might be early signs of schizophrenia; only time would tell. Psychological testing is helpful in evaluating hallucinations in an adolescent.

SPECIAL SUICIDE OBSERVATION

Hospitals commonly have two or three levels of special suicide observation and precautions. The most stringent level is "one on one," in which a specific person is designated to be in constant attendance on the individual patient and to keep the patient in sight at all times. The question of how bathroom privacy should be managed is controversial, and is best left to the policy makers of each separate unit. A second level consists of observational checks on the whereabouts of the patient every 15 minutes, and a third level may consist of checks every 30 minutes. It is helpful to have a special form that can be initialed by the staff member to indicate that the observation has been made at each required time. It is the doctor's responsibility to specify in the doctor's orders the exact level of special suicide observation that he or she considers correct. Other members of the staff, such as nurses, should take the responsibility of instituting suicide precautions only in an unusual and dramatic emergency. Since the purpose of special observation goes beyond security to providing information about what is on the patient's mind, it is the responsibility of staff members to talk with the patient, in order to explore the meaning to the patient of being in the hospital and of having suicidal plans and ideas. The staff should try to help the patient achieve better relationships and more hope.

It is also the doctor's responsibility to specify "privileges" for the patient, such as where meals can be taken, what clothes can be worn, whether the patient can be off the ward, and when passes can be issued. The doctor also authorizes the use of restraints or seclusion. Each decision calls for consideration of the benefits versus the risks, and may require consultation among the staff members. Pauker and Cooper (1990) discuss maximal observation as "psychiatric life support," meaning that these are procedures that help keep psychiatric patients alive, but are not directed at ameliorating psychopathology. For example, maximum observation can actually be harmful for some patients, leading them to increase their acting out in order to challenge the alertness and dedication of the observers.

There is a limit to how long maximum observation can be effective, and at some point the observation measures must be relaxed and then discontinued. Discussion with the patient can be helpful in reaching the decision to discontinue. A reasonably competent patient who has formed some therapeutic relationship with the staff and/or the doctor will usually be able to cooperate in this decision, especially after the first week in the hospital. However, certain types of patients are extremely difficult to monitor. Rapidly cycling manic–depressives, for example can go from elation to deep suicidal depression, sometimes in a few hours or even minutes. Paranoid schizophrenics often react very badly to maximum observation, becoming first suspicious and distrustful, then frightened and desperate. Some patients who are both psychotic and depressed are always at high risk for suicide.

In general, the presence of other people is the most powerful antisuicide measure. Sometimes when the patient is first admitted, or if there is a brief period of increased suicide ideation, a member of the family can be used to provide company for the patient (at least during daytime hours). Once again, this is a considered decision on the part of the clinician, because sometimes family members can be toxic to the patient. Being visited by a rejecting spouse, or receiving other types of bad news, can precipitate suicide attempts in hospitals.

Some people advocate the use of seclusion rooms for disturbed and agitated suicidal patients. But the use of such rooms calls for extreme caution and nearly constant observation, because people are able to devise ingenious ways of hurting themselves when they are alone. In general, it is better to have the observation out in the open. Sometimes acutely psychotic persons must be restrained with belts or other types of restraining devices; these can be effective in limited emergency situations for brief periods of time.

The decision to discontinue special observation and precautions is based chiefly on the feedback from the observer team. This feedback is used to evaluate the total adjustment of a patient to the unit and the degree of comfort he or she is showing. Also, it is important to evaluate the degree to which the patient has developed a therapeutic alliance or a working alliance with doctors and other members of the staff. If there is a need for some extra precautions short of special observation, it is recommended that a patient, especially a new patient, be placed in a room that is easily observable from the nurses' station.

SECURITY

There is controversy over what patients should be allowed to wear. For example, should they be allowed to wear their belts and their shoelaces? In many states there is a "patients' bill of rights," which includes the provision that patients should have their own clothes unless there is some special reason for them not to. For example, persons who are suspected of trying to elope from the hospital may be put in hospital garments to make them more conspicuous if they run out into the halls or streets. Some hospital suicides do occur when patients elope from the ward and then jump from a height, but I doubt that their clothing makes any difference. Within the unit itself, hanging is the most common method of suicide; the most important element that enables people to hang themselves is not the belt or the cord that holds their pants up, or the shoelaces that keep their shoes on, but rather the opportunity to be alone (usually in the bathroom). When people in hospitals and jails hang themselves, they generally use articles of clothing such as a shirt, pants, or robe, or sometimes strips of sheets and blankets.

It has been advocated that breakaway shower bars and hooks should be placed in bathrooms, so that people can not suspend themselves from these devices. But I wonder whether the benefit is worth the cost, since people often hang themselves from a doorjamb or doorknob. Many people asphyxiate themselves in a sitting position, without being suspended off the ground at all. They put their necks through a noose (made, for instance, from a shirt sleeve), tie the shirt to the bed, and lean forward so that the weight of their bodies causes them to lapse quickly into unconsciousness and then death.

HOSPITAL POLICIES

Most hospitals have policy guidelines for the staff concerning many of the patient care matters I have just discussed. According to a leading textbook (Kaplan, Freedman, & Sadock, 1980), in the 1970s specific suicide management policies were required for accreditation of a psychiatric hospital by the Joint Commission on Accreditation of Hospitals, but when I reviewed this subject for the committee on hospital accreditation of the American Association of Suicidology in 1985 I discovered that all such requirements had been dropped. The reason for this is that the structures and operations of different psychiatric units are so different that no standard set of requirements really fits them all. I talked to the Joint Commission about this and was invited to submit a set of my own proposals, but it was difficult to meet the challenge.

My recommendation (Litman, 1982) is that hospitals should ask themselves whether they treat persons at special risk for suicide. If they do, there must be policies for the management of suicidal persons. These policies are best determined by a committee representing the hospital staff, the medical staff, and the administration. The committee establishes written guidelines after surveying the security areas, and talking with staff and patients. *Suicide management policies are then incorporated into the training and supervision of staff.* A reasonable performance requires that each patient be evaluated for suicide risk, that a treatment plan be formulated, and that staff members follow the treatment plan according to the hospital's own policies.

THE TREATMENT PLAN

The treatment plan is individualized according to the patient's diagnosis and according to the circumstances that led to the hospital admission. In general, there is an effort to relieve stress, improve support, and strengthen the patient's vulnerabilities. For crisis patients the general principles of crisis treatment apply. The staff tries to be understanding, empathic, supportive, and optimistic, and to help the patient toward improved relationships, increased problem solving, and increased self-confidence. The work is primarily reparative. The staff offers an environment of friendship and structure, and emphasizes patients' strengths rather than their weaknesses. I feel that confrontation techniques with suicidal people are more dangerous than helpful. For example, encouraging helpless and dependent patients to get in touch with their anger at the families upon whom they depend is not helpful unless the unit is prepared to hold these patients for many months or years of character strengthening. My recommendation is for flexible supportive therapy along the lines of cognitive therapy and/or interpersonal therapy models. I save the deeper psychodynamic interpretations for long term-therapy usually in outpatient practice.

Standard treatment of suicidal patients in hospitals usually includes medication—often antidepressants or antipsychotics, or both where they are appropriate. (For an excellent review, see Joyce & Paykel, 1989.) I have already mentioned the optimal use of the interdisciplinary team. It is important to emphasize that discharge planning should start early during the hospitalization and should continue as the patient's stay goes on. One of the main roles of the team leader is to track the progress of the patient and to evaluate the effectiveness of the different treatment modalities. Modern treatment in hospitals emphasizes short-term hospital stays, and there is no evidence that prolonging hospitalization is effective as a form of suicide prevention, although it may be necessary for other reasons (Yamamoto, Roath, & Litman, 1973).

DISCHARGE PLANNING AND DISCHARGE

There is some mortality by suicide directly following the discharge of patients of all types from psychiatric units. Motto, Heilbron, and Juster (1985), Roy (1982), Pokorny (1983), and Fawcett et al. (1987), all report that 0.2–0.5% of all patients discharged from psychiatric hospitals commit suicide within a year, with a decreasing but noticeable suicide rate thereafter. The problem is how to reduce the suicide rate to a minimum. Ideally, the decision to discharge the patient should be a team decision, and it should be made when the patient has achieved maximum benefit from hospitalization. There are many advantages to a smooth transition from the inpatient to the outpatient status.

More often than not, a new outpatient doctor will take over treatment of the patient from the hospital doctor. In the current psychiatric scene in metropolitan areas, it is common for inpatients to be treated by hospital psychiatrists who make hospital work their chief specialty, while other psychiatrists are outpatient specialists. One reason for this is that in order to be an effective inpatient psychiatrist one needs to be acquainted with the nurses and the staff personnel, to know the hospital policies, and to attend numerous staff meetings. If an outpatient psychiatrist only has one patient in the hospital, it is not an effective use of his or her time to become acquainted with the staff and attend all the staff conferences. So, although it might be closer to the ideal for the same doctor to follow the patient out of the hospital, there usually has to be a transition. It is preferable for the outpatient therapist to visit with the patient once or twice while the patient is in the hospital; certainly there should be communication between the hospital doctor and the outpatient doctor.

It is important to prepare the patient and family for the transition out of the hospital. During this transition period, passes out of the hospital to visit home are useful for testing how the patient does, and it is important to get feedback from the family or friends concerning what happens during a visit. Giving patients passes means taking risks, since more than a third of hospital suicides occur on pass (Krammer, 1984). Both the patient and family should be given a realistic appraisal of the patient's progress and need for follow-up treatment.

OUTPATIENT TREATMENT

General Considerations

Often, for patients who have been in a true crisis, the hospitalization and a brief follow-up are sufficient. They readjust and go on with their lives. They usually return to fairly normal functioning, or the patient may elect to continue in therapy in order to strengthen himself of herself, so as to be able to handle some future stressful event more effectively.

The chronically suicidal patients are the ones who present special problems for long-term outpatient treatment (Litman, 1989a). Examples are many: dysthymic persons suffering from chronic apathy and anhedonia; schizophrenic persons who feel abandoned to their persecutors; alcoholic persons who face the reality of trying to be sober; borderline personality patients who use the threat of suicide to control their environments. These patients feel trapped in a hostile milieu with inadequate resources and limited hope, and so they fantasize about death—not only as an escape from pain, but also often as a final vindication. Chronically suicidal patients often express appreciation for the doctor's efforts, while still maintaining an inner conviction that sooner or later they will commit suicide.

I estimate that 20-25% of these chronically suicidal individuals eventually terminate their lives. But in any one year the suicide rate for chronically suicidal patients is only 1-3%, even for high-risk patients. I use this statistic when I treat suicidal persons. For example, when I am talking with persons who have recently made another suicide attempt after being suicidal much of their lives, I may say something like this: "According to the statistics, you are a patient at high risk for suicide. This means that there is a 2-5% chance that you will commit suicide in the next 2 to 5 years. However, there is a 95%

chance that 5 years from now you will not have committed suicide, and that you will still be alive. I am gearing this treatment toward that 95% chance." Note that I am already thinking in terms of a 5 year survival; recognizing that we are dealing with malignant, potentially life-threatening disease processes, and our efforts may only postpone suicide rather than prevent it.

Chronic Depression

Generally recommended in the treatment of chronic depression is a flexible combination of medication and psychotherapy. I employ a variety of psychotherapy tactics, depending on the patient's needs. For patients sunk in passivity and apathy, I prescribe specific activities and participation diaries, along with continuing re-education efforts to break the habit of negative thoughts and pessimism and to substitute more realistic and optimistic appraisals of self and the world based on a cognitive therapy model. I also encourage efforts to improve interpersonal relationships and to melt the affective blocks that tend to freeze these persons out of the warmth they might obtain from personal relationships. These patients have often failed to respond to extensive trials of antidepressant drug therapy, but I usually continue trying other drugs, seeking a combination that will work, and offering hope that perhaps a new product will be successful. Several years ago, trazodone became available and helped some chronically depressed patients. More recently, fluoxetine has been successful for others.

There is a subpopulation of dysthymic patients who respond well to dextroamphetamine (20 mg/day) over a long period of time. Unlike most people, these patients sleep better with dextroamphetamine and do not lose weight; it improves their energy and mental concentration and does not precipitate mania. Most importantly, they do not develop tolerance and the need for increased amounts of medication to produce the same effect. A trial of dextroamphetamine will quickly reveal its suitability for a patient.

A Team Approach

Ordinarily psychiatric treatment, especially psychotherapy, is a two-person confidential relationship between patient and doctor. But when suicide has become an important chronic issue, the doctor must avoid feeling isolated with the patient. Psychiatrists retain responsibility for treatment, but they share responsibility for suicide prevention, mainly with their patients and also with the social network and the treatment team. The team includes many people, not just the psychiatrist. I usually talk with the family, especially the spouse, and sometimes others who can be of help. I hope that they will be available if needed to act as ancillary therapists, and to communicate information that the index patient may not reveal-for example, that the patient is not taking prescribed medicine, or that family tension has increased.

Because suicides often occur when the therapist goes on vacation or is otherwise absent or unavailable, it is prudent to arrange for backup therapists who are acquainted with the patient to serve as substitutes or consultants. The team concept helps to dilute the transference dependency which becomes dangerous if it is too intense and too ambivalent. Intensity is generally not desirable in the treatment of these patients. To use another sports metaphor, we are involved in a marathon and not a sprint, so endurance, consistency, and steadiness are the essential parameters.

Monitoring the Transference and the Countertransference

Dysthymic patients form stable, positive dependency transferences and persist in treatment. Countertransference problems arise when a therapist becomes weary with the treatment's lack of success. The transference problem with suicidal schizophrenic patients is that they become totally dependent on and then paranoid toward the treating psychiatrist. The countertransference problem is that the psychiatrist becomes terrified by the psychotic projections. Therapists treating suicidal borderline patients find themselves feeling responsible for the lives of the patients as suicidal threats and attempts escalate. The antidotes are consultation, case review, and sometimes transfer of the patient. Brief hospitalization is a creative option during a transference–countertransference suicidal crisis.

Record Keeping

Early in outpatient treatment, the doctor should record the patient's history, mental status, and suicidal ideas, fantasies, and plans. The diagnostic impression and treatment plan should also be included. Later in treatment the notes may record only significant changes or significant events in the patient's life and therapy, and the results of periodic reassessments. After several years of treatment these records will enable the clinician to reevaluate the original complaints, to check the effectiveness of medications, and to determine seasonal variations in symptoms. The records will reinforce the therapist's reminder to the patient that there has been progress or that there have been "up" periods as well as "downs." Finally, the records provide assurance to the clinician that his or her decisions and treatments have been carried out in a careful, competent, and prudent manner.

REFERENCES

Berman, A. L., & Cohen-Sandler, R. (1982). Suicide and the standard of care: Optimal vs. acceptable. *Suicide and Life-Threatening Behavior, 12*(2), 114–122.

Brent, D. A., Kupfer, D. J., Bromet, E. J., and Dew, M. A. (1988). The assessment and treatment of patients at risk for suicide. In A. J. Frances, & R. E. Hales (Eds.), *Review of psychiatry* (Vol. 7, pp. 353-385). Washington, DC: American Psychiatric Press.

Conroy, R. W., & Smith, E. K. (1983). Family loss and hospital suicide. *Suicide and Life-Threatening Behavior, 13*(3), 179-194.

Fawcett, J. (1988). Predictors of early suicide: Identification and appropriate intervention. *Journal of Clinical Psychiatry, 49*(Suppl.), 7-8.

Fawcett, J., Scheftner, W., Clark, D., Hedeker, D., Gibbons, R., & Coryell, W. (1987). Clinical predictors of suicide in patients with major affective disorders. *American Journal of Psychiatry, 144*(1), 35-50.

Gutheil, T. G., Burszt, A. H., & Brodsky, A. (1986). The multidimensional assessment of dangerousness: Competence assessment in patient care and liability prevention. *Bulletin of the American Academy of Psychiatry and Law, 14*(2), 123-129.

Joyce, P. R., & Paykel, E. S. (1989). Predictors of drug response in depression. *Archives of General Psychiatry, 46*, 89-99.

Kaplan, H. I., Freedman, A. M., & Sadock, B. J. (Eds.). (1980). *Comprehensive textbook of psychiatry* (3rd ed.). Baltimore: Williams & Wilkins.

Krammer, J. L. (1984). The special characteristics of suicide of hospital inpatients. *British Journal of Psychiatry, 145*, 460-463.

Litman, R. E. (1974). Models for predicting suicide risk. In C. Neuringer (Ed.) *Psychological assessment of suicidal risk*, (pp. 177-185). Springfield, IL: Charles C Thomas.

Litman, R. E. (1982). Hospital suicides: Lawsuits and standards. *Suicide and Life-Threatening Behavior, 12*(4), 212-220.

Litman, R. E. (1989a). Long term treatment of chronically suicidal patients. *Bulletin of the Menninger Clinic, 53*(3), 215-228.

Litman, R. E. (1989b). Suicides: What do they have in mind? In D. J. Jacobs, & H. N. Brown (Eds.), *Suicide: Understanding and responding* (pp. 143-156), Madison, CT: International Universities Press.

Litman, R. E., & Farberow, N. L. (1966). The hospital's obligation toward suicide-prone patients. *Hospitals, 40*, 64-68.

Maris, R. W. (1981). *Pathways to suicide: A survey of self-destructive behaviors*. Baltimore: Johns Hopkins University Press.

Motto, J. A., & Bostrom, A. (1990). Empirical indications of near-term suicide risk. *Crisis, 11*(1), 52-59.

Motto, J. A., Heilbron, D., & Juster, R. (1985). Development of an instrument to estimate suicide risk. *American Journal of Psychiatry, 142*, 680-686.

Pauker, S. L., & Cooper, A. M. (1990). Paradoxical patient reactions to psychiatric life support: Clinical and ethical considerations. *American Journal of Psychiatry, 147*(4), 488-491.

Pokorny, A. D. (1983). Prediction of suicide in psychiatric patients: Report of a prospective study. *Archives of General Psychiatry, 40*, 249-257.

Rich, C. L., Young, D., and Fowler, R. C. (1986). San Diego Suicide Study: I. Young vs. old subjects. *Archives of General Psychiatry, 43*, 577-582.

Roy, A. (1982). Risk factors for suicide in psychiatric patients. *Archives of General Psychiatry, 39*, 1089–1095.

Weissman, M. M., Klerman, G. L., Markovitz, J. S., and Ouellette, R. (1989). Suicidal ideation and suicide attempts in panic disorder and attacks. *New England Journal of Medicine, 321*(18), 1209–1214.

Yamamoto, J., Roath, M., & Litman, R. E. (1973). Suicides in the new" community hospital. *Archives of General Psychiatry, 28*, 101–102.

CHAPTER 22

Clinical and Cognitive Predictors of Suicide

Marjorie E. Weishaar, Ph.D.
Brown University
Aaron T. Beck, M.D.
University of Pennsylvania

Whereas epidemiological factors identify groups at risk for suicide, the identification of clinical factors may help avert suicide in individual cases. Such identification may guide clinical decision making and direct a choice of therapeutic intervention. With the establishment of a classification system of suicidal behaviors (Beck et al., 1973), research has determined psychological and proximate factors that influence suicidality, from ideation to overt self-destructive behavior. This chapter reviews clinical risk factors—those pertaining to the individual's psychological state and immediate environment—and discusses cognitive characteristics of suicidal individuals. A model of suicidal behavior, with hopelessness as the key psychological variable, is presented.

Much of this chapter is based on cognitive therapy research. Cognitive therapy itself arose from research on depressed patients, whose thoughts and images were found to be negatively biased in systematic and habitual ways (Beck 1964). The cognitive triad characteristic of depression reflects the patient's negative view of the self, the world, and the future (Beck, 1967/1972). Both the hopelessness associated with a pessimistic view of the future and, more recently, the negative view of self reflected in low self-concept (Beck & Stewart, 1989) have been found to be precursors of suicidal ideation and intent.

Concomitant with the development of cognitive therapy as a treatment for depression (and, later, for anxiety and personality disorders), has been a continuing generation of research, including research on suicide risk assessment and prediction. Such investigations have yielded scales to assess suicidal ideation, suicide intent, and hopelessness, which can be used in prospective studies, thereby enhancing their clinical utility. Additional research by a number of investigators has identified other cognitive factors in suicide risk.

CLASSIFICATION OF SUICIDAL BEHAVIOR

To clarify terminology, to identify commonalities and differences among those labeled as suicidal, and to facilitate research on suicide risk, the task force of the National Institute of Mental Health (NIMH) Center for Studies of Suicide Prevention developed a tripartite classification system consisting of suicide ideation, suicide attempt, and completed suicide (Beck et al. 1973). Suicide intent, medical lethality, and method of attempted or completed suicide are subdivisions of these categories. Suicide ideators are defined as those who have thoughts and wishes of suicide, but have not yet acted on a plan to cause self-injury. Suicide ideation includes suicide threats, suicide preoccupations, direct expressions of the wish to die, and indirect indicators of suicide planning (Beck 1986).

Suicide intent, a subcategory of suicide ideation, attempts, and completed suicide, refers to the "intensity and pervasiveness of the wish to die" (Beck, 1986; pp. 91–92). Intent cannot always be inferred from outcome, for those who have seriously injured themselves may have had a relatively low wish to die, and vice versa. Lethality and intent are positively correlated only when the suicide attempter has reasonably accurate knowledge of the probable medical lethality of his or her chosen means (Beck, Beck & Kovacs, 1975).

Method is a subcategory for attempted and completed suicide. Knowing the method used in a suicide attempt identifies a likely method for any future attempt and may allow others to reduce future access to that method (e.g., by restricting prescribed medication). Recent work by Beck and Steer (1989) suggests that patients who have taken precautions against discovery at the time of the index attempt are likely to use similar methods in the ultimate attempt. Thus, awareness of a method may warn of a pattern.

ASSESSMENT SCALES

Beck Depression Inventory

The Beck Depression Inventory (BDI; Beck & Steer, 1987) is a 21-item self-report questionnaire that asks respondents to assess depressive symptoms over the previous week. Each item contains four statements reflecting increasing levels of severity. Items are scored from 0 to 3, and summed for an overall depression score potentially ranging from 0 to 63. A score of indicates severe depression. The psychometric properties of the BDI have been reviewed by Beck and Steer (1987).

The BDI has been found to correlate with suicide intent when a broad heterogeneous population is studied, such as a general clinic population. When a more homogeneous population is studied—specifically, a highly depressed population, such as a sample of inpatient suicide ideators or highly d—ssed outpatients—the Beck Hopelessness Scale (BHS; Beck, Weissman, Lester, & Trexler, 1974) and the Beck Self-Concept Test (BST; Beck, Steer, Epstein, & Brown, 1990) are better correlates of suicidal intent.

Scale for Suicide Ideation

The Scale for Suicide Ideation (SSI; Beck, Kovacs, & Weissman, 1979) assesses the degree to which someone is currently thinking about suicide. Nineteen items are answered in a structured clinical interview, with ratings made on a 3-point scale. Items include the frequency and duration of and ability to control suicidal wishes, characteristics of a contemplated attempt (e.g., preparations or final acts), the purpose of a contemplated attempt, availability and opportunity of method, and the relative strengths of the person's wish to live and wish to die. Studies of reliability, construct validity, and concurrent validity have demonstrated the usefulness of the SSI (Beck, Kovacs, & Weissman, 1979).

Suicide Intent Scale

The Suicide Intent Scale (SIS; Beck, Schuyler, & Herman, 1974) is a 15-item structured clinical interview with a 3-point rating scale that assesses the severity of the person's psychological intent to die at the time of a recent suicide attempt. Items include pertinent aspects of the attempter's thoughts and behavior before, during, and after the suicidal act, including purpose of the attempt, attitudes toward living and dying, and relationship of drug or alcohol intake (when drugs are not the method employed) to the attempt. The SIS has been consistently validated as a measure of seriousness of intent of a suicide attempt (Beck, Schuyler, & Herman, 1974; Beck, Kovacs, & Weissman, 1975; Beck & Lester, 1976; R. W. Beck, Morris, & Beck, 1974; Minkoff, Bergman, Beck, & Beck, 1973; Silver, Bohnert, Beck, & Marcus, 1971).

Although the SIS has largely been used as a dependent variable, Pallis, Gibbons, and Pierce (1984) employed this measure to predict eventual suicide. A modified SIS was found to improve the predictability of estimating suicide risk when combined with two additional measures developed by Pallis and colleagues. More recently, Beck and Steer (1989) found that the Precautions subscale of the SIS was predictive of eventual suicide among suicide attempters.

Beck Hopelessness Scale

The BHS (Beck, Weissman, et al., 1974) is a 20-item true–false, self-report questionnaire that assesses the degree of pessimism or negative view of the future held by the respondent. The psychometric properties of the BHS have been presented by Beck, Kovacs, and Weissman (1975). Correlations ranging from .56 to .68 between the BHS and the BDI have been reported in studies of hospitalized suicide attempters (Nekanda-Trepka, Bishop, & Blackburn, 1983) and depressed patients (Beck, Kovacs, and Weissman 1975).

Clinicians' ratings of hopelessness have also been demonstrated to be useful predictors of eventual suicide (Fawcett et al., 1987; Drake & Cotton, 1986; Beck, Brown, & Steer, 1989). In an examination of concordance between the self-report BHS and the clinical rating, the Clinician's Hopelessness Scale (CHS; Beck, Weissman, et al., 1974), the CHS was found to be comparable to the BHS in terms of sensitivity (the proportion of suicide attempters correctly identified as eventually committing suicide) for both inpatients and outpatients. However, the specificity rate (the proportion of nonsuiciders identified as not committing suicide) of the CHS was lower than that of the BHS for inpatients and outpatients (Beck et al., 1989).

CLINICAL FACTORS

Suicide risk for an individual (as opposed to a population) is more strongly related to clinical and proximate risk factors than to demographic characteristics. Clinical factors include presence of a psychiatric disorder, intensity of suicide ideation, level of suicide intent, degree of hopelessness, history of previous suicide attempts, family history of suicide, and abuse of alcohol or other drugs. Proximate risk factors include access to lethal means, knowledge of lethal dosage when drugs are used, precautions against discovery during previous attempts, correct conception of the probability of medical rescuability after an attempt, and the presence of people who might intervene to save the person's life after a suicide attempt.

Alcohol consumption at the time of a suicide attempt adds to risk. Large numbers of suicides studied by Morris, Kovacs, Beck, and Wolffe (1970) showed blood ethanol levels above the legal definition of intoxication, suggesting that individuals with suicidal intentions are more likely to act under the influence of alcohol. Further evidence of the association between alcohol intake and suicidal action has been presented by Chiles, Strosahl, Cowden, Graham, and Linehan (1986). Suicide attempters were found to be more likely than other psychiatric patients to have used alcohol in the 24 hours before hospitalization. Alcohol use may be considered both an important epidemiological risk factor and a clinical one. The association between alcoholism and suicide has long been noted, and a recent longitudinal study (Beck & Steer, 1989) found that a diagnosis of alcoholism at the time of index admission increased the risk of eventual suicide at least five times. Even if a person is not an alcoholic, use of alcohol at the time of suicidal ideation may increase the probability of poor judgment, lack of control, and mood changes.

COGNITIVE FACTORS AND SUICIDAL RISK
Hopelessness

Hopelessness may be conceptualized as a state of negative expectancies. A number of studies have demonstrated its role in suicide intent and behavior. Lester, Beck, and Mitchell (1979) found that depression and hopelessness were related to a wish to die. Nekanda-Trepka et al. (1983) found that, among psychiatric outpatients, hopelessness was associated with increases in suicidal wishes. Fawcett et al. (1987) reported hopelessness, loss of pleasure or interest, and mood fluctuations as factors which discrminated those who committed suicide from those who did not.

Hopelessness has been found to be more strongly related to suicidal intent than depression per se has been for both suicide ideators (Bedrosian & Beck, 1979; Wetzel, Margulies, Davis, & Karam, 1980) and suicide attempters (Beck, Kovacs, and Weissman, 1975; Beck, Weissman, & Kovacs, 1976; Dyer & Kreitman, 1984; Goldney, 1979; Minkoff et al., 1973; Petrie & Chamberlain, 1983; Weissman, Beck, & Kovacs, 1979; Wetzel, 1976a). A study of depressed and nondepressed (schizophrenic) patients found that even nondepressed patients who had high levels of hopelessness had high levels of suicide intent (Minkoff et al. 1973). Kovacs, Beck, and Weissman (1975) found that hopelessness was a better indicator of current suicidal ideation among suicide attempters than depression was; and Beck, Kovacs, and Weissman (1975) reported that among suicide attempters, hopelessness mediated the relationship between depression and suicide intent. Hopelessness has also been found to play a major role in the relationship between alcoholism and suicide attempts (Beck et al., 1976) and is a more powerful determinant of suicide intent among drug abusers than is either depression (Emery, Steer, & Beck, 1981) or drug use per se (Weissman et al. 1979).

Hopelessness as a suicide risk factor has been most strongly supported by prospective studies of inpatients and outpatients (Beck, Brown, Berchick, Stewart, & Steer, 1990; Beck et al., 1989; Beck, Steer, Kovacs, & Garrison, 1985; Drake & Cotton, 1986; Fawcett et al., 1987). Longitudinal work by Beck and associates (Beck et al., 1985, 1989, 1990) demonstrates the predictive utility of hopelessness. In addition to self-report ratings of hopelessness, clinicians' ratings of hopelessness have also been found to be predictive of eventual suicide (Beck et al., 1989; Drake & Cotton, 1986; Fawcett et al., 1987).

Longitudinal research conducted over a 10-year period found that, for inpatients initially hospitalized for suicidal *ideation*, BHS scores at index hospitalization were strong predictors of eventual suicide. Of the 165 patients studied, 11 eventually committed suicide. A cutoff score of 9 on the BHS distinguished between suicide completers and noncompleters. Only 1 (9.1%) of the completers had obtained a score less than 9; the other 10 (90.9%) of the completers had obtained a score of 9 or more (Beck et al., 1985, 1989). Alcohol and drug abuse histories did not differentiate between completers and noncompleters in this sample. Furthermore, the BDI total score was not predictive of eventual suicide, and length of follow-up was not related to detecting more eventual suicides.

In a replication study of 1,958 psychiatric outpatients, the mean BHS score of those eventually killing themselves was significantly higher than that of those not committing suicide. Again, a BHS cutoff score of 9 or more identified 16 (94.2%) of the 17 eventual suicides. The high-risk group identified by this cutoff score was 11 times more likely to complete suicide than the rest of the outpatients were (Beck et al., 1990).

The BHS had less predictive validity in a study of suicide *attempters* (Beck & Steer, 1989). In that study, a diagnosis of alcoholism predicted eventual suicide. Hopelessness, however, was assessed *after* the suicide attempt. Some patients actually experience an uplift in mood following an unsuccessful suicide attempt (Stengel, 1964; Maris, 1981). Dyer and Kreitman (1984) found hopelesssness to be highest and most strongly related to suicidal intent when attempters were asked to describe the severity of their hopelessness just before the attempt as compared to following the attempt. In addition, the sample of ideators who eventually committed suicide (Beck et al., 1985) had significantly higher BHS scores than the group of suicide attempters who eventually committed suicide (Beck & Steer, 1989). Thus, the predictive valiadity of the BHS in this study may not have been adequately assessed because of the timing of its administration.

According to Beck's cognitive theory, hopelessness can be conceptualized as a stable schema incorporating negative expectations. During psychiatric distress, such as a depressive episode, hopelessness escalates and then subsides with the course of the illness. The level of hopelessness in one episode is indicative of the level of hopelessness in subsequent episodes (Beck, 1988). Thus, hopelessness is a potentially recurring state of negative expectancies. For some individuals, hopelessness appears to have trait characteristics (Beck, 1987). These chronically hopeless individuals often have alcoholism, personality problems, and other difficulties that predispose them to poor interpersonal interactions. Their low self-concept or negative view of self is often reinforced by society. For them, the schemas generating hopelessness are quite resistant to change. Such individuals may be chronically prone to suicidal behavior (Beck, 1987; Beck et al., 1990).

Despite the chronicity of hopelessness in some types of individuals, hopelessness among most depressed patients is a risk factor that can be reduced. Depressed patients treated with cognitive therapy showed a more rapid reduction in hopelessness than did a group treated with antidepressant medication (Rush, Beck, Kovacs, Weissenburger, & Hollon, 1982).

Other Cognitive Factors in Suicide Risk

The past decade has seen increasing interest in and effort directed toward identifying cognitive characteristics of suicidal individuals. Cognitive differences have been demonstrated to exist between suicidal and nonsuicidal persons even when level of depression and degree of pathology have been controlled for. In addition to hopelessness, the cognitive characteristics of suicidal persons include dysfunctional assumptions (Bonner & Rich, 1987; Ellis & Ratliff, 1986), dichotomous thinking and cognitive rigidity (Neuringer & Lettieri, 1971; Patsiokas, Clum, & Luscomb, 1979), poor problem-solving ability (Cohen-Sandler & Berman, 1982; Levenson, 1974; Linehan, Camper, Chiles, Strosahl, & Shearin, 1987; McLeavey, Daly, Murray, O'Riodan, & Taylor, 1987; Orbach, Rosenheim, & Hary, 1987; Schotte & Clum, 1987), and negative self-concept (Beck & Stewart, 1989). The cognitive matrix of negative expectations generating hopelessness may interact with these cognitive deficits, creating a mindset in which suicide appears to be the only recourse to insoluble problems. Specific cognitive deficits related to suicidal behavior are described below.

Dysfunctional Assumptions

Ellis and Ratliff (1986) administered a battery of cognitive inventories to a group of suicide attempters and to a group of equally depressed nonsuicidal psychiatric patients. The suicide attempters were found to score higher in terms of irrational beliefs, depressogenic attitudes, and hopelessness than the nonsuicidal patients. Bonner and Rich (1987) found that dysfunctional assumptions played an important role in predicting the suicidal ideation of college students. Other factors operating in this college sample were emotional alienation and deficient adaptive resources, such as family cohesion and reasons for living. The role of reasons for living is noteworthy. Linehan, Goodstein, Nielsen, and Chiles (1983) similarly found that those who thought of and attempted suicide stated fewer reasons for living than did psychiatric and normal controls, even when levels of stress were held constant. Thus, the presence of dysfunctional assumptions and the absence of positive reasons for living may both be considered cognitive variables or attitudes influencing suicidal behavior. Cognitive distortions may intensify stress, whereas lack of adaptive resources may leave the individual unprepared to cope (Bonner & Rich, 1987).

Dichotomous Thinking

Dichotomous or "all-or-nothing" thinking is a cognitive distortion characteristic of depression and present in other disorders (see Beck, Rush, Shaw, & Emery, 1979, for a review of cognitive distortions). Currently, it is the only cognitive distortion specifically linked to suicidal ideation and behavior, although any systematic errors in logic may contribute to the mental gridlock of suicide.

Early studies by Neuringer (1961, 1967, 1968) found that suicidal individuals rated certain concepts such as life and death more extremely than did nonsuicidal ones on semantic differential tests. Differential ratings were attributed to extremeness as a cognitive style. Later work (Neuringer & Lettieri, 1971) supported the notion of extremeness as a cognitive style, for the tendency persisted over time. Wetzel (1976b), however, has interpreted differences on semantic differential ratings as reflecting attitudes toward specific concepts (i.e., life, death, self) rather than a generalized style of dichotomous thinking.

Dichotomous thinking categorizes experience into one of two polar extremes and is a form of rigid thinking. It has therefore been subsumed under "cognitive rigidity" in some research.

Problem-Solving Deficits

Several studies have found that rigid or dichotomous thinking distinguishes suicide ideators and/or suicide attempters from both normal and psychiatric control groups. Initially, cognitive rigidity was measured by tests of impersonal tasks, such as map reading, arithmetic, and word association. More recently, interpersonal problem solving ("social cognition") has been the research focus, for the two may be inherently different (Arffa, 1983; Schotte & Clum, 1982). Interpersonal problem solving may also be more clinically relevant, for suicide attempters report greater difficulty with interpersonal problems than do suicide ideators, nonsuicidal psychiatric patients, and general population controls (Linehan, Chiles, Egan, Devine, & Laffaw, 1986).

Suicidal adults and children have been found to demonstrate a limited ability to find solutions to impersonal problems. They are less able to produce new ideas and think flexibly (Orbach et al., 1987; Patsiokas et al., 1979) or to consider alternatives (Cohen-Sandler & Berman, 1982; Levenson, 1974), and they may persist in ineffective problem solving even when a more effective strategy is presented to them (Levenson & Neuringer, 1971). In regard to interpersonal problem solving, suicidal children appear less able to generate alternatives to life-and-death dilemmas portrayed in stories than are normal or chronically ill children (Orbach et al., 1987). They are also less able than nonsuicidal children to generate active cognitive coping strategies in the face of stressful life events (Asarnow, Carlson, & Guthrie, 1987). Active cognitive coping strategies include self-comforting statements and instrumental problem solving.

Lack of active problem solving has also been found among suicide attempters as compared to suicide ideators and nonsuicidal medical patients (Linehan et al., 1987). The suicide attempters in this study were found to employ a passive approach to interpersonal problem solving, either letting problems solve themselves or enlisting someone else to arrive at a solution. In this sample, the level of expectancy that suicide would effectively solve one's problems was associated with higher suicidal intent.

Schotte and Clum (1987) found that inpatients who had expressed suicide ideation or had made suicide attempts lacked problem solving skills for both impersonal and interpersonal tasks, as compared to nonsuicidal patients. They described these problem solving skills deficits in terms of D'Zurilla and Goldfried's (1971) model of problem solving: (1) Suicidal individuals lack an appropriate general orientation to problems; (2) they have difficulty generating potential alternative solutions to problems once the problems have been identified; (3) they tend to focus on potential negative consequences of implementing the alternatives generated; and (4) they do not adequately implement viable alternatives (Schotte & Clum 1987, p. 53)

McLeavey et al. (1987) similarly found a number of problem-solving deficits among self-poisoning patients compared to nonsuicidal patients and nonpatient controls. These deficits were noted on both impersonal and interpersonal problem solving measures, but were more striking on measures with greater interpersonal content. The suicide attempters were less able to conceptualize the means of solving a problem than were either of the other two groups. They were less capable of generating alternative solutions and less able to anticipate consequences of various courses of action. A self-report measure to assess how well subjects were dealing with problems in their own lives found that the suicidal group did significantly worse than either control group. These authors concluded that suicide attempters are less flexible in social cognition than are other psychiatric patients or normal individuals. They argued that repetition of suicide attempts becomes likely as this type of solution is established as part of such a limited repertoire.

Finally, a study by Beck and Brown (1987) demonstrated the relationship between impaired problem solving and suicidal intent. This study of 48 pyschiatric outpatients found that the combination of the BDI, the BHS, and the Problem-Solving Scale (a self-report measure of problem solving ability) accounted for 43% of the variation in suicide intent.

View of Suicide as a "Desirable" Solution

Beck, Rush, et al. (1979) reported the clinical observation that those prone to suicide have a unique cognitive deficit in solving interpersonal problems:

When their usual solutions do not work, they become paralyzed and view suicide as a way out. Suicide appears as a relief and an escape from problems. Recent research supports the notion that attraction to death may be a cognitive characteristic of suicidal individuals. Linehan et al. (1987) found that belief in suicide as a solution to interpersonal problems was related to higher levels of suicide intent. More directly, Orbach et al. (1987) found that the interaction of inability to generate solutions to life-and-death dilemmas and attraction to death was unique to suicidal children. Among chronically ill and normal children, there was no interaction between ability to generate alternatives and attraction to death. In this study, the combination of cognitive rigidity and attraction to death posed a risk of suicide.

Models of Suicidal Behavior

Explanatory models of suicidal behavior have been developed that incorporate factors found to correlate independently with suicidal ideation and behavior. These include the cognitive factors discussed above.

Clum and his colleagues (Clum, Patsiokas, & Luscomb, 1979; Schotte & Clum, 1982) developed a model of suicidal behavior in which poor problem solving mediates between life stress and suicide attempts. In a college student sample of suicide ideators, it was found that at low levels of suicidal ideation, depression was the best predictor of suicide intent. At high levels of suicide ideation, hopelessness was the best predictor of intent. Clum and his colleagues hypothesized that the combination of life stress and poor problem solving ability leads to hopelessness, which in turn discourages the person from trying to solve problems. A test of this model (Schotte & Clum 1987) with suicidal psychiatric patients found no relationship between hopelessness and levels of interpersonal problem solving skill, indicating that hopelessness and problem solving deficits are independent factors in suicide risk.

Bonner and Rich (1987), on the basis of results from a college student sample, developed a model in which alienation, cognitive distortions, and deficient reasons for living predispose an individual to suicidal behavior, whereas stress and increased hopelessness are more immediate precipitants to a suicide attempt. A follow-up study (Rich & Bonner, 1987) validated the roles of these factors in self-predicted future suicide probability.

The Relationship of Hopelessness to Problem-Solving Deficits

The exact nature of the relationship between hopelessness and other cognitive characteristics in suicide is not clear. Some researchers have considered hopelessness to be a consequence of dichotomous thinking, cognitive rigidity, and problem-solving deficits (Ellis, 1987; Patsiokas & Clum, 1985), and in a study by Patsiokas and Clum (1985), problem-solving training decreased hopelessness among suicide attempters. Subsequent research, however, has found hopelessness to be unrelated to problem-solving skill (McLeavey et al., 1987; Schotte & Clum, 1987), suggesting that hopelessness is an independent risk factor that interacts with and may exacerbate other cognitive vulnerabilities.

Beck's (1987) longitudinal research on suicide ideators and suicide attempt "repeaters" helps articulate the relationship between hopelessness and problem solving skills. The suicide ideators studied were primarily patients hospitalized for depression. Their suicidal ideation and hopelessness were present during their clinical episodes of depression, but were resolved when the depression remitted. This group demonstrated impaired problem-solving skills when depressed, but regained their abilities when the depression resolved completely. In this group, problem-solving deficits were state-dependent.

The suicide attempt "repeaters," however, appeared much more trait-like in their problem-solving deficits. This group was made up of individuals suffering from alcoholism, personality disorders, and antisocial behavior problems. This group distorted reality, but their negative views of themselves were also reinforced by society. Moreover, their negative perceptions of themselves persisted between suicidal crises, although not always at the same level of intensity. Although some depressive symptoms were present, suicide attempts were usually reactions to very recent life events. This group was further characterized by cognitive rigidity, impulsivity, and poor problem-solving ability, all of which persisted between suicidal episodes. At the time of suicidal crisis, both groups had elevated levels of hopelessness and showed problem-solving deficits, but these characteristics had different "causes."

In addition, a recent study of outpatients who ultimately killed themselves found that negative self-concept contributed to suicide risk, independently of depression and hopelessness (Beck & Stewart, 1988). On the basis of these findings, it appears that elevated levels of hopelessness and negative self-concept are acute risk factors when they accompany a major depression. In other cases, they represent more chronic risk factors. Nevertheless, hopelessness and self-concept can be treated by psychotherapeutic (Rush et al., 1982) and pharmacological means.

DISCUSSION OF THE FIVE CASE EXAMPLES

In his review of the background and clinical characteristics relevant to estimating suicide risk, Hawton (1987) arrived at the following factors: presence of a psychiatric disorder, hopelessness, alcoholism, drug abuse, recent loss of a close interpersonal relationship, poor health, recent bereavement, a history of familial suicide, unemployment, sex, age, previous attempts, marital status, and the lethality of the method employed. The five clinical cases presented in Chapter 12 and discussed throughout this volume all illustrate some of these risk factors.

Heather B, the 13-year-old girl, was exhibiting warning signs in her behavior (e.g., drop in grades, isolation, rebellion), cognitions (self-hate, suicidal ideation, personal writings with self-destructive themes, low self-confidence), and affect (anhedonia, sadness, depression, sense of loss, aimlessness). She had had a traumatic loss in the death of her father, and had experienced familial instability since. Heather would probably score low on the BST (Beck et al., 1990), which is related to suicidal ideation. Hopelessness was apparent in her writings. Regardless of her history of being "provocative," we would recommend taking Heather's suicidal ideation and hints of self-injury seriously, and assessing these factors with the BHS and the SSI.

Ralph F, the 16-year-old boy, had several clinical risk factors for suicide: depression, hopelessness, persistent suicidal ideation over which he had little control, and alcohol abuse. In addition, he had a family history of suicide attempts, health problems, immediate and severe family stressors, and poor problem solving (as reflected by his conscious solution of turning his anger at his grandfather on himself). His auditory hallucinations were also a danger, as was his "obsession with the notion of suicide." Furthermore, his "considerable ambivalence about suicide" would not reduce his risk, for Kovacs and Beck (1977) found that 50% of the suicide attempters studied had, at the time of their attempts, wanted both to live and to die.

Levy and Deykin (1989) reported that in a nonclinical population of 16- to 19-year-olds, major depression and substance abuse were independent and interactive risk factors for suicidal ideation and attempts, and that substance abuse had an especially deleterious effect on males. They also found that a prolonged desire to be dead was a more specific risk factor for a suicide attempt than was a thought of suicide. Ralph's profile suggests that concern for a lethal attempt would be justified, according to these findings. His case also illustrates Bonner and Rich's (1987) model of the effects of social alienation and deficient adaptive resources on suicidal ideation.

John Z, the 39-year-old man, also had severe depression, immediate stressors, negative self-concept, and a family history of suicide attempts. He reported two attempts himself, and these reports would certainly need to be assessed more closely. Lester, Beck, and Narrett (1978) reported data indicating that suicide intent increases with successive suicide attempts. We would recommend assessing John with the SIS, as well as the BHS and the SSI. John also demonstrated impaired problem solving when he enrolled in a graduate program without anticipating the length of the degree program or considering whether his goals would be served by this alternative.

Faye C, the 49-year-old woman, was vulnerable to suicidal ideation because of her depression and psychosis. According to her case history, she was capable of being a reliable informant, and thus could complete the BHS and SSI.

José G, the 64-year-old man, had the demographic risk factors of age, sex, unemployment, alcoholism, and poor health. Some of these characteristics could also be conceptualized as clinical factors, for they were losses: job loss, the loss of health, and the loss of pleasure in recreational hunting. He would score high on the BDI and the BHS, and should be given the SSI as well.

In all these cases, hopelessness and self-concept would be better indicators of suicide risk than depression alone. As mentioned above, in a highly depressed group the BHS and BST are more useful; the BDI is useful as a screening device in a heterogeneous population. In addition, Schotte and Clum (1982) have reported that the relative importance of hopelessness to depression increases as intent increases. Measures of self-concept and problem-solving ability would also facilitate clinical judgment in these cases: They not only would aid in the prediction of suicide risk, but would identify targets for therapeutic intervention. One of the most striking findings of the clinical research is that cognitive characteristics predisposing an individual to suicidal ideation and behavior often persist between suicidal episodes. They should be addressed directly and systematically in psychotherapy, not just at the time of crisis.

REFERENCES

Arffa, S. (1983). Cognition and suicide: A methodological review. *Suicide and Life-Threatening Behavior, 13*, 109–122.

Asarnow, J. R., Carlson, G. A., & Guthrie, D. (1987). Coping strategies, self-perceptions, hopelessness, and perceived family environments in depressed and suicidal children. *Journal of Consulting and Clinical Psychology, 55*, 361–366.

Beck, A. T. (1964). Thinking and depression: 1.Idiosyncratic content and cognitive distortions. *Archives of General Psychiatry, 9*, 324–333.

Beck, A. T. (1972) *Depression: Causes and Treatment. Philadelphia: University of Pennsylvania Press.* (Originally published as *Depression: Clinical, experimental, and theoretical aspects.* NY: Harper & Row, 1967.)

Beck, A. T. (1986). Hopelessness as a predictor of eventual suicide. *Annals of the New York Academy of Sciences, 487*, 90–96.

Beck, A. T. (1987). *Cognitive approaches to hopelessness and suicide.* Paper presented at the annual meeting of the Association for Advancement of Behavior Therapy, Boston.

Beck, A. T. (1988). [Continuity of hopelessness over repeated episodes of depression]. Center for Cognitive Therapy. Unpublished raw data.

Beck, A. T., Beck, R. W. & Kovacs, M. (1975). Classification of suicidal behaviors: I. Quantifying intent and medical lethality. *American Journal of Psychiatry, 132*, 285–287.

Beck, A. T. & Brown, G. (1987). *Incremental validity of the problem-solving Scale in the prediction of suicide intent.* Poster session presented at the Department of Psychiatry, University of Pennsylvania.

Beck, A. T., Brown, G., Berchick, R. J., Stewart, B. L., & Steer, R. A. (1990). Relationship between hopelessness and ultimate suicide: A replication with psychiatric outpatients. *American Journal of Psychiatry, 147*(2), 190–195.

Beck, A. T., Brown, G., & Steer, R. A. (1989). Prediction of eventual suicide in psychiatric inpatients by clinical ratings of hopelessness. *Journal of Consulting and Clinical Psychology, 57*(2), 309–310.

Beck, A. T., Davis, J. H., Frederick, C. J., Perlin, S., Pokorny, A. D., Schulman, R. E., Seiden, R. H., & Wittlin, B. J. (1973). Classification and nomenclature. In H. L. P. Resnik & B. C. Hathorne (Eds.), *Suicide prevention in the seventies.* (DHEW Publication No. HSM 72-9054, pp. 7–12). Washington, DC: U.S. Government Printing Office.

Beck, A. T., Kovacs, M., & Weissman, A. (1975). Hopelessness and suicidal behavior: An overview. *Journal of the American Medical Association, 234*(11), 1146–1149.

Beck, A. T., Kovacs, M. & Weissman, A. (1979). Assessment of suicidal intention: The Scale for Suicide Ideation. *Journal of Consulting and Clinical Psychology, 47*(2), 343–352.

Beck, A. T., & Lester, D. (1976). Components of suicidal intent in completed and attempted suicides. *Journal of Psychology, 92*, 35–38.

Beck, A. T., Rush, A. J., Shaw, B., & Emery, G. (1979). *Cognitive therapy of depression.* New York: Guilford Press.

Beck, A. T., Schuyler, D., & Herman, I. (1974). Development of suicidal intent scales. In A. T. Beck, H. C. P. Resnik, & D. J. Lettieri (Eds.), *The prediction of suicide* (pp. 45–56). Bowie, MD: Charles Press.

Beck, A. T., & Steer, R. A. (1987). *Manual for the revised Beck Depression Inventory.* San Antonio, TX: Psychological Corporation.

Beck, A. T., & Steer, R. A. (1989). Clinical predictors of eventual suicide: A 5- to 10-year prospective study of suicide attempters. *Journal of Affective Disorders, 17*, 203–209.

Beck, A. T., Steer, R. A., Epstein, N., & Brown, G. (1990). The Beck Self-Concept Test. *Psychological Assessment: A Journal of Consulting and Clinical Psychology, 2*(2), 191–197.

Beck, A. T., Steer, R. A., Kovacs, M., & Garrison, B. (1985). Hopelessness and eventual suicide: A ten-year prospective study of patients hospitalized with suicidal ideation. *American Journal of Psychiatry, 142*(5), 559–563.

Beck, A. T., & Stewart, B. (1989). *The self-concept as a risk factor in patients who kill themselves.* Unpublished manuscript.

Beck, A. T., Weissman, A., & Kovacs, M. (1976). Alcoholism, hopelessness and suicidal behavior. *Journal of Studies on Alcohol, 37*(1), 66–77.

Beck, A. T., Weissman, A., Lester, D., & Trexler, L.(1974). The measurement of pessimism: The Hopelessness Scale. *Journal of Consulting and Clinical Psychology, 42*, 861–865.

Beck, R. W., Morris, J. B., & Beck, A. T. (1974). Cross-validation of the Suicide Intent Scale. *Psychological Reports, 34*, 445–446.

Bedrosian, R. C., & Beck, A. T. (1979). Cogntive aspects of suicidal behavior. *Suicide and Life-Threatening Behavior, 9*(2), 87–96.

Bonner, R. L., & Rich, A. R. (1987). Toward a predictive model of suicidal ideation and behavior: Some preliminary data in college students. *Suicide and Life-Treatening Behavior, 17*, 50–63.

Chiles, J. A., Strosahl, K., Cowden, L., Graham, R., & Linehan, M. (1986). The 24 hours before hospitalization: Factors related to suicide attempting. *Suicide and Life-Threatening Behavior, 16*, 335–342.

Clum, G. A., Patsiokas, A. T., & Luscomb, R. L. (1979). Empirically based comprehensive treatment program for parasuicide. *Journal of Consulting and Clinical Psychology, 47*, 937–945.

Cohen-Sandler, R. & Berman, A. L. (1982). *Training suicidal children to problem-solve in nonsuicidal ways.* Paper presented at the annual meeting of the American Association of Suicidology, New York.

Drake, R. E., & Cotton, P. G. (1986). Depression, hopelessness, and suicide in chronic schizophrenia. *British Journal of Psychiatry, 148*, 554–559.

Dyer, J. A. T., & Kreitman, N. (1984). Hopelessness, depression and suicidal intent in parasuicide. *British Journal of Psychiatry, 144*, 127–133.

D'Zurilla, T. J., & Goldfried, M. R. (1971). Problem- solving and behavior modification. *Journal of Abnormal Psychology, 78*, 107–126.

Ellis, T. E. (1987). A cognitive approach to treating the suicidal client. In P. A. Keller & L. G. Ritt (Eds.), *Innovations in clinical practice: A sourcebook* (pp. 93–107). Sarasota, FL: Professional Resource Exchange.

Ellis, T. E., & Ratliff, K. G. (1986). Cognitive characteristics of suicidal and nonsuicidal psychiatric patients. *Cognitive Therapy and Research, 10*, 625–634.

Emery, G. D., Steer, R.A., & Beck, A. T. (1981). Depression, hopelessness and suicidal intent among heroin addicts. *International Journal of the Addictions, 16*(3), 425–429.

Fawcett, J., Schefter, W., Clark, D., Hedeker, D., Gibbons, R., & Coryell, W. (1987). Clinical predictors of suicide in patients with major affective disorder: A controlled prospective study. *American Journal of Psychiatry, 144*, 35–40.

Goldney, R. D. (1979). *Attempted suicide: correlates of lethality.* Unpublished doctoral dissertation. University of Adelaide, Australia.

Hawton, K. (1987). Assessment of suicide risk. *British Journal of Psychiatry, 150*, 145–153.

Kovacs, M., & Beck, A. T. (1977). The wish to die and the wish to live in attempted suicides. *Journal of Clinical Psychology, 33*, 361–365.

Kovacs, M., Beck, A. T., & Weissman, A. (1975). Hopelessness: An indicator of suicidal risk. *Suicide and Life-Threatening Behavior, 5*(2), 98–103.

Lester, D., Beck, A. T., & Mitchell, B. (1979). Extrapolation from attempted suicides to completed suicides: A test. *Journal of Abormal Psychology, 88*, 78–80.

Lester, D., Beck, A. T., & Narrett, S. (1978). Suicidal intent in successive suicidal actions. *Psychological Reports, 43*, 110.

Levenson, M. (1974). Cognitive characteristics of suicide risk. In C. Neuringer (Ed.),

Psychological assessment of suicide risk (pp. 150–163). Springfield, IL: Charles C Thomas.

Levenson, M., & Neuringer, C. (1971). Problem-solving behavior in suicidal adolescents. *Journal of Consulting and Clinical Psychology, 37,* 433–436.

Levy, J. C., & Deykin, E. Y. (1989). Suicidality, depression, and substance abuse in adolescence. *American Journal of Psychiatry, 146*(11), 1462–1467.

Linehan, M. M., Camper, P. Chiles, J., Strosahl, K., & Shearin, E. (1987). Interpersonal problem solving and parasuicide. Cognitive Therapy and Research, *11,* 1–12.

Linehan, M. M., Chiles, J. A., Egan, K. J., Devine, R. H., & Laffaw, J. A. (1986). Presenting problems of parasuicides versus suicide ideators and nonsuicidal psychiatric patients. *Journal of Consulting and Clinical Psychology, 54,* 880–881.

Linehan, M. M., Goodstein, J. L., Nielsen, S. L., & Chiles, J. A. (1983). Reasons for staying alive when you are thinking of killing yourself: The Reasons for Living Inventory. *Journal of Consulting and Clinical Psychology, 51,* 276–286.

Maris, R. W. (1981). *Pathways to suicide: A survey of self-destructive behaviors.* Baltimore: Johns Hopkins University Press.

McLeavey, B. C., Daly, R. J., Murray, C. M., O'Riodan, J., & Taylor, M. (1987). Interpersonal problem-solving deficits in self-poisoning patients. *Suicide and Life-Threatening Behavior, 17,* 33–49.

Minkoff, K., Bergman, E., Beck, A. T., & Beck, R. W. (1973). Hopelessness, depression, and attempted suicide. *American Journal of Psychiatry, 130*(4), 455–459.

Morris, J. B., Kovacs, M., Beck, A. T., & Wolffe, A. (1970). Notes towards an epidemiology of urban suicide. *Comprehensive Psychiatry, 127,* 764–770.

Nekanda-Trepka, C. J. S., Bishop, S., & Blackburn, I. M. (1983). Hopelessness and depression. *British Journal of Clinical Psychology, 22,* 49–60.

Neuringer, C. (1961). Dichotomous evaluations in suicidal individuals. *Journal of Consulting Psychology, 25,* 445–449.

Neuringer, C. (1967). The cognitive organization of meaning in suicidal individuals. *Journal of General Psychology, 76,* 91–100.

Neuringer, C. (1968). Divergencies between attitudes towards life and death among suicidal, psychosomatic, and normal hospitalized patients. *Journal of Consulting and Clinical Psychology, 32,* 59–63.

Neuringer, C., & Lettieri, D. J. (1971). Cognition, attitude, and affect in suicidal individuals. *Suicide and Life-Threatening Behavior, 1,* 106–124.

Orbach, I., Rosenheim, E., & Hary, E. (1987). some aspects of cognitive functioning in suicidal children. *Journal of the American Academy of Child and Adolescent Psychiatry, 26*(2), 181–185.

Pallis, J. J., Gibons, J. S., & Pierce, D. W. (1984). Estimating suicidal risk among attempted suicides: II. Efficacy of predictive scales after the attempt. *British Journal of Psychiatry, 144,* 139–148.

Patsiokas, A. T., & Clum, G. A. (1985). Effects of psychotherapeutic strategies in the treatment of suicide attempters. *Psychotherapy, 22,* 281–290.

Patsiokas, A. T., Clum, G. A., & Luscomb, R. L. (1979). Cognitive characteristics of suicide attempters. *Journal of Consulting and Clinical Psychology, 47,* 478–484.

Petrie, K., & Chamberlain, K. (1983). Hopelessness and social desirability as moderator variables in predicting suicidal behavior. *Journal of Consulting and Clinical Psychology, 51*, 485–487.

Rich, A. R., & Bonner, R. L. (1987). Concurrent validity of a stress vulnerability model of suicidal ideation and behavior: A follow-up study. *Suicide and Life-Threatening Behavior, 17*(4), 265–270.

Rush, A. J., Beck, A. T., Kovacs, M., Weissenburger, J., & Hollon, S. (1982). Comparison of the differential effects of cognitive therapy and pharmacotherapy on hopelessness and self-concept. *American Journal of Psychiatry, 139*, 862–866.

Schotte, D. E., & Clum, G. A. (1982). Suicide ideation in a college population: A test of a model. *Journal of Consulting and Clinical Psychology, 50*, 690–696.

Schotte, D. E., & Clum, G. A. (1987). Problem-solving skills in suicidal psychiatric patients. *Journal of Consulting and Clinical Psychology, 55*, 49–54.

Silver, M. A., Bohnert, M., Beck, A. T., & Marcus, D. (1971). Relation of depression of attempted suicide and seriousness of intent. *Archives of General Psychiatry, 25*, 573–576.

Stengel, E. (1964). *Suicide and attempted suicide.* Harmondsworth, England: Penguin.

Weissman, A., Beck, A. T., & Kovacs, M. (1979). Drug abuse, hopelessness, and suicidal behavior. *International Journal of the Addictions, 14*, 451–464.

Wetzel, R. D. (1976a). Hopelessness, depression and suicide intent. *Archives of General Psychiatry, 33*, 1069–1073.

Wetzel, R. D. (1976b). Semantic differential ratings of concepts and suicide intent. *Journal of Clinical Psychology, 32*, 4–13.

Wetzel, R. D., Margulies, T., Davis, R., & Karam, E. (1980). Hopelessness, depression, and suicide intent. *Journal of Clinical Psychology, 41*, 159–160.

CHAPTER 23

Demographic Predictors of Suicide

Carol Z. Garrison, Ph.D.
University of South Carolina

Suicide is currently a serious public health problem in the United States. In 1987 alone (the most recent year for which national data are available), 30,796 individuals committed suicide (National Center for Health Statistics [NCHS], 1990). This represents a rate of 12.7 completed suicides per 100,000 population. Suicide is the eighth leading cause of death, accounting for 1.5% of total deaths when all age groups are combined (NCHS, 1990). Among adolescents and young adults, suicide is an even more prominent cause of death (the second or third leading cause), whose impact is intensified in terms of potential years of life lost, as these younger individuals have lived little of their expected lives. An informed perspective on the issue is gained if one considers the fact that over the last three decades, more expected years of life were lost annually to violent deaths (a category including suicides, homicides, and accidents) than to either cancer or cardiovascular disease (Holinger, 1980). Taken alone, suicide is the fourth leading cause of potential years of life lost.

An international view of the problem can be provided by comparing rates in this country with those published in the World Health Organization's 1982 (WHO's) study of suicide rates (for 1975–1980) in 24 European countries (WHO, Regional Office for Europe, 1982). Had the United States been included in the study, it would have ranked 15th with a suicide rate of 12 per 100,000. In comparison, Hungary had the highest rate (45.2 per 100,000). Czechoslovakia, Denmark, Austria, Finland, Germany, Sweden, and Switzerland were next (in that order), with rates exceeding 24 per 100,000. France, Poland, and Bulgaria had rates above 15 but below 24 per 100,000. The Netherlands, Norway, Scotland, England, and Wales had rates similar to that of the United States (between 10 and 12 per 100,000). Italy, Spain, Northern Ireland, and Greece all reported rates below 5 per 100,000. Since the mid-1980s the overall suicide rate has remained stable in the United States. In the same period rates in England and Wales have decreased, and those in Belgium, The Netherlands, and Ireland have risen precipitously (Diekstra, 1985). Suicide rates vary in other parts of the world as well. They are high in Japan, and although the figures are not too reliable for Third World countries, the rates are thought to be fairly low in these nations within all but the emerging middle and upper classes (Grinspoon, 1986).

PROBLEMS IN REPORTING AND CLASSIFYING SUICIDE DEATHS

This chapter focuses on the observed variation in completed suicide rates in the United States by gender, race, age, method, and geographic location. The emphasis is on current rates. The data reported are based on death certificates for all 50 states and the District of Columbia, as compiled by the NCHS and reported in *Vital Statistics of the United States, 1987: Volume 2* (NCHS, 1990). All deaths classified as falling within the *International Classification of Diseases* (ICD) codes for suicide and self-inflicted injury (E950–E959) are included. These data should be interpreted with consideration of the problems associated with accurately ascertaining and reporting suicide as a cause of death. Suicide is believed to be underreported (Jobes, Berman, & Josselsen, 1986). Several factors contribute to this underreporting: the reluctance to classify deaths as suicide, the nonuniformity of ascertainment procedures, and the variability in the background and training of those responsible for certifying the cause of death.

Hirschfeld and Davidson (1988) have pointed out that a coroner's or medical examiner's determination of suicide necessitates establishing that the death was both self-inflicted and intentional. The latter criterion may not be met if suspicion of suicide is tempered by personal biases, incomplete information, and pressure from the family or community. Conversely, deaths preceded by mental illness or suicidal threats are more likely to be coded as suicide. Uniform criteria for the classification of suicide have not been implemented (see Maris, Chapter 4, this volume). In some cases the certifier may require the presence of an unambiguous suicide note; in other instances a death may be classified as a suicide on the basis of autopsy evidence and interviews with the decedent's family. Litman, Curphey, Shneidman, Farberow, and Tabachnick (1963) have suggested that only about one-third of all completers leave suicide notes. Thus, requiring a note may decrease rates of reported suicide by as much as two-thirds, especially among those with lower educational attainment. Similarly, the thoroughness of a postmortem examination can affect the accuracy with which a death is classified. In 1987, only 52.2% of male and 35.8% of female suicides were autopsied. Autopsies were performed on similar proportions of accidental deaths (51.9% in males and 42.0% in females). Clearly, suicides that are disguised as accidents may not be autopsied, and therefore carry a greater likelihood of being misclassified.

Kleck (1988) reviewed 1980 U.S. mortality statistics to estimate the effect of misclassifying death by suicide. Utilizing data for the 10 most common causes of death by suicide (i.e., firearms, hanging, tranquilizers, barbiturates, car exhaust, other carbon monoxide, falls from man-made structures, drowning, and cutting–piercing instruments), he estimated that if *all* deaths associated with these methods were suicides, the true number of suicides would exceed the official count by 46%. If drowning deaths were excluded from this count, the true number of suicides would be 22% higher. However, given that "overcounting" (i.e., incorrect certification of false suicides) can also occur, Kleck postulated that the net undercount of suicides would not exceed 10% and concluded that there was little hard evidence to support the claims that suicides are seriously underreported in the United States. These findings are in line with those of most other empirical studies, which have indicated that suicide underestimates are small in magnitude and most often result from legal evidentiary requirements rather than naiveté (Clark, 1989).

Brent, Perper, and Allman (1987) specifically looked at the undercounting of suicides among youths by examining coroner's records in Allegheny County, Pennsylvania, for the period from 1960 to 1983. Deaths among 10–19-year-olds that were classified as accidental or due to undetermined causes were reviewed by a panel of experts. Insufficient data prevented classification of 86% of the accidental deaths and 18% of the deaths by undetermined causes. Eight of the accidental deaths and 30 of the deaths by undetermined causes with sufficient data were reclassified as suicides. Although more deaths were reclassified from the earlier years (31% from 1960 to 1962) than from the later years (11% from 1978 to 1983), major increases (exceeding 200%) in the youth suicide rate persisted even after all appropriate adjustments were made. Reclassified subjects were somewhat more apt to have disguised the events or activities that led to their deaths and to have made past indications of suicidal intent.

Wide variations exist regarding the qualifications and procedures for selecting persons responsible for certifying deaths. Monk (1987) has suggested that certifiers who are medically (as opposed to legally) trained may certify more suicides, and that a medical examiner system in which a forensic pathologist certifies sudden and unexpected deaths is likely to be least affected by social or political pressures. Certification procedures differ sufficiently that comparisons of rates in different regions or localities must be made carefully. Furthermore, death certificates provide little information related to the etiology of suicide. They do not list the decedent's socioeconomic status, nor do they provide data regarding history of mental illness, family history of mental illness or suicide, family structure (other than marital status), or history of drug or alcohol use (Centers for Disease Control, 1986). Both of these factors limit the usefulness and generalizability of results based on vital statistics data alone.

VARIATION IN SUICIDE RATES BY RACE AND GENDER

Table 23.1 displays rates of completed suicide by race and gender for 1987. Rates are four to five times higher in men than in women, and approximately two times greater in whites than in nonwhites. The highest rates are found in white males, who comprise 72% of all reported suicides. The lowest rates are in black females, who account for fewer than 1% of all suicides. Although overall rates of suicide have increased over the last 30 years (from 9.8 per 100,000 in 1957 to 12.7 per 100,000 in 1987), the magnitude of the observed male– female differences has been consistent in all but the youngest age group (15-19 years old). Since 1900 the ratio of male to female suicides among adolescents fell to a low of 0.7:1.0 in 1911, then rose to a high of 4.7:1.0 in 1980 (Rosenberg, Smith, Davidson, & Conn, 1987). At the same time the white –nonwhite ratio has declined, in part because of sharp increases in suicide rates among black males and females aged 15-44.

Much speculation has occurred regarding the consistently lower rates of suicide among blacks than among whites. Bush (1976) has contended that intragroup cohesion is a validating force for blacks and buffers them against suicide. Along these same lines, Comer (1973) contends that as a result of their connections with community institutions, such as the black church, black women have lower rates of suicide. The connectedness of blacks to community institutions, such as the Southern black church, has also been offered as an explanation for the lower rates of black suicide in the South than in the North. However, Griffith and Bell (1989) challenge the plausibility of these arguments. They observe that southern blacks have high

TABLE 23.1. Rates of Completed Suicide per 100,000 Population by Race and Gender for 1987

Race–gender group	Number of suicides	Rate per 100,000
White males	22,188	22.1
White females	6,029	5.7
Black males	1,635	11.6
Black females	328	2.1
Other males[a]	449	11.6
Other females[a]	167	2.5

*Note.*The data are from NCHS (1990).
[a]Includes American Indian, Chinese, Hawaiian, Japanese, Filipino, other Asian or Pacific islander, and other.

homicide rates and that it is unclear why "solid black community institutions should selectively protect against suicide and not homicide"(p.2267). Others have suggested that suicide and homicide may be related, in that both may be types of self-inflicted death (Holinger, Offer, & Ostrov, 1987; Cheek, 1985). Homicide is viewed as a more subtle manifestation of self-destructive tendencies and risk-taking behaviors. In this paradigm, homicide may be "victim precipitated and self-inflicted in that some victims may provoke their own deaths by being in the wrong place at the wrong time" (Holinger et al., 1987, p. 215). Such a model gains a limited measure of support from the fact that suicide rates are highest among whites, whereas homicide rates are highest among blacks.

Hispanic ethnicity has not been widely investigated as a risk factor for suicide, because until recently national mortality statistics could not identify deaths of Hispanics as a specific ethnic subgroup. Two fairly recent investigations (Smith, Mercy, & Rosenberg, 1986; Sorenson & Golding, 1988) have provided insight into this issue. Smith et al. (1986) looked at the incidence of suicide among Mexican-Americans in Arizona, California, Colorado, New Mexico, and Texas from 1976 through 1980. Sixty percent of all Hispanics in the United States live in these five states, and 85% of the Hispanics residing there are Mexican-Americans. The suicide rate for Hispanics (9.0 per 100,000) was less than the national rate for whites (13.2 per 100,000) and half that of the non-Hispanic whites living in the same area (19.2 per 100,000). These trends were apparent in all but the young male subgroup, where the rates were similar in both ethnic groups. A higher proportion of male to female suicides was observed for each age group among Hispanics as compared to Anglos.

Sorenson and Golding (1988) utilized data from the Los Angeles site of the Epidemiologic Catchment Area study to look at suicidal behaviors among 3,125 Hispanics. Rates of self-reported suicidal ideation and attempts among Hispanics were approximately 50% lower than those of non-Hispanic whites residing in the same area. Suicide attempts were more frequent among women and better-educated Hispanics. Similar risk factors for suicide were identified when the Hispanic and non-Hispanic white groups were compared; these included low religiosity, psychiatric disorder (especially depression), marital status (separated or divorced), female gender, and higher education status.

VARIATION IN SUICIDE RATES BY AGE

Table 23.2 displays completed rates of suicide by age for 10-year intervals beginning in 1957. Some general trends deserve comment. Total rates have increased over time, with the largest increase occurring between 1957 and 1977. Rates have been consistently higher among those over 45 years than

TABLE 23.2. Rates of Completed Suicide per 100,000 Population by Year and Age

Age[a]	Year			
	1957	1967	1977	1987
5–14	0.2	0.3	0.5	0.7
15–24	4.0	7.0	13.6	12.9
25–34	8.6	12.4	17.7	15.4
35–44	12.8	16.6	16.8	15.0
45–54	18.0	19.5	18.9	15.9
55–64	22.4	22.4	19.4	16.6
65–74	25.0	19.8	20.1	19.4
75–84	26.8	21.0	21.5	25.8
>85	26.3	22.7	17.3	22.1
Total	9.8	10.8	13.3	12.7

Note. The 1987 data are from NCHS (1990); the 1957, 1967, and 1977 data are from National Office of Vital Statistics (1959, 1969) and NCHS (1980), respectively.
[a] No suicides reported for individuals under 5 years of age.

among those 44 years of age and younger. Among the older age groups there has been a decline in rates over time, whereas among younger individuals rates have increased fairly consistently, with a slight decline followed by a leveling off in the 1980s. The greatest relative increase is found among those between 15 and 24 years of age (323%). This increase is largely attributable to the sharp rise in suicide rates among young white males, whose current rates reach 17.6 per 100,000 in those aged 15–19 and 27.5 per 100,000 in those aged 20–24. Large increases have also been noted among black males, whose 1987 rates were 8.9 per 100,000 in those aged 15–19 and 17.2 per 100,000 in those aged 20–24. Rates for young white females and for females of black and other races are approximately equal and have been relatively stable over time. It is the relative magnitude of the increase noted among adolescents and young adults that has caused so much attention to be paid this particular age group. Smaller but important increases are apparent for the 25–34 group (179%) and the 35–44 group (117%).

Recently, there have been efforts to ascertain whether there is a cohort effect in suicide rates—that is, whether the elevated rates observed in the younger individuals will remain constant throughout the group's lifetime (Monk, 1987). Murphy and Wetzel's (1980) analysis of U.S. data from 1949 to 1970 suggests that the high rates may persist through middle age. Similar results have been found in two Canadian studies (Solomon & Hellon, 1980; Reed, Camus, & Last, 1985). However, inspection of more recent rates (from 1980 on) in this country indicates that the projected elevations have not persisted (NCHS, 1990).

Holinger et al. (1987) have suggested that age-related changes in reported suicide rates may in part reflect changes in the proportion of the population occupied by a particular age group or in the ratio of younger to older individuals. The concepts of competition, political power, and economic attainment are central to this conceptualization. Such a model highlights the discrepancy between means and aspirations experienced by members of larger cohorts; it suggests, for instance, that with increases in the proportion of 15–24-year-olds in the population, increased competition for and inability to secure desired jobs, college positions, academic and athletic honors, and external sources of self-esteem occur. Conversely, adults in the 35–64-year-old groups have more experience, opportunities, economic attainment, and political power; therefore, suicide rates should tend to fall when the population of older individuals increases. These assertions are supported by the work of Ahlburg and Shapiro (1984), who found relative cohort size to be positively correlated with the suicide rate for young males and negatively correlated with the suicide rate for older males. Whether large cohort size differentially affects blacks versus whites has not been studied.

Lester (1984), on the other hand, has suggested that within every cohort a certain number of persons will commit suicide. His theory suggests that cohorts with greater rates of suicide in the younger years will experience lower rates in later years, since the pool of potential suicide candidates will have been exhausted. Lindsay (1989) tested Lester's hypothesis by examining gender-specific suicide rates in England and Wales for each 5-year age group between the ages of 15 and 69 and at 5-year intervals between 1921 and 1980. Lindsay's findings did not support Lester's hypothesis. Among women, there was a drop in female suicide rates at the ages most often associated with pregnancy and motherhood, followed by increasing rates in middle age. Clark (1990) has noted that this observation supports previous work indicating that responsibility for children is related to a lower suicide risk. In men, suicide rates were positively related at intervals of 5, 20, 25, and 30 years, but negatively related at intervals of 10 and 15 years. A marked period effect was present during World War II, with lower rates for both genders and for all but the youngest individuals.

Kreitman (1988) has pointed out that the investigation of age–gender effects should not be undertaken without consideration for other demographic characteristics. Kreitman used data obtained from the Registrar General of Scotland for the years 1973 to 1983 to explore the association between marital status and suicide rates for both genders by age. Results indicated that married individuals of both genders had the lowest suicide rates at all ages. Younger widowed persons evidenced the highest suicide rates (200% more than divorced and 700% more than married individuals). In older individuals the increase associated with widowhood was less apparent.

When age was controlled for, widowhood emerged as an even more important predictor of suicide. Kreitman suggested that marital status is a stronger correlate of suicide than age, and that widowhood may explain the higher rates of suicide among the elderly.

A number of other investigators have attempted to link changes in suicide rates to concomitant historical changes or period effects that influence the behavior of all or most living generations for a specific period of time. The impact of economic conditions has been studied widely, with unemployment being used as a common indicator of economic standing. Findings at both national and local levels have associated unemployment and high rates of suicide (Brenner, 1979; Platt, 1984; Wasserman, 1984; Platt & Kreitman, 1985). However, many of these studies have been ecological in nature (i.e., they have simply shown correlations between rates of unemployment and suicide across broad geographic areas), and significant associations have most often been found in time- series rather than cross-sectional analyses. Robins and Kulbok (1988) have suggested that more compelling support for an etiological relationship would be the finding that a national rise in unemployment is always followed by an increased suicide rate, which is reversed when the employment situation brightens.

Economic indicators other than employment have been studied including (1) changes in disposable income (Barnes, 1975); (2) stock market indices (Pierce, 1967); (3) per capita income as a percentage of the gross national product (Brenner, 1976, 1979, 1983); and (4) poverty levels (McCall & Land, 1989). Most existing analyses have focused on white males. Little is known about how these economic factors affect other groups (i.e., females and nonwhites) or whether the impact varies with age. Furthermore, the timing and duration of economic factors in relation to suicide require more careful consideration, as the nature and directionality of the observed associations are unclear (Monk, 1987). For example, those with a psychiatric disorder may be more likely to be unemployed (self-selection) and may be affected more seriously by that unemployment.

VARIATION IN SUICIDE RATES
BY CHOICE OF METHOD

Table 17.4 of this volume (see Maris, Chapter 17), which draws on the same data source as that employed here (NCHS, 1990), displays the percentage of completed suicides by method and gender. The method most frequently employed by both sexes (64.0% in males and 39.8% in females) is the use of firearms. In males, hanging (13.5%) and carbon monoxide, primarily motor vehicle exhaust (9.6%), are other frequently used methods. In females, drugs/medications (25.0%), as well as carbon monoxide (12.6%) and hanging

(9.4%) are common. The relative frequency with which the more common methods are selected varies little by race, with perhaps the exception of carbon monoxide, which is somewhat less frequently employed by blacks (2.9% in males and 4.4% in females). Trends over time (i.e., the last 30 years) indicate increasing use of firearms by males (up 14%) and females (up 18%). In males the use of firearms has consistently been the most popular method, whereas in females it has only been in the last decade that firearms have surpassed medications and poisons in popularity. Other secular changes are that the proportion of suicides attributable to hanging has decreased by a factor of one-third in men and two-fifths in women, and that domestic gas is now rarely (0.2% of the time) used. A major issue (whose detailed treatment is beyond the scope of this chapter) is whether the availability of method influences the number of completed suicides or simply the way in which suicide is committed. Examples of historical events that have been hypothesized as being related to changes in both the method and rate of suicide have been the selective prescription of less lethal sedatives (benzodiazepines instead of barbiturates; Oliver & Hetzel, 1973) and the enactment of legislation that considerably alters access to ways of committing suicide (e.g., the removal of carbon monoxide from cooking gas and the institution of gun control statutes) (Lester & Murrell, 1980; Kreitman, 1976).

Given that a firearm is used in 57% of all suicides in the United States, the availability of guns (particularly handguns) and gun control is an essential parameter to consider. Sloan, Rivara, Reay, Ferris, & Kellerman (1990) recently examined suicide rates for the years 1985 through 1987 in two similar urban areas with different firearm control regulations—King County (Seattle), Washington, and Vancouver, British Columbia. King County requires a 7-day waiting period before a handgun can be purchased and a 30-day waiting period before a permit can be obtained to carry a handgun as a concealed weapon. Rifles and shotguns may be purchased without a waiting period or any registration. In Vancouver, handguns cannot be used for self- protection or carried in public as concealed weapons, and individuals are required to obtain certificates in order to purchase rifles and shotguns. Although the most common method of suicide varied, with the rate of suicide by handgun being almost six times higher in King County, findings indicated similar overall age- and gender-adjusted rates of suicide. Conversely, suicide rates in King County residents aged 15–24 were 1.4 times higher than in Vancouver. The divergence in rates was attributable largely to a much greater use of handguns (almost 10 times higher) in King County, which was not offset by other means in Vancouver residents of similar age. Sloan et al. (1990) suggested that adolescent and young adult suicide may include a large number of impulsive/opportunistic acts, which could be prevented through the institution of stricter gun control laws; they noted, however, that stricter gun control laws would not cause a decrease in the *overall* suicide rate, because persons intent on suicide can always use alternate methods to kill themselves.

Boyd and Mościcki (1986) specifically investigated the relationship of firearms and youth suicide. They noted that between 1933 and 1982 the firearm suicide rate for persons aged 10-24 increased 139%, from 2.3 per 100,000 to 5.5 per 100,000. Over the same 50-year interval, the suicide rate by methods other than firearms rose only 32%, from 2.5 to 3.3 per 100,000. The greatest increases in overall suicide rates and rates of suicide involving firearms were found since 1970 for males aged 15-24. This rise in firearm suicide rates corresponds to a substantial increase in the number of civilian firearms produced in the United States during the 1960s and 1970s. The proportion of families possessing a firearm has remained constant at approximately 50% from 1959 to 1977, suggesting that families who have previously owned firearms now own more of them. The unanswered question is whether an increase in the number of firearms per family increases access to firearms, especially among adolescents and young adults.

Several researchers have speculated that there may be an association between alcohol and/or drug use and suicide by firearms (Brent et al., 1987; Rich, Young, & Fowler, 1986). In examining coroner's records for all youths aged 10-19 years in Allegheny County, Pennsylvania, whose deaths were classified as accidental or suicides, Brent et al. (1987) noted that the suicide by firearms rate increased more rapidly than the rate for suicide by other means. During the same 24- year study period, the incidence of positive blood alcohol tests among suicide victims rose from 13% to 46%. Findings further indicated that the higher the blood alcohol concentration, the greater the probability that a firearm was utilized as the method of suicide. Interestingly, during the same period the rate of positive drug findings remained fairly constant, ranging from 10% to 17%. The investigators speculated that the rise in youth suicide may be a consequence of an increase in the frequency of adolescent alcohol abuse, and that the role of other drug abuse or combined drug and alcohol use may not be as important.

In contrast Rich et al. (1986) found a high frequency (66%) and variety of substance abuse diagnoses in individuals below 30 years of age in their psychological autopsy study of consecutive cases of suicide in San Diego County for the years 1981 to 1983. Substance abuse was implicated in more youthful deaths by suicide than was depressive illness. Significantly more subjects under 30 had a drug use disorder than did subjects over 30. Among the older suicides, 60% under the age of 40 and 14% aged 40 or older had drug abuse disorders. Furthermore, subjects in the under-30 group had a mean of 2.8 classes of drugs per suicide as opposed to 2.4 classes per suicide in the older group. The investigators concluded that their findings were consistent with previous assertions identifying drug usage as the most important factor explaining the increased rate of suicide among youths in the United States.

VARIATION IN SUICIDE RATES
BY GEOGRAPHIC LOCATION

Table 23.3 displays rates of suicide according to geographic divisions of the United States. Nine separate regions are represented:

1. New England—Maine, New Hampshire, Vermont, Massachusetts, Rhode Island, Connecticut.
2. Middle Atlantic—New York, New Jersey, Pennsylvania.
3. East North Central—Ohio, Indiana, Illinois, Michigan, Wisconsin.
4. West North Central—Minnesota, Iowa, Missouri, North Dakota, Nebraska, Kansas.
5. South Atlantic—Delaware, Maryland, District of Columbia, Virginia, West Virginia, North Carolina, South Carolina, Georgia, Florida.
6. East South Central—Kentucky, Tennessee, Alabama, Mississippi.
7. West South Central—Arkansas, Louisiana, Oklahoma, Texas.
8. Mountain—Montana, Idaho, Wyoming, Colorado, New Mexico, Arizona, Utah, Nevada.
9. Pacific—Washington, Oregon, California, Alaska, Hawaii.

The highest rates are found in the Mountain (18.7 per 100,000) and Pacific (14.1 per 100,000) regions. The lowest rate is found in the Middle Atlantic states (9.0 per 100,000). Although this differential between the Atlantic and Pacific coasts has existed for over three decades, the magnitude of the difference has narrowed substantially as a result of increasing rates along the Atlantic coast. Substantial intraregion variation in suicide rates occurs. For example in the South Atlantic region, rates range from a low of

TABLE 23.3. Rates of Completed Suicide (1987) per 100,000 Population by Geographic Region

Region	Rate per 100,000
Mountain	18.7
Pacific	14.1
South Atlantic	13.9
West North Central	13.6
West South Central	12.9
East South Central	12.1
East North Central	11.7
New England	11.0
Middle Atlantic	9.0

Note. The data are from NCHS (1990).

7.1 per 100,000 in the District of Columbia to a high of 16.8 in Florida. Similarly, in the New England region, rates range from a low of 9.3 per 100,000 in Connecticut to a high of 16.8 in Vermont. The individual states with the lowest suicide rates are New York (7.0 per 100,000), the District of Columbia (7.1 per 100,000), and New Jersey (8.1 per 100,000). The individual states with the highest rates are Nevada (26.4 per 100,000), Arizona (20.2 per 100,000), and New Mexico (20.1 per 100,000). Although suicide is more common among men, in the state of Nevada the suicide rate among women is 16 per 100,000, which is greater than the male rate for suicide in New Jersey (Stevenson, 1988). Rates of suicide have also been found to be higher in persons in standard metropolitan statistical areas than in nonmetropolitan and rural areas. Variations in the accuracy of reporting may explain these differences, as the high rate of suicide in some metropolitan areas may reflect the high rate of autopsy examinations performed there.

APPLICATION OF DEMOGRAPHIC FACTORS TO THE FIVE CLINICAL CASES

The demographic factors discussed in this chapter (age, race, gender, marital status, and geographic location) provide a general indication of those groups of individuals at highest risk for suicide. A number of these factors were reflected in the five case studies described in Chapter 12 and discussed throughout the text: the upsurge in adolescent suicides (Heather B and Ralph F), the preponderance of male completers (Ralph, John Z, and Jos G), the overrepresentation of whites versus nonwhites (the first four cases vs. Jos), and the significance of marital status (Faye C) and employment (John and Jos). However, even when considered simultaneously, this group of demographic factors provides little indication regarding a specific individual's probability of attempting or completing a suicide. Consideration of additional types of information (e.g., family history of suicide, presence of psychiatric disorder, drug and alcohol use/abuse, chronic medical illness) is necessary and improves prediction.

Still, the ability to identify in advance those individuals who will complete a suicide in the future remains marginal. Murphy (1972) has suggested that although considerable progress has been made in identifying groups at high risk for suicide, the existing risk profile" is too general to be of practical predictive use (i.e., it identifies large groups of individuals never at risk, and misses a large proportion of those who will commit suicide). The problem becomes one of predicting relatively infrequent events and events that are predicated on a far from constant underlying intent. However, available risk profiles and descriptions can provide the structure with which to begin to identify high-risk groups and individuals, and to target them for appropriate preventive and clinical interventions.

SUMMARY

Analyses of the patterns of suicide utilizing death certificate data indicate the marked effect of gender, race, age, and geographic residence on suicide rates. Rates are higher for men than women, for whites than nonwhites, for residents of the western United States, and for those over 45 years of age. However, suicide rates for young people have increased dramatically over the last three decades. Although death certificate data can provide insights regarding the frequency and distribution of suicide, their usefulness is impaired by the underreporting of suicide deaths and by the absence of information on pertinent risk factors. The challenge for future research is to investigate demographic trends in suicide within a multifactorial etiological framework that allows for complex relationships, direct and intervening causes, and improved predictive models.

REFERENCES

Ahlburg, D. A., & Shapiro, M. D. (1984). Socioeconomic ramifications of changing cohort size: An analysis of U.S. postwar suicide rates by age and sex. *Demography, 21*, 97-105.

Barnes, C. B. (1975). The partial effect of income on suicide is always negative. *American Journal of Sociology, 80*, 1454-1462.

Boyd, J. F., & Mościcki, E. K. (1986). Firearms and youth suicide. *American Journal of Public Health, 76*, 1240-1242.

Brenner, M. H. (1976). *Estimating the social costs of national economic policy: Implications for mental and physical health and criminal aggression.* Paper No. 5, Joint Economic Committee, Congress of the United States. Washington, DC: U.S. Government Printing Office.

Brenner, M. H. (1979). Mortality and the national economy: A review, and the experiences of England and Wales, 1936-1976. *Lancet, ii,* 568-573.

Brenner, M. H. (1983). Unemployment and health in the context of economic change. *Social Science Medicine, 17,* 1125-1138.

Brent, D. A., Perper, J. A., & Allman, C. J. (1987). Alcohol, firearms, and suicide among youth: Temporal trends in Allegheny County Pennsylvania, 1960 to 1983. *Journal of the American Medical Association, 257,* 3369-3372.

Bush, J. A. (1976). Suicide and blacks: A conceptual framework. *Suicide and Life-Threatening Behavior, 6,* 216-222.

Centers for Disease Control. (1986). *Youth suicide in the United States, 1970-1980: Youth suicide surveillance.* Atlanta, GA: Author.

Cheek, W. A. (1985). Homicide, suicide, other violence gain increasing medical attention. *Journal of the American Medical Association, 254,* 721-730.

Clark, D. (1989). Official misclassification. *Suicide Research Digest, 3,* 7.

Clark, D. (1990). Age effects on suicide rates. *Suicide Research Digest, 4,* 12.

Comer, J. P. (1973). Black suicide: A hidden crisis. *Urban Health, 2,* 41-44.

Diekstra, R. F. W. (1985). Suicide and suicide attempts in European Economic

Community: An analysis of trends, with special emphasis upon trends among the young. *Suicide and Life-Threatening Behavior, 15,* 27-42.

Griffith, E. E. H., & Bell, C . C. (1989). Recent trends in suicide and homicide among blacks. *Journal of the American Medical Association, 262,* 2265-2269.

Grinspoon, L. (1986). Suicide—Part I. *Harvard Medical School Mental Health Letter, 2*(8), 1-4.

Hirschfeld, R. M. A., & Davidson, L. (1988). Risk factors for suicide. In A. J. Frances & R. Hales (Eds.), *Review of psychiatry* (Vol. 7). Washington, DC: American Psychiatric Press.

Holinger, P.C. (1980). Violent deaths as a leading cause of mortality: An epidemiologic study of suicide, homicide and accidents. *American Journal of Psychiatry, 137,* 472-476.

Holinger, P. C., Offer, D., & Ostrov, E. (1987). Suicide and homicide in the United States: An epidemiologic study of violent death, population changes, and the potential for prediction. *American Journal of Psychiatry, 144,* 215-219.

Jobes, D. A., Berman, A. L., & Josselsen, A. R. (1986). The impact of psychological autopsies on medical examiners' determination of manner of death. *Journal of Forensic Science, 31,* 177-189.

Kleck, G. (1988). Miscounting suicides. *Suicide and Life-Threatening Behavior, 18,* 219-236.

Kreitman, N. (1976). The coal gas story: United Kingdom suicide rates, 1960-1971. *British Journal of Preventive and Social Medicine, 30,* 86-93.

Kreitman, N. (1988). Suicide, age and marital status. *Psychological Medicine, 18,* 121-128.

Lester, D. (1984). Suicide risk by birth cohort. *Suicide and Life-Threatening Behavior, 14,* 132-136.

Lester, D., & Murrell, M. E. (1980). The influence of gun laws on suicidal behavior. *American Journal of Psychiatry, 137,* 121-122.

Lindsay, J. (1989). Age, sex and suicide rates within birth cohorts in England and Wales. *Social Psychiatry and Psychiatric Epidemiology, 24,* 249-252.

Litman, R. E., Curphey, T. J., Shneidman, E. S., Farberow, N. L., & Tabachnick, N. (1963). Investigations of equivocal suicides. *Journal of the American Medical Association, 184,* 924-929.

McCall, P. L., & Land, K. (1989, March). *Trends in adolescent, young adult and elderly suicide: Are there common underlying structural factors?* Paper presented at the annual meetings of the Population Association of America, Baltimore.

Monk, M. (1987). Epidemiology of suicide. *Epidemiologic Reviews, 9,* 51-69.

Murphy, G. E. (1972). Clinical identification of suicidal risk. *Archives of General Psychiatry, 27,* 356-359.

Murphy, G. E., & Wetzel, R. D. (1980). Suicide risk by birth cohort in the United States, 1949-1974. *Archives of General Psychiatry, 37,* 519-23.

National Center for Health Statistics (NCHS). (1980). *Vital statistics of the United States, 1977: Vol. 2. Mortality* (Part A). Washington, DC: U.S. Government Printing Office.

National Center for Health Statistics (NCHS). (1990). *Vital statistics of the United States, 1987: Vol. 2. Mortality* (Part A). Washington, DC: U.S. Government Printing Office.

National Office of Vital Statistics (1959). *Vital statistics of the United States, 1957: Vol. 2. Mortality* (Part A). Washington, DC: U.S. Government Printing Office.

National Office of Vital Statistics. (1969). *Vital statistics of the United States, 1967: Vol. 2. Mortality* (Part A). Washington, DC: U.S. Government Printing Office.

Oliver, R. G., & Hetzel, B. S. (1973). An analysis of recent trends in suicide rates in Australia. *International Journal of Epidemiology, 2*, 91-101.

Pierce, A. (1967). The economic cycle and the social suicide rate. *American Sociological Review, 51*, 523-540.

Platt, S. (1984). Unemployment and suicide behavior: A review of the literature. *Social Science and Medicine, 19*, 93-115.

Platt, S., & Kreitman, N. (1985). Parasuicide and unemployment among men in Edinburgh 1968-1982. *Psychological Medicine, 15*, 113-123.

Reed, J., Camus, J., & Last, J. M. (1985). Suicide in Canada: Birth-cohort analysis. *Canadian Journal of Public Health, 76*, 43-47.

Rich, C. L., Young, D., & Fowler, R. C. (1986). San Diego Suicide Study: I. Young vs. old subjects. *Archives of General Psychiatry, 43*, 577-582.

Robins, L. N., & Kulbok, P. A. (1988). Epidemiologic studies in suicide. In A. J. Frances & R. Hales (Eds.), *Review of psychiatry* (Vol. 7). Washington, DC: American Psychiatric Press.

Rosenberg, M. L., Smith, J. C., Davidson, L. E., & Conn, J. M. (1987). The emergence of youth suicide: An epidemiologic analysis and public health perspective. *Annual Review of Public Health, 8*, 417-440.

Sloan, J. H., Rivara, F. P., Reay, D. T., Ferris, J. A., & Kellermann, A. L. (1990). Firearm regulations and rates of suicide: A comparison of two metropolitan areas. *New England Journal of Medicine, 322*, 369-373.

Smith, J. C., Mercy, J. A., & Rosenberg, M. L. (1986). Suicide and homicide among Hispanics in the Southwest. *Public Health Reports, 101*, 265-270.

Solomon, M. I., & Hellon, C. P. (1980). Suicide and age in Alberta, Canada, 1951 to 1977: A cohort analysis. *Archives of General Psychiatry, 37*, 511-513.

Sorenson, S. B., & Golding, J. M. (1988). Suicide ideation and attempts in Hispanics and non-Hispanic whites: Demographic and psychiatric disorder issues. *Suicide and Life-Threatening Behavior, 18*, 205-218.

Stevenson, J. M. (1988). Suicide. In J. A. Talbott, R. E. Hales, & S. C. Yudofsky (Eds.), *Textbook of psychiatry*. Washington, DC: American Psychiatric Press.

Wasserman, I. M. (1984). The influence of economic business cycles on United States suicide rates. *Suicide and Life-Threatening Behavior, 14*, 143-156.

World Health Organization (WHO), Regional Office for Europe. (1982). *Changing patterns in suicide behavior: Report on WHO working group*. Copenhagen: European Reports and Studies.

CHAPTER 24

Suicide and the Media

David P. Phillips, Ph.D.
Katherine Lesyna, M.A.
Daniel J. Paight, M.A.
University of California at San Diego

Most people contemplating suicide are at some point ambivalent in the face of such a fateful decision (Weisman & Worden, 1972; Shneidman, 1985). This suggests a question seldom asked in the literature: What factors lead a distressed person to suicide rather than to some alternative solution to distress? We have no complete answers to this question, but much research suggests that one of the factors leading a distressed individual to suicide is the publicizing of "model" suicides in the mass media. These publicized suicide stories seem to function as "natural advertisements" for suicide. It may be possible to reduce the effectiveness of these "advertisements" by drawing on findings in various fields, including decision making and advertising. Some research in these fields also suggests ways for constructing effective "antisuicide stories"—advertisements for alternatives to suicide. Thus, although studies on suicide stories appear at first sight to have gloomy implications, they also suggest some positive conclusions: Modeling processes can lead ambivalent individuals toward suicide or toward alternatives.

We begin this chapter with a review of the literature on the impact of suicide stories publicized in the mass media. (The focus here is on the mass media's effects, so we do not review a smaller body of related research on suicide "epidemics" and time–space clustering. For a recent example of this approach to the study of suicide modeling, see Gould, Wallenstein, & Kleinman, 1990.) We then address the question of how the effects of suicide stories might be mitigated, consulting the literature in the fields of advertising and decision making. Finally, we suggest a list of research topics that remain to be addressed, and some ways in which public health agencies, mental health professionals, and the mass media can facilitate this research.

REVIEW OF THE LITERATURE ON THE IMITATION OF PUBLICIZED SUICIDES

Studies on the Effects of Nonfictional Suicide Stories

Effect of Newspaper Stories

In the first modern study of the topic, Motto (1967) approached the problem indirectly by assuming that during a newspaper strike there would be a reduction in the publicity accorded to suicide stories. In a study of seven U.S. cities, he compared the suicide rate during a newspaper strike to the mean rate for the previous 5 years, controlling for population increase, population characteristics, seasonal variation, and yearly trends. He found no evidence to support his hypothesis that suicides would decline during strikes. However, in a later study, in which he compared the suicide rate during a 268-day newspaper strike in Detroit with the mean rates for the same calendar period of the previous 4 years and the subsequent year, Motto (1970) found a significant reduction in the number of suicides by females, (especially those under age 35), during the newspaper strike. Blumenthal and Bergner (1973) replicated Motto's Detroit study using New York City data, and found no significant change in the suicide rate during the strike period for any age- or sex-specific group. They noted that the different findings may have resulted from the fact that New York City's strike, unlike Detroit's, affected only half of the city's newspapers.

These early studies had several methodological problems. First, they neglected the effect of radio, television news, and newspapers brought in from out of town during the newspaper strikes. Second, there may not have been any noteworthy suicides during the strike; with no suicides to report, a newspaper strike could hardly be expected to affect the suicide rate. Third, a newspaper strike introduces many changes in a city; some of these changes (such as the cessation of suicide stories) may decrease the suicide rate, some may increase it, and some may make no difference. Until these methodological problems can be resolved, Motto's study design is inherently inconclusive.

Phillips (1974) used a different study design to provide a more direct estimate of the impact of suicide stories. Using *Facts on File* (1946–1968) and the *New York Times Index* (1946–1968), Phillips compiled a list of suicide stories appearing on page 1 of the *New York Times*. He then examined official U.S. monthly suicide statistics to estimate the effect of front-page suicide stories, from 1947 to 1967 (after correction for the effects of trends and seasons on suicides). U.S. suicides rose significantly just after front-page suicide stories. Phillips named this poststory rise in suicide "the Werther effect," after Goethe's fictional hero whose suicide was thought by contemporary observers to have triggered imitative acts. To increase confidence in the hypothesis that publicized suicide stories elicit a rise in U.S.

suicides, Phillips tested additional predictions that should hold if suicide stories trigger imitative behavior. If the Werther effect occurs because of imitation, then (1) suicides should peak after the publicized story, but not before; (2) the more publicity given to a story, the larger the suicide peak should be; and (3) suicides should peak mainly in the geographic area where the suicide story is publicized. The data were consistent with all of these predictions.

Phillips then assessed six competing explanations (of which the four most plausible are summarized here):

1. The "coroner explanation" asserts that the publicized suicide prompts the coroner to shift ambiguous deaths into the category of suicide from the competing categories of accident, homicide, and undetermined death. Deaths in competing categories should then decrease after a suicide story; however, no such decrease was found.

2. The "precipitation explanation" asserts that publicized suicides merely hasten suicides that would have occurred anyway, even in the absence of a suicide story. The poststory peak in suicides, then, should be followed by an equally large drop in suicides, caused by suicides' "moving up" their death dates; however, no such drop was seen.

3. The "prior-conditions explanation" asserts that a prior change in social conditions—for example, an economic recession—produces a rise in both publicized and unpublicized suicides. This hypothesis, however, cannot explain the observed correlation between the rise in suicides after a suicide story and the amount of publicity devoted to that story.

4. The "bereavement explanation" asserts that suicide stories elicit grief rather than imitation, and that this grief prompts additional suicides. But if this is the case, we would expect celebrity deaths to trigger additional suicides, even if these deaths are not themselves suicides. This prediction was inconsistent with the data.

After assessing these and other alternative explanations, Phillips concluded that the best available explanation of the Werther effect is that it is caused by processes related to imitation or suggestion. The detailed psychological processes involved could not be precisely identified with the mortality statistics he was studying.

In a pair of sequels, Phillips (1977, 1979) sought to estimate the influence of publicized suicide stories on motor vehicle fatalities (MVFs) in California, from 1966 to 1973. Many researchers have suspected some motor vehicle crashes to have a suicidal component; if this is so, MVFs, like overt suicides, should peak after publicized suicides. Controlling for weekday and monthly fluctuations in MVFs, holiday weekends, and yearly linear trends, Phillips found a significant rise after (but not before) publicized suicides, with a 31% peak in MVFs on the third day following the story. He also found that the amount of publicity given to a suicide and the size of the increase in MVFs were positively correlated, and that the increase occurred mainly in the area where the suicide was publicized. Furthermore, he found that single-vehicle crashes increased more than other types just after the suicide story, and that drivers, but not passengers, dying just after a suicide story were similar to the person described in that story. Stories about murder-suicides tended to be followed by multiple-vehicle crashes involving passenger deaths, whereas stories about suicide alone tended to be followed by single-vehicle crashes involving driver deaths. Phillips assessed alternative explanations for the findings and concluded that the best available explanation is that publicized suicides elicit a rise in suicides, some of which are disguised as MVFs. Bollen and Phillips (1981) replicated the principal California findings, using data for Detroit, from 1973 to 1976.

The study of California MVFs indicated that murder–suicide stories and "pure" suicide stories have different effects. Prompted by this observation, Phillips (1978, 1980) examined the impact of U.S. murder–suicide stories on U.S. noncommercial airplane crashes and found a peak in suicides lasting 9 days. The size and geographic location of the peak varied with the amount of publicity given to murder–suicides.

Wasserman (1984) re-examined Phillips's (1974) findings, extending the time period from 1946–1968 to 1946–1977. Using multivariate time-series analyses to control for seasonal effects, economic cycles, and war, Wasserman found that the U.S. suicide rate rose significantly after stories about celebrity suicides, but not after noncelebrity suicide stories. However, Stack (1984), adding more than 10 publicized stories that Wasserman had inadvertently overlooked, found a significant effect both for celebrity and for noncelebrity stories. Phillips and Carstensen (1988) uncovered similar findings with a different data set. Stack (1987) also tried to estimate whether some types of celebrity suicide stories had an unusually large effect on U.S. monthly suicide rates from 1948 to 1983. The U.S. suicide rate rose significantly after suicide stories about U.S. political and entertainment celebrities, but not after stories about other types of celebrities. Consistent with earlier findings, Stack found a correlation between the publicity accorded a suicide and the increase in suicide following it.

Thus far, we have confined the discussion to U.S. studies, which make up most of the literature. The evidence from European studies, however, is more equivocal. An English study (Barraclough, Shepherd, & Jennings, 1977) sought to determine whether Portsmouth suicides were preceded by an unusually large number of news reports on suicide inquests. In contrast to the U.S. studies, however, the English study did not confine attention to front-page reports of suicide. Indeed, nearly all the inquest stories were carried on inside pages of the newspaper. This failure to restrict attention to front-page stories also characterized Littman's (1985) study of Canadian subway suicides. Failure to find peaks in suicide after such stories is not surprising, since earlier work on U.S. data found no evidence linking suicide rates with inside-page reports of suicide. Jonas (in press) examined suicides in Baden-Württemberg, Germany, from 1968 to 1980. Using the binomial analysis employed by Phillips (1974), Jonas found statistically significant evidence of the Werther effect. However, when he applied regression analysis to the data, he found nonsignificant increases in suicides after suicide stories; thus, results of this study must be regarded as inconclusive.

A team of Dutch researchers conducted two careful studies, which replicated the U.S. methodology in many respects. Most notably, they restricted attention to front-page stories. In the first of these studies (Ganzeboom & de Haan, 1982), the authors reported their results to be inconclusive: "For suicide and traffic accidents, mortality rates tend to rise 3-8% on a monthly basis (about the same amount as Phillips revealed), but this is not significant at conventional significance levels (though very near so)" (p. 55). The second study (Kopping, Ganzeboom, & Swanborn, 1990) did reveal a statistically significant relationship between the appearance of front-page suicide stories and monthly increases in the Dutch suicide rate. Stories in which the headline explicitly conveyed the idea of suicide showed a significantly greater impact than did stories in which the headline failed to mention suicide. Similarly, long suicide stories appeared to elicit a greater rise in suicide than short suicide stories. However, because neither the presence of a picture nor the celebrity status of the suicide appeared to have any impact, and because an analysis of a subset of daily suicides (1974–1984) failed to provide evidence of imitation, the authors judged their findings to be inconclusive.

Nevertheless, nearly all the Dutch findings (both positive and negative) are consistent with earlier reports in the literature and need not reduce confidence in the hypothesis of imitative suicide. The U.S. and the Dutch studies failed to find associations between either (1) the celebrity status of the victim and the subsequent rise in suicides (Phillips & Carstensen, 1988; Stack, 1987) or (2) the presence of a photograph of the victim and the subsequent rise in suicides (Phillips & Carstensen, 1988). Similarly, positive Dutch findings linking the length of the newspaper story with the subsequent rise in suicides is consistent with much earlier U.S. work (Phillips, 1974, 1977, 1978, 1979, 1980; Stack, 1987), which also showed a dose-response relationship.

These Dutch studies are particularly interesting not only for their methodological similarities to U.S. studies, but also for the instructive differences they reveal between Dutch and U.S. suicide stories. First, whereas U.S. newspapers almost always explicitly convey the idea of suicide in the headline, Dutch newspapers are more circumspect. Kopping et al. (1990) found that only half of the Dutch reports explicitly referred to suicide in the headlines. Since newspaper readers often scan a headline and do not read the rest of the story, to mention suicide explicitly in the headline is to communicate the idea of suicide to a greater number of persons. In the first Dutch study, Ganzeboom and de Haan (1982) did not distinguish between explicit-headline and ambiguous-headline suicide stories; as we have seen, however, Kopping et al. (1990) did make this distinction in their monthly analysis and found a significantly greater impact for explicit-headline stories. In their daily analysis, however, in which they found no evidence of imitation, they did not distinguish between explicit- and ambiguous-headline stories. This, and the authors' failure to correct for the known effects of holidays on suicides (Phillips & Wills, 1987), casts some doubt on the validity of these negative findings.

Second, whereas U.S. newspapers report the name of the suicide victim, Dutch newspapers typically do not; Kopping et al. (1990) found that only 45% of the Dutch reports revealed the name of the suicide victim. Readers may be relatively unmoved by the narrative if the suicidal victim is presented as an anonymous individual. Finally, about 50% of the Dutch suicide stories involved multiple victims—these were typically stories about murder followed by suicide (Kopping et al., 1990). In contrast, this percentage was much smaller in the typical U.S. study.

The European findings suggest some modifications to conclusions based on U.S. studies: (1) Suicides peak after front-page suicide stories in which the idea of suicide is explicitly conveyed in the headline; (2) the more publicity given to the suicide story, the greater the peak in suicides thereafter; (3) the rise in suicides is particularly large in the areas where the suicide story is most heavily publicized.

Effect of Television Stories

Researchers have paid less attention to television news stories about suicide than to newspaper suicide stories. The first investigations of the topic (Phillips, 1978, 1980) examined the impact of both TV and newspaper stories on U.S. airplane accidents. Phillips (1980) found that "the correlation between newspaper coverage and crashes ($r = .734$) is almost as high as the multiple correlation between newspaper–television coverage and crashes ($R = .737$). . . . Evidently, newspaper coverage alone predicts . . . crashes almost as well as newspaper and television coverage combined" (p. 1007).

Bollen and Phillips (1982) sought to replicate the findings from Phillips's (1974) research using TV rather than newspaper stories. They restricted attention to heavily publicized stories—those appearing on two or more network evening news programs. Applying regression techniques to daily suicide statistics, they found a significant increase in the number of U.S. suicides after TV news reports about suicides. Their findings indicated that the effect of a given suicide story lasts at most 10 days. Thus, the duration of the story effect seems to be about the same for suicides, auto accidents, and airplane accidents. Baron and Reiss (1985) claimed that the results of Bollen and Phillips (1982) could be an artifact of heteroscedasticity (which was not corrected for in Bollen and Phillips's original paper). In response, Phillips and Bollen (1985) showed that their original findings remained statistically significant after heteroscedasticity was corrected for. Baron and Reiss (1985) also suggested that Bollen and Phillips (1982) had only partially corrected for the confounding effects of holidays on suicides. In reply, Phillips and Bollen (1985) noted that their results remained statistically significant after they omitted suicide stories occurring near the holidays.

Phillips and Carstensen (1986) studied the the daily suicide rate of U.S. teens (1973-1979) after 38 U.S. TV news or feature stories about suicide. Teen suicides rose significantly in the week after a suicide story appeared on TV; the adult rate also rose, but not significantly. The more publicity given the suicide story, the more the teen suicide rate went up. In a sequel, Phillips and Carstensen (1988) expanded their work on network TV news, nearly tripling the time period under analysis (from 1973-1979 to 1968-1985). Restricting their attention to heavily publicized stories, they applied a time-series regression model to California data. This analysis uncovered a significant increase in both male and female suicides 0-7 days after multiprogram suicide stories. Phillips and Carstensen's findings indicate that the Werther effect is not stronger for those groups that are already predisposed to suicide: males, whites, the unmarried, and people of retirement age.

In a study sponsored by the NBC television network, Kessler, Downey, Milavsky, and Stipp (1988) examined the fluctuation of U.S. suicides after TV suicide stories from 1973 to 1984. The NBC study replicated Phillips and Carstensen's (1986) earlier finding of a statistically significant increase in teen suicides after TV stories from 1973 to 1979. However, after adding many stories for 1980-1984 (most of which appeared only once), the NBC study found a nonsignificant rise in suicides after suicide stories from 1973 to 1984. This NBC study had two important methodological defects. First, and most important, the NBC study did not restrict attention to multiprogram suicide stories, despite the evidence that only these stories are known to affect suicides. Second, in contrast to all recent studies on the topic, the NBC investigation failed to test for the effects of autocorrelation and heteroscedasticity, which are known to bias significance tests.

In a thoughtful critique of the NBC study, Clark (1989) notes a finding that is tabulated by the NBC authors, but not discussed in the text of their study: "celebrity suicides were significantly associated with subsequent teen suicides over the period 1973-1984" (p. 2). Clark conjectured that "by expanding the number of suicides included in their analysis with one-time broadcasts on programs like 'The Today Show,' 'CBS Morning News,' or '60 Minutes,' the likelihood is that Kessler and colleagues inadvertently diluted their sample with noncelebrity cases and feature stories, and thus diluted the observed association between news broadcasts and teen suicide rates" (p. 2).

After making several methodological criticisms in addition to those mentioned above, Clark raised "a question of how neutral a major force in network news broadcasting can remain when responding (scientifically or otherwise) to evidence that certain kinds of news reports may have a damaging impact. There is an appearance that the network is refuting studies which criticize its news policies" (p. 2).

Kessler, Downey, Stipp, and Milavsky (1989) later republished their earlier findings. This time they tested for the effects of autocorrelation and, using the Nielsen television program ratings data, controlled for the amount of coverage stories received (either "high" or "low"). In separate analyses of "high-exposure" and "low-exposure" stories, the authors observed a statistically significant 10% rise in teen suicides following "high-exposure" stories and no rise following "low-exposure" stories for the years 1973–1984. However, because there was no increase in the years 1981–1984 for either "high-" or "low-exposure" stories, the authors suggested the "possibility . . . that the increased public sensitivity to teenage suicide in the 1980s could have created a context in which teenagers are more resistent [sic] to the effects of television" (p. 555).

As in their previous study, however, Kessler et al. (1989) failed to restrict attention to multiprogram stories. Although Nielsen ratings tell us something about how many persons viewed a particular story, they tell us nothing about how often persons saw the story. Researchers in the advertising industry have repeatedly found that repetition is a crucial component of a successful advertisement (for a review, see Comstock, Chaffee, Katzman, McCombs, & Roberts, 1978). Thus, it is common to see the same advertisement repeated during the same television program; this has the effect of exposing the same audience to the same message more than once. If suicide stories, in effect, "advertise" suicide, then the effectiveness of these "advertisements" should depend on the same factors as advertisements for Toyotas and light beer. We have more to say about this later. For now, it is enough to point out that from 1981 to 1984 the overwhelming majority of those suicide stories Kessler et al. (1989) examined aired only once.

We conclude this section with a discussion of some recent work by Sonneck, Nagel-Kuess, Etzerdorfer, Smeh, and Hauer (in press). These investigators have provided what seems to be the first experimental evidence for the Werther effect. After reviewing the evidence linking suicide stories with a subsequent rise in suicides, the Austrian Association for Suicide Prevention, Crisis Intervention, and Conflict Resolution persuaded the two largest-circulation Viennese newspapers on June 16, 1987 to curtail drastically the publicity they accorded to Viennese subway suicides. Sonneck et al. tabulated the number of Viennese subway suicides before and after this change in publication policy, and their findings are displayed in Figure 24.1. It is evident that there was an abrupt decline in the incidence of

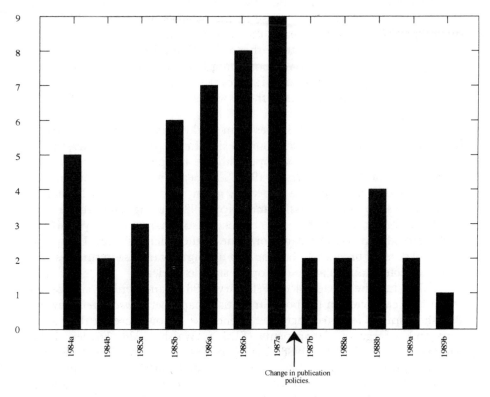

FIGURE 24.1. Number of Viennese subway suicides (in 6-month periods) before and after two major Viennese newspapers curtailed their coverage of subway suicides. The figure is based on data from Sonneck et al. (in press).

Viennese subway suicides immediately after the change in publication policy, and that this incidence has remained low ever since. No such marked decline is evident for other types of suicides in Vienna.

Studies on the Effects of Fictional Suicide Stories

We have seen that studies of highly publicized nonfictional suicide stories generally report a poststory rise in suicides. When we turn to fictional suicide stories, however, evidence for a story effect is less clear. Holding (1974, 1975), who conducted the first empirical studies on the effects of fictional suicide stories, investigated the effect of an 11-episode weekly TV series broadcast in 1972 (*The Befrienders*) on the parasuicide rate in Edinburgh, Scotland. The series dramatized the work of a suicide prevention service there. Holding found a rise in the number of people visiting the suicide prevention center during the running time of the series and the 4 weeks thereafter, but he found neither a significant decrease in the number of people admitted to a regional poisoning treatment center for attempted suicide (Holding, 1974) nor any significant change in the number of suicides and undetermined deaths in the 10 weeks of the series or the 10 weeks afterward (Holding, 1975).

After identifying suicide stories from weekly newspaper summaries of soap opera plots, Phillips (1982) found a significant peak in suicides, MVFs and nonfatal accidents after soap opera suicide and parasuicide stories were broadcast in the United States in 1977. The peaks were larger for females than for males, as would be expected, given the predominantly female audience of soap operas. Kessler and Stipp (1984), using data provided by the TV industry, noted that the newspaper summaries used by Phillips (1982) provided inaccurate dates for some of the suicide stories. Using the corrected dates of broadcast, they found a nonsignificant rise in suicides and motor vehicle fatalities after soap opera suicide stories.

Following the broadcast on February 1986 of an overdose suicide attempt by a character on the popular British soap opera *EastEnders*, several British hospitals reported increased attendance for overdoses at their accident and emergency departments (Ellis & Walsh, 1986; Fowler, 1986; Sandler, Connell, & Welsh, 1986). Platt (1987) examined data from 63 British hospitals on the numbers of cases the hospitals treated for deliberate overdoses in the week after the broadcast and in a control period of the week preceding it. Although he found a statistically significant peak in the incidence of parasuicides by overdose for persons aged 45 and over, he suggested that it was an unreliable finding, noting that the television program primarily appealed to young people and that identification with the parasuicidal character would presumably be greater for people in the character's age group (30–44). Williams, Lawton, Ellis, Walsh, and Reed (1987, n.d.) drew similarly cautious conclusions. Although Williams et al. found increases in overdoses after the broadcast at the two hospitals they studied, the increases were part of a trend, which preceded and outlasted the period under investigation.

Ostroff and colleagues (Ostroff, Behrends, Lee, & Oliphant, 1985; Ostroff & Boyd, 1987) provided stronger evidence for imitation of a fictional suicide. From October 1984 through February 1985, four television movies dealing with suicide were broadcast in the United States. Ostroff et al. (1985) reported an increase in the number of adolescents admitted to a Connecticut hospital for attempted suicide after the February broadcast of the fourth movie, which depicted the suicide of a teenage couple. In a subsequent study of the same hospital, Ostroff and Boyd (1987) looked at data for the entire year and found that whereas the mean number of suicide attempts per month was 1.9, in February there were 16 attempts, 14 of them in the period after the fictional suicide. All the adolescents involved had watched the movie. And in one case, a teenage couple planned their suicide attempt immediately after watching the movie together.

Gould and Shaffer (1986) studied the effects of all four television movies on the number of teen attempted suicides in the greater New York area; they also examined the effects of three of the four movies on completed suicides by the same group. Both attempted and completed suicides rose significantly after the broadcasts. Phillips and Paight (1987) replicated Gould and Shaffer's (1986) work on completed suicide. Using data on all teen suicides in California and Pennsylvania, and applying the statistical methods of Gould and Shaffer, they found no evidence that teen suicides peaked after the three broadcasts; this result held even after Gould and Shaffer's New York data were combined with the California and Pennsylvania data. Berman (1988) also replicated part of Gould and Shaffer's (1986) study. He examined a nationwide sample of more than 6,000 suicides and found no significant increase in the total number of suicides after the broadcasts of three fictional accounts of suicide; he did, however, find some evidence suggesting that suicides were prompted to use the specific methods portrayed on the television programs. Gould, Shaffer, and Kleinman (1988) then expanded their earlier study by analyzing the effects of the three broadcasts on teen suicides in four urban areas—New York, Cleveland, Dallas, and Los Angeles. Teen suicides peaked significantly after broadcasts in the New York and Cleveland areas, but not in Dallas or Los Angeles. The authors suggested that this discrepancy might be due to differences in the educational programs accompanying the movies in the different cities.

To date, the strongest evidence for imitation of a fictional suicide comes from an ingenious German study by Schmidtke and Häfner (1988). In 1981 and again in 1982, West German television broadcast a six-episode series about a 19-year-old male student who killed himself by jumping in front of a train. Using nationwide data, Schmidtke and Häfner found a significant increase in railway suicides after the broadcasts. The increase was strongest in young males, who were most similar to the suicidal model. Schmidtke and Häfner assessed the possibility that only the method of suicide had shifted to that of the model, whereas the overall number of suicides had not increased, but they found that the evidence was not consistent with this alternative explanation. The study by Schmidtke and Häfner is unique in focusing on a multiprogram fictional story (each of the episodes in the German television series repeated a segment showing the train suicide of the teenage boy). It is noteworthy that the strongest evidence of imitation of fictional suicide stories comes from a study of a multiprogram story. Studies of both fictional and nonfictional television suicide stories support the view that multiprogram stories elicit imitative behavior, whereas single-program stories do not.

"Scholars dispute, but the case is still before the court," said Horace some 2,000 years ago. Few literatures in social science are free from controversy, and the literature on imitative suicide is no exception. However, although some of the investigations reviewed above reported no imitative effects, these were almost always studies that failed to focus on multiprogram stories. When attention has been focused on explicit suicide stories that are clearly labeled and repeated, studies have consistently supported the following conclusions: (1) Overt and covert suicides increase significantly after nonfictional stories; (2) the more publicity given the story, the greater the increase in suicides thereafter; (3) the increase is largest in the geographic areas where the story is most heavily publicized; (4) the increase is proportionally largest for teens, but also evident in other demographic groups; and (5) although the evidence strongly suggests that nonfictional suicide stories elicit imitative suicides, when we turn to the impact of fictional suicide stories evidence of imitation is weaker, though still suggestive.

IMPLICATIONS FROM OTHER FIELDS FOR THE COVERAGE OF SUICIDE STORIES AND ANTISUICIDE STORIES

The studies we have examined are in the epidemiological tradition, which assesses the effect of environmental factors on mortality. Many epidemiological studies are concerned with the effects of physical features, such as polluted water or polluted air. By contrast, the studies we are examining are concerned with cultural factors, particularly the mass media. Relatively few moral questions are raised when governmental agencies seek to purify the air or the water, but the situation is quite different with regard to the cultural environment. How can one reduce the impact of suicide stories without at the same time infringing on freedom of speech or freedom of the press? Although censorship would be unacceptable to almost everyone, there is already some evidence of voluntary restraint on the part of the news media and others involved with suicide stories. Some public health investigators will no longer talk to reporters about incipient suicide clusters because of a fear of imitation (Centers for Disease Control, 1988), and some media representatives have voluntarily decided not to run certain suicide stories (Pell & Watters, 1982). As more news editors learn about the detrimental effects of publicity, some may choose to reduce the coverage they give to suicide stories; others may choose to change the way they present these stories. Suicide and antisuicide stories can vary on at least four dimensions: (1) the nature of the message; (2) the frequency, timing, and length of the message; (3) the placement of the message in the media; and (4) the nature of the messenger. Varying a story's position on each of these dimensions may affect its impact.

Nature of the Message

Nearly all advertisements convey a homogeneous, focused message. To inform the consumer of several alternatives is to reduce the probability that he or she will select any one of them. This suggests that the effect of a suicide story can be reduced if the story "advertises" several alternatives to suicide. Many print advertisements display the equivalent of a newspaper headline, which catches the reader's attention and summarizes the advertiser's message. Advertisers write these headlines to be focused, clear, and unqualified. This suggests that headlines about antisuicide stories should have these qualities, but that suicide story headlines should have the opposite qualities. Vague story headlines should trigger relatively fewer suicides. Indeed, we have already seen from Dutch data (Kopping et al., 1990) that headlines failing to mention suicide explicitly also fail to trigger imitative suicide.

Tversky and Kahneman (1981) found that people lose their enthusiasm for an option when the option is linked with negative outcomes. Most suicide stories do not stress (or even report) the suffering suicides bring upon themselves, their relatives, and their friends. Were these negative consequences reported, some readers might be dissuaded from committing suicide. An epidemic of female suicides in ancient Sparta was reportedly ended by an official proclamation that henceforth all female suicides would be displayed naked in the marketplace. Some 2,500 years before Tversky and Kahneman's article the Spartan government changed the preference for the suicide option by linking it to an additional negative outcome. Commercial messages frequently link an advertised product to such things as sex, freedom, or patriotism. Similarly, news stories about teen suicides sometimes present them in a romantic and idealized light; for example, one television story about a teen suicide pact presented a shot of a yellow rose as the last scene in the story. Romantic treatment of this sort enhances the effect of advertisements and seems likely to enhance the effect of suicide stories as well.

Frequency, Timing, and Length of the Message

As we have noted earlier, many advertising studies (see Comstock et al., 1978) indicate that the repetition of an advertisement increases its effect. These findings are consistent with the literature on imitative suicide (Phillips, 1974,1979; Phillips & Carstensen, 1988). Thus, studies in advertising and elsewhere suggest that the impact of a suicide story can be reduced if the story is not repeated, either from day to day or from network to network. These studies also indicate that longer advertisements on television result in greater recall of the messages. And newspaper research suggests that longer stories attract more readers (Bogart, 1984) and have a greater effect (Kopping et al., 1990). These findings suggest that suicide stories, "natural advertisements" for suicide, should be short. On the other hand, to increase the effectiveness of antisuicide stories, these stories should be repeated—especially following suicide stories. In addition, they should be more frequent during periods with a high suicide rate (e.g., after some holidays; Phillips & Wills, 1987).

Placement of the Message

Front-page stories in newspapers are read more often than those on any other page (Bogart, 1984). This suggests that suicide stories should be confined to the inside pages of the newspaper, and that antisuicide stories should be placed on the front page or in places where the targeted audience is most likely to see them. A further consideration is the format of the message. Print advertisements are commonly presented in single, compact rectangles; presumably advertisers prefer this format because it is effective. In contrast, some newspaper stories are continued from page to page, so that some effort is required to follow up the story, disentangle it from other accounts, and read it in its entirety. The effect of a suicide story will probably be reduced if it is presented in a straggling rather than a compact format.

Advertisers are reluctant to place their messages close to advertisements for competing products. The competing messages distract the consumer and remind him or her of options. This suggests that the effectiveness of a suicide story could be reduced by placing it next to a story about an alternative to suicide (e.g., Alcoholics Anonymous, a suicide prevention center, etc.). Conversely, some types of placement may actually magnify the effect of the suicide story. Asch's (1955/1973) classic work showed that a person who perceived that he or she was the sole deviant in a sea of conformists was unlikely to engage in a deviant act. The person became more likely to behave deviantly if one other person modeled the deviant act, and still more likely to behave deviantly if two model deviants were presented. These considerations suggest that the effect of the suicide story will be enhanced if it is placed adjacent in time or space to another suicide story. In addition, the suicide story is likely to have an amplified effect if it alludes to a "suicide epidemic" or to other, unrelated suicides. If at all possible, then, a suicide story should not be presented as if it were just another example in a general category of "epidemic suicides."

Nature of the Messenger

Advertisements commonly use several types of spokespersons, including the trustworthy expert and the "person who is just like you or me." If at all possible, television suicide stories should not be conveyed by either type of person (Andreoli & Worchel, 1978). The effect of a suicide story might be reduced if reporters exclude justifications of suicide from sympathetic, ordinary people. Conversely, since some research on imitation of publicized suicides suggests that demographic characteristics (e.g., sex, race, and age) mediate imitation of the suicide model, the people conveying antisuicide messages should be *similar* to the members of the targeted audience whenever possible (Phillips 1977, 1979; Stack, 1987; Schmidtke & Häfner, 1988). Messages aimed at teens, for example, might feature teen celebrities who were once suicidal talking about how suicide is not the answer, about how they sought help, and about how glad they are to be alive today. And in view of Asch's (1955/1973) findings, a single antisuicide advocate seems likely to have relatively little effect (especially if suicidal members of the audience believe that suicide is widespread). A more effective approach might involve several advocates, each of whom says that suicide is rare and that constructive solutions to distress are preferable.

RESEARCH TOPICS FOR THE FUTURE, AND WAYS OF FACILITATING THIS RESEARCH

Recommendations for Future Research

Replications and Generalizations

The studies reviewed in this chapter were conducted in only six countries—the United States, Great Britain, The Netherlands, Germany, Austria, and Canada. We need more studies to learn which media effects are peculiar to a cultural group and which are relatively universal. In addition, the studies we have reviewed have almost always focused on stories in traditional newspapers and on national television programs; we need to learn about the effects of stories appearing in other media.

Studies on the Effects of Different Types of Suicide Stories

Most studies on the topic have dealt with nonfictional rather than fictional suicide stories; future work should seek to redress this imbalance. Research in the area is also likely to be most useful if it is restricted to repeated stories. Furthermore, the U.S. Centers for Disease Control (1988) have suggested that the precise method used by a publicized suicide should not be released to the media. When the details are included in the suicide story (e.g., the name and dosage of the poison used), does the story have an unusually large effect? Conversely, when the suicide story focuses primarily on the grief-stricken survivors of the suicide, does this diminish the effect of the story on imitation? In general, is the effect of a story reduced when the suicide story contains negative comments about suicide?

Studies Identifying Behaviors Affected by Suicide Stories

The vast majority of studies have examined the effects of suicide stories on completed suicides. Future studies should also examine the effects of publicized suicides on types of parasuicidal behavior. Some studies, for example, indicate that fatal car crashes increase after suicide stories. Do nonfatal car crashes also increase? Is this increase larger for serious than for minor car crashes? Is there also a poststory increase in other types of accidents and in various types of undetermined deaths?

Studies on Media Owners and Managers

Pell and Watters (1982) found that most Canadian editors in their sample had formal policies on the coverage of suicide stories. Is this true in other countries? What features of a suicide story determine whether it is considered worth placing on the front page? In general, we need to learn more about the extent to which editors change their policies about suicide stories after they have been educated about the impact of suicide stories.

Studies on Antisuicide Stories and Advertisements

We need research on whether suicide and parasuicide rates do in fact drop after stories and advertisements about suicide prevention centers. When should these advertisements run? Are they most effectively placed on television, on billboards, on the radio, in magazines, or in pamphlets distributed at schools?

Some types of stories are not explicitly aimed at reducing the general suicide rate, but may nonetheless have this effect. For example, syndicated advice columns are extremely popular. What happens to the suicide rate after a survivor of a suicide attempt writes to an advice columnist expressing happiness that he or she did not die? What happens after a grieving family member writes to describe the pain he or she has felt after a child committed suicide? Does the suicide rate decline after the advice columnist lists alternatives to suicide and provides telephone numbers for suicide prevention centers? So far, too, we have limited discussion to alternatives to suicide (e.g., counseling) that are provided by mental health professionals. Other alternatives to suicide are provided by religious leaders. What happens to the suicide rate when an evangelist like Billy Graham brings a religious crusade to town?

Studies on Readers, Listeners, and Viewers

Little is known about the reading, listening, and viewing habits of suicidal people. Knowledge of these habits would help to enhance the impact of antisuicide stories, and perhaps to reduce the effect of suicide stories.

Studies on Psychological Mechanisms Producing the Werther Effect

The evidence linking suicide stories with imitative suicides is persuasive, and there is no obvious alternative explanation that accounts for the cumulative findings reported here, especially the finding that the rise in suicides after the suicide story is correlated with the amount of publicity devoted to the story. Nonetheless, all these studies have suffered from two deficiencies that need to be addressed in future research. First, no one has yet demonstrated that the "excess" people who killed themselves after a given publicized suicide had in fact heard about the suicide (although this seems likely). Second, the detailed psychological mechanisms connecting the suicide story with the subsequent rise in suicides are not yet known, and cannot be determined with the death certificate data under study.

Most studies on imitative suicide have been epidemiological. The researchers have typically examined large samples of decedents and have collected only a small amount of information per decedent. Investigations of this type are suitable for establishing the existence of an effect, but not for elucidating the detailed mechanisms that produce it. In addition to more epidemiological studies, we also need psychological research conducted in a clinical fashion. That is, we need to examine small samples of people, on each of whom we have collected a great deal of information. Only in this way can we learn the nature of the psychological processes that mediate individuals' reactions to the suicide story, as well as the poststory rise in deaths.

Recommended Data Collection Activities for Media Organizations, Health Professionals, and Governmental Agencies

Many of the questions described in the preceding section cannot be answered with records that are currently available. Indices and abstracts of televised nonfictional news stories have been made public by various organizations (the Vanderbilt TV News Archives, CBS News, and ABC News), and these sources have been invaluable in research on the effects of suicide stories. Unfortunately, no index or abstract of televised fictional stories is available. A document of this sort would be of extraordinary value to the study of imitative suicide. Similarly, it would be helpful if NBC News released to the public its own index/abstract of NBC News stories; NBC is the only major network that treats its index/abstract as a private resource.

Government agencies need to publish daily or weekly suicide statistics (not just monthly data). Official mortality tables should also be classified by date of injury as well as by date of death; this would allow researchers to pinpoint the relationship between the appearance of a suicide story and a subsequent rise in suicidal behavior. Moreover, research on imitative suicide would be greatly facilitated if health professionals could document and publish information on the number of suicidal people who contact them each day. In addition, it would be useful for health professionals to publish more information on factors that might precipitate suicidal thoughts. With data of this sort, reseachers could estimate the effects of suicide stories not only on suicides, but also on parasuicidal behavior.

SUMMARY AND CONCLUSION

Many studies indicate that heavily publicized suicide stories are followed by significant increases in imitative suicides. The more publicity given to the stories, the greater the increase in suicides thereafter. For nearly every demographic group, suicide stories have a large effect compared with other temporal variables. The effect of a story is small when compared with demographic variables; however, unlike either other temporal or demographic variables, the publicizing (even romanticizing) of suicide in the mass media is readily manipulable. We have offered some guidelines for the news media that may help to diminish the harmful effects of suicide stories. The weight of the evidence on imitative suicide has already prompted some news editors to limit the publicity they give suicide stories and to change the way they report them. The findings of Sonneck et al. (in press) offer encouraging evidence that adherence to such guidelines might help to reduce the incidence of suicide. In addition, we have suggested some ways in which health professionals can design antisuicide stories and advertisements that may counteract the imitative effects of suicide stories.

Much more research is needed before we can be sure of the precise effects of different kinds of suicide stories on different kinds of people. We have suggested several research topics that remain to be addressed. This research would be greatly facilitated if media organizations published more detailed information on the content of their stories, if government agencies published daily suicide statistics, and if health professionals published information on the suicidal clients with whom they work. When some of these steps are taken, it seems likely that we will be able to make progress on what is now recognized as a recalcitrant public health problem in all countries—reducing the incidence of suicide.

ACKNOWLEDGMENTS

This research was supported by a grant from an anonymous private foundation for unrestricted research, awarded to David P. Phillips. We gratefully acknowledge the assistance of Josie van Dijk, who translated Dutch articles for us. As always, we are grateful for outstanding support from Michael O'Hagan and Michael Corrigan of the University of California at San Diego Social Science Computing Facility.

REFERENCES

Andreoli, V., & Worchel, S. (1978). Effects of media, communicator, and message position on attitude change. *Public Opinion Quarterly, 42,* 59–70.

Asch, S. E. (1973). Opinions and social pressure. In E. Aronson (Ed.), *Readings about the social animal.* San Francisco: W. H. Freeman. (Original work published 1955)

Baron, J. N., & Reiss, P. C. (1985). Same time next year: Aggregate analyses of the mass media and violent behavior. *American Sociological Review, 50,* 347–363.

Barraclough, B., Shepherd, D., & Jennings, C. (1977). Do newspaper reports of coroners' inquests incite people to commit suicide? *British Journal of Psychiatry, 131,* 528–532.

Berman, A. L. (1988). Fictional depiction of suicide in television films and imitation effects. *American Journal of Psychiatry, 145,* 982–986.

Blumenthal, S., & Bergner, L. (1973). Suicide and newspapers: A replicated study. *American Journal of Psychiatry, 130,* 468–471.

Bogart, L. (1984). The public's use and perception of newspapers. *Public Opinion Quarterly, 48,* 709–719.

Bollen, K. A., & Phillips, D. P. (1981). Suicidal motor vehicle fatalities in Detroit: A replication. *American Journal of Sociology, 87,* 404–412.

Bollen, K. A., & Phillips, D. P. (1982). Imitative suicides: A national study of the effects of television news stories. *American Sociological Review, 47,* 802–809.

Centers for Disease Control. (1988). CDC recommendations for a community plan for the prevention and containment of suicide clusters. *Morbidity and Mortality Weekly Report, 37*(Suppl. S-6).

Clark, D. C. (1989). Impact of television news reports. *Suicide Research Digest, 3,* 1–2.

Comstock, G., Chaffee, S., Katzman, N., McCombs, M., & Roberts, D. (1978). *Television and human behavior.* New York: Columbia University Press.

Ellis, S. J., & Walsh, S. (1986). Soap may seriously damage your health. *Lancet, i*(8482), 686.

Fowler, B. P. (1986).Emotional crises imitating television. *Lancet, i*(8488), 1036–1037.

Ganzeboom, H. B. G., & de Haan, D. (1982). Gepubliceerde zelfmoorden en verhoging van sterfte door zelfmoord en ongelukken in Nederland 1972–1980. *Mens en Maatschappij, 57,* 55–69.

Gould, M. S., & Shaffer, D. (1986). The impact of suicide in television movies. *New England Journal of Medicine, 315,* 690–694.

Gould, M. S., Shaffer, D., & Kleinman, M. (1988). The impact of suicide in television movies: Replication and commentary. *Suicide and Life-Threatening Behavior, 18,* 90–99.

Gould, M. S., Wallenstein, S., & Kleinman, M. (1990).Time-space clustering of teenage suicide. *American Journal of Epidemiology, 131,* 71–78.

Holding, T. A. (1974). The B.B.C. "Befrienders'" series and its effects. *British Journal of Psychiatry, 124,* 470–472.

Holding, T. A. (1975). Suicide and "The Befrienders'". *British Medical Journal, 3*(5986), 751–752.

Jonas, K. (in press). Modeling and suicide: A test of the Werther effect hypothesis. *Crisis.*

Kessler, R. C., Downey, G., Milavsky, J. R., & Stipp, H. (1988). Clustering of teenage suicides after television news stories about suicide: A reconsideration. *American Journal of Psychiatry, 145,* 1379–1383.

Kessler, R. C., Downey, G., Stipp, H., & Milavsky, R. (1989). Network television news stories about suicide and short-term changes in total U.S. suicides. *Journal of Nervous and Mental Disease, 177,* 551–555.

Kessler, R. C., & Stipp, H. (1984). The impact of fictional television suicide stories on American fatalities. *American Journal of Sociology, 90,* 151–167.

Kopping, A. P., Ganzeboom, H. B. G., & Swanborn, P. G. (1990). *Verhoging van suicide door navolging van kranteberichten.* Unpublished manuscript.

Littman, S. K. (1985). Suicide epidemics and newspaper reporting. *Suicide and Life-Threatening Behavior, 15,* 43–50.

Motto, J. A. (1967). Suicide and suggestibility: The role of the press. *American Journal of Psychiatry, 124,* 252–256.

Motto, J. A. (1970). Newspaper influence on suicide. *Archives of General Psychiatry, 23,* 143–148.

Ostroff, R. B., Behrends, R. W., Lee, K., & Oliphant, J. (1985). Adolescent suicides modeled after television movie. *American Journal of Psychiatry, 142,* 989.

Ostroff, R. B., & Boyd, J. H. (1987). Television and suicide. *New England Journal of Medicine, 316,* 876–877.

Pell, B., & Watters, D., (1982, December). Newspaper policies on suicide stories. *Canada's Mental Health, 30,* 8–9.

Phillips, D. P. (1974). The influence of suggestion on suicide: Substantive and theoretical implications of the Werther effect. *American Sociological Review, 39,* 340–354.

Phillips, D. P. (1977). Motor vehicle fatalities increase just after publicized suicide stories. *Science, 196,* 1464–1465.

Phillips, D. P. (1978). Airplane accident fatalities increase just after stories about murder and suicide. *Science, 201,* 148–150.

Phillips, D. P. (1979). Suicide, motor vehicle fatalities, and the mass media: Evidence toward a theory of suggestion. *American Journal of Sociology, 84,* 1150–1174.

Phillips, D. P. (1980). Airplane accidents, murder, and the mass media: Towards a theory of imitation and suggestion. *Social Forces, 58,* 1001–1024.

Phillips, D. P. (1982). The impact of fictional television stories on American adult fatalities: New evidence on the effect of the mass media on violence. *American Journal of Sociology, 87,* 1340–1359.

Phillips, D. P., & Bollen, K. A. (1985). Same time last year: Selective data dredging for negative findings. *American Sociological Review, 50,* 364–371.

Phillips, D. P., & Carstensen, L. L. (1986). Clustering of teenage suicides after television news stories about suicide. *New England Journal of Medicine, 315,* 685–689.

Phillips, D. P., & Carstensen, L. L. (1988). The effect of suicide stories on various demographic groups, 1968-1985. *Suicide and Life-Threatening Behavior, 18,* 100-114.

Phillips, D. P., & Paight, D. J. (1987). The impact of televised movies about suicide. *New England Journal of Medicine, 317,* 809-811.

Phillips, D. P., & Wills, J. S. (1987). A drop in suicides around major national holidays. *Suicide and Life-Threatening Behavior, 17,* 1-12.

Platt, S. (1987). The aftermath of Angie's overdose: Is soap (opera) damaging to your health? *British Medical Journal, 294,* 954-957.

Sandler, D. A., Connell, P. A., & Welsh, K. (1986). Emotional crises imitating television. *Lancet i*(8485), 856.

Schmidtke, A., & Häfner, H. (1988). The Werther effect after television films: New evidence for an old hypothesis. *Psychological Medicine, 18,* 665-676.

Shneidman, E. S. (1985). *Definition of suicide.* New York: John Wiley.

Sonneck, G., Nagel-Kuess, S., Etzersdorfer, E., Smeh, E., & Hauer, B. (in press). Subway-suicide in Vienna: A contribution to the imitation effect in suicidal behavior (1984-1989). *Crisis.*

Stack, S. (1984). *The effect of suggestion on suicide: A reassessment.* Paper presented at the annual meeting of the American Sociological Association, San Antonio, TX.

Stack, S. (1987). Celebrities and suicide: A taxonomy and analysis, 1948-1983. *American Sociological Review, 52,* 401-412.

Tversky, A., & Kahneman, D. (1981). The framing of decisions and the psychology of choice. *Science, 211,* 453-458.

Wasserman, I. (1984). Imitation and suicide: A reexamination of the Werther effect. *American Sociological Review, 49,* 427-436.

Weisman, A. D., & Worden, J. W. (1972). Risk-rescue rating in suicide assessment. *Archives of General Psychiatry, 26,* 553-560.

Williams, J. M. G., Lawton, C., Ellis, S. J., Walsh, S., & Reed, J. (1987). Copycat suicide attempts. *Lancet, ii*(8550), 102-103.

Williams, J. M. G., Lawton, C., Ellis, S. J., Walsh, S., & Reed, J. (n.d.) *Imitative parasuicide by overdose.* London: Research Department, Independent Broadcasting Authority.

Economy, Work, Occupation, and Suicide

Ira M. Wasserman, Ph.D.
Eastern Michigan University

DURKHEIM'S ANOMIE MODEL OF SUICIDE

A useful initial perspective for examining the impact of the economy on suicidal behavior is Durkheim's "anomie" model of suicide. As Durkheim defined it (see Orru, 1987, pp. 57–59), anomie represents a state of moral decay caused by a breakdown of the moral order (e.g., religious, kinship) and its social regulation. In his early study of this process (Durkheim 1893/ 1933) he related the growth of social anomie to the changing forms of the division of labor in society, which affected the social regulation of professional and occupational groups. One illustration of this shift is the decreased time allowed for personal bereavement in the modern industrial order (Platt, 1981).

In his application of this anomie model to the study of suicide, Durkheim (1897/1951, pp. 241–258) defined "economic anomie,"and differentiated "acute" economic anomie, which involve a short term disruption of the economic order, from "chronic" economic anomie, which involves a gradual weakening of social regulation. Acute economic anomie, as exemplified by significant swings in the economy, creates an imbalance between human needs and desires, and subsequently stimulates suicidal behavior. By contrast, chronic economic anomie decreases the regulation of occupational groups in society and increases their suicidal propensity.

A number of empirical studies have provided partial support for the anomie model. For example, Halbwachs (1930/1978, p. 127) found in Europe that there were greater suicide levels in areas with higher levels of urbanization. However, he also found that economic depression, rather than economic prosperity, was more likely to increase suicide (1930/1978, pp. 231–244). For the United States, Pierce (1967) found that all economic shifts increased suicide, but a more precise analysis of his findings (Marshall & Hodge, 1981) showed that only downward shifts increased suicide.

The Durkheimian anomie model provides a useful general outline for examining shifts in suicidal behavior in relation to the economy, work, and occupations. However, it has limited usefulness for developing specific testable hypotheses, since it fails to provide adequate measures for "social regulation" (Pope, 1976, pp. 116–124). Without such measures, it is impossible to specify the social processes that cause economic shifts to influence the social suicide rate. The model is also limited by its assumption that the total population is suicide-prone. Empirical studies (Kramer, Pollock, Redlick, & Locke, 1972; Miles, 1972) have shown that only a small subset of individuals in society is suicide-prone. These individuals are mentally disturbed, suffer severe depression, and may tend to overuse alcohol and drugs. It is this portion of the population that may be swayed toward suicide by short- and long-term economic shifts.

CURRENT FINDINGS REGARDING ACUTE ECONOMIC ANOMIE

A number of cross-sectional (Boor, 1982; Travis, 1983) and longitudinal (Hamermesh, 1974; Hamermesh & Soss, 1974; Brenner, 1976, 1977; Vigderhaus, 1977; Adams, 1981; Wasserman, 1983) studies of suicidal behavior have established a statistical linkage between suicide and unemployment. Even the fall in suicide during "great" or "major" wars (Rojcewicz, 1971; Lunden, 1977) has been explained not only in terms of war per se (which is assumed to increase political integration, thereby decreasing suicide), but in terms of the decline in unemployment caused by the wartime expansion of the economy (Marshall, 1981). Some empirical studies have not shown this statistical linkage, but these findings may be due to special historical circumstances. For example, examining suicide data for Norway between 1951 and 1980, Stack (1989) found no statistical linkage between suicide and unemployment. He concluded that this lack of statistical linkage might have been caused by Norway's welfare economy, which mitigates the impact of unemployment on individuals. Similarly, a cross-sectional study in Canada between 1979 and 1981 (Sakinofsky & Roberts, 1985) found that the Maritime provinces (Nova Scotia, New Brunswick, Newfoundland and Prince Edward Island) had a high unemployment rate and a low suicide rate. The study concluded that the anomaly might be explained by the facts that unemployment is less stigmatized in these provinces, and that kinship ties in these provinces provide economic support for the unemployed.

Examining both parasuicide and completed suicide studies, Platt (1984) concluded that there is a statistical linkage between unemployment and suicide. However, he argued that there is no causal linkage between the two variables, in that one cannot conclude that being unemployed automatically causes an individual to commit suicide. Rather, he contended that individuals with mental disorders are more likely to suffer a loss of employment, and are also more likely to commit suicide. This explanation stresses the importance of selection by the mechanism of "psychiatric morbidity."

A serious problem in interpreting statistical findings on suicide is related to the rareness of the event. In examining any causal linkage employing statistical data, it is always necessary to be aware of the "ecological fallacy" (Robinson, 1950), which involves making individual-level inferences from aggregate-level data. With suicide behavior the problem is even more serious, since the rarity of the event (e.g., on the average there are 12 suicides per 100,000 population in the United States population) makes any individual-level interpretation almost impossible unless the units of analysis (e.g., counties, neighborhoods) are relatively homogeneous (Selvin, 1965). As one moves to larger, less homogeneous aggregation units, individual-level interpretations become impossible, as illustrated by the interpretations in a recent study on social stress in the United States (Linsky & Strauss, 1986). The only way to make an individual level causal interpretation from such aggregate-level findings is to use additional information.

There are some empirical studies that provide some of this side information. For example, a number of studies (Breed, 1963; Shepherd & Barraclough, 1980) suggest that long-term unemployment increases suicidal propensity. An attitudinal study of suicidal ideation among a randomly selected southern California population between 1975 and 1982 (Dooley, Catalano, Rook, & Serxner, 1989b) found that long-term unemployment increased social stress. Similarly, Maris (1981) found that suicide was more likely to occur among individuals who experienced serious career difficulties. A monthly study of completed suicides in southern California (Dooley, Catalano, Rook, & Serxner, 1989a) found that economic downturns had their greatest impact on males 50–64 years of age, and on females in general. With regard to the males in this study, it is likely that they had become marginal to the economy but were too young to retire. With regard to the females, it may have been the case that increased male unemployment raised the level of "wife abuse" in society. Some cross-cultural studies (e.g., Counts, 1987) suggest a causal linkage of wife abuse and suicide. Further individual-level studies are required to verify this hypothesis.

CURRENT FINDINGS REGARDING OCCUPATIONAL SUICIDE PATTERNS

The findings regarding occupational status and suicide are inconsistent, with different patterns being observed in different studies. In part, this inconsistency is caused by the difficulties with classifying many occupational statuses into clearly defined categories (Bogue, 1969, pp. 431–437) and linking this classification with occupational suicide behavior. Death certificates list the last occupation of the deceased, and numerous studies (e.g., Breed, 1963; Shepherd & Barraclough, 1980; Platt, 1984) have shown that individuals who commit suicide have serious career difficulties. In general, there is an inverse connection between occupational status and suicide (Lampert, Bourque, & Kraus, 1984), but there are significant variations in suicide within occupational groups. For example, without controls, medical personnel have above-average suicide rates (Labovitz & Hagedown, 1971); furthermore, within this group psychiatrists tend to have high suicide rates, but surgeons and pediatricians tend to have low suicide rates (Arnetz, Harte, Hedberg, Theorel, Allander, & Malker, 1987; Chemtob, Bauer, Hamada, & Pelowski, 1989). A major difficulty with determining a causal explanation for occupational suicide patterns is the lack of a causal framework for examining occupational suicide patterns.

Figure 25.1 provides a general heuristic model that can be employed to examine the multicausal nature of occupational suicide patterns. It can be seen from Figure 25.1 that psychiatric morbidity influences both occupa-

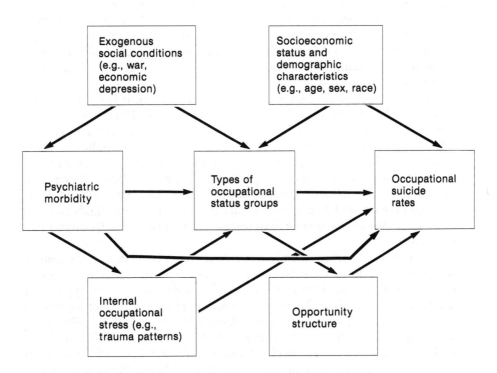

FIGURE 25.1. Model linking occupational status to suicide.

tional suicide rates and the characteristics of individuals in various occupations. For example, a study of completed suicides in two New Hampshire counties between 1968 and 1970 (Sanborn, Sanborn, & Cimbolic, 1974) found a high level of psychiatric morbidity among individuals who committed suicide, regardless of their occupational status. Other studies (e.g., Berman, 1982, p. 217) have suggested that the high suicide rates found among psychiatrists may be related to psychiatric selection, in that highly educated individuals with depressive disorders may tend to select this specialty.

Exogenous social conditions, such as economic depressions or recessions and wars, may also have an impact on the suicide patterns of occupational groups. As noted earlier, Marshall (1981) maintains that total war reduces the unemployment rates of all occupational groups, and that this in turn may lower their suicide rates. Changing social conditions in general may significantly influence the level of social anomie, and this may affect the suicide rates of different occupational groups (Powell, 1958). Araki and Murata (1987) found that in Japan between 1950 and 1980, suicides increased during periods preceding economic crises and decreased during periods of economic prosperity. The recent economic farm crisis in the United States has increased personal depression among farmers, and may have raised their suicide rates (Ragland & Berman, 1990–1991; Stallones, 1990). I explore this issue further in this chapter by considering long-term cohort patterns of suicide in relation to exogenous social conditions (e.g., changes in economic opportunities for different age groups in different historic periods).

In examining variations in suicide by occupation, it is usually necessary to control for variations in socioeconomic status within various occupations. For example, the suicide rate in the volunteer military services is relatively low in relation to that of a comparable civilian population (Datel & Johnson, 1979; Rothberg & Jones, 1987). Moreover, as was not the case in the 19th century, officers have a significantly lower rate than enlisted men. However, in the modern military most officers are married, with their spouses present, and it is a known fact that married individuals have an appreciably lower suicide rate than unmarried or divorced individuals (Trovato, 1986a).

The issue of socioeconomic controls is partially related to the controversial issue of the suicidal behavior of physicians and psychiatrists. In an early study, Craig and Pitts (1968) found that physicians had an apparently higher suicide rate than the general populace. However, further analysis of their occupational suicide patterns (Ross, 1973; Brauchitsch, 1976; Bergman, 1979; Rich & Pitts, 1980; Arnetz et al., 1987; Rimpela, 1989) found that both the socioeconomic status characteristics of physicians and the methods of enumerating their suicide influenced the findings. Physician suicides include the suicides of medical students—individuals who experience high stress levels and have high suicide rates. Also, relatively few women and members of minority groups are physicians, and these two status groups have relatively low suicide rates. Since World War II many foreign immigrants have entered the medical profession in the United States, and foreign medical personnel have a relatively high suicide rate. Also, the average age of physicians is higher than that of many other occupations, and suicide increases with age. In general, the socioeconomic status and demographic characteristics of physicians and psychiatrists tend to inflate their suicide rate, independently of the other factors in the model in Figure 25.1.

Internal occupational stress may also influence occupational suicide patterns. Hilliard-Lysen and Riemer (1988) examined the personal attitudes of 25 dentists in the Midwest, and found that they suffered high levels of daily stress (e.g., time schedules, hostile patients) that might influence their suicide behavior, although they also found that 21 of the 25 dentists stated that they never thought of suicide. A problem with linking stress measures to occupational suicide rates is that most studies do not specify the type of social stress that is most likely to lead to suicide. With regard to physician suicide, there is strong empirical evidence that women physicians have a significantly higher suicide rate than the general female population (Pitts, Schuller, Rich, & Pitts, 1979); it may be the case that they suffer occupational stress because of competing household demands on their time. A study of completed female suicides in a series of states between 1975 and 1979 (Alston, 1986) found that women in traditional female occupations (e.g., nursing, teaching, social work) had a lower suicide rate than women employed in nontraditional occupations. Gifted women in nontraditional occupations may suffer occupational stress, and this may increase their suicide propensity (Tomlinson-Keasey, Warren, & Elliott, 1986). With regard to the relatively high suicide behavior of psychiatrists, it has been shown (Chemtob, Hamada, Bauer, Kinney, & Torigoe, 1988) that many patients of psychiatrists attempt and complete suicide, and that this behavior of their patients is likely to increase trauma and stress among psychiatrists.

In the London Underground, suicides that involve jumping under railway trains produces a post-traumatic syndrome among train drivers (Cocks, 1989). For the state of Washington between 1950 and 1979, the use of standardized mortality ratios for occupations (Milham, 1983, p. 69) found that sheepherders tended to have an elevated suicide ratio. Sheepherders are alone for long periods of time in remote areas, and may suffer severe social stress because of their social isolation, although one must not exaggerate the influence of a single predictor apart from others. In any case, one must specify the relevant dimensions of social stress that lead to suicide before one can employ this factor in the model in Figure 25.1.

The final factor in the model concerns the opportunity structure in a social order for suicide to occur. The next section of this chapter examines this structure in greater detail, since it is related to the linkage of parasuicide and suicide, as well as to the relationship between substance use and suicide. For example, physicians have greater access to drugs, and this greater access may influence their level of drug abuse, which is causally linked to suicide (Bressler, 1976). The previously cited study of the state of Washington (Milham, 1983, p. 69) found an elevated suicide rate for dentists, veterinarians, physicians, and medical and dental technicians, all of whom have access to drugs that may be used to commit suicide. Members of these occupational groups also have knowledge of how to use the drugs effectively. Also, in cases when these individuals use drugs to commit suicide, coroners are more likely to classify the act as a suicide rather than as an accidental overdose, since they are assumed to have knowledge concerning the consequences of drug use.

Figure 25.1 illustrates the complicated nature of occupational suicides, as well as the difficulties of disentangling the various factors that may play a role in such suicides. Without the controls shown in Figure 25.1, it is impossible to establish a causal linkage between occupational behavior and suicide. The rarity of the event and the difficulty of obtaining accurate data have further limited the ability of researchers to establish causal relationships in this area.

ROUTINE ACTIVITY, OPPORTUNITY STRUCTURE AND SUICIDE

The "routine-activity" or "opportunity-structure" model has been employed in the field of criminology (Cohen & Felson, 1979) to explain temporal and spatial shifts in deviant behavior. The model hypothesizes that shifts in the social structure may influence the level of deviant behavior in society. For example, more lightweight products (e.g., televisions, computers) are being produced by the American capitalist system, and this shift is related to the growth of property crimes, since these products are easier to steal. Similarly, the greater use of checks and credit cards by women, as well as their greater use of the welfare system, is causally related to the acceleration of property crimes among women. With regard to suicide, shifts in opportunity are likely to influence the social suicide rate. A recent study of Great Britain and The Netherlands (Clarke & Mayhew, 1989) discovered that the detoxification of the gas supply in these two nations eliminated gas suicides, and thus caused a decline in overall suicide rates. Many individuals began to use substitute methods (e.g., drugs, firearms), but the rate remained lower than it did prior to the gas detoxification. States in the United States (e.g., Alaska; Hlady & Middaugh, 1988) that have high levels of firearms per capita are likely to have higher suicide rates than states with low levels (e.g., Vermont). The opportunity structure in any society influences the causal linkage between parasuicides and completed suicides.

The opportunity structure also influences the suicide patterns of different occupational groups. Access to the means of self-destruction influences the probability of suicide for various occupations. For example, as noted above, the relatively high suicide rate of medical personnel in relation to other high-socioeconomic-status occupations is partially related to their greater access to drugs (Bressler, 1976; Rimpela, 1989). Similarly, the high suicide rates of police officials during periods of occupational stress (e.g., police officials in New York City from 1934 to 1940, when previous scandals were being prosecuted by the city authorities; Heiman, 1975) is related to their access to firearms. Also, the recent increase in female suicides appears to be related to their greater access to firearms (Alston, 1986, p. 111).

One important opportunity factor related to suicide is the changing level of alcohol consumption. A number of macro-level studies (Sullivan, 1900; DeLint & Schmidt, 1976; DeLint, 1981; Poikolainen, 1983; Gliksman & Rush, 1986) have demonstrated a statistical linkage between levels of alcohol consumption and suicide. The enactment of national prohibition in the United States between 1920 and 1933 resulted in a noteworthy decrease in the national suicide rate (Wasserman, 1989). There is a causal linkage between alcoholism and suicide (Kessel & Grossman, 1961; Englebrecht, 1983; Roy & Linnoila, 1986), since alcohol is a depressant, and a causal linkage has been established between depression and suicide (Sainsbury, 1980). Alcoholism also has an association with destructive behavior (Goodwin, 1973; Hertzman & Bendit, 1975; Abel & Zeidenberg, 1985), which may be involved in suicide. For example, the high level of suicide among Native Americans is causally related to the high levels of alcoholism and drug abuse among them, which tend to increase their level of violence (May, 1986).

Alcoholism is more prevalent among certain occupations, and this prevalence influences the suicide rates of these occupations. An early study of attempted suicides in England (East, 1913) found that members of occupations with greater access to alcohol (e.g., bartenders) were likely to have more suicide attempts. Levels of alcoholism vary among occupations (Plant, 1977), and this variation affects the suicide rates of these occupations. For example, alcoholism is common among male physicians in comparison to members of similar high-status occupations (Roy & Linnoila, 1986), and this high level of alcoholism influences the suicide behavior of physicians. Alcohol is employed as a coping mechanism by many individuals (Pearlin & Radebaugh, 1976), but its overuse may have serious long-term consequences, including suicide and homicide. Occupational stress may cause individuals to abuse alcohol (Herold & Conlon, 1981), and this abuse may in turn influence their levels of suicide.

Downward shifts in the economy may increase the levels of social stress, which may in turn influence levels of alcohol consumption (Brenner, 1975;

Smart, 1979; Layne & Whitehead, 1985) and the levels of suicide. For males in American society, work is one of their main sources of social identity and economic support (Tausky & Piedmont, 1967–1968; Maris, 1981), and a loss of employment is likely to increase their levels of social stress. In order to cope with this increased social stress, many unemployed individuals consume more alcohol, which increases their vulnerability to suicide. Also, increased alcoholism is statistically related to wife abuse, which increases the suicide vulnerability of women (Counts, 1987).

In summary, routine activity influences the probability that a parasuicide will become a completed suicide. Occupations with access to firearms (e.g., police officials) and drugs (e.g., medical personnel) possess more lethal means of self-destruction, and thus are likely to have fewer parasuicides and more completed suicides. Alcohol use also influences suicide behavior. Occupations with greater access to alcohol and drugs (e.g., bartenders, entertainers, medical personnel) are more likely to abuse drugs, which increases their disposition toward suicide. Also, alcohol and drugs are coping mechanisms; increases in their use are likely to occur during economic downturns, and this increased use is likely to increase suicide.

DEMOGRAPHIC FACTORS RELATED TO WORK AND OCCUPATION

As an earlier section of this chapter has shown, the linkage of work settings and social stress that may induce suicide is a complicated relationship. For example, a study that examined types of illness related to social stress (e.g., coronary heart disease, hypertension, suicide, and homicide) and industrial settings (manufacturing, agriculture, forestry) found no consistent relationship between these stress-induced illnesses and these settings (Kercher & Linden, 1982). Although suicide does not vary consistently with work settings, an inverse relationship was found between the suicide rate and the relative growth of both occupation and industries for all time periods (Reinhart & Linden, 1982, p. 40). These findings can be understood within the framework of the "relative-cohort-size" model.

Easterlin (1978, 1980) developed a causal demographic model in which he argued that the relative size of a demographic cohort will influence its members' life chances in general, and thus will influence their long-term work patterns and suicide rates. For example, the age cohort born in the United States during the Great Depression was a relatively numerically small one, and individuals in a smaller cohort should have more economic opportunities than members of a numerically larger cohort should have. As a result, the smaller cohort's members should suffer lower levels of social stress and suicide. By contrast, numerically larger age cohorts (e.g., individuals born in the United States from 1945 to 1954 during the "baby boom") should have fewer economic opportunities, which should raise their level of social stress and their suicide rates.

A number of empirical findings would appear to support the relative-cohort-size model. A study of suicide rates in the United States in the postwar period (Ahlburg & Schapiro, 1984) found that numerical increases in the size of cohorts were positively related to the suicide rates of the larger cohorts. Similarly, a U.S. study covering a longer time period (1933-1982; Holinger, Offer, & Ostrov, 1987) obtained similar findings: "The suicide rates . . . increased among 15-24 year olds as the proportion of the 15-24 year olds in the population increased, and the rate decreased as the proportion of 15-24 olds decreased" (p. 216).

The Easterlin relative-cohort-size model argues that competition for college admission, employment opportunities, and other status honors will be a function of the relative size of the cohorts. Cohorts deprived of these rewards will suffer higher levels of social stress, which will increase their vulnerability to suicide. The weakness of the model is that it fails to control adequately for age and period effects. Age effects involve changes related to the individual aging process (e.g., role changes), whereas period effects involve historic events (e.g., war, economic depression) that impinge on all social actors in a society. It is usually mathematically difficult to separate out these three effects, since they are statistically related to one another (Palmore, 1978). A recent study of age, period and cohort effects for the United States between 1933 and 1978 (Wasserman, 1987) did specify the strength of cohort effects, but the study had to make special assumptions regarding the constraints. Converse (1976) demonstrated that when one is dealing with these three effects simultaneously, it is necessary to employ additional information to separate out the three effects. Another difficulty with this type of analysis is that period effects are usually specified by dummy variables, and not by the changing strength of historic period effects (e.g., war effects are specified by dummy variables rather than by measures of the consequences of war; Marshall, 1981).

If long-term historic changes have a negative impact on occupational and work groups, it is likely that these social groups will experience an increase in their suicide rates, especially if these effects cause a downward occupational movement for these work groups (e.g., farmers, automobile workers). However, the actual consequences of these historic effects will depend on the manner in which they influence the total social environment of the actors. For example, a number of empirical studies (e.g., Newman, Whitemore, & Newman, 1973; Davis, 1981) have shown a positive statistical linkage between female labor force participation and female suicide rates. However, a study in British Columbia (Ornstein, 1983) found that women participating in the work force were less likely to commit suicide than were unemployed or economically inactive (e.g., housewives) women. The previous findings suggest that increased female economic activity triggers certain social changes (e.g., increased divorce, spouse abuse) that causally increase female suicide rates. Further studies are needed to specify the causal mechanism that links changes in the numerical size of cohorts and their suicide rates.

EMPIRICAL ILLUSTRATIONS LINKING THE ECONOMY, WORK, OCCUPATIONS, AND SUICIDE

In this section of the chapter, two illustrations of the findings discussed above are provided. First, changing suicide rates for males and females in Quebec, Canada, in relation to changing unemployment rates and standardized divorce rates are provided. Second, the relative occupational suicide rates for white males in the state of Washington between 1950 and 1979 are presented.

Changing Male and Female Suicide Rates in Quebec

Quebec is the French Canadian province within Canada. It began with the colony of New France in 1534 and slowly expanded throughout southeastern Canada. The Roman Catholic Church was politically, socially, and economically dominant within the province from the time of its founding until the 1960s. The church dominated and controlled the early economic growth of the province (Ryan, 1966). Prior to the "quiet revolution" in the 1960s there was an extended kinship system with large families in the province (Queen, Habenstein, & Quadagno, 1985, pp. 360–378). Economic development occurred continuously throughout the 19th and 20th centuries in the province, although this development was controlled by capital from English-speaking Canada and the United States (Economic Research Corporation, 1960). The opening of the St. Lawrence Seaway in April 1959 made the midwestern American economic market more accessible to Quebec, and significantly expanded the economy of the province.However, even with this expansion there was still a split labor market in the province, since the English-speaking population of the province (approximately 20% of the population) controlled the private economic means of production and dominated the private sector of the economy in the province (Porter, 1965; Fenwick, 1982).

Beginning in 1960, a "quiet revolution" began in Quebec that brought about the political modernization of the province. For example, in 1964 the Public Ministry of Education was established in the province, reducing the Catholic Church's control of education (Fenwick, 1982, p. 3). The effect of this quiet revolution was a shrinking role for the Catholic Church.

> For the majority [of Quebec's population during the 1960s], estrangement from religious practice developed as a result of the church's growing irrelevance in meeting their everyday needs. Schools were no longer linked to the Catholic

parish; teachers were more apt to be lay than clerical; hospitals and clinics were professionally administered by specialists. (Guindon, 1988, pp. 137–138)

One would expect these changes to influence the suicide patterns in the province. Table 25.1 gives the suicide rates for males and females in Quebec between 1969 and 1983; the ratio of male to female suicide rates; the standardized divorce rate (divorce rate/[divorce rate + marriage rate]), which is utilized because yearly divorce rates will vary in relation to yearly marriage rates (Stack, 1989); and the unemployment rate. Consistent with the results from other studies (e.g., Dyck, Newman, & Thompson, 1988), an increase in the suicide rates of both sexes in the province from 1969 to 1983 was found. This growth in suicide rates was statistically related to the increasing unemployment rates in the province (Cormier & Klerman, 1985), as well as to an increased standardized divorce rate. Both sexes experienced an increase in suicide, but the rate of increase was greater for males than for females, as illustrated by the changing ratio of male to female suicide rates from 1969 to 1983. The findings are consistent with Trovato's (1986b, p. 42) time-series analysis for Canada between 1950 and 1982, which found that unemployment strongly influenced male suicide rates, but had weak impact on female suicide rates. The split labor market in the province may also have influenced the impact of male suicide rates, since the French-speaking residents of the province were (and still are) highly aware of their income inequalities relative to the English-speaking residents (Laczko, 1987).

White Male Occupational Suicide Patterns in Washington State

Occupational suicide patterns for white males in the state of Washington between 1950 and 1979 are also presented to illustrate the findings discussed earlier in this chapter. The occupational suicide data were kindly supplied by Dr. Samuel Milham, Jr. of the Washington State Department of Social and Health Services (Milham, 1983). Table 25.2 indicates the proportionate mortality ratio (PMR) for suicide for various occupations in the state between 1950 and 1979. PMR is calculated as follows (Milham, 1983, p. 96):

$$PMR = \frac{\text{Tabulated deaths for an occupation–cause–color group}}{\text{Expected deaths for an occupation–cause–color group}} \times 100$$

By employing this measure, Milham (1983) was able to standardize for the age, sex, and racial characteristics of the various occupationnal groups

TABLE 25.1. Male and Female Suicide Rates, Standardized Divorce Rates, and Unemployment Rates for the Province of Quebec, Canada, 1969–1983

Year	Male suicide rate (per 100,000)	Female suicide rate (per 100,000)	Ratio of Male to female suicide rates	Standardized divorce rate[a]	Average unemployment rate
1969	18.0	6.1	2.55	.058	6.9
1970	13.3	4.6	2.89	.089	7.9
1971	13.8	4.6	3.00	.095	8.2
1972	15.0	5.0	3.00	.107	8.3
1973	16.4	6.3	2.60	.135	7.4
1974	16.1	4.9	3.29	.192	7.3
1975	13.4	5.3	2.53	.219	8.8
1976	15.8	5.4	2.93	.230	8.7
1977	18.3	6.5	2.82	.231	10.3
1978	21.8	6.8	3.21	.244	10.9
1979	23.3	8.1	2.88	.237	9.6
1980	23.3	6.9	3.38	.237	9.8
1981	25.2	7.8	3.23	.279	10.3
1982	25.4	7.9	3.22	.318	13.8
1983	28.7	8.6	3.34	.318	13.9

Note. The data were kindly supplied by Statistics Canada.
[a]Standardized divorce rate = divorce rate/(divorce rate + marriage rate).

TABLE 25.2. Proportionate Mortality Ratios for Various Occupational Categories for the State of Washington, 1950–1979

Occupational category	Proportionate mortality ratio
Sheepherders and wool workers	264*
Dentists	236*
Hairdressers and cosmetologists	227
Veterinarians	223*
Tool and die makers and setters	194*
Physicians	175*
Mechanical engineers	175
Medical and dental technicians	163
Draftsmen	160
Body and fender repairmen and auto painters	152
Barbers	151*
Students	125*
Army/Air Force/Marine Corps officers and enlisted men	86
Cooks, candymakers, and chefs	79
Navy/Coast Guard officers and enlisted men	78
Road graders, pavers, machine operators	76*
Building and construction contractors and foremen	64*
Lumber/log/sawmill truck drivers	63
Purchasing agents and buyers (not exclusive category), sales managers	41*
Airplane pilots and navigators	40
Disabled, retarded, institutionalized, and unemployable persons	31*
Clergymen	25*

Note. The data are from Milham (1983).
*$p < .01$.

The results suggest the possible influence of the various factors specified in Figure 25.1 on occupational suicide patterns in the state of Washington between 1950 and 1979. The relatively high suicide rates for physicians, dentists, veterinarians, and medical and dental technicians were probably related to their access to drugs and other means of self-destruction. By contrast, the relatively low suicide rate for disabled, retarded, institutionalized and unemployable persons was probably related to their lack of access to efficient means of self-destruction, as well as the close supervision of this group. The relatively high suicide rates for sheepherders and wool workers and for students may have been related to the social stress and isolation experienced by these groups. The relatively low suicide rates for military personnel were probably related to the present selection procedures for these occupations, with individuals with severe psychiatric morbidity being eliminated from these occupations. The relatively low suicide rates for clergymen may well have been related to the influence of religious belief systems on this occupation. All of these hypotheses of course are speculative, and higher quality data are required to verify them.

SUMMARY

The purpose of this chapter has been to examine the impact of the economy, work, and occupation on suicide. Although a number of studies have shown a statistical linkage between unemployment and suicide, one must be cautious in interpreting these findings. The rareness of the event (there are approximately 12 per 100,000 suicides per year in the United States) makes individual-level interpretations impossible (i.e., one cannot causally conclude from the collective statistical findings that unemployed *individuals* are more likely to commit suicide; Selvin, 1965). Rather, it is necessary to assume that unemployment triggers certain social processes that increase the likelihood of suicide for individuals with high levels of psychiatric morbidity. Two social groups that are significantly affected by increased unemployment are older, nonretired male workers, who have difficulty obtaining employment during periods of economic downturns, and women, who may suffer increased family abuse as a result of increased use of alcohol by unemployed spouses.

With regard to the causal linkage of occupation and suicide, Figure 25.1 has presented some of the factors that may influence occupational suicide patterns. Occupational suicide is related to exogenous conditions, the opportunity of various occupational categories to commit suicide, occupational stress (e.g., loneliness, trauma events), selection for occupation linked with psychiatric morbidity, and the socioeconomic characteristics of individuals within various occupations. Any comprehensive social theory of occupational suicide must consider all these factors. The chapter has shown the difficulties with establishing causal relationships between the economy, work, and occupation. From the results presented, it is clear that better data and controls are required to test causal models in this area.

REFERENCES

Abel, E. L., & Zeidenberg, P. (1985). Age, alcohol and violent death: A postmortem study. *Journal of Studies on Alcohol, 46,* 228–231.

Adams, O. B. (1981). *Health and economic activity: A time-series analysis of Canadian mortality and unemployment rates 1950–77.* Ottawa: Statistics Canada.

Ahlburg, D. A., & Schapiro, M. O. (1984). Socioeconomic ramifications of changing cohort size: An analysis of U.S. postwar suicide rates by age and sex. *Demography, 21,* 97–105.

Alston, M. H. (1986). Occupation and suicide among women. *Issues in Mental Health Nursing, 8,* 109–119.

Araki, S., & Murati, K. (1987). Suicide in Japan: Socioeconomic effects of its secular and seasonal trends. *Suicide and Life-Threatening Behavior, 17,* 64–71.

Arnetz, B. B., Harte, L. G., Hedberg, A., Theorel, T., Allander, E., & Malker, H. (1987). Suicide patterns among physicians related to other academicians and well as to the general population. *Acta Psychiatrica Scandinavica, 75,* 139–143.

Bergman, J. (1979). The suicide rate among psychiatrists revisited. *Suicide and Life-Threatening Behavior, 9,* 219–229.

Berman, A. G. (1982). Suicide and occupation: A review. *Journal of Vocational Behavior, 21,* 206–223.

Bogue, D. J. (1969). *Principles of demography.* New York: Wiley.

Boor, M. (1982). Relationship of anomie to perceived changes in financial status, 1973–1980. *Journal of Clinical Psychology, 38,* 891–892.

Brauchitsch, H. V. (1976). The physician's suicide revisited. *Journal of Nervous and Mental Disease, 162,* 40–45.

Breed, W. (1963). Occupational mobility and suicide among white males. *American Sociological Review, 29,* 179–188.

Brenner, M. H. (1975). Trends in alcohol consumption and associated illness: Some effects of economic change. *American Journal of Public Health, 65,* 1279–1292.

Brenner, M. H. (1976). Estimating the social cost of national economic policy: Implications for mental and physical health and criminal aggression. In *Achieving the goals of the Employment Act of 1946: Thirtieth anniversary review* (Vol. 1). Washington, DC: U.S. Government Printing Office.

Brenner, M. H. (1977). Personal stability and economic security. *Social Policy, 8,* 2–4.

Bressler, B. (1976). Suicide and drug abuse in the medical community. *Suicide and Life-Threatening Behavior, 6,* 169–178.

Chemtob, C. M., Hamada, R. S., Bauer, G., Kinney, B., & Torigoe, R. (1988). Patients' suicide: Frequency and impact on psychiatrists. *American Journal of Psychiatry, 145,* 224–228.

Chemtob, C. M., Bauer, G. B., Hamada, R. S., & Pelowski, S. (1989). Patient suicide: Occupational hazard for psychologists and psychiatrists. *Professional Psychology: Research and Procedure, 20,* 294–300.

Clarke, R. V., & Mayhew, P. (1989). Crime as opportunity: A note on domestic gas suicide in Britain and the Netherlands. *Journal of Criminology, 29,* 35–46.

Cocks, R. A. (1989). Trauma in the tube: The problem of railway suicide and its consequences. *Stress Medicine, 5,* 93–97.

Cohen, L., & Felson, M. (1979). Social change and crime trends: A routine activity approach. *American Sociological Review, 44,* 588–607.

Converse, P. E. (1976). *The dynamics of party support: Cohort-analyzing party identification.* Beverly Hills, CA: Sage.

Cornier, H. J., & Klerman, G. L. (1985). Unemployment and male–female participation as determinants of changing suicide rates of males and females in Quebec. *Social Psychiatry, 20,* 109–114.

Counts, D. A. (1987). Female suicide and wife-abuse: A cross-cultural perspective. *Suicide and Life-Threatening Behavior, 17,* 194–204.

Craig, A. G., & Pitts, A. W. (1968). Suicide by physicians. *Disease of the Nervous System, 29*, 763-772.

Datel, W. E., & Johnson, A. W., Jr. (1979). Suicide in United States army personnel, 1975-76. *Military Medicine, 144*, 239-244.

Davis, R. A. (1981). Female labor force participation, status integration and suicide, 1950-1969. *Suicide and Life-Threatening Behavior, 11*, 111-123.

DeLint, J. (1981). The influence of much increased alcohol consumption on mortality rates: The Netherlands between 1950 and 1976. *British Journal of Addiction, 76*, 77-83.

DeLint, J., & Schmidt, W. (1976). Alcoholism and mortality. In B. Kissin & H. Begleiter (Eds.), *Social aspects of alcoholism* (pp. 275-305). New York: Plenum Press.

Dooley, D., Catalno, R., & Serxner, S. (1989a). Economic stress and suicide: Multi-level analyses. Part I: Aggregate time-series analysis of economic stress and suicide. *Suicide and Life-Threatening Behavior, 19*, 321-336.

Dooley, D., Catalano, R., & Serxner, S. (1989b). Economic stress and suicide: Multi-level analyses. Part 2: Cross-level analyses of economic stress and suicidal ideation. *Suicide and Life-Threatening Behavior, 19*, 337-351.

Durkheim, E. (1933) *The division of labor in society* (G. Simpson, Trans.). Glencoe, IL: Free Press. (Original work published 1893).

Durkheim, E. (1951). *Suicide: A study in sociology* (J. A. Spaulding & G. Simpson, Trans.). Glencoe, IL: Free Press (Original work published 1897).

Dyck, R. J., Newman, S. C., & Thompson, A. H. (1988). Suicide trends in Canada, 1956-1981. *Acta Psychiatrica Scandinavica, 77*, 411-419.

East, W. N. (1913). On attempted suicide with an analysis of 1000 consecutive cases. *Journal of Mental Sciences, 59*, 428-478.

Easterlin, R. A. (1978). What will 1984 be like? Socioeconomic ramifications of recent twists in age structure. *Demography, 15*, 397-432.

Easterlin, R. A. (1980). *Birth and fortune: The impact of numbers on personal welfare.* New York: Basic Books.

Economic Research Corporation. (1960). *The economy of Quebec: An appraisal and forecast.* Montreal: Author.

Englebrecht, G. K. (1983). Alcohol as a possible variable in suicide. *Humanitas, 9*, 61-68.

Fenwick, R. (1982). Ethnic culture and economic structure: Determinants of French-English earnings inequality in Quebec. *Social Forces, 61*, 1-23.

Gliksman, L., & Rush, B. R. (1986). Alcohol availability, alcohol consumption and alcohol-related damage: II. The role of sociodemographic factors. *Journal of Studies on Alcohol, 47*, 11-18.

Goodwin, D. W. (1973). Alcohol in suicide and homicide. *Quarterly Journal of Studies on Alcohol, 34*, 144-156.

Guindon, H. (1988). *Quebec society: Tradition, modernity and nationhood* (R. Hamilton & J.L. McMullan, Eds.). Toronto: University of Toronto Press.

Halbwach, M. (1977). *The causes of suicide.* Trans. H. Goldblatt. New York: Free Press. (Original work published 1930)

Hamermesh, D. S. (1974). The economics of black suicide. *Southern Economic Journal, 41*, 188-199.

Hamermesh, D. S., & Soss, N. N. (1974). An economic theory of suicide. *Journal of Political Economy, 82,* 83–98.

Heiman, M. F. (1975). Police suicide revisited. *Suicide and Life-Threatening Behavior, 5,* 5–20.

Herold, D. M., & Conlon, E. J. (1981). Work factors as potential causal agents of alcohol abuse. *Journal of Drug Issues, 11,* 337–356.

Hertzman, M., & Bendit, E. A. (1975). Alcoholism and destructive behavior. In A. P. Roberts (Ed.), *Self-destructive behavior* (pp. 164–187). Springfield, IL: Charles C Thomas.

Hilliard-Lysen, J., & Riemer, J. W. (1988). Occupational stress and suicide among dentists. *Deviant Behavior, 9,* 333–346.

Hlady, W. G., & Middaugh, J. P. (1988). Suicide in Alaska: Firearms and alcohol. *American Journal of Public Health, 78,* 179–180.

Holinger, P. C., Offer, D., & Ostrov, E. (1987). Suicide and homicide in the United States: An epidemiologic study of violent death, population changes and the potential for prediction. *American Journal of Psychiatry, 144,* 215–218.

Kercher, C., & Linden, L. L. (1982). Is work conducive to self-destruction? *Suicide and Life-Threatening Behavior, 12,* 151–173.

Kessel, N., & Grossman, G. (1961). Suicide in alcoholics. *British Medical Journal* (51), 1671–1672.

Kramer, M., Pollock, E. S., Redlick, R. W., & Locke, B. Z. (1972). *Mental disorder/ suicide.* Cambridge, MA: Harvard University Press.

Labovitz, S., & Hagedown, R. (1971). An analysis of suicide rates among occupational categories. *Sociological Inquiry, 47,* 67–72.

Laczko, L. S. (1987). Perceived communal inequalities in Quebec: A multidimensional analysis. *Canadian Journal of Sociology, 12,* 83–110.

Lampert, D. I., Bourque, L. B., & Kraus, J. F. (1984). Occupational status and suicide. *Suicide and Life-Threatening Behavior, 14,* 254–269.

Layne, N., & Whitehead, P. C. (1985). Employment, marital status and alcohol consumption by young Canadian men. *Journal of Studies on Alcohol, 46,* 538–540.

Linsky, A. S., & Straus, M. A. (1986). *Social stress in the United States.* Dover, MA: Auburn House.

Lunden, W. A. (1977). *The suicide cycle.* Montezuma, IA: Sutherland.

Maris, R. W. (1981). *Pathways to suicide: A survey of self-destructive behavior.* Baltimore: John Hopkins University Press.

Marshall, J. R. (1981). Political integration and the effect of war on suicide; United States, 1933–1976. *Social Forces, 59,* 771–786.

Marshall, J. R., & Hodge, R. W. (1981). Durkheim and Pierce on suicide and economic change. *Social Science Research, 10,* 101–114.

May, P. A. (1986). Alcohol and drug measure prevention programs for American Indians: Needs and opportunities. *Journal of Studies on Alcohol, 47,* 187–195.

Miles, C. P. (1972). Conditions predisposing to suicide: A review. *The Journal of Nervous and Mental Disease, 164,* 231–246.

Milham, S., Jr. (1983). *Occupational mortality in Washington State 1950–1979.* Olympia: Washington State Department of Social and Health Services.

Newman, J. F., Whitemore, K. P., & Newman, H. G. (1973). Women in the labor force and suicide. *Social Problems, 21,* 220–235.

Ornstein, M. D. (1983). The impact of marital status, age and employment on female suicide in British Columbia. *The Canadian Review of Sociology and Anthropology, 20*, 96–100.

Orru, M. (1987). *Anomie: History and meanings.* Boston: Allen & Unwin.

Palmore, E. (1978). When can age, period, and cohort be separated? *Social Forces, 57*, 282–295.

Pearlin, L. I., & Radebaugh, C. W. (1976). Economic stress and the coping function of alcohol. *American Journal of Sociology, 82*, 652–663.

Pitts, F. N., Schuller, A. B., Rich, C. L., & Pitts, A. F. (1979). Suicide among U.S. women physicians, 1969–1972. *The American Journal of Psychiatry, 136*, 694–696.

Pierce, A. (1967). The economic cycle and the social suicide rate. *American Sociological Review, 32*, 457–462.

Plant, M. A. (1977). Alcoholism and occupation: A review. *British Journal of Addiction, 72*, 309–316.

Platt, L. (1981). Business temporal norms and bereavement behavior. *American Sociological Review, 46*, 317–333.

Platt, S. (1984). Unemployment and suicidal behavior: A review of the literature. *Social Science and Medicine, 19*, 93–115.

Poikolainen, K. (1983). Increasing alcohol consumption correlated with hospital admission rates. *British Journal of Addiction, 78*, 305–309.

Pope, W. (1976). *Durkheim's* Suicide: *A classic analyzed.* Chicago: University of Chicago Press.

Porter, J. (1965). *The vertical mosaic.* Toronto: University of Toronto Press.

Powell, E. (1958). Occupational status and suicide: Toward a redefinition of anomie. *American Sociological Review, 23*, 131–139.

Queen, S. A., Habenstein, R. W., & Quadagno, J. S. (1985). *The family in various cultures* (5th ed.). New York: Harper & Row.

Ragland, J. D., & Berman, A. L. (1990–1991). Farm crisis and suicide: Dying on the vine? *Omega: Journal of Death and Dying, 22*, 173–185.

Reinhart, G. R., & Linden, L. L. (1982). Suicide by industry and occupation: A structural change approach. *Suicide and Life-Threatening Behavior, 12*, 34–45.

Rich, C. L., & Pitts, F. N., Jr. (1980). Suicide by psychiatrists. *Journal of Clinical Psychiatry, 41*, 261–263.

Rimpela, A. (1989). Death amongst doctors. *Stress Medicine, 5*, 73–75.

Robinson, W. S. (1950). Ecological correlations and the behavior of individuals. *American Sociological Review, 15*, 351–357.

Rojcewicz, S. J. (1971). War and suicide. *Suicide and Life-Threatening Behavior, 1*, 46–54.

Ross, M. (1973). Suicide among physicians. *Diseases of the Nervous System, 34*, 145–150.

Rothberg, J. M., & Jones, F. D. (1987). Suicide in the U.S. Army: Epidemiological and periodic aspects. *Suicide and Life-Threatening Behavior, 17*, 119–132.

Roy, A., & Linnoila, M. (1986). Alcoholism and suicide. *Suicide and Life-Threatening Behavior, 16*, 244–273.

Ryan, W. F. (1966). *The clergy and economic growth in Quebec (1896–1914).* Quebec City: Les Presses de L' Universite Laval.

Sainsbury, P. (1980). Suicide and depression. *Psychiatria Fennica, 1*(Suppl.), 259–266.

Sakinofsky, I., & Robert, P. (1985). *The correlates of suicide in Canada, 1979–1981.* Paper presented at the annual meeting of the American Psychiatric Association, Dallas.

Sanborn, D. E., Sanborn, C. J., & Cimbolic, P. (1974). Occupation and suicide: A study of two counties in New Hampshire. *Diseases of the Nervous System, 35,* 7–12.

Selvin, H. C. (1965). Durkheim's *Suicide:* Further thoughts on a methodological classic. In R. A. Nisbet (Ed.), *Emile Durkheim* (pp. 113–136). Englewood Cliffs, NJ: Prentice-Hall.

Shepherd, D. M., & Barraclough, B. M. (1980). Work and suicide: An empirical investigation. *British Journal of Psychiatry, 136,* 463–478.

Smart, R. G. (1979). Drinking problems among employed and unemployed workers. *Journal of Occupational Medicine, 136,* 469–478.

Stack, S. (1989). The impact of divorce on suicide in Norway, 1951–1980. *Journal of Marriage and the Family, 51,* 229–238.

Stallones, L. (1990). Suicide mortality among Kentucky farmers, 1979–1985. *Suicide and Life-Threatening Behavior, 20,* 156–163.

Sullivan, W. C. (1900). The relation of alcoholism to suicide in England, with special reference to recent statistics. *Journal of Mental Sciences, 46,* 260–280.

Tausky, C., & Piedmont, E. B. (1967–1968). The meaning of work and unemployment: Implications for mental health. *The International Journal of Social Psychiatry, 14,* 44–49.

Tomlinson-Keasey, C., Warren, L. W., & Elliott, J. E. (1986). Suicide among gifted women: A prospective study. *Journal of Abnormal Psychology, 95,* 123–130.

Travis, R. (1983). Suicide in northwest Alaska, White Cloud. *Journal of American Indian Mental Health, 3,* 23–30.

Trovato, F. (1986a). The relationship between marital dissolution and suicide: The Canadian case. *Journal of Marriage and the Family, 48,* 341–348.

Trovato, F. (1986b). A time series analysis of international immigration and suicide mortality in Canada. *International Journal of Social Psychology, 32,* 38–46.

Vigderhaus, G. (1977). Forecasting sociological phenomena: Applications of Box-Jenkins methodology to suicide rates. In K. F. Schuessler (Ed.), *Sociological Methodology 1978* (pp. 20–51). San Francisco: Jossey-Bass.

Wasserman, I. M. (1983). Political business cycles, presidential elections, and suicide and mortality patterns. *American Sociological Review, 48,* 711–720.

Wasserman, I. M. (1987). Cohort, age and period effects in the analysis of United States suicide patterns, 1933–1978. *Suicide and Life-Threatening Behavior, 17,* 179–193.

Wasserman, I. M. (1989). The effects of war and alcohol consumption patterns on suicide: United States, 1910–1933. *Social Forces, 68,* 513–530.

CHAPTER 26

Marriage, Family, Religion, and Suicide

Steven Stack, Ph.D.
Wayne State University

The literature on the impacts of marriage, family, and religion on suicide has pursued a number of themes: social integration/regulation (e.g., Trovato, 1987), status integration (e.g., Stafford & Gibbs, 1988), and network theory (Pescosolido & Georgianna, 1989). This chapter reviews the main theoretical arguments and representative research studies on each of these streams. The main body of the chapter is divided into two broad sections: "Marriage, the Family, and Suicide," and "Religion and Suicide." The chapter then turns to a problematic application of the work reviewed to the five case studies serving as a unifying element in the present book. A concluding discussion stresses the need for new directions in future work; these directions include the testing of a synthetic theory of social individualism and suicide, as well as more attention to the growing numbers of people living alone—a domestic factor neglected in the work on assessing suicide potential, yet very potent.

MARRIAGE, THE FAMILY, AND SUICIDE

Work on the influence of marriage and family variables on suicide has been guided primarily by Durkheim's (1897/1951) classic perspective, and secondarily by the status integration view (Gibbs & Martin, 1964). I have compared these two orientations at some length elsewhere (Stack, 1990a, pp. 119–121). Durkheim contended that the subordination of the individual to the needs of others in the family unit lowers the destructive potential of the drive toward individualism. The fact that divorced persons, for example, have much higher suicide rates is explained in terms of their reduction in family-based interaction and responsibilities. More recent work has contended that divorce also increases economic anomie, since two households have to be supported. In contrast to the social integration/regulation view, Gibbs and Martin's (1964) status integration view contends that marital statuses that are statistically infrequent will tend to be marked by high role conflict, and hence, by a high risk of suicide. People will tend to avoid status sets that are marked by high levels of conflict, thereby making the sets statistically infrequent. Conceivably, for example, in a society where only a small minority of the population was married and a majority was divorced, the married would be high in suicide and the divorced would be low in suicide. This would be the opposite of what Durkheimians would predict. The high proportion divorced would be taken as a clear sign of little conflict, although this might in fact not be the case.

Research in the Durkheimian Tradition

A decade review of the 1970s work strongly supported Durkheim's theory as it relates to the domestic institution (Stack, 1982). More recent work has consistently supported it as well, although some studies have suggested that it works best under certain contextual factors. Recent data at the individual level confirm that, for each marital status group by both age and gender, married persons have the lowest suicide rate (Smith, Mercy, & Conn, 1988). For example, with all races, ages, and sexes combined, the suicide rate for the divorced was 34.9 per 100,000, compared to only 11.9 per 100,000 for the married. Table 26.1 provides 1979 U.S. suicide rates by marital status for

TABLE 26.1. Suicide Rates by Gender and Selected Age and Marital Status Groups: Whites, 1979, United States

Age	Marital status				Coefficient of aggravation (divorced/married)
	Single	Married	Widowed	Divorced	
A. Males					
25–29	43.3	15.8	186.6	70.1	4.44
35–39	43.1	15.3	188.2	67.0	4.37
45–49	49.5	17.5	100.5	72.6	4.15
55–59	50.0	19.0	86.3	76.3	4.02
65–69	53.3	25.0	74.6	74.2	2.90
B. Females					
25–29	12.2	4.7	26.4	19.5	4.15
35–39	15.8	7.3	17.7	25.6	3.51
45–49	15.1	9.1	23.0	28.1	3.09
55–59	9.9	8.0	15.7	21.4	2.68
65–69	8.6	6.1	11.1	14.4	2.36

Note. The data are from Stack (1990a). Rates per 100,000 population.

selected age groups of males and females. The data are from Stack (1990a). For example, for divorced males between 25 and 29 the suicide rate (this and all subsequent rates are rates per 100,000) was 70.1; for married males in that age group, the suicide rate was only 15.8. The ratio of the suicide rate of the divorced to that of the married is termed the "coefficient of aggravation" (COA). For males in their late 20s the COA was 4.44. That is, divorced males in this age group were 4.44 times more likely to commit suicide than married males in the group.

Turning to the females in this sample, one notices that the suicide rates were much lower than those of males for all specific marital status and age groups. Nevertheless, divorced females were also more likely to commit suicide than married females. For example, the suicide rate for divorced females aged 25–29 was 19.5; for married females in the same age bracket, the suicide rate was only 4.7. The COA was 4.15, nearly as high as that of males in their late 20s. Clearly, marriage appears to protect both males and females from self-destruction. One qualification is that in these data the COAs declined more for females than for males over the age spectrum. For example, for elderly females the COA was 2.36. In contrast, elderly males were 2.90 times more likely to commit suicide than their married counterparts.

In ecological, cross-sectional studies, the incidence of divorce was found to be a leading predictor of county suicide rates (e.g., Kowalski, Faupel, & Starr, 1987; Breault, 1986) and state suicide rates (Breault, 1986). Time-series analyses have confirmed the divorce–suicide relationship for other nations, including Canada (Trovato, 1987), Norway (Stack, 1989), and Denmark (Stack, 1990c). In Sweden, however, divorce trends were related only to the suicide rates of young people (Stack, 1991).

Two studies have revealed that the divorce–suicide relationship works best under two contexts: urbanism, which provides better structural conduits for influencing suicide than rural areas (Kowalski et al., 1987); and gun availability, which provides an efficient means or opportunity for committing suicide for a population marked by low marital integration (Gundlach, 1990). The Gundlach (1990) paper combined the traditional Durkheimian perspective with an opportunity theory. The latter has been badly neglected in suicidology generally. A key factor that facilitates suicide is the availability of lethal means of self-destruction. These "opportunities" include lethal gas, such as that in England before the detoxification of natural gas, and firearms. Gundlach contended that in areas with high gun availability, the impact of low family integration should be especially strong; in areas with low gun availability, the effect of family integration should be relatively weak. That is, people should have more opportunities for quick suicides in cities where the population is more heavily armed. In his analysis of suicide rates for 77 metropolitan areas, Gundlach found strong support for his contextual model: In cities with high gun availability, there was a stronger relationship between family variables and suicide rates than in cities with low gun availability. The associations were much stronger for males than females—a finding interpreted in terms of males' being more familiar with firearms than females.

Status Integration Research

Compared to the Durkheimian model, the status integration theory, as noted in a decade review (Stack, 1982, p. 57), continues to be surrounded by controversy. Divergent findings have included the notion that marital status is irrelevant in explaining suicide rates among U.S. age groups; this has been especially true for women since 1960 (Stafford & Gibbs, 1985, 1988). In contrast, when "within-column" tests were used, strong support was found for the theory (Stafford, Martin, & Gibbs, 1990). That is, when the marital status integration scores for each of four marital statuses were correlated with their respective suicide rates, support was found for the status integration theory for all 15 correlations (one each for 15 age groups); this was true for both males and females. The results based on "within-column" tests were not fully replicated for "between-columns" tests, however. In between-columns tests, only two correlations were computed: one for males and one for females. The suicide rates for 15 age groups were then correlated with their 15 respective status integration scores. Here the results broke down, especially for females. Hence, the vitality of the theory depends on the type of test deemed more appropriate.

Research that has attempted to test both the status integration and the Durkheimian model has been rare. A recent exception is an over-time study exploring the COA—the ratio of the suicide rate of the divorced to that of the married (Stack, 1990a). At the heart of status integration theory is the notion of the statistical frequency of status sets. The status configurations involving the divorced increased 174% between 1960 and 1980, from 3.1% of the population in 1960 to 8.5% in 1980. Hence, we would anticipate a decline in both role conflict and suicide. This was the case between 1960 and 1980: The COA declined for 11 of 15 male age groups, and for 12 of 15 female age groups. The remaining differences in suicide rates were, however, substantial, with divorced people generally having suicide rates triple those of married persons. I concluded that both theories are supported by the data. Divorced people are not quite as suicidal today as a generation ago (compared to married people). Yet the remaining differences are so large that it would seem that Durkheim must also be right—that divorce may be an inherently stressful life event, no matter how statistically frequent it may be.

Status integration theory has been applied to explanations of a link between female labor force participation (FLFP) and suicide through the concept of role conflict between work and family responsibilities (Stack, 1978, 1982). Recent work has argued that the FLFP–suicide link is influenced by the cultural support given working women (Stack, 1987). For example, given the antipathy surrounding FLFP in 1948–1963, increases in FLFP were associated with suicide increases for both males and females. In contrast, for the emancipation era of 1964–1980—a period marked by cultural support for working women—increases in FLFP were unrelated to female suicide, whereas they remained directly related to male suicide. For females the benefits of work appear to outweigh the costs in an emancipation period, but this is evidently not true for males.

For the case of Australia, Hassan and Tan (1989) reported that for 1901–1985 FLFP was positively—not negatively, as found in an earlier study through 1972 (Stack & Danigelis, 1985)—related to the male–female suicide ratio. They contended that the discrepancy was due to the previous study's not introducing a trend variable. However, in an analysis not reported here, the introduction of a trend variable did not change the findings through 1972. The discrepancy was due, in fact, to the addition of the years 1973–1986—a period when female suicide was falling, possibly in part because of the increasing social support for FLFP noted (Stack, 1987) in the United States.

RELIGION AND SUICIDE

Elsewhere (Stack, 1983, pp. 363–366), I have compared and contrasted the social integration theory with the religious commitment theory of religion and suicide. Basically, the social integration theory is based on two dimensions of religion: the number of shared religious beliefs and practices (Durkheim, 1897/1951, pp. 152–170). The greater the number of such beliefs and practices, the greater the subordination of the individual to group life; the lower the chances of alleged destructive individualism and free inquiry; and, as such, the lower the risk of suicide. The actual content of religious dogma and rites is viewed as secondary; the sheer numbers of the dogmas and rites are central (Durkheim, 1897/1951, p. 170). In contrast to the classic integration view, the theory of religious commitment holds that just a few life-saving religious beliefs may be all that are necessary to lower suicide risk. Vast numbers of rituals and beliefs may not be necessary. Belief in an afterlife, for example, may make worldly suffering more endurable and less life-threatening. The provision of idealistic role models, an alternative stratification system for building self-esteem, glorification of the state of poverty (a key risk factor in suicide), and so on, are seen as life-saving aspects of American religions.

Research on Religion and Suicide

As Maris (1981, pp. 246–247) notes, individual-level data on religion and suicide are very limited. Some data do exist, however, and these do indicate that Catholics have a lower suicide rate than Protestants. For example, in the case of The Netherlands during 1900–1910, Catholics had a suicide rate of 7.0 compared to 17.1 for Protestants (Gargas, 1932). (Again, all suicide rates given are rates per 100,000 population.) More recent data often confirm the Durkheimian position on religious affiliation and suicide; even these data are over 20 years old, however. Table 26.2 provides data on suicide rates by broad religious groups for Chicago (Maris, 1981, p. 248). For example, for both males and females aged 25–44, the suicide rate for Protestants was greater than that of Catholics. For males, Catholics had a suicide rate of 11 compared to 16 for Protestants. For females, Catholics had a suicide rate of 8 compared to 10 for Protestants.

Some caution needs to be exercised in interpreting micro-level data wherein all Protestant denominations are lumped together. This may mask variations in suicide that correspond to relevant variations in religious practices and beliefs among denominations. Data from New Zealand (Gibbs, 1971) provide a further breakdown of Protestantism into various denominations. Table 26.3 provides these data. Five Protestant denominations had suicide rates higher than that of Catholics; Congregationalists, for example, had a suicide rate of 15.1 compared to 7.3 for Catholics. Only the Church of Christ had a suicide rate lower than that of Catholics. These data are, however, for 1946–1951, a period before modern-day convergence between the faiths in orthodoxy and religious practice.

Other studies, however, often find no difference between Catholic and Protestant suicide rates. Sometimes, in fact, Catholics have a higher suicide rate than Protestants. An earlier review of a series of studies (Stack, 1980) found the following negative evidence for the Durkheimian position. For Toronto during 1928–1935, the rate for Catholics (11.0) was more than double that for Protestants (4.5). Another study of Newcastle-upon-Tyne, England, for 1962–1964 also found the reverse of the Durkheimian position. Two studies of Brisbane, Australia, and a review of college student suicides found no significant difference in the suicide rates of Catholics and Protestants.

TABLE 26.2. Suicide Rates by Religious Affiliation, Age, and Gender: Whites, Chicago, 1966–1968

| | Age and gender | | | | | | | |
| | 24 and under | | 25–44 | | 45–64 | | 65 and over | |
Religion	M	F	M	F	M	F	M	F
Protestants	25	12	16	10	28	13	40	14
Jews	22	—	15	—	28	—	26	—
Catholics	13	7	11	8	16	6	24	8

Note. The data are from Maris (1981). Rates per 100,000 population.

TABLE 26.3. Suicide Rates by Religions Affiliation:
New Zealand, 1946–1951

Affiliation	Suicide rate
Catholic	7.3
Congregationalist	15.1
Methodist	12.9
Church of Eng- land	9.7
Baptist	9.5
Presbyterian	9.5
Church of Christ	6.9

Note. The data are from Gibbs (1971). Rates per 100,000
population.

The inconsistencies in the findings on religious affiliation and suicide
are indicative of a normative change taking place in Catholicism. A review
of the literature of the 1970s found that, given a convergence in religious
beliefs and practices between Catholics and Protestants, religious integration was no longer a significant determinant of suicide; this was taken as a
refutation of Durkheim (Stack, 1982).

Little work has documented differences, if any, between Catholics and
Protestants in their attitudes toward suicide. If the Catholics still have a
lower suicide rate than Protestants in the U.S. it would appear reasonable to
expect that Catholics would be less accepting of suicide than Protestants. A
recent study (Stack & Lester, 1991) fills this void in the research. This study
presented data on 1,687 individuals who were part of a national poll during
1988–1989. Suicide ideation was measured in terms of a "no" or "yes"
response to the question "Do you think a person has the right to end his or
her own life if this person has an incurable disease?" Responses were almost
evenly split, with 821 replying "no" and 866 replying "yes." The percentage
of Catholics who responded "yes" was not significantly different from the
percentage of Protestants responding in the affirmative. A further analysis,
which introduced controls for socioeconomic variables, supported the nil
effect of religious affiliation on suicide attitudes.

Work from the 1980s often continues to refute Durkheim. In a study of
214 standard metropolitan statistical areas, Stark, Doyle, and Rushing
(1983, p. 126) found that when church membership rates (a measure of basic
religious commitment) were controlled for, the proportion of church
members who were Catholic had no impact on urban suicide. Pescosolido
and Mendelsohn (1986) studied 404 county groups and found that the
percentage of Catholics was not significantly related to suicide, but that a
control for the percentage of Baptists was sometimes significant. Extending
the analysis to all 3,108 U.S. counties and controlling for numerous social

and economic conditions (including the percentage of Protestants), Kowalski et al. (1987, p. 92) also found no impact of religious affiliation on suicide.

Other studies have found an impact, but have tended to fail to introduce a key control for religious denominations other than Catholic. For example, using the same data set and nearly the same long list of control variables, Faupel, Kowalski, and Starr (1987, p. 528) reported that the percentage of Catholics was a leading predictor of county suicide rates. However, they mysteriously left out the control for the percentage of Protestants that was employed in their related article (Kowalski et al., 1987). Breault (1986), employing data on 414 large counties and using analysis of covariance, reported a mean suicide rate of 11.6 for Catholic counties and a mean of 13.0 for non-Catholic counties.

Work on the religious commitment perspective on suicide has proven more fruitful than work on the classic Durkheimian model based on religious affiliation. This work typically finds that religion is still a significant predictor of suicide. Stark et al. (1983) found that church membership rates lowered suicide rates in large American cities. For a sample of 25 nations, I found (Stack, 1983) that the higher the religiosity (measured as religious books produced as a proportion of all books), the lower the incidence of suicide. This was especially true for females, a group higher in religiosity levels than males. Finally, Breault (1986) found that church membership rates lowered suicide rates in both American counties and states.

Work at the individual level on suicide ideation also confirms the religious commitment view. Our study of national attitudes toward suicide (Stack & Lester, 1991) determined that the greater the church attendance, the lower the approval of suicide as a solution to life's problems. Furthermore, church attendance was the variable most closely tied to the variation in suicide attitudes. It was more important to the explanation of such attitudes than marital status, age, education, or gender.

The Network Approach

Pescosolido and Georgianna (1989) have offered a clarification and elaboration of Durkheim's theory; they argue that religious affiliation reflects the vitality of network ties. They have developed topologies of religious strength and social bonds. In an analysis of data from 404 county groups, denominations with a hierarchical structure (i.e., a passive role for the rank-and-file members), such as Episcopalians, had a higher suicide rate. Ecumenical churches and ones with little tension between themselves and the greater sociocultural environment also fostered higher suicide rates.

In contrast, denominations that are in tension with societal culture, conservative, and nonecumenical, and whose power structures are nonhierarchical, should have lower suicide rates. For example, Pescosolido and

Georgianna found that the greater the percentage of Evangelical Baptists, Reformed Church members, or Seventh-Day Adventists, the lower the county's suicide rate. The theoretical interpretation of this finding is that these are precisely the kinds of church structures that facilitate friendship ties among members of their congregations. These ties act as important sources of social support; social support, in turn, reduces suicide risk.

This study truly breaks new ground in the investigation of exactly what kinds of religions and religious organization will promote the kinds of networking among people that should reduce suicide potential.

APPLICATIONS TO THE FIVE CASE STUDIES

I hesitate to apply sociological theories to case studies. Since the former, technically speaking, deal with groups, they probably should not be applied to individuals. In addition, the case descriptions provided in Chapter 12 contain no information regarding some critical sociological variables, such as intensity of religious involvement. Other factors (such as gun availability, known to interact with sociological variables) are also not addressed in many of the case descriptions. Finally, as a sociologist, I do not have the expertise to interpret the various cognitive and psychological test scores reported in the case studies. Given these reservations, I can only offer very weak and tentative assessments of suicide risk.

1. *Heather B.* At 13, Heather was in an age cohort with a very low suicide risk. Possibly her rather negative life experiences in her early teenage years would increase her risk of suicide during her latter teen years—years where the suicide rate is multiplied. Heather's loss of her father through death would not contribute to suicide (e.g., Lester, 1983), but if it had been a loss through divorce, the reverse would be true. More generally, however, her low family attachment/integration would certainly increase her risk. We are told nothing about her religiosity level. If she were to fit the broader American pattern of synergy between family and religious individualism, however, she would be low in both—a state further contributing to suicide risk.

2. *Ralph F.* Ralph's social integration level in both religious and family life was clearly low, increasing the propensity toward suicidal behavior.

3. *John Z.* Inadequate information is provided on John's religiosity or family life. His alleged suicide attempts would seem to place him in a high-risk group.

4. *Faye C.* As an unmarried woman of 49, Faye was located in a status configuration with a relatively high female suicide rate. Her level of marital/family integration was low both as an adult and as a child, to judge from her own reports.

5. *José G.* Once again, Core marital/religion variables are left largely undescribed. At 64, his combined problems of disability and involuntary job loss, as well as his access to firearms, would place Jose in a high-risk male group.

NEW DIRECTIONS FOR FUTURE RESEARCH

An analysis of American time-series data (Stack, 1985) indicated that trends in religiosity and family life are virtually inseparable. The correlation between them, for example, was in excess of .90. I suggest that the two institutions represent a common tendency in the social fabric: collectivism versus individualism. The family and religious institutions are the two most collectivistic ones in the contemporary United States. Trends in one are reflected in the other. Trovato and Voss (1990) have recently replicated my results for the case of youth suicide in Canada. Nevertheless, most cross-sectional research has been able to analyze religion and family trends as separate entities, indicating that they represent somewhat independent influences on suicide (e.g., Breault, 1986; Kowalski et al., 1987). Some time-series work on other nations has also found independence between these two factors (Stack, 1989, 1990c). I speculate that in these latter societies (Norway and Denmark), religion is highly secularized; as such, it will be less apt to prevent suicide and less apt to be dependent on trends in family life.

Some family-related variables are often absent from most empirical work. Parenting or the presence–absence of children is routinely left out, often because of data availability problems. Work on the impact of children on suicide would fit both the Durkheimian and the status integration models of suicide. Such work will require funding in order for the necessary data to be collected.

A variable that has received little systematic attention, but that often is entered into the analysis and then lost track of, is the proportion of the population living alone. This clearly represents low integration in domestic life—isolation from both marriage and the family. This variable may in fact be the most important determinant of suicide, as witnessed in recent analyses (Kowalski et al., 1987). Most work, however, continues to focus on divorce as a primary measure of domestic integration.

Comparative work on family organization is needed to unravel the influence of different patterns of family organization on suicide. A key question is this: To what extent does American theorizing fit domestic patterns found in very different cultural contexts? For example, in Japan, households containing members of three generations (three-generation households; or 3GH) are more common than in the United States. Dodge and Austin (1990) tested two different theories: (1) 3GH should increase elderly suicide; they are more traditional and as such will encourage altruistic suicide among the elderly. (2) 3GH will contribute to a lower elderly suicide rate, given that the 3GH lowers social isolation and provides social support for the elderly. A multivariate statistical model supported the second hypothesis, involving "egoistic" suicide, but not the first, involving widespread assumptions regarding Japanese "altruistic" suicide.

The domestic factor can make a contribution to the growing literature on media impacts on suicide. For example, given that suicidal people need to identify with the victim involved in a suicide news story, stories on persons with marital problems should be apt to trigger "copycat" suicide. That is, since suicidal people are high in marital troubles, it is likely that they will identify with such stories, as opposed to stories about victims far removed from their everyday lives (e.g., political villains, foreign artists, and rich corporate executives). Indeed, the one study that has followed these lines of reasoning has found strong support for them (Stack, 1990b). Stories on divorced victims, victims with marital problems, and even spouse murderers who committed suicide after murdering their spouses all had a significant impact on suicide rates. Other stories, lumped together, did not. Further work, with additional stories to draw on, might develop a more refined classification scheme for stories about marital life, and ways in which still more relevant social types might affect suicide rates.

Finally, the pioneering work of Gundlach (1990) suggests that the impact of domestic factors on suicide is mediated by opportunities for suicide. Future work needs to add this contextual factor, when possible, to the analysis. Many aggregated data sets, including those I have used in my work are amenable to this task. The percentage of suicides involving firearms can be used as a proxy measure of gun availability. This has long been the case in homicide research, and it may be time for suicide researchers to rework their models to take this neglected variable into account.

REFERENCES

Breault, K. (1986). Suicide in America: A test of Durkheim's theory of religious and family integration, 1933-1980. *American Journal of Sociology*, *92*(3), 628-656.

Dodge, H. Austin, R. L. (1990). Household structure and elderly Japanese female suicide. *Family Perspective*, *24*(1), 83-97.

Durkheim, E. (1951). *Suicide: A study in sociology* (J. A. Spaulding & G. Simpson, Trans.). Glencoe, IL: Free Press. (Original work published 1897).

Faupel, C., Kowalski G., and Starr, P. (1987). Sociology's one law: Religion and suicide in the urban context. *Journal for the Scientific Study of Religion*, *26*(4), 523-534.

Gargas, S. (1932). Suicide in the Netherlands. *American Journal of Sociology*, *37*, 697-713.

Gibbs, J. P. (1971). Suicide. In R. Merton & R. Nisbet (Eds.), *Contemporary social problems* (pp. 271-312). New York: Harcourt Brace Jovanovich.

Gibbs, J., & Martin, W. T. (1964). *Status integration and suicide.* Eugene: University of Oregon Press.

Gundlach, J. (1990). Absence of family support, opportunity, and suicide. *Family Perspective, 24*(1), 7–14.

Hassan, R., & Tan, G. (1989). Suicide trends in Australia, 1901–1985: An analysis of sex differentials. *Suicide and Life-Threatening Behavior, 19*(4), 362–380.

Kowalski, G., Faupel, C., & Starr, P. (1987). Urbanism and suicide: A study of American counties. *Social Forces, 66*(1), 85–101.

Lester, D. (1983). *Why people kill themselves.* (2nd ed.). Springfield, IL: Charles C Thomas.

Maris, R. (1981). *Pathways to suicide: A survey of self-destructive behaviors.* Baltimore: Johns Hopkins University Press.

Pescosolido, B., & Georgianna, S. (1989). Durkheim, suicide and religion: Toward a network of suicide. *American Sociological Review, 54*, 33–48.

Pescosolido, B., & Mendelsohn, R. (1986). Social causation or social construction of suicide? An investigation of the social construction of official rates. *American Sociological Review, 51*(1), 80–100.

Smith, J., Mercy, J., & Conn, J. (1988). Marital status and the risk of suicide. *American Journal of Public Health, 78*(1), 78–80.

Stack, S. (1978). Suicide: A comparative analysis. *Social Forces, 57*, 644–653.

Stack, S. (1980). Religion and suicide: A reanalysis. *Social Psychiatry, 15*, 65–70.

Stack, S. (1982). Suicide: A decade review of the sociological literature. *Deviant Behavior, 4*, 41–66.

Stack, S. (1983). The effect of religious commitment on suicide: A cross national analysis. *Journal of Health and Social Behavior, 24*, 362–374.

Stack, S. (1985). The effect of domestic/religious individualism on suicide, 1954–1978. *Journal of Marriage and the Family, 47*, 431–447.

Stack, S. (1987). The effect of female participation in the labor force on suicide: A time series analysis, 1948–1980. *Sociological Forum, 2*(2), 257–277.

Stack, S. (1989). The impact of divorce on suicide in Norway. *Journal of Marriage and the Family, 51*, 229–238.

Stack, S. (1990a). New micro level data on the impact of divorce on suicide, 1959–1980: A test of two theories. *Journal of Marriage and the Family, 52*, 119–127.

Stack, S. (1990b). Divorce, suicide and the mass media: An analysis of differential identification, 1948–1980. *Journal of Marriage and the Family, 52*, 553–560.

Stack, S. (1990c). The impact of divorce on suicide in Denmark, 1950–1980. *Sociological Quarterly, 31*(3), 359–370.

Stack, S. (1991). The effect of religiosity on suicide in Sweden. *Journal for the Scientific Study of Religion, 30*(4), 462–468.

Stack, S., & Danigelis, N. (1985). Modernization and the sex differential in suicide, 1919–1972. *Comparative Social Research, 8*, 203–216.

Stack, S., & Lester, D. (1991). The effect of religion on suicide ideation. *Social Psychiatry and Psychiatric Epidemiology, 26*, 168–170.

Stafford, M., & Gibbs, J. P. (1985). A major problem with the theory of status integration. *Social Forces, 63*, 643–660.

Stafford, M., & Gibbs, J. P. (1988). Change in the relation between marital integration and suicide. *Social Forces, 66*(3), 643–660.

Stafford, M., Martin, W. T., & Gibbs, J. P. (1990). Marital status and suicide: Within column tests of the status integration theory. *Family Perspective, 24*(1), 15–32.

Stark, R., Doyle, D., & Rushing, J. (1983). Beyond Durkheim: religion and suicide. *Journal for the Scientific Study of Religion, 22*(2), 120–131.

Trovato, F. (1987). A longitudinal analysis of divorce and suicide in Canada. *Journal of Marriage and the Family, 49*, 193–203.

Trovato, F., & Voss, R. (1990). Domestic/religious individualism and youth suicide in Canada. *Family Perspective, 24*(1), 69–82.

Suicide, Stress, and Coping with Life Cycle Events

Robert I. Yufit, Ph.D.
Northwestern University Medical School
Bruce Bongar, Ph.D.
Pacific Graduate School of Psychology
and
Department of Psychiatry
University of Massachusetts Medical School

Despite the enormous amount of empirical and clinical research on the subject, completed and attempted suicides are not precisely understood phenomena. There is a consensus that most suicide completers suffer from a major psychiatric illness in the period immediately prior to their death. However, there is a distinct lack of consensus on specific causal pathways and on the weight and significance to be ascribed to various psychological, psychodynamic, biological, social-relational, and epidemiological factors (i.e., on how each factor contributes to the completion or attempt and how the factors interact). It *is* generally agreed that suicidality must be viewed as a highly complex biopsychosocial phenomenon with multiple pathways and determinants, all of which must be fitted into the assessment–management equation (Blumenthal, 1990). Many authorities also agree that certain psychiatric illnesses, including depression, alcohol or other substance abuse, and schizophrenia, are the most common diagnostic categories among completed suicides. To demonstrate the rapidly changing and dynamic quality of the knowledge base, an important recent study has reported that those who suffer from panic disorder and attacks exhibit a very high rate of suicide ideation and attempts (Weissman, Klerman, Markowitz, & Ouellette, 1989). There are also clear differences between the profiles of those who attempt and those who complete suicide, especially with regard to age, sex, and race.

One of the most basic facts about suicide in the United States is that its risk increases with age (Vaillant & Blumenthal, 1990), and although in the last 30 years we have seen a great increase in the rate of suicide amoung youths, "80-year-olds are still twice as likely to commit suicide as 20-year-olds" (Vaillant & Blumenthal, 1990, p. 1). Maris (1988) comments that although there has been a recent emphasis on the tragedy of youth suicide, suicidologists need to study the entire range of the life cycle, including the middle-aged and the elderly. In his opinion,

> it is probably true that the longer one lives, the more likely it is that problems will develop. Most suicide tolerance thresholds are gradually breached by accumulated stresses and developmental strains . . . and youthful suicides often result from relatively few factors' acutely overwhelming the young person. (p. xv)

Thus, as human beings live through each day of their lives, they encounter new experiences. They absorb and react to these experiences in many different ways—at times drawing on their own resources, at times drawing upon help from others, most often relying on a combination of inner and outer resources. As these experiences accumulate, individuals develop distinctive ways of thinking and reacting, which eventually become formalized in their personality makeup. Each person can also develop specific cognitive, dynamic, and behavioral strengths and weaknesses in dealing with these accumulated life experiences and their concomitant demands for change. These abilities and deficits can be viewed definitionally as "coping skills" and "specific vulnerabilities," respectively (Yufit, 1988). How people use these skills to deal with adversity and to combat vulnerability is a measure of how they gain a sense of self and of how they learn to cope with the stress of life (Selye, 1976; Vaillant & Blumenthal, 1990). As Motto (1979) points out, we must never forget that the understanding of suicide depends on our understanding of both the patient's unique capabilities and tolerances for stress and uncertainty, and his or her social matrix. Smith (1985) has also noted that serial assessments over time can be a superior method for evaluating risk. This method allows for the vicissitudes of clinical symptoms, changing life stress, and long-standing problems in the person's character structure.

In addition, Maltsberger (1988) believes that one of the specific components in the general formulation of suicide risk must be assessing the patient's past responses to stress, especially to losses. Bongar (1991) emphasizes that it is also critical to consider whether the patient has suffered any stressful recent and important losses in his or her life (e.g., job, relationships, residence), or whether the patient has suffered more subtle recent psychological losses (e.g., humiliation, shame, or self-hate) (H. Block-

Lewis, personal communication, November 15, 1985; Lazare, 1987; Blumenthal, 1990; Peterson & Bongar, 1989; Shneidman, 1986a, 1986b).

Thus, in this chapter we state that the ability to cope with stressful life events and losses, particularly during stressful critical periods of the life cycle, is a major factor in the development of coping and adaptational skills in general. Conversely, we contend that the absence of this ability is an important factor in vulnerability to suicidal behavior. Continued success in such coping behavior may lead to a sense of mastery, to a positive attitude toward life, and to a sense that life is worthwhile. The lack of the capacity to cope and to adapt can create doubt as to whether life is really worthwhile, or even possible.

The ideas and proposals contained in the present chapter are based for the most part on our accumulated clinical experience in diagnosing and treating a large number of suicidal persons over the course of many years. Where pertinent, we also draw upon relevant psychological theory and relevant empirical studies; however, at the present time there is not a large body of empirical research in this specific area. Therefore, we adopt a nomothetic approach in our attempt to integrate clinical experiences into a proposed working model that may help contribute to our understanding of the impact of stress and critical life events on a person's view of life— and, in particular, the way in which such experiences can affect an individual's decision to end his or her own life.

AN OVERVIEW OF THE RESEARCH LITERATURE

Paykel (1989) has surveyed the literature on stress and life events as they relate to suicidal behavior. The results of this survey confirm that high rates of early loss, broken homes, and academic pressure resulting from overachievement are frequent correlates of suicidal behavior (both attempts and completions) in adolescents. However, it is difficult to ascertain the extent to which these life stresses are specific to suicide per se, as opposed to particular psychiatric disturbances. For, as noted previously, it is fairly well established that a psychiatric history is highly correlated with subsequent suicidal potential and suicidal behavior. Unfortunately, there are few studies of recent stressful life events and subsequent suicidal behavior that use a controlled empirical methodology. Nonetheless, Paykel (1989) notes that life stress events frequently do precede suicide attempts and suicidal ideation.

Using a sample of 202 college students, Rich and Bonner (1987) conducted a follow-up study to test the concurrent validity of their stress–vulnerability model of suicidal ideation and behavior. In this research, the subjects completed self-report measures of life stress, loneliness, depression, dysfunctional cognitions, reasons for living, hopelessness, current suicide ideation, and predictions of future suicide probability. A multiple-regression analysis indicated that 30% of the variation in suicide ideation scores could be accounted for by the linear combination of negative life stress, depression, loneliness, and a paucity of reasons for living. The linear combination of current suicide ideation, hopelessness, dysfunctional cognitions, and few reasons for living explained 56% of the variance in self-predicted future suicide probability. Rich and Bonner concluded that the results in general supported their proposed model.

Another study by the same authors, using a sample of 186 undergraduates (Rich & Bonner, 1988), examined the effects of problem-solving self-appraisal (PSSA) and negative life stress on hopelessness. Subjects completed a problem-solving inventory, the Life Experiences Survey, the Zung Self-Rating Depression Scale, and the Hopelessness Scale. The results showed that PSSA and its interaction with negative life stress emerged as significant independent predictors of hopelessness. The findings also suggest that PSSA and negative life events may interact to produce hopelessness.

Linehan, Goodstein, Nielsen, and Chiles (1983) studied 65 adults who generated 72 distinct reasons for not committing suicide. These were reduced to 48 by factor analyses performed on two additional samples, and the items were arranged into the Reasons for Living Inventory (RFL), which requires a rating of how important each reason would be for living if suicide were contemplated. In addition, factor analyses indicated six primary reasons for living: Survival and Coping Beliefs, Responsibility to Family, Child-Related Concerns, Fear of Suicide, Fear of Social Disapproval, and Moral Objections. Linehan et al. subsequently administered the RFL to two additional samples: 197 Seattle shoppers (mean age, 36 years) and 175 psychiatric inpatients (mean age, 31 years). Both samples were divided into several groups—suicidal (ideators and parasuicides) and nonsuicidal. Separate multivariate analyses of variance indicated that the RFL differentiated suicidal from nonsuicidal subjects in both samples. In the subjects from the shopping center, the Fear of Suicide scale further differentiated previous ideators and previous parasuicides. In the clinical sample, the Child-Related Concerns scale differentiated between current suicide ideators and current parasuicides. In both samples, the Survival and Coping Beliefs, the Responsibility to Family, and the Child-Related Concerns scales were most useful in differentiating groups.

In the area of family interaction, Aldredge (1984) has reviewed a number of research studies that have investigated suicidal behavior within the context of the family. A subculture of distress seems to develop in some families—not from random deviations, but from familial and cultural expectations of how distress can be managed. Suicide potential is marked by a pattern of marked hostility or role disturbance and failure; a process of escalation when developmental crises occur in the management of family life cycle transitions; a symbiotic attachment between partners that tolerates no autonomy; an intolerance of crisis; a crisis management family conflict-family organization relationship; and suicidal behavior as a pattern of communication. The critical variables seem to be suicidal behavior as communication, and a family tradition of crisis management by symptoms in the presence of intrafamilial conflict.

Another family-based study (Friedman, 1984) examined the history of family illness (including attempted and completed suicide) among two groups of 13- to 19-year-olds: 16 depressed, seriously suicidal adolescents, and 18 severely depressed adolescents who had never attempted suicide or been considered immediately suicidal by clinicians. The results showed that the chronic illness of a parent during a suicidal subject's childhood or latency years, particularly a history of parental depression, may have influenced the subject to engage in seriously suicidal behavior. These findings suggest that identification with a depressed parent may lead to a hopeless-helpless view of the self and to a suicidal stance, particularly when adaptation to adverse circumstances is required.

In a classic study, Shneidman (1971) analyzed 30 cases for whom longitudinal personality data were available from 1921 to 1960. The subjects were all Caucasian males with high IQs. Five of the subjects had committed suicide (all by gunshot); 10 (matched) individuals had died natural deaths from cancer or heart disease; and 15 were still living. Shneidman conducted a blind clinical analysis primarily in terms of two guiding theoretical concepts (i.e., perturbation and lethality), using a Meyerian "life chart" and "psychological autopsy." His results indicated that four of the five cases deemed to be most suicidal had in fact committed suicide (a chance probability of 1 out of 1,131). In a discussion of the prodromal clues, the role of the "significant other" and the "burning out" of affect seemed to be paramount. For the completed suicides, their deaths could be seen as a discernible part of their lifestyles by the time the persons were 30 years of age, and as a predictable outcome by the time they were 50.

Thus, one of the primary conclusions that can be drawn from this literature and from our own clinical experience— and a central premise in the proposal contained in this chapter—is that although recent (as well as long-standing) life stresses can be important catalytic events in an individual's subsequent suicide, these stressful events must be contextualized within the larger overall picture of the individual's personality structure and life-long characterological ability to cope with (or to be vulnerable to) stress, failure, and loss. We now examine various elements in the individual's lifestyle as one theoretical element in conceptualizing a "coping versus vulnerability" model.

ADAPTATION TO CHANGE

The changes a human being encounters in life are likely to be especially stressful at points of significant life events. These can occur at both planned and unplanned intervals. For example, physical development, different school environments, puberty, marriage, parenthood, personal or occupational loss, and serious illness are all life events that present the need to confront extreme change and to adapt to new experiences (even new life-styles)—often with even greater versatility than a person has shown in the past. Here, a major thesis is that versatility or flexibility facilitates adaptability, assists problem solving, and tends to minimize persistent feelings that life is not worthwhile (when thoughts of suicide as the *only* way out become prominent in the person's mind). More specifically, in relation to the experience of failure and to loss, the concept of "buoyancy" (i.e., the ability to bounce back) becomes a major technique of both coping and adapting to change.

"Coping" is defined as behavior that facilitates adaptation to change and helps to maintain a continued level of previously adequate functioning. The term "vulnerability" signifies a weakness in coping skills—a soft area (or areas) of behavior that allow a stressful event to overwhelm the person in spite of his or her attempts to cope with it (e.g., the person's defenses are soft, and the level of good functioning declines). That is to say, the more capable people become in making such adaptations, the more they learn to cope and eventually to adapt to life changes. When their attempts to cope fail, they may stagnate or even regress to a prior pattern of behavior that served them well in the past, but that may not be appropriate to the present period (Antonovsky, 1981). If people continually fail to adapt to change, they eventually start to lose confidence and begin to lose an inner sense of trust, as well as hope. The continual loss of trust in self can frequently lead to an erosion of hope, and the loss of hope is considered a primary factor in the loss of a positive future time perspective (see "A Time Model," below). Sequentially, the loss of hope and of a positive future time perspective is often a major precipitating factor in the eventual loss of a sense of significance and meaning in life, as well as of the desire to continue life itself (Yufit, 1977).

It is at this juncture that thoughts about the significance of life, and even thoughts of ending one's life, can become prominent. The individual's thoughts on ending his or her life may become a major preoccupation, especially if there is a lack of resiliency or buoyancy in his or her attempts to adapt to an unexpected change or to solve a particular problem or fill a void; most often, such a deficiency is due to a loss of the ability (or the inability) to absorb or to defend oneself against a failure or a humiliating experience. The handling and working through of positive and negative life changes, or the feelings of shame and/or guilt, constitute a difficult task for many people (Piers & Singer, 1953). When an individual is placed under such demands, his or her previous psychological equilibrium may become destabilized, with vulnerability increasing when previously existing ego defenses either sag or become rigid and brittle. Such rigidity can severely limit buoyancy, and can contribute to a sense of personal stagnation, boredom, and hopelessness.

PSYCHOLOGICAL EQUILIBRIUM: A SERIES OF PROPOSALS

In representing these concepts, we present our proposals in the form of equations. These proposed equations are not necessarily causal; rather, they are a method of presenting a nomothetic conceptual framework for adaptation to change.

Proposal 1: Psychological Equilibrium, or a Healthy Adaptation to Change, Is a Function of Adequate Coping Skills Predominating over the Vulnerability to Stress

Our first proposal—again, not a mathematical equation, but an explanatory proposition or "explanation sketch"—is being evaluated by current research efforts (Yufit, 1989). The converse of this proposal is that a rigid cognitive style, developed over the years in dealing with different life experiences (especially during critical life cycle events), is one of the major deterrents to not being able to develop suitable options for problem solving (Neuringer, 1974). When the inability to develop such viable coping options is combined with a loss of hope, diminished internal resources, and weakened ego defenses (and further combined with an inadequate interpersonal support system), coping behavior is often diminished and a sense of vulnerability may become overwhelming. It is at this point that suicidal ideation may make its initial incursion into the thinking process. Since such cognitive rigidity narrows the person's chance of developing effective options, continuing or increasing psychological pain may become unbearable, and a more desperate option (i.e., suicide) can then become a final choice (Neuringer, 1974).

During significant life cycle events (e.g., separation from parents at the beginning of school, rejection by peers, first intimate relationship, school graduation, the first job, marriage, loss of loved ones, aging, etc.), the balance between coping and vulnerability can assume varying degrees of amplitude; one's ability to maintain a balance during these "ups" and "downs," or to improve the control of mastery of this balance, may become a source of concern. The success of problem resolution, or lack of it, will often be a major factor contributing to how effectively an individual's present problems are solved, and how future life cycle changes and challenges are met and resolved.

Erikson's Theoretical Model

As most readers know, Erik Erikson's model of human development and change over the life cycle indicates how a coping and vulnerability balance can be represented as psychological equilibrium, as well as how this equilibrium may be developed (Erikson, 1982). This model presents a view of sequential ego growth in defined stages; although it has been criticized by some as being an oversimplification of personality development, it does offer a unique, time-related, epigenetic schema for illustrating the development of critical personality variables and their subsequent integration into the formation of the total personality. This schema is presented in the format of the balance between two opposing personality characteristics, which can readily be related to establishing the vital balance between the "coping and vulnerability" concept. Erikson's eight-stage framework of ego development over the life cycle is shown in Table 27.1.

The manner is which an ego stage of development is resolved is a manner of integration (i.e., of fashioning a sense of who one is, where one wants to go, and how one is hoping to get there), thus helping to evolve an identity. These tasks emphasize the need for resiliency and adaptability. Their accomplishment will relate directly to establishing an equilibrium of coping versus vulnerability in dealing with future unfolding life cycle events. For example, the adolescent, in developing a sense of self, needs to know what his or her inner feelings are and how to achieve his or her future goals. This young person is building vital components in the mechanism that will enable him or her to deal with the vicissitudes of everyday stress and change, as well as to face and master the tasks of future significant life changes.

TABLE 27.1. Erikson's Eight Stages

Psychosocial Crisis	Time (age) period
1. Basic trust versus mistrust	Infancy
2. Autonomy versus shame, doubt	Early childhood
3. Initiative versus guilt	Play age
4. Industry versus inferiority	School age
5. Identity versus identity diffusion	Adolescence
6. Intimacy versus isolation	Young adulthood
7. Generativity versus stagnation, self-absorption	Adulthood
8. Ego integrity versus disgust, despair	Old age

On the other hand, a failure to make progress toward the establishment of one's identity can lead to difficulty in adequate coping with concomitant increases in vulnerability— often with the consequences of varying symptomatology, such as uncertainty, anxiety, and rigidity. Here, it is not uncommon to see signs of depression, hopelessness, and despair (Beck, Resnik, & Lettieri, 1974). When such feelings occur and are accompanied by the loss of perspective in viewing a particular crisis, constricted thinking often results. Yufit (1969) notes that self-harm or self-destructive thoughts may develop and be acted upon, especially by the burdened and confused adolescent who lacks trust and has not yet had the needed experience of intimacy to help in coping with stress.

Adaptation to Life Events

To further illustrate the application of Erikson's developmental framework with regard to a significant, often stressful life cycle event, let us consider the stressful life event of beginning school (usually kindergarten). Here the immediate issue is separation from parents and/or siblings, which for some children may be occuring for the first time. The manner in which the separation is handled (both by the child and by his or her parents, siblings, and members of other support systems) will determine to a large extent not only how the child will handle future separations, but how he or she will adapt to new kinds of separation and change experiences. Success in such adaptation will lead to a sense of accomplishment and to the development of flexibility. A lack of success often leads to doubt, uncertainty, anxiety, and a narrowing of problem-solving ability, with the real possibility of increased rigidity in the individual's future attempts at coping. The lessening of the likelihood of successful coping further increases the person's doubt, uncertainty, and even despair.

In a similar manner, passages through more elective life cycle benchmark events (e.g., marriage and divorce) or unexpected changes (e.g., the sudden loss of significant loved ones, unexpected job termination, or negative change in health status) will be either aided or thwarted by the kinds of personal resolutions that the individual has made during earlier basic developmental periods, such as the extent to which a sense of trust has or has not been established. A sense of trust can lead to autonomy, which can provide another pathway to assist in coping with change. Achieving such coping skills can help in the development of a sense of personal freedom, and can create a desire to take the initiative in one's behavior and to be productive in one's life. All of this can greatly assist a person in coping with change and can help to further strengthen the overall picture of the individual's character development. Such sequential development provides a form of inner continuity—the essence of developing a well-integrated, resilient ego identity—which in turn enables the person to continue using coping skills to deal with life changes, whether these are expected or not. The person who learns how to "roll with the punches" (i.e., who internalizes "buoyancy") will be less likely to become submerged by the stresses of such demands to change.

On the other hand, the failure to resolve basic developmental tasks minimizes the creation and integration of inner resources. This often leads to far greater reliance on external resources (such as existing external support systems) or on internal, highly elaborated fantasized support systems, in order to help with coping. When such support systems are unavailable or inaccurately perceived, or when mistrust and doubt dilute or prevent their use, withdrawal from life's challenges becomes a common pathway of "adapting." Continued failure often leads to a sense of self-absorption, then to despair, and eventually to stagnation, hopelessness, and "giving up." From our clinical perspective, it is at this point that suicidal behavior is often considered the means to escape from such a painful dilemma. The person determines that it is in effect a situation of "endgame"—that no solution can be found and that the psychological pain is too much to bear (Yufit & Benzies, 1973).

This constriction of perception, as noted above, is accompanied by feeling states of hopelessness and helplessness. These further severely deplete the individual's energy to engage in coping, and they also promote self-absorption and stagnation—thus increasing the person's sense of vulnerability and inability to adapt to any kind of change, and certainly his or her inability to adapt to major life cycle events. When such vulnerability becomes all-encompassing, the person often loses both his or her immediate and long-term time perspective. He or she determines that life itself has lost its significance. This determination may be accompanied by a psychological regression to an earlier time, by a withdrawal into a depression, or by thoughts of escape from continuing psychological pain via death. The person may act out by making a suicide attempt in order to gain needed attention, so as to bolster low self-esteem or to alleviate guilt or shame. However, if the attempt is physically damaging, it can create further practical problems in adaptation; it can also result in severe economic loss from decline of productivity, and eventually in a need for support systems (e.g., governmental supports) (Committee on Trauma Research, 1985).

Erikson himself has stated:

> The suicidal act must first be viewed as a form of total self-destructive action in a life situation in which positive alternatives of action seem to have lost their credence. . . . In assessing suicide potential, one must remember that there is often a mix-up in the simplest and the deepest things. The sense of "I" would have much to do with, for example, a sense of being active. Those are big words. The opposite of that would be to become inactivated (not just to be "passive"). If someone feels totally inactivated, suicidal ideas may become inevitable as a

way to restore some sense of being "in control." (Quoted in Jacobs & Brown, 1989, pp. xi–xiii)

Shneidman's Model

Shneidman believes that the central feature of suicide is pain, and that

> the key to suicide prevention lies in the reduction of that individual's psychological pain. All else—demographic variables, family history, previous suicidal history—is peripheral except as those factors bear on the presently felt pain. Ultimately, suicide occurs when there is the co-existence of intolerable pain, intense negative press, and extreme perturbation with perceptual constriction and an irresistible penchant for life-ending action. (Shneidman, 1987, pp. 176–177)

Shneidman (1984, 1986a) believes that clinicians also must exercise extreme caution with every patient who is perturbed and who has a lethal means of attempting suicide available. This would include clinical work with patients with poor impulse control who are in crisis and are unable to decrease their level of perturbation in the therapeutic encounter. Shneidman (1987) has presented a theoretical cubic model of suicide, which includes the combined effects of psychological pain, perturbation, lethality, and what he calls "press" to attempt to identify those individuals most at risk for suicide. (For a depiction of the model, see Figure 3.1 in Shneidman, Chapter 3, this volume.) Here "press," a term originated by Murray (1938), refers to those aspects of the inner or outer world or environment that touch, move, impinge on, or affect an individual, and to which he or she reacts. "Press" can be either positive or negative.

A Time Model

Temporal perspective also provides a useful dimension to explore in the examination of a person's adaptation to stress and his or her ability to cope with change (Cottle, 1976). The ability to maintain a future time perspective is vital to maintaining a sense of perspective in times of crisis, as well to providing a goal orientation for the present (Yufit, 1977). An adaptive time profile is usually characterized by a predominant orientation to the present and to the future, with minimal involvement in the past. A maladaptive time profile, which is very frequently found to characterize the suicidal person, is exemplified by a predominant orientation to the past, with a minimal (usually negative) present time orientation and a minimal to nonexistent future time perspective. A heavy involvement in the past usually creates a negative time equilibrium (Van Kalder, 1980; Yufit & Benzies, 1978).

Proposal 2: Negative Time Equilibrium Is a Function of Fear of the Future, Plus Nostalgia for the Past

Many well-functioning individuals may, in times of heavy stress or after a sudden loss, experience brief and transient suicidal thoughts; however, these thoughts are then typically displaced by other, more adaptive options and solutions. When a lack of confidence or a lack of resiliency (e.g., cognitive rigidity) prevents such shifts in adaptation, more enduring thoughts of self-harm or self-destruction may persist, with overt action at time occurring very precipitously. The feelings of pain, anxiety, and depression may become too painful to endure, and a "permanent way out" becomes a plausible "solution" to the rigid, despairing, hopeless, frightened, or angry affective state. Depending on the levels of either intentionality or ambivalence that are present, such an overt action may take the form of a carefully planned, nonlethal suicide attempt, geared toward gaining attention, inflicting self-punishment, or creating shame and guilt for another; in this case, the result is intended to be survival. Or the overt behavior selected may be highly lethal in nature, and the chances of rescue may be carefully planned to be negligible; in this case, the result sought is cessation of psychological pain via death (Farber, 1968; Shneidman, 1985).

A Sense of Belonging and Connectedness

From our clinical perspective, suicidal ideation is often observed in individuals who lack a sense of belonging or connectedness. "Belonging" generally refers to external activity systems (e.g., a person's career, recreation, club, religion, significant other, etc.). However, a lack of belonging can also occur when a person's sense of inner continuity to himself or herself is lost, diluting perhaps the most important of all relationships—the relationship with the self.

"How do you *really* feel about yourself?" is a critical question to ask in any suicide assessment interview. Being connected to one's inner feelings promotes a sense of continuity in self-knowledge and in one's inner workings (identity), as well as knowledge of how much one can rely on one's own abilities in a self-sufficient manner (autonomy). These inner connections can provide the necessary continuity to achieve accurate self-appraisals, so that a person can maintain his or her identity even in times of great stress and change. When the person's self-perceptions are congruent with the perceptions that others have about him or her, then there is a coalescence of inner and outer perceptions, and ego identity is enhanced. Coping and adaptation resources are more readily available as a result of this important coalescence of inner and outer perceptions. The person thus feels more connected internally.

The inability to maintain such inner and interpersonal connections has a tendency to dissolve positive self-esteem, to lower self-confidence, and to diminish trust and hope. In a severe instance the person's connections with reality may be severed, to be replaced by a withdrawal into a depression or by a regression into a psychosis. Such an escape presumes that these destinations serve as a haven of safe refuge from environmental (or internal) unbearable stress (Yufit, 1977). By contrast, when a person's sense of belonging is well established, the resulting connections (both internal and external) provide the necessary basis for establishing and maintaining an identity. This identity, along with a developed future time perspective, is a vital deterrent to developing a sense of hopelessness—a most ominous vulnerability in dealing with crisis situations.

The Future in Coping

A desired future event—a new relationship, a new job, travel to new places, a sought-after retirement—can create a sense of pleasurable anticipation. It can thus provide an inner connectedness to a feeling of day-to-day continuity and control, and can help to develop a solid identity, often with a perception of having a meaningful life. Who cannot tolerate a "bad week" more readily if a weekend of planned pleasurable events is being awaited? On the other hand, the prospect of an empty weekend devoid of positive anticipated experiences often makes it more difficult to manage the daily stresses of a week's day-to-day events. There is no "balance" available (i.e., anticipation of pleasures) to provide energy and initiative to deal with the current stress. Depressed persons often describe "Blue Sunday" as the day before another dreaded week of jobs or school.

It is not uncommon for human beings to feel that they remain connected to the past through commemorating anniversaries and nostalgically reminiscing about prior events, usually forming fantasies that may be further stimulated by music, stories, travel, or old friends. People tend to make their most important connections with the present, for that is where they commonly reside psychologically when they are not making plans for the future or reminiscing via music or important memories at anniversary times. Finally, the development of specific plans for the future tends to provide some sense of control over the unknown ahead, and also furnishes blueprints of happy endings and new beginnings.

Proposal 3: Positive Time Equilibrium Is a Function of a Planned Future Time Orientation and an Acceptance and Integration of Past Events

A plausible, meaningful connection to past, present, and future time periods enhances the coping strengths of a person under more-than-usual stress. This is even more so during critical life cycle events. Being able to shift to the past in recalling previous methods of successful problem resolution, or to shift to the future in anticipation of an ego-enhancing event, provides an important inner resource or perspective in coping with problems or conflict situations. Such a resource is especially needed in dealing with major life changes in the life cycle. The degree of basic trust, autonomy, and initiative bolsters the ego and allows various levels of deeper involvement in events or with people; as a result, the person eventually gains a greater inner strength and skill in dealing with significant benchmarks in the life cycle (Yufit, 1969). As each life cycle event is successfully resolved (even partially), a renewed feeling of competence and eventual mastery can develop, leading to a more solid sense of self-actualization (Maslow, 1973).

Coping itself can be conceptualized as a form of resiliency that facilitates adaptation to change. The ability to be resilient facilitates the needed buoyancy to keep one's head "above water" when flooded with stress or engulfed by loss. By contrast, the lack of such resiliency can breed a sense of rigidity and self-absorption—critical precursors to the development of a vulnerability to stressful events (Antonovsky, 1981).

Proposal 4: Maintaining a Vital Balance during Critical Life Cycle Events Is a Function of Resilient and Buoyant Coping and Adaptation Abilities Predominating over Vulnerability and the Loss of Future Time Perspective

The loss of meaning and perspective in life can narrow the possibilities for the development of alternative solutions, and may in due time reduce or curtail the desire to live. Loss of meaning may increase the possibility of self-harm (to punish the self or others) or self-destruction (to permanently stop the pain of psychological suffering). As psychotherapists who have worked with many suicidal persons over the years, we have consistently noted that this sequence is present in both self-harming and self-destructive persons.

Ego Strengths

In each of the five clinical cases discussed in this book, we can see an absence of what Erik Erikson called "basic strengths." These strengths can be viewed as the core elements in the ability to cope effectively. The basic strengths listed by Erikson (1982) as components of the eight developmental stages are hope, will, purpose, competence, fidelity, love, care, and wisdom. It is noteworthy that the absence of these strengths or the presence of their basic antipathies—namely, withdrawal, compulsion, inhibition, inertia, repudiation, exclusivity, rejectivity, and disdain—is frequently a key element underlying suicidal vulnerability. The existence of many of these debilitating attributes is often correlated with an increased likelihood of worthlessness, helplessness, hopelessness, and despair; in many vulnerable persons, the emergence of suicidal ideation and behaviors is the result.

If we wish to help people cope more effectively by making them more aware of how to develop good ego strengths, and of how to anticipate and curb weaknesses via understanding and insight, we must help them to learn problem solving, conflict resolution, stress reduction, and broader time perspectives—in other words, effective mechanisms to handle major events in the life cycle. The development of these skills needs to take place early in life—certainly by the onset of adolescence at the latest—in order to have its greatest impact. These skills can be taught by parents, teachers, and (when necessary) by psychotherapists. The interaction of different coping skills based on these basic strengths helps to develop a sense of coherence, inner connection, and wholeness in the personality, as well as competence and a sense of mastery (the basic qualities of a good ego identity).

The capacity for intimacy is necessary for eventually choosing major life involvements—career, marriage, leisure-time pursuits. Any of these choices can have a positive as well as a negative resolution. Or the person may choose isolation, with minimal involvement with others. Whatever choice is made, there occurs an emerging pattern of enduring and characteristic ways of behaving, which will affect the manner in which future life cycle events are resolved. The capacity for intimacy often facilitates a sense of belonging and broadens the feeling of connectedness to self and to others, which is considered an asset to coping and a vital deterrent to considerations of self-harm or self-destructive behaviors when major stress is encountered (Yufit, 1969).

Although personality structure can shift over time with new experiences and with consequences of the experience of new life cycle events, there usually remain some enduring characteristics, termed "personality traits," that serve to enhance or to dilute methods of coping with change. Such traits as hopelessness, doubt, uncertainty, lack of confidence, and mistrust may weaken adaptation by increasing, the specificity of vulnerability and lowering self-esteem; if the continuing stress remains too high, they may lead to regression.

Measurement of Coping and Vulnerability

Suicide attempts or completed suicides are most likely during times of extreme vulnerability, which usually result from a lack of resiliency and from weakened and inadequate ego defenses. The person often succumbs to a loss of self, which may lead to a subsequent loss of desire to live—a desire to end the continuing psychological pain, which is too much to endure (Shneidman, 1985). We still need to define more clearly those coping qualities that allow most persons to adapt to traumatic events or negative life cycle changes, and not to choose suicide as an immediate option. A number of these coping skills are represented in the Coping Abilities Questionnaire (CAQ), which was constructed in an attempt to assess quantitatively how people do cope with stress mediated by change (Yufit, 1988). The Suicide Screening Checklist (SSC) has also been developed to evaluate vulnerability and the potential for suicidal behavior (Yufit, 1989).

The SSC (Yufit, 1989) was commissioned by the Centers for Disease Control. It consists of 60 items, each of which is considered to be correlated with suicidal behavior. The items are scored on the basis of responses to relevant questions in a focused clinical interview. Certain items are differentially weighted on the basis of supporting empirical evidence as to their degree of correlation with suicidal behavior. Many of the items in the SSC are related to critical life cycle events and to the stressors of everyday life. The CAQ consists of 15 items, also differentially weighted in terms of presumed relevance to coping ability. Each CAQ item is keyed to a presumed component of coping ability; the components are based on both the theoretical framework presented above and empirical data. Both the CAQ and the SSC are currently being field-tested to ascertain their sensitivity and specificity.

APPLICATION OF THIS CHAPTER'S PROPOSALS TO THE BOOK'S CLINICAL CASE MATERIAL: THE VITAL BALANCE IN ACTION

We now discuss the five clinical cases presented in this volume. A lack of interpersonal connectedness was evident in Heather B's reaction at age 7 to her father's death (she went out to play in the snow, "showing no strong emotional reaction"). Even if her denial was prevalent at that time, her inability to express feelings in response to the loss of a parent would seem to indicate both a loss of connection with her own feelings and a lack of awareness of (or even caring about) the feelings of other family members. Such withdrawals could set a dangerous precedent for continued distancing, as well as for inadequate coping with future stressful events. It might not necessarily be a direct correlate to suicide, but it would tend to increase Heather's vulnerability in stressful situations. Even more alarming was the lack of both inner and outer connectedness shown by John Z. The patient lost connection with sustenance via food (as evidenced by a 20-pound weight loss in 2 months) and was becoming increasingly self-absorbed with his own ruminations, experiencing a loss of time connection and time continuity. All of these might be equally important signs in the examination of any desire to end his life.

Numerous other details in the case descriptions illustrate the importance of assessing individuals' ability to cope, as well as their specific personality vulnerabilities. For example, Heather often expressed strong self-condemnation, losing any sense of the positive connections she had or of her own abilities to do well in school. Her Rorschach responses indicated a decline in interests relating to interpersonal relations, together with an extreme sense of destruction, which she projected in seeing "the collision of two alien worlds." Her Thematic Apperception Test themes also portrayed conflict through interaction, safety and protection via isolation, and many other areas of vulnerability as she struggled to see something meaningful in life. The paucity of coping abilities to be found anywhere in the case material suggests that Heather was a youngster with increasing suicide potential.

The case of Ralph F reveals the effects of early traumatic ruptures in a child's ability to trust (i.e., the disclosure of several female relatives' sexual molestation by his grandfather). The subsequent anxiety and discomfort (perhaps including strong guilt) were exacerbated by the loss of a significant relative, his molested aunt. Seen together, these elements can be seen as precipitants to Ralph's obsession with suicide; they increased his sense of hopelessness and his vulnerability to subsequent suicidal impulses.

As noted earlier, John also exhibited increasing levels of vulnerability. He lost his connection to the occupational world when he was laid off. He tried to strengthen himself via further education to gain more of a sense of mastery and control, but as his depression deepened it interfered with his attempts to cope and to re-establish a sense of accomplishment. John also exhibited evidence of a decline in eating (as noted above) and in many other areas of primary functioning (sleep, sexual drive, intellectual skills, etc.). These declines in primary functioning no doubt exacerbated the deficiencies in whatever coping abilities might still exist and intensified his feelings of depression and despondency. That is, as his sense of trust and hope became seriously reduced, John became less and less able to tolerate the level of psychological pain; his two reported suicide attempts may be seen as efforts to end the pain. John's case illustrates the inability, most often found in high-status males, to handle the failure, humiliation, and shame often associated with loss. In our clinical experience, women appear to be able to reach out and share their loss more easily than do men (i.e., to talk with other women and work through their feelings via candid, involved interactions with their same-sex peers).

In the case of Faye C, the patient was overprotected as an adolescent and made a strong (perhaps too strong) connection to certain important figures in her life. Her overdependence on her father would appear to have inhibited her own growth and sense of autonomy (one questions whether she ever really belonged to herself in terms of understanding her own feelings). She was also apparently unable to develop an adequate therapeutic alliance in psychotherapy, which would have alerted the careful clinician to the presence of a major risk factor (Bongar, 1991).

The case of José G illustrates the importance of an occupational connection (his career with the railroad). Yet the patient showed both a high degree of externalized anger toward his job with the railroad and an increasing sense of self-depreciation, which increased over time. José also maintained an important connection to his "habits" (smoking and drinking), which served his high-dependency needs and may have served as poor substitutes for developing more meaningful interpersonal relationships.

CONCLUSION

An individual's previous success in resolving life's difficulties is a major factor in his or her ability to handle current problems. Through successful problem solving, the person develops an inner sense of self-trust; this sets the stage for developing a sense of mastery, of control, of the ability to solve life's problems, and of the capacity to adapt to change over the life cycle. This sense of mastery and achievement can be enhanced by maintaining a future-oriented time perspective (Van Kalder, 1980; Yufit, 1977).

Menninger (1938) wrote extensively about the deeper dynamic and dyadic motives for suicide. He held that suicide must be regarded as a peculiar type of death that entails three internal elements: the element of dying, the element of killing, and the element of being killed. He also emphasized that people remain alive through the mechanism of a vital balance in the self (Menninger, 1938; see also Brown & Jacobs, 1989) In Menninger's view, the self is composed of component subselves. A weakness in the ability to integrate these subselves and balance them is one measure of a person's vulnerability to suicide (Litman, 1989). Menninger has also noted that although there are some psychological pains so severe as to evoke the act of suicide, the role of the psychotherapist is to persuade the person to cling to hope, to "try life a while longer. . . . One has to be a very strong persuader to dissuade people set on suicide because it is a strong impulse. That's why Freud thought it was an instinct" (quoted in Brown & Jacobs, p. 484). Menninger has further urged that the patient be brought to a sense of connectedness to others—that is, a sense that all of us are struggling to cope effectively with stress and change over the life cycle. The therapist's task is to encourage and develop the patient's sense of trust and hope: to encourage the patient not to give up, but to cling to hope a bit longer. Finally, Brown and Jacobs (1989) note that Menninger's exhortations on hope recall Erikson's thoughts about activity and continuity: "everybody has to recover his own sense of actuality" (p. 485). Here the clinical challenge is to find and enhance a sense of personal identity, coping abilities, and staying power—to lessen vulnerability and to facilitate a faith in the future.

REFERENCES

Aldredge, D. (1984). Family interaction and suicidal behavior: A brief review. *Journal of Family Therapy, 6*(9), 304-322.

Antonovsky, A. (1981). *Health, stress and coping.* San Francisco: Jossey-Bass.

Beck, A. T., Resnik, H. L. P., & Lettieri, D. J. (Eds.). (1974). *The prediction of suicide.* Bowie, MD: Charles Press.

Blumenthal, S. J. (1990). An overview and synopsis of risk factors, assessment, and treatment of suicidal patients over the life cycle. In S. J. Blumenthal & D. J. Kupfer (Eds.), *Suicide over the life cycle: Risk factors, assessment, and treatment of suicidal patients* (pp. 685-734). Washington, DC: American Psychiatric Press.

Bongar, B. (1991). *The suicidal patient: Clinical and legal standards of care.* Washington, DC: American Psychological Association.

Brown, H. N., & Jacobs, D. G. (1989). Concluding remarks. In D. G. Jacobs & H. N. Brown (Eds.), *Suicide: Understanding and responding. Harvard Medical School perspectives on suicide* (pp. 485-486). Madison, CT: International Universities Press.

Committee on Trauma Research. (1985). Injury in America. Washington, DC: National Academy Press.

Cottle, T. J. (1976). *Perceiving time.* New York: Wiley.

Erikson, E. H. (1982). *Life cycle completed.* New York: Norton.

Farber, M. L. (1968). *Theory of suicide.* New York: Funk & Wagnalls.

Friedman, R. C. (1984). Family history of illness in seriously suicidal adolescents: A life-cycle approach, *American Journal of Orthopsychiatry, 54*(3), 390-397.

Jacobs, D. G., & Brown, H. N. (1989). Dialogue with Erik H. Erikson. In D. G. Jacobs & H. N. Brown (Eds.), *Suicide: Understanding and responding. Harvard Medical School perspectives on suicide* (pp. xi-xiv). Madison, CT: International Universities Press.

Lazare, A. (1987). Shame and humiliation in the medical encounter. *Archives of Internal Medicine, 147*, 1653-1658.

Linehan, M. M., Goodstein, J. L., Neilsen, S. L., & Chiles, J. K. (1983). Reasons for staying alive when you are thinking of killing yourself: The Reasons for Living Inventory. *Journal of Consulting and Clinical Psychology, 51*(2), 276-286.

Litman, R. E. (1989). Suicides: What do they have in mind? In D. G. Jacobs & H. N. Brown (Eds.), *Suicide: Understanding and responding. Harvard Medical School perspectives on suicide* (pp. 233-244). Madison, CT: International Universities Press.

Maltsberger, J. T. (1988). Suicide danger: Clinical estimation and decision. *Suicide and Life-Threatening Behavior, 18*(1), 47-54.

Maris, R. W. (1988). Preface: Overview and discussion. In R. W. Maris (Ed.), *Understanding and preventing suicide: Plenary papers of the first combined meeting of the AAS and IASP* (pp. vii-xxiii). New York: Guilford Press.

Maslow, A. H. (1973). *The further reaches of human nature.* New York: Viking Press.

Menninger, K. (1938). *Man against himself.* New York: Harcourt, Brace, & World.

Motto, J. A. (1979). Guidelines for the management of the suicidal patient. *Weekly Psychiatry Update Series Lesson, 20*(3), 3-7. (Available from Biomedia, Inc., 20 Nassau Street, Princeton, NJ 08540).

Murray, H. (1938). *Explorations in personality.* New York: Oxford University Press.

Neuringer, C. (Ed.). (1974). *Psychological assessment of suicide.* Springfield, IL: Charles C Thomas.

Paykel, E. S. (1989). Stress and life events. In L. Davidson & M. Linnoila (Eds.), *Report of the Secretary's Task Force on Youth Suicide: Vol. 2. Risk factors for youth suicide* (DHHS Publication No. ADM 89-1622). Washington, DC: U. S. Government Printing Office.

Peterson, L. G., & Bongar, B. (1989). The suicidal patient. In A. Lazare (Ed.), *Outpatient psychiatry: Diagnosis and treatment* (2nd ed., pp. 569-584). Baltimore: Williams & Wilkins.

Piers, G., & Singer, M. B. (1953). *Shame and guilt.* Springfield, IL: Charles C Thomas.

Rich, A. R., & Bonner, R. L. (1987). Concurrent validity of a stress–vulnerability model of suicidal ideation and behavior: A follow-up study. *Suicide and Life-Threatening Behavior, 17*(4), 265-270.

Rich, A. R., & Bonner, R. L. (1988). *Negative life stress, social problem solving, self appraisal and hopelessness.* Unpublished manuscript, U. S. Penitentiary, Lewisburg, PA.

Selye, H. (1976). *The stress of life.* New York: McGraw-Hill.

Shneidman, E. S. (1971). Perturbation and lethality as precursors of suicide in a gifted group. *Suicide and Life-Threatening Behavior, 1*(1), 23-45.

Shneidman, E. S. (1984). Aphorisms of suicide and some implications for psychotherapy. *American Journal of Psychotherapy, 38*(3), 319-328.

Shneidman, E. S. (1985). *Definition of suicide.* New York: Wiley.

Shneidman, E. S. (1986a). Some essentials of suicide and some implications for response. In A. Roy (F.d.), *Suicide* (pp. 1-16). Baltimore: Williams & Wilkins.

Shneidman, E. S. (1986b). Suicidal logic. In W. S. Sahakian, B. J. Sahakian, & P. L. Sahakian-Nunn (Eds.), *Psychopathology today: The current status of abnormal psychology* (3rd ed. pp. 267-281). Itasca, Il: Peacock Press.

Shneidman, E. S. (1987). A psychological approach to suicide. In G. R. VandenBos & B. K. Bryant (Eds.), *Cataclysms, crises, and catastrophes: Psychology in action* (pp. 147- 183). Washington, DC: American Psychological Association.

Smith, K. (1985). Suicide assessment: An ego vulnerabilities approach. *Bulletin of the Menninger Clinic, 48*(5), 489-499.

Vaillant, G. E., & Blumenthal, S. J. (1990). Introduction—Suicide over the life cycle: Risk factors and life-span development. In S. J. Blumenthal & D. J. Kupfer (Eds.), *Suicide over the life cycle: Risk factors, assessment, and treatment of suicidal patients* (pp. 1-16). Washington, DC: American Psychiatric Press.

Van Kalder, C. (1980). *Achievement and time perspective.* Louvain, Belgium: Institute of Time Perspective, University of Louvain.

Weissman, M. M., Klerman, G. L., Markowitz, J. S., & Ouellette, R. (1989). Suicidal ideation and suicide attempts in panic disorder and attacks. *New England Journal of Medicine, 321,* 1209-1214.

Yufit, R. I. (1969). Variations of intimacy and isolation. *Journal of Projective Techniques, 3*(4), 49–58.

Yufit, R. I., & Benzies, B. (1973). Assessment of suicide potential by time perspective. *Suicide and Life-Threatening Behavior, 3*(4), 270–282.

Yufit, R. I. (1977). Suicide, bereavement and time perspective. In B. L. Danto & A. H. Kutscher (Eds.), *Suicide and bereavement* (pp. 138–143). New York: Arno Press.

Yufit, R. I., & Benzies, B. (1978). *Scoring manual for the Time Questionnaire.* Palo Alto, CA: Consulting Psychologists Press.

Yufit, R. I. (1988). *Manual of procedures—assessing suicide potential: Suicide assessment team.* Unpublished manuscript. (Available from Robert I. Yufit, Department of Psychiatry and Behavioral Sciences, Division of Clinical Psychology, Northwestern University Medical School, Chicago, IL).

Yufit, R. I. (1989). Developing a suicide screening instrument for adolescents and young adults. In M. Rosenberg & K. Baer (Eds.), *Report of the Secretary's Task Force on Youth Suicide: Vol. 4. Strategies for prevention of youth suicide* (DHHS Publication No. 89-1622, pp. 129–141). Washington, DC: U. S. Government Printing Office.

CHAPTER 28

Genetics, Biology, and Suicide in the Family

Alec Roy, M.D.
Hillside Hospital, Glen Oaks, New York

Over the last 10 to 15 years a number of lines of evidence have led to the suggestions that familial/genetic and biological determinants may play a role in the multidetermined act that is suicide for reviews, see Roy, 1982, 1985a, 1985b, 1989). The purpose of this chapter is to review some of these data briefly. Their possible implications for the difficult task of identifying individuals who may be at increased risk for further suicidal behavior are also discussed.

FAMILY HISTORY OF SUICIDE

There are five lines of evidence about the possibility that there may be family/genetic factors in suicide. These are as follows: clinical, twin, Iowa 500, Amish, and Copenhagen adoption studies.

Clinical Studies

Pitts and Winokur (1964) found that among 748 consecutively admitted patients, 37 reported a possible or definite suicide in a first-degree relative (4.9%). In 25 of these 37 cases (68%), the diagnosis was an affective disorder. The statistical probability of this distribution's occurring by chance was less than .02. When the probable diagnoses in the cases of the first-degree relatives who committed suicide were considered, in 24 of the 37 patient-relative pairings both members had affective disorders. Pitts and Winokur estimated that 79% of the suicides of the first-degree relatives were associated with probable affective disorder.

I (Roy, 1983) found that a family history of suicide significantly increased the risk of a suicide attempt in a wide variety of diagnostic groups.

Almost half (48.6%) of 243 patients with a family history of suicide had themselves attempted suicide. More than half (56.4%) of all the patients with a family history of suicide had a primary diagnosis of an affective disorder, and more than a third (34.4%) had a recurrent unipolar or bipolar affective disorder. In a Belgian study, Linkowski, de Maertelaer, and Mendlewicz (1985) found that 123 of 713 depressed patients (17%) had a first- or second-degree relative who had committed suicide. A family history of suicide particularly increased the risk for a violent suicide attempt. Linkowski et al. concluded: "A positive family history for violent suicide should be considered as a strong predictor of active suicide attempting behavior in major depressive illness" (1985, p. 237).

Murphy and Wetzel (1982) studied suicide attempters. Seventeen percent of those with a primary diagnosis of primary affective disorder had a family history of suicide, and 17% had a family history of suicide attempts. Because individuals with affective disorders comprise a larger proportion of suicides than individuals with personality disorders do, Murphy and Wetzel predicted that more of their patients with affective disorder could be expected to present a significant suicide risk in the future. They concluded that a "systematic family history of such behavior coupled with modern clinical diagnosis would prove useful in identifying those attempters at increased risk for suicide" (1982, p. 90).

Twin Studies

Kallman and colleagues (Kallman & Anastasio, 1947; Kallman, DePorte, DePorte, & Feingold, 1949) encouraged the application of classic twin methodology in studies of suicide: "[I]f hereditary factors play a decisive role, we should find a concordant tendency to suicide more frequently in one-egg than in two-egg pairs" (Kallman & Anastasio, 1947, p. 54). Twenty years later, Haberlandt (1965, 1967) reviewed the accumulated data in the literature on 149 sets of twins in which at least one twin committed suicide. Among these 149 twin pairs, 9 sets of twins were concordant for suicide. Interestingly, all of these 9 twin pairs were found among the 51 monozygotic (MZ) twin pairs. In contrast, concordance for suicide did not occur among the 98 dizygotic (DZ) twin pairs. This difference between MZ and DZ pairs for concordance for suicide was statistically significant (Fisher's exact test, $p = .001$).

We recently reported on 176 twin pairs in which one twin had committed suicide (Roy, Segal, Centerwall, & Robinette, 1990). In 9 of these twin pairs, both twins had committed suicide. Seven of these 9 twin pairs concordant for suicide were found among the 62 MZ twin pairs, while the other 2 twin pairs were found among the 114 DZ twin pairs. This twin group difference for concordance for suicide (11.3% vs. 1.8%) was statistically significant (Fisher's exact test, $p = .01$). Combining our 176 twin pairs with the

149 twin pairs reviewed by Haberlandt, the 73 twin pairs (none of which were concordant for suicide) reported by Juel-Nielsen and Videbech (1970), and the 1 concordant MZ twin pair reported by Zair (1981) yields 399 twin pairs: 129 MZ twin pairs (17 of 129, or 13.2%, concordant for suicide) and 270 DZ twin pairs (2 of 270, or 0.7%, concordant for suicide). These combined data further demonstrate that MZ twin pairs show significantly greater concordance for suicide than do DZ twin pairs (Fisher's exact test, $p = .001$).

However, we (Roy et al., 1990) also examined for the presence of psychiatric disorder in twins, and their families in a subsample of 11 twin pairs, 2 of which were concordant for suicide. Eleven of these 13 twin suicide victims had been treated for psychiatric disorder, as had 8 of their 9 surviving cotwins. In addition, twins in 10 pairs had other first- or second-degree relatives who had been treated for psychiatric disorder. Thus, these twin data suggest that genetic factors related to suicide may largely represent a genetic predisposition to the psychiatric disorders associated with suicide. However, they leave open the question of whether there may be an independent genetic component for suicide.

The Iowa 500 Study

In a recent follow-up study, Tsuang (1983) found that the first-degree relatives of the psychiatric patient in the Iowa 500 study had a risk of suicide almost eight times greater than the risk in the relatives of normal controls. The risk of suicide was significantly greater among the first-degree relatives of depressed patients than it was among the relatives of either schizophrenic or manic patients. Among the first-degree relatives of the psychiatric patients in the Iowa 500 study who had committed suicide, the suicide risk was four times greater than the risk in the relatives of patients who did not commit suicide. Here the suicide risk was equally high among the relatives of both depressed and manic patients.

The Amish Study

Egeland and Sussex (1985) reported on the suicide data obtained from the study of affective disorders among the Older Order Amish community of Lancaster County in southeast Pennsylvania. Several of the important social risk factors for suicide among individuals in the general population, such as unemployment, divorced or separated marital status, social isolation, and alcoholism, are not commonly found among these Amish. Of the 26 suicide victims among these Amish over the 100 years from 1880 to 1980, 24 met Research Diagnostic Criteria for a major affective disorder. Eight of the suicide victims had bipolar I disorder, 4 had bipolar II disorder, and 12 had unipolar affective disorder. A further case met diagnostic criteria for a minor depression. Furthermore, most of the suicide victims had a heavy family loading for affective disorders. For example, among the 8 bipolar I suicide victims, the morbidity risk for affective disorders among their 110 first-degree relatives was 29%, compared with the 1–4% found among the general population.

Almost three-quarters of the 26 suicide victims were found to cluster in four family pedigrees, each of which contained a heavy loading for affective disorders and suicide (Figures 28.1 and 28.2). Interestingly, the converse was not true, as there were other family pedigrees with heavy loadings for affective disorder but without suicides. It is also of note that the morbidity risk for affective disorders among 170 first-degree relatives in other bipolar I family pedigrees without suicide was similar to that found in bipolar family pedigrees with suicide, also in the 20% range. Thus, a family loading for affective disorders was not in itself a predictor for suicide. Egeland and Sussex concluded:

> Our study replicates findings that indicate an increased suicidal risk for patients with a diagnosis of major affective disorder and a strong family history of suicide. The number not receiving adequate treatment for manic–depressive illness (among the suicides) supports the common belief that intervention for these patients at risk is recommended. . . . It appears most warranted in those families in which there is a family history of suicide. The clustering of suicides in Amish pedigrees follows the distribution of affective illness in the kinship and suggests the role of inheritance. (1985, p. 918)

Copenhagen Adoption Studies

The strongest evidence for the presence of genetic factors in suicide comes from the adoption studies carried out in Denmark by Schulsinger, Kety, Wender, and Rosenthal reviewed in Kety (1986) and in Schulsinger, Kety, Rosenthal, and Wender (1979). The Psykologisk Institut has a register of the 5,483 adoptions that occurred in greater Copenhagen between 1924 and 1947. A screening of the registers of causes of death revealed that 57 of these adoptees eventually committed suicide. They were matched with 57 adopted controls for age, sex, social class of the adopting parents, and time spent both with their biological relatives and in institutions before being adopted. Searches of the causes of death revealed that 12 of the 269 biological relatives (4.5%) of these 57 adopted suicides had themselves committed suicide, compared with only 2 of the 269 biological relatives (0.7%) of the 57 adopted controls ($p. < .01$). None of the adopting relatives of either the suicide group or the control group had committed suicide.

Wender, Kety, Rosenthal, & Schulsinger (1986) went on to study the 71 adoptees identified by the psychiatric case register as having suffered from an affective disorder. They were matched with 71 control adoptees without

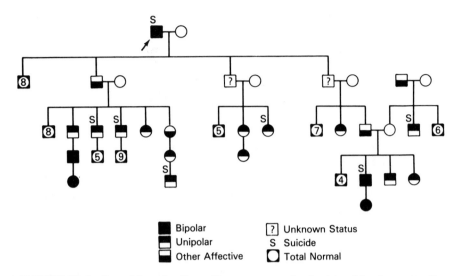

FIGURE 28.1. One of four family pedigrees among the Amish with a heavy loading for affective disorder and suicide. All seven suicides were found among individuals with a definite affective disorder. From "Suicide and Family Loading for Affective Disorders" by J. Egeland and J. Sussex, 1985, *Journal of the American Medical Association, 254,* 915–918. Copyright 1985 by the American Medical Association. Reprinted by permission.

affective disorder. Significantly more of the biological relatives of the adoptees with affective suicide disorder had committed suicide than their controls (Table 28.1). In particular, adoptee suicide victims with the diagnosis of "affect reaction" had significantly more biological relatives who had committed suicide than controls (Table 28.2). This diagnosis is used in Denmark to describe an individual who has affective symptoms accompanying a situational crisis (often an impulsive suicide attempt). These findings led Kety (1986) to suggest that a genetic factor in suicide may be an inability to control impulsive behavior, which has its effect independently of (or additively to) that of psychiatric disorder. Affective disorder and/or environmental stress may serve "as potentiating mechanisms which foster or trigger the impulsive behavior, directing it toward a suicidal outcome" (Kety, 1986).

Summary

Suicide, like so much else in psychiatry, tends to run in families. The family member who has committed suicide may serve as a role model when the option of committing suicide becomes one possible "solution" to intoler

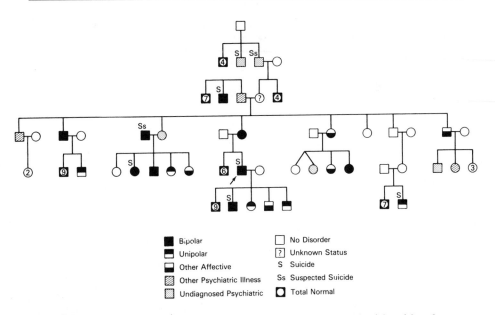

FIGURE 28.2. A second of four family pedigrees among the Amish with a heavy loading for affective disorder and suicide. Five of the six suicides were found among individuals with definite affective disorder. From "Suicide and Family Loading for Affective Disorders" by J. Egeland and J. Sussex, 1985, *Journal of the American Medical Association, 254*, 915–918. Copyright 1985 by the American Medical Association. Reprinted by permission.

able psychological pain. However, the family, twin, Amish, and adoption studies reviewed here suggest that there may be family/genetic factors in suicide. In many suicide victims, these will be the genetic factors involved in the genetic transmission of bipolar disorder, schizophrenia, and alcoholism. However, the Copenhagen adoption studies strongly suggest that there may be a genetic factor for suicide that is independent of, or additive to, the genetic transmission of affective disorder. Kety's (1986) suggestion that this may be an inability to control impulsive behavior is compatible with the data to be reviewed next, suggesting that diminished central serotonin turnover may be associated with poor impulse control.

BIOLOGICAL FACTORS IN SUICIDE

Cerebrospinal Fluid Studies

The possibility that a genetic factor in suicide may be related to impulsivity is of interest, as a larger body of data from studies of individuals attempting

TABLE 28.1. Incidence of Suicide in the Relatives of Adoptees Who Had Suffered a Depressive Illness and Their Controls

Adoptees	Biological relatives	Adoptive relatives
71 adoptees with depression	$\dfrac{15}{407}$ (3.7%)	$\dfrac{1}{187}$ (0.5%)
71 matched control adoptees	$\dfrac{1}{360}$ (0.3%)	$\dfrac{2}{171}$ (1.2%)
	$p < 0.01$	

Note. From "Genetic Factors in Suicide" by S. Kety, 1986, in A. Roy (Ed.), *Suicide* (pp. 41–45). Baltimore: Williams & Wilkins. Copyright 1986 by Williams & Wilkins Co. Reprinted by permission.

suicide, violent offenders, and arsonists suggests that impulsivity and anti-social personality traits may be related to deficient central serotonin function (for reviews, see Roy, Nutt, Virkkunen, & Linnoila, 1987, and Roy & Linnoila, 1988). These studies have reported reduced cerebrospinal fluid (CSF) levels of the serotonin metabolite 5-hydroxyindoleacetic acid (5-HIAA) compared with controls.

Depressed Patients

This line of inquiry was begun in 1976 by Asberg, Traskman, and Thoren, who reported a bimodal distribution of levels of 5-HIAA in the lumbar CSF of 68 depressed patients. Asberg et al. noted that significantly more of the depressed patients in the "low" CSF 5-HIAA group had attempted suicide in comparison with those in the "high" CSF 5-HIAA group. Subsequently, a number of other studies have reported that low CSF levels of 5-HIAA are significantly associated with suicidal behavior in depressed, personality-disordered, and schizophrenic patients, although there have been some negative reports as well (for a review, see Asberg, Nordstrom, & Traskman-Bendz, 1986). Although CSF levels of 5-HIAA are an imprecise indicator of central serotonin, these data, along with those from postmortem neuro-chemical and receptor studies (see below), have led to the suggestion that reduced central serotonin metabolism may be associated with suicidal behavior for reviews, see Roy & Linnoila, 1988, 1990).

Violent Suicide Attempters

It is of note that low CSF 5-HIAA levels have been found to be particularly associated with violent suicide attempts. In fact, Traskman, Asberg, Bertils-

TABLE 28.2. Incidence of Suicide in the Biological Relatives of Depressive and Control Adoptees

Diagnosis in adoptee	Incidence of suicide in biological relatives	p
Affective reaction	$\dfrac{5}{660}$ (7.6%)	0.0004[a]
Neurotic depression	$\dfrac{3}{127}$ (2.4%)	0.056[a]
Bipolar depression	$\dfrac{4}{750}$ (5.3%)	0.0036[a]
Unipolar depression	$\dfrac{3}{139}$ (2.2%)	0.067[a]
No mental illness	$\dfrac{1}{360}$ (0.3%)	

Note. From "Genetic Factors in Suicide" by S. Kety, 1986, in A. Roy (Ed.), *Suicide* (pp. 41–45). Baltimore: Williams & Wilkins. Copyright 1986 by Williams & Wilkins Co. Reprinted by permission.
[a]Compared with biological relatives of control adoptees with no known history of mental illness.

son, and Sjostrand (1981) reported that CSF 5-HIAA levels were significantly lower only among those patients who had made a violent suicide attempt (hanging, drowning, shooting, gassing, several deep cuts), and that levels were not reduced among those who had made a nonviolent suicide attempt (overdosage). (Figure 28.3). More recently, Banki and Arato (1983), studying 141 psychiatric patients suffering from depression, schizophrenia, alcoholism, or adjustment disorder, found that levels of CSF 5-HIAA were significantly lower among the violent suicide attempters in all four diagnostic categories. (For a further discussion of possible biological factors in aggression, violence, and impulsivity, see Brown, Linnoila, & Goodwin, Chapters 29, this volume.)

Postmortem Studies

Over the years, most postmortem studies of the brains of suicide victims have focused on the serotonin system. Some (but not all) of the neurochemical studies have reported modest decreases in serotonin itself, or in its metabolite 5-HIAA, in either the brain stem or frontal cortex. The few studies that have examined norepinephrine, dopamine, or the dopamine metabolite homovanillic acid (HVA) have tended to be negative (for a review, see Stanley, Mann, & Cohen, 1986). There have been few postmortem brain studies of the enzymes involved in catecholamine metabolism. No

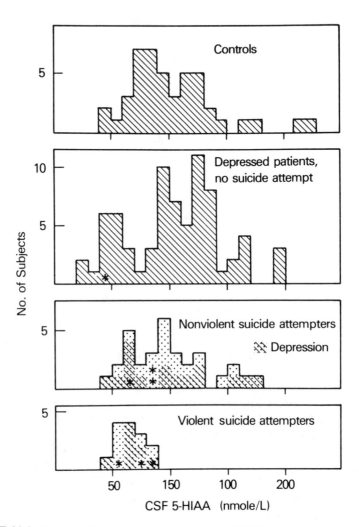

FIGURE 28.3. Levels of 5-hydroxyindoleacetic acid (5-HIAA) in cerebrospinal fluid (CSF) of all subjects in a short-term study of suicide "attempters" and a follow-up study. Controls, $n = 45$; depressed patients, no suicide attempt during the index period, $n = 73$; nonviolent suicide attempters, $n = 32$; and violent suicide attempters, $n = 14$. Each asterisk represents a patient who subsequently committed suicide. From "Monomine Metabolites in CSF and Suicidal Behavior" by L. Traskman, M. Asberg, L. Bertilsson, and L. Sjostrand, 1981, *Archives of General Psychiatry, 38,* 631–636. Copyright 1981 by the American Medical Association. Reprinted by permission.

changes in monomine oxidase activity have been reported (for a review, see Mann, McBride, & Stanley, 1986).

Four of five postmortem brain receptor studies, using [³H]imipramine as the ligand, have reported significant decreases in the presynaptic binding of this ligand to serotonin neurons in suicide victims (for a review, see Stanley et al., 1986). Stanley et al., using [³H]spiroperidol as the ligand, have also reported a significant increase in postsynaptic serotonin-2 binding sites among suicide victims who used violent methods to end their lives. Taken together, these postmortem neurochemical and receptor studies tend to support the hypothesis that diminished central serotonin metabolism (as evidenced by reduced presynaptic imipramine binding, reduced levels of serotonin and 5-HIAA, and up-regulation of the postsynaptic serotonin-2 receptor) is associated with suicide.

PREDICTION OF SUICIDE

A previous suicide attempt is the best long-range predictor that an individual may be at increased risk of committing suicide (although most suicide completers die by their first attempts). Studies show that about 40% of depressed patients who commit suicide have made a previous suicide attempt. Also, about 30% of suicide victims in the general population have made a previous suicide attempt. Furthermore, follow-up studies show that approximately 1% of individuals who attempt suicide commit suicide during the subsequent year, and approximately 10% do so over the subsequent 10 years.

However, unfortunately, no combination of demographic or clinical variables has proven very useful in predicting suicide. For example, Pokorny (1983) reported a prospective study to try to identify which psychiatric patients would commit suicide (see Chapter 6, this volume). A consecutive series of 4,800 patients admitted to the Houston Veterans Administration Medical Center was examined and rated on a battery of instruments that were thought to be useful in predicting suicide. Twenty-one items were used to identify a subsample of 803 patients, about 15% of the total group, who were thought to be at high risk for suicide. All of the 4,800 patients were followed up over an average of 5 years. Sixty-seven committed suicide during the follow-up period. However, only 30 of the 67 suicides were patients from the subsample of 803 patients thought to be at high risk. Thus, 37 of the eventual suicides—over 50%—were not identified earlier as being at risk (false negatives), whereas 766 of the 803 patients identified as being at risk did not commit suicide (false positives). Pokorny concluded that "we do not possess any item of information or any combination of items that permit us to identify to a useful degree the particular persons who will commit suicide, in spite of the fact that we do have scores of items available, each of which is significantly related to suicide. (1983; again, see Chapter 6, this volume, for the full presentation).

Cohen (1986), a statistician, reviewed the limitations of future improvements in statistical approaches to increase the predictability of suicidal behavior using psychosocial risk factors alone. He concluded: "If to the psychosocial factors now employed we can add relevant biological factors and their interactions with psychosocial factors, we may be able to develop the causal models necessary for the understanding, prediction, and prevention of suicide" (p. 41). Thus, the hope is that a combination of clinical and biological variables may better predict individuals at increased risk of suicidal behavior.

Traskman et al. (1981) carried out the first follow-up study of patients who had attempted suicide and who had had a lumbar puncture for determination of CSF levels of 5-HIAA. They found that within a year of leaving the hospital 21% of the patients who had both a suicide attempt and a CSF level of 5-HIAA below 90 nmol/liter had committed suicide. To put it another way, among patients who had made a suicide attempt, those with low CSF levels of 5-HIAA were 10 times more likely to die of suicide than the remainder.

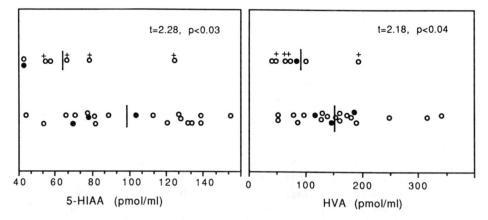

FIGURE 28.4. Depressed patients who reattempted suicide during follow-up ($n = 7$), compared with all other patients for CSF levels of 5-HIAA and HVA ($n = 20$). Patients who reattempted had significantly lower CSF levels of both 5-HIAA ($p < .03$) and HVA ($p < .04$). Plus signs indicate completed suicides. Filled circles indicate men; open circles indicate women. From "Cerebrospinal Fluid Monomine Metabolites and Suicidal Behavior in Depressed Patients" by A. Roy, J. DeJong, and M. Linnoila, 1989, *Archives of General Psychiatry, 46,* 609–612.

Recently, my colleagues and I carried out a 5-year follow-up study of suicidal behavior among depressed patients who had earlier had determinations of CSF levels of monoamine metabolites (Roy et al., 1986; Roy, DeJong, & Linnoila, 1989). Patients who reattempted suicide during the follow-up period had significantly lower CSF levels of both the serotonin metabolite 5-HIAA and the dopamine metabolite HVA. The findings were most striking among depressed patients with melancholia. For example, 11 (91.7%) of 12 melancholics with a CSF level of 5-HIAA below 80 pmol/ml had attempted suicide before their index admission; 6 (54.5%) of those 11 reattempted suicide during the follow-up period. Nine (90%) of the 10 melancholics with a CSF level of HVA below 100 pmol/ml had attempted suicide before their index admission; 6 (66.6%) of these 9 reattempted suicide during follow-up (Figures 28.4, 28.5, and 28.6). There were also striking findings in relationship to committing suicide during the follow-up. Three (25%) of the 12 depressed patients who had made a past attempt and who had a CSF level of 5-HIAA below 80 pmol/ml committed suicide during the first year of follow-up. This 25% is similar to the 21% rate of suicides reported by

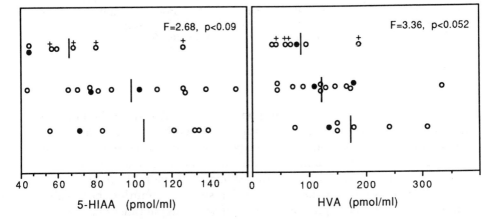

FIGURE 28.5. Scattergrams showing analysis of variance (ANOVA) comparison of CSF 5-HIAA and HVA levels of depressed patients who did ($n = 7$) or did not ($n = 13$) reattempt suicide during follow-up and patients who never attempted suicide ($n = 7$). Patients who reattempted had significantly lower CSF levels of HVA than patients who never attempted ($p < .05$) (analysis of covariance) [ANCOVA] $F = 3.55$, $df = 2, 22$, $p < .046$). Plus signs indicate completed suicides. Filled circles indicate men; open circles indicate women. From "Cerebrospinal Fluid Monomine Metabolites and Suicidal Behavior in Depressed Patients" by A. Roy, J. DeJong, and M. Linnoila, 1989, *Archives of General Psychiatry, 46*, 609–612.

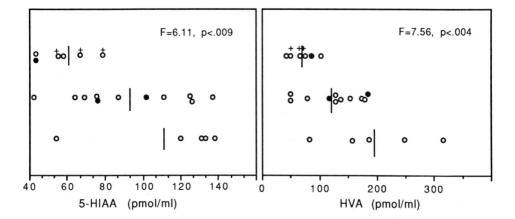

FIGURE 28.6 Scattergram showing ANOVA comparison of CSF 5-HIAA and HVA levels of depressed patients with melancholia who did ($n = 6$) or did not ($n = 11$) reattempt suicide during follow-up or who never attempted suicide ($n = 5$). Melancholics who reattempted had significantly lower CSF levels of both 5-HIAA ($p < .01$) and HVA ($p < .01$) than melancholics who never attempted, and lower levels of 5-HIAA than melancholics who did not reattempt ($p < .05$). Melancholics who did not reattempt had significantly lower CSF levels of HVA than melancholics who never attempted ($p < .05$) (ANCOVA $F = 5.28$, $df = 2$, 17, $p < .016$, and $F = 7.18$, $df = 2$, 17, $p < 0.005$, respectively). Plus signs indicate completed suicides. Filled circles indicate men; open circles indicate women. From "Cerebrospinal Fluid Monomine Metabolites and Suicidal Behavior in Depressed Patients" by A. Roy, J. DeJong, and M. Linnoila, 1989, *Archives of General Psychiatry, 46*, 609–612.

Traskman et al. (1981) as occurring within a year of leaving the hospital among their previous attempters with a CSF level of 5-HIAA below 90 nmol/liter. These follow-up results suggest that among depressed patients who have previously attempted suicide, these measures may be predictive markers of an increased risk of further suicidal behavior. However, further such follow-up studies are needed, as well as studies examining the possible predictive utility of peripheral measures of serotonergic function.

REFERENCES

Asberg, M., Nordstrom, P., Traskman-Benz, L. (1986). Biological factors in suicide. In A. Roy (Ed.), *Suicide* (pp. 47–71). Baltimore: Williams & Wilkins.

Asberg, M., Traskman, L., & Thoren, P. (1976). 5-HIAA in the cerebrospinal fluid: A biochemical suicide predictor? *Archives of General Psychiatry, 33*, 1193–1197.

Banki, C., & Arato, M. (1983). Amine metabolites and neuroendocrine responses related to depression and suicide. *Journal of Affective Disorders, 5*, 223-232.

Cohen, J. (1986). Statistical approaches to suicidal risk factor analysis. *Annals of the New York Academy of Sciences, 487*, 34-41.

Egeland, J., & Sussex, J. (1985). Suicide and family loading for affective disorders. *Journal of the American Medical Association, 254*, 915-918.

Haberlandt, W. (1965). Der suizid als genetisches problem (zwillings and familien analyse). *Anthropologischer Anzeiger 29*, 65-89.

Haberlandt, W. (1967). Aportacion a la genetica del suicide. *Folia Clinica Internacional, 17*, 319-322.

Juel-Nielsen, N., & Videbech, T. (1970). A twin study of suicide. *Acta Geneticale Medicae et Gemellologiae, 19*, 307-310.

Kallman, F., & Anastasio, M. (1947). Twin studies on the psychopathology of suicide. *Journal of Nervous and Mental Disease, 105*, 40-55.

Kallman, F., DePorte, J., DePorte, E., & Feingold, L. (1949). Suicide in twins and only children. *American Journal of Human Genetics, 2*, 113-126.

Kety, S. (1986). Genetic factors in suicide. In A. Roy (Ed.), *Suicide* (pp. 41-45). Baltimore: Williams & Wilkins.

Linkowski, P., de Maertelaer, V., & Mendlewicz, J. (1985). Suicidal behavior in major depressive illness. *Acta Psychiatrica Scandinavica, 72*, 233-238.

Mann, J., McBride, A., & Stanley, M. (1986). Postmortem monoamine receptor and enzyme studies in suicide. *Annals of the New York Academy of Sciences, 487*, 114-121.

Murphy, G., & Wetzel, R. (1982). Family history of suicidal behavior among suicide attempters. *Journal of Nervous and Mental Disease, 170*, 86-90.

Pitts, F., & Winokur, G. (1964). Affective disorder: Part 3. Diagnostic correlates and incidence of suicide. *Journal of Nervous and Mental Disease, 139*, 176-181.

Pokorny, A. (1983). Prediction of suicide in psychiatric patients: Report of a prospective study. *Archives of General Psychiatry, 40*, 249-257.

Roy, A. (1982). Risk factors for suicide in psychiatric patients. *Archives of General Psychiatry, 39*, 1089-1095.

Roy, A. (1983). Family history of suicide. *Archives of General Psychiatry, 40*, 971-974.

Roy, A. (1985a). Suicide: A multidetermined act. *Psychiatric Clinics of North America, 8*, 243-250.

Roy, A. (1985b). Suicide and psychiatric patients. *Psychiatric Clinics of North America, 8*, 227-241.

Roy, A. (1989). Suicide. In H. Kaplan & B. Sadock (Eds.), *Comprehensive textbook of psychiatry* (5th ed., pp. 1414-1427). Baltimore: Williams & Wilkins.

Roy, A., Agren, H., Pickar, D., Linnoila, M., Doran, A., Cutler, N., & Paul, S. (1986). Reduced CSF concentration of homovanillic acid and homovanillic acid to 5-hydroxyindoleacetic acid ratios in depressed patients: Relationship to suicidal behavior and dexamethasone nonsuppression. *American Journal of Psychiatry, 143*, 1539-1545.

Roy, A., DeJong, J., & Linnoila, M. (1989). Cerebrospinal fluid monoamine metabolites and suicidal behavior in depressed patients. *Archives of General Psychiatry, 46*, 609-612.

Roy, A., & Linnoila, M. (1988). Suicidal behavior, impulsiveness and serotonin. *Acta Psychiatrica Scandinavica, 78,* 529-535.

Roy, A., & Linnoila, M. (1990). Monoamines and suicidal behavior. In H. van Praag (Ed.), *Monoamine regulation of aggression and impulse control* (pp. 141-183). New York: Brunner/Mazel.

Roy, A., Nutt, D., Virkkunen, M., & Linnoila, M. (1987). Serotonin, suicidal behaviour and impulsivity. *Lancet, ii,* 949-950.

Roy, A., Segal, N., Centerwall, B., & Robinette, D. (1990). Suicide in twins. *Archives of General Psychiatry, 48,* 29-32.

Schulsinger, F., Kety, S., Rosenthal, D., & Wender, P. (1979). A family study of suicide. In M. Schou & E. Stromgren (Eds.), *Origin, prevention and treatment of affective disorders* (pp. 277-287). London: Academic Press.

Stanley, M., Mann, J., & Cohen, L. (1986). Serotonin and serotonergic receptors in suicide. *Annals of the New York Academy of Sciences, 487,* 122-127.

Traskman, L., Asberg, M., Bertilsson, L., & Sjostrand, L. (1981). Monoamine metabolites in CSF and suicidal behavior. *Archives of General Psychiatry, 38,* 631-636.

Tsuang, M. (1983). Risk of suicide in the relatives of schizophrenics, manic depressives and controls. *Journal of Clinical Psychiatry, 44,* 396-400.

Wender, P., Kety, S., Rosenthal, D., & Schulsinger, F. (1986). Psychiatric disorders in the biological and adoptive families of adopted individuals with affective disorders. *Archives of General Psychiatry, 43,* 923-929.

Zair, K. (1981). A suicidal family. *British Journal of Psychiatry, 139,* 68-69.

CHAPTER 29

Impulsivity, Aggression, and Associated Affects: Relationship to Self-Destructive Behavior and Suicide

Gerald L. Brown, M.D.
Markku I. Linnoila, M.D., Ph.D.
National Institute on Alcohol Abuse and Alcoholism
Frederick K. Goodwin, M.D.
Alcohol, Drug Abuse and Mental Health Administration, Rockville, MD

Hypotheses for aggressive behavior emanating from within have been inherently deterministic. Psychoanalytic theory (Freud, 1917/1957), ethological theory (Lorenz, 1963), and early work on the neurobiological bases of emotional behavior (Darwin, 1872; Papez, 1937, 1958; MacLean, 1949, 1952, 1954) have shared deterministic bases. By contrast, hypotheses for aggressive behavior emanating from without have been largely environmental or interactional and have depended heavily on psychological, social, and/or economic theories. The latter foci have been clearly predominant with regard to suicidality, often associated with aggressive/impulsive behavior and always with self-destructive behavior, until the seminal work of Asberg, Thoren, and Traskman (1976) and Asberg, Traskman, and Thoren (1976).

A stimulus for recent biochemical studies has been the renewal of interest in the relationship between human aggression and suicide. In psychoanalysis, aggression and suicide have been thought to be closely related, as stated by Freud (1917/1957): "We have long known, it is true, that no neurotic harbours thoughts of suicide which he has not turned back upon himself from murderous impulses against others, but we have never been able to explain what interplay of forces can carry such a purpose through to execution" (p. 252). Asberg and colleagues, in their two 1976 papers, reported that suicide attempts related to violent behavior were most likely to be associated with lower levels of cerebrospinal fluid (CSF)

5-hydroxyindoleacetic acid (5-HIAA). Brown, Goodwin, Ballenger, Goyer, and Major (1979) and Brown et al. (1982) later showed that aggressive/impulsive behavior per se, including some suicidal behaviors, was also associated with lower levels of CSF 5-HIAA. This latter work was largely consistent with earlier assessments of aggression and serotonin (5-HT) in animals (Eichelman & Thoa, 1973), as well as with animal and human pharmacological research (Sheard, 1971, 1975, 1988; Sheard, Marini, & Bridges, 1976; Leventhal, 1984; Tyrer & Seivewright, 1988).

The relationship between animal and human studies with regard to aggression/impulsivity, suicide, and 5-HT has been reviewed elsewhere (Eichelman, 1979; Valzelli, 1981; Soubrie, 1986). Difficulties in measuring aggressive behavior in humans (Brown, Linnoila, & Goodwin, 1990; Brown and Linnoila, 1990), as well as in measuring suicidal behavior (Stanley, Traskman-Bendz, & Stanley, 1986), have also been reviewed elsewhere. There are special concerns related to trait and state in both humans and animals (Brown et al., 1990). Most laboratory-controlled animal studies focus on a highly controlled "state." Examples of animal studies that have focused on trait characteristics include selective breeding for aggressive behavior and biochemical characteristics (Lamprecht, Eichelman, Thoa, Williams, & Kopin, 1972; Ciaranello, Lipsky, & Axelrod, 1974); examples that have focused on state characteristics include the induction of aggressive behavior via shock, isolation, introduction of an intruder, diet manipulations, drugs, and localized central nervous system (CNS) lesions (Eichelman, 1979; Valzelli, 1981; Soubrie, 1986).

Human studies that may elucidate a trait include studies of individuals with a history of repeated aggressive and impulsive behaviors in varied environments (Brown et al., 1979, 1982, 1986; Brown & Goodwin, 1984), and genetic studies indicating that antisocial and suicidal behavior may be independent heritable characteristics, though often associated with mental disturbances (Schulsinger, Kety, Rosenthal, & Wender, 1979; Kety, 1979). Even when a trait can be demonstrated, an overlying state (e.g., that produced by an episode of a mood disorder) may confound the understanding. Examples of human emotional disturbances that may be state-related are those associated with the menstrual cycle (Dalton, 1961, 1964) and pharmacological manipulations (Leventhal, 1984), though results of such studies may also be related to differences in genetic predisposition or vulnerability. Multiple repeated measures in longitudinal small-n studies may help discriminate state–trait issues, which can be further investigated in large populations, wherein testable hypotheses may lead to the establishment of more solid findings. Some data do not easily lend themselves for a distinction between "trait" and "state" (e.g., Asberg and colleagues' categories of "violent" and "nonviolent" suicide). It is not clear whether the violent behavior reflects an isolated "state" or an episode in a longitudinal history of similar behaviors, only some of which have been associated with self-destructive or suicidal behavior.

Some literature suggests a "serotonergic" trait in animals (Jouvet, 1969; Depue & Spoont, 1986), children (Brown et al., 1986; Brown, Goodson, Rodriguez, Belmont, & Yarrow, 1991; Reimherr, Wender, Ebert, & Wood, 1984; Stoff, Pollock, Vitiello, Behar, & Bridger, 1987; Kruesi et al., 1990, and adults (Brown et al., 1979, 1982; Linnoila et al., 1983). Characteristics of such a trait include sleep difficulties, impulsivity and disinhibition (including seizure activity), headaches, pain-proneness, evidence of glucocorticoid abnormalities, conduct disorders, mood volatility, suicidal behaviors, and poor peer relationships. Because these characteristics have been related with varying specificities in animals and humans to CNS 5-HT, which varies with both age and sex and may be inherited, one might entertain the possibility that longitudinal observation of these characteristics in children and assessment of the psychiatric status of their parents might add to current understanding. Data indicate that offspring of mothers with either unipolar or bipolar major affective disorder (as defined by the Research Diagnostic Criteria; Spitzer, Endicott, & Robins, 1978) are more likely than the offspring of control mothers to evince suicidal behaviors by adolescence (Free, Brown, Rawlins, & Yarrow, 1990), though a predisposition may manifest itself prior to adolescence in the form of disturbances in impulsivity, conduct, mood, and sleep. Furthermore, suicidality ratings (ideation and behavior) are more variable in children of disturbed mothers, and both variability and frequency of suicidal behaviors increase with age in the offspring of bipolar mothers (Free et al., 1990).

GENETICS AND DEVELOPMENT: CLINICAL ASSESSMENT AND PREDICTION

Of particular and understudied importance is the relationship between genetic and developmental data with regard to suicidal behaviors and/or those behaviors that may be associated with CNS 5-HT. For example, suicidality is known to have a genetic component (Schulsinger et al., 1979), which may be more closely related to certain personality characteristics (aggression, impulsivity) than to the incidence of specific psychopathology (antisocial personality, alcoholism, and/or major affective disorder). Though one may view genes as constant compared to environmental factors, the clinical manifestation of a genetic predisposition is a matter of age, among other factors; that is, it may manifest itself from physiological and pathological conditions, drug-induced or otherwise.

Of special interest is the fact that the incidence of suicide is very low in preadolescent children (Pfeffer, 1985), begins a steep rise in early adolescence, and reaches a peak in late adolescence; it then plateaus or rises slightly during adult life until approximately age 65, at which time it begins another dramatic rise (Blumenthal & Kupfer, 1990) (see Figure 29.1). It has been shown from within-group studies in late adolescence, middle adult life, and the elderly that lower levels of CSF 5-HIAA are associated with suicidal behavior (Jones et al., 1990). Figure 29.1 does raise the question that age-controlled within-group lower levels of CSF 5-HIAA may be no more important than the "rate" of change that is occurring during adolescence, in which the level of suicide rises strongly in close proximity to the time at which CSF 5-HIAA decreases relatively rapidly to its nadir. One

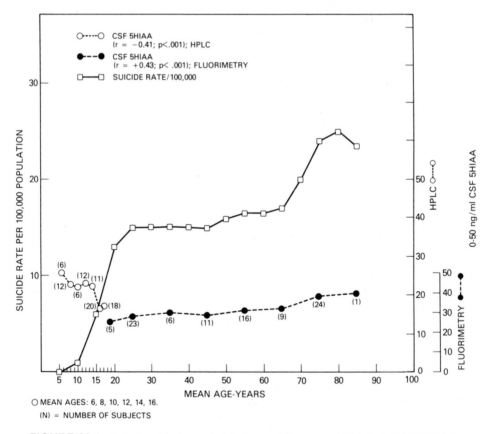

FIGURE 29.1. Relationship between lifetime suicide rate and lifetime CSF 5-HIAA. HPLC, high pressure liquid chromatography; O, calculated from Kruesi et al. (1990); ●, adapted from Gottfries et al. (1971); □, data from the National Center for Health Statistics, adapted from Blumenthal and Kupfer (1990).

might also wonder whether the rapidity of environmental and life changes in older individuals may not be as important a predisposing variable for suicidal behavior as alteration in CNS 5-HT.

A number of relatively predictable environmental factors accompany the life cycle. However, some information is also available regarding CNS functional maturational changes (e.g., myelinization; Yakovlev & Lecours, 1967; Yakovlev, 1959), as well as maturation-associated biochemical changes (5-HT is of specific interest here) in both primates and humans (Sperry, 1959; Higley, Suomi, & Linnoila, 1990a, 1990b; Lawlor et al., 1989). As noted above, lifetime changes in CSF 5-HIAA may be related to the lifetime incidence of suicide. CSF 5-HIAA is relatively high in children (Kruesi et al., 1990) and decreases significantly through midadolescence to its nadir in late adolescence (Brown et al., 1979, 1982) before rising again significantly in middle-aged and older adults (Asberg, Thoren, & Traskman, 1976; Bowers & Gerbode, 1968; Gottfries et al., 1971) (see Figure 29.1).

Relatively less is known about the 5-HT changes of old age (Sunderland, Tariot, & Newhouse, 1988). Some studies report lower CSF 5-HIAA in patients with Alzheimer's disease (Soininen, MacDonald, Rekonen, & Riekkinen, 1981; Lawlor, 1990), but others (Kay et al., 1986) report no significant differences in CSF 5-HIAA between older controls and those with Alzheimer's disease. Of course, many other biological changes occur throughout the life cycle; interestingly, however, "trait" characteristics are often studied with regard to early development, as opposed to attempting to understand some commonality of trait manifestations that might be gleaned from the much longer individual "data base" that the elderly, with their relatively high suicide rate, provide. As noted above, in addition to biological changes, the elderly must deal with many major (often negative) environmental changes, such as loss of occupational status and loss of social and emotional support. However, immediate, traumatic, and unexpected change (e.g., an illness) or an increased rate of environmental change (e.g., the type of change expected in adolescence) is certainly accompanied by major psychological adjustments for any person at any age. Nevertheless, why most individuals who undergo rapid and/or apparently negative environmental changes show no propensity toward self-destructive behaviors, whereas a relative few do, has yet to be explained satisfactorily.

COMMENTS ON THE FIVE CLINICAL CASES

The following comments on the five cases described in Chapter 12 and discussed throughout this volume are based primarily on our clinical experiences, though there are clinical data in the case reports that can be related to areas of research with which this chapter deals. Comments from other areas of research that seem pertinent to us are provided where appropriate.

In order for our comments on clinical material to be useful to clinicians of different orientations, the comments are specifically tied to the clinical data, with research information interspersed where available. We have commented upon all cases, even though our clinical and research expertise may be greater in some areas than in others. The cases do represent suicidality in both sexes and over a broad spectrum of ages, circumstances, and environments.

Case 1: Heather B

Most CSF 5-HIAA studies on suicidal subjects have been conducted on men, though some, especially those whose subjects had mood disorders, have contained women; however, even in those studies, the age range of the women has been primarily between 20 and 60. Though aggressive/impulsive behaviors in relationship to biochemical variables have been little studied in women, some of Heather's reported aggressive/impulsive and rebellious behaviors—lying, violating restrictions and curfews, sneaking out at night, making unauthorized and extensive long-distance telephone calls, and being "sexually precocious" (the mother may have been denying or unaware of sexual promiscuity despite some evidence for it from Heather's reported social activities)—were like those noted in males of similar age who go on to exhibit suicidal behaviors. Furthermore, the case material contains a number of indications of mood disturbance: Heather's referring to herself as "manic–depressive" (see also her letter to Babs), her low self-esteem ("I'm stupid . . . I hate myself"), her suicidal ideation, and her boredom (often the childhood and early adolescent equivalent of the adult's psychological feeling of depression). Her deteriorating school performance and peer relations indicated a progressive loss of age-appropriate psychosocial functioning, though the final outcome of such deterioration would not necessarily have any direct relationship to suicidal behavior.

The case material also contains a number of indications of just how strongly Heather felt the loss (of her father) and wished for a replacement (the 33-year-old president of a rock star's fan club; see also Thematic Apperception Test cards 2, 3GF, 5, 6BM, 8GF, 13MF, and 14). Her stick-figure drawing ("Dimehead" in Figure 12.1) was like the drawing of a much younger child, and the name she chose to sign to the drawing ("Zelda Q. Pinwheel") might indicate some knowledge of F. Scott Fitzgerald's disturbed wife, Zelda. Of further interest are the several indications that her mother did not realize the seriousness of the problem (the mother's provision of history, the letter to Babs, and the first of the two journal entries). The apparent discrepancy between a patient's report of his or her condition and the patient's mother's understanding of the same has recently been reported by Walker, Moreau, and Weissman (1990) and Free et al. (1990).

Case 2: Ralph F

Ralph would appear to be fairly similar to some of the subjects reported by Brown et al. (1979, 1982). Though he did not demonstrate enough aggressive/impulsive behavior to justify a diagnosis of antisocial personality disorder, some of the behaviors he did exhibit (alcohol abuse, drug abuse, suicidal ideation/aggressive plans, homicidal ideation, and promiscuous sexual behavior) are often associated with such a diagnosis. Furthermore, though he also did not clearly qualify for a diagnosis of borderline personality disorder, some of his characteristics—such as hallucinatory experiences, some of which were associated with alcohol and others with depressive moods; some of the above-listed antisocial and suicidal behaviors; and no indication of sustained, mature relationships with peers—are often associated with borderline personalities.

Ralph's *Diagnostic and Statistical Manual of Mental Disorders*, third edition, revised (DSM-III-R) Axis I and II diagnoses (Axis I—major depression, single episode, and alcohol abuse, episodic, secondary; Axis II—none) would seem to be well substantiated by the historical data provided. There is no clear association between rheumatoid arthritis (Ralph's DSM-III-R Axis III diagnosis) and 5-HT metabolism. The history of a suicide attempt by his mother and a completed suicide by her sister, both associated with significant psychopathology, is further consistent with reported data on the familial occurrence of suicide attempts (Roy, 1989). Ralph's scores on his validating Minnesota Multiphasic Personality Inventory (MMPI) scales, though conventionally and generally thought to invalidate the clinical scale profile, nevertheless are highly consistent with MMPI scores reported (Brown & Goodwin, 1984; Brown et al., 1990) for young males who were aggressive/impulsive and/or suicidal, with low levels of CSF 5-HIAA and a DSM-III-R diagnosis of borderline personality disorder.

Case 3: John Z

The case of John Z does not bear very directly on the aggressive/impulsive behavioral and psychobiological aspects of suicidality: In terms of the generally expected lifetime curve of CSF 5-HIAA, John would clearly have passed his nadir. However, John's case, like Ralph's, illustrates the importance of a family history of suicide attempts and completions (Roy, 1989). Though the sniper episode from John's Vietnam experience and his reactions to his more recent life reversals are perhaps included in Chapter 12 to give some basis for the development of this man's psychodynamic status, these personal characteristics of the patient would also play an important part in the ultimate hoped-for reconstitution of an emotionally healthy and functional state.

Perhaps the most practical point to be made regarding the management of the case is that John would need considerable structure (i.e., hospitalization and close monitoring of his pharmacological therapy) to prevent suicide. Pharmacological therapy could be viewed as a necessary, but not sufficient, condition from which he might work toward gaining the healthiest, most functional status of which he might be capable. Though one cannot necessarily provide a rule of thumb for hospitalizations (or psychotherapy!), even with all the information that one might be able to acquire in the clinical situation, for the management of such a patient, it is obviously more dangerous to err on the side of trying to keep the patient out of the hospital than on that of what might be seen in retrospect as too hasty an admission.

Case 4: Faye C

Faye's immediate history indicated a functional, acute psychosis—probably some form of schizophrenia, particularly in view of the thought control symptomatology. The history of her mother indicated some sort of schizoid personality, or perhaps an ambulatory, mild psychotic condition. The subject matter of her mother's jokes (i.e., urination and defecation) also revealed the psychological primitiveness and perhaps marginal control of her mother's thought processes. Like the cases of Ralph and John, Faye's case illustrates the clinical importance of obtaining a good family history in all patients, particularly with regard to enhanced suicide risk.

Faye's first hospitalization would appear to have been related to depression and not necessarily to a thought process disorder (though the use of electroconvulsive therapy [ECT] indicated the possibility, among others, that this depressive episode might have been of psychotic proportions). However, her emergency room visit would seem to indicate an episode of further deterioration. The patient's attribution to ECT of a number of other problems (temporal lobe epilepsy, etc.) indicated the unreliability of her cognitive processes, although her strong negative emotional response to the treatment should not be discounted. Temporal lobe epilepsy has been associated with psychotic experiences (Laidlaw & Richens, 1982). Epilepsy has also been associated with low CSF 5-HIAA, and CSF 5-HIAA has been shown to be elevated by anticonvulsants, particularly phenytoin (Dilantin) (Chadwick, Jenner, & Reynolds, 1975). Finally, epilepsy has been associated with suicide (Matthews & Barabas, 1981). Carbamazapine (Tegretol), another anticonvulsant, has also been used for the treatment of aggressive behaviors (Tunks & Dermer, 1977; Hakola & Laulumaa, 1982; Neppe, 1982; Garbutt & Loosen, 1983; Yassa & Dupont, 1983; Luchins, 1983; Gardner & Cowdry, 1986; Yathma & McHale, 1988; Foster, Hillbrand, & Chi, 1989; Fichtner, Kuhlman, Gruenfeld, & Hughes, 1990); if its apparent antiaggressive effect for some patients is associated with 5-HT function, the mechanism is unclear. Faye's treatment history might very well have been instrumental in facilitating the accomplishments she attained during her "well" episodes. This patient would clearly need not only careful psychiatric assessment, but neurological assessment as well.

Case 5: José G

In many respects, José was a well-functioning man prior to his injury. For example, he had no family history of psychiatric illness and no disordered developmental history; he had been honorably discharged from military service (a kind of functional diagnostic test in itself); he had a good, sustained job history, with increasing levels of productivity and responsibility; and he had an apparently stable family life, with good functioning as a husband and father. His drinking history might indicate an area of vulnerability: Increased suicidal behavior has been associated with alcohol use and abuse (Roy & Linnoila, 1986; Flavin, Franklin, & Frances, 1990). His apparently episodic alcohol use might have met the diagnostic criteria for acute alcohol abuse, but probably not dependence; nor did he evince any indications of organic complications from alcohol.

Both José's recent increase in drinking and his depression would seem to be reactions to the injury that ultimately led to his being declared disabled. Not only did the injury compromise his physical functioning, but it and the declaration of disability were severe insults to his psychological self-concept. As a further insult during this period, his long-term case of adult-onset diabetes, requiring insulin, had recently resulted in a diagnosis of "widespread diabetic retinopathy"—an indication that he had had abnormal glucose metabolism for an extended period of time. His use of alcohol would have exacerbated the diabetic disorder. Though the relationship between glucose metabolism and 5-HT is complicated (Linnoila, Virkkunen, Roy, & Potter, 1990). José may have been somewhat more biologically vulnerable to suicidal tendencies than he would have been had he not had this illness. However, the review of MacKenzie and Popkin (1990) does not indicate increased risk among groups of diabetics in whom suicidal behaviors have been recorded.

In any case, since José (now 64 years old) had probably had little contact with mental health professionals during his life, very close monitoring would be advisable at this time. During the last several weeks, he had developed clear signs of clinical depression with some suicidal ideation; he had probably not had to contend consciously with such feelings during his life prior to the accident. The close monitoring would allow for hospitalization, should he deteriorate further, and perhaps some level of supportive psychotherapy could help him understand his new situation in life and learn coping techniques to deal with it more adequately and less self-destructively. Collaboration with an internist would clearly be indicated.

GENERAL COMMENTS ON ASSESSMENT

Evidence continues to accumulate that psychiatric and medical conditions contribute to or create a vulnerability to suicidality in individuals, though this statement is not meant to imply that every suicide attempt (e.g., that of a kamikaze pilot) can be convincingly linked to such conditions. Sometimes, in the acutely suicidal individual, psychological and environmental assessments and decisions may take precedence over immediate formal psychiatric and medical diagnostic assessments; however, one cannot unduly postpone such assessments. Though suicidal behavior has long been associated with depression (Pokorny, 1964), it has also been linked with a number of other psychiatric conditions (personality disorders, psychoses, alcoholism, drug abuse, dementia, etc.; Black & Winokur, 1986).

Until recent years, personality disorders have often been overlooked as important concomitant factors in many suicidal individuals. Though the psychological limitations and inflexibilities in adaptation found in any individual who would meet the diagnostic criteria for a DSM-III-R Axis II personality disorder would be significant disadvantages in dealing with environmental stress and provocation, those personality disorders that include aggression, impulsivity, and mood volatility as predominant features seem particularly to increase the risk for suicidal behavior, as has been shown by Brown et al. (1979, 1982), Linnoila et al. (1983), and Coccaro et al. (1989).

Until the pioneering work of Asberg and colleagues (Asberg, Thoren, & Traskman, 1976; Asberg, Traskman, & Thoren, 1976), suicidal behavior was viewed almost entirely from a psychosocial perspective, thus leading to an assumption that the "cause" of suicide lies somewhere within the psychosocial realm and not within a biological or medical realm. In light of current research, however, it seems clear that suicide is a final outcome of a number of provocations and vulnerabilities. Among possibilities that may contribute to an individual's vulnerabilities are medical conditions. Any medical condition that is perceived as life-threatening or severely physically compromising may be associated with depressive or hopeless mood and suicidal ideation. For example, are the depressive affects and suicidal ideation and behaviors sometimes seen in patients with parkinsonism due to the stress and the realities of the medical condition, or due to the alterations of CNS 5-HT, dopamine, and other neurotransmitters that characterize the neurological disease itself (Hohman, 1922; Johansson & Ross, 1967; Bunney et al., 1969; Brown & Wilson, 1972; Brown, Wilson, & Green, 1973)?

Some data indicate that a number of conditions associated with glucose metabolism, corticosteroid metabolism, 5-HT metabolism, or neurological disorders may make more direct contributions. Glucose metabolic conditions include diabetes or insulin secretion disturbances (Linnoila et al., 1990). Corticosteroid metabolic conditions include Cushing's disease or a major disturbance in cortisol metabolism (Cohen, 1980; Starkman &

Schteingart, 1981; Lewis & Smith, 1983). 5-HT metabolic disturbances include carcinoid syndrome (Sjordsma et al., 1970; Major, Brown, & Wilson, 1973) and Lesch–Nyhan syndrome (Mizuno & Yugari, 1975; Ciaranello, Anders, Barchas, Berger, & Cann, 1976; Anders, Cann, Ciaranello, Barchas, & Berger, 1978; Castells et al., 1979). Neurological conditions (which may also include disturbances in 5-HT metabolism) include epilepsy, Parkinson's disease, Cornelia de Lange syndrome (Bryson, Sakati, Nyhan, & Fish, 1971; Singh & Pulman, 1979), and Gilles de la Tourette syndrome (Cohen, Shaywitz, Caparulo, Young, & Bowers, 1978; Cohen et al., 1979). In individuals with these medical conditions, one cannot always distinguish between self-injurious behavior and suicidality, or determine what role 5-HT may play, or tell whether subclinical (but genetically present) disturbances are contributing to the self-destructive behavior. In any case, it seems clear that the assessment of an individual who may be suicidal should include a medical assessment for both ethical and medical–legal reasons.

Along with the assessment of an individual's current psychiatric and medical state, the childhood emotional and behavioral developmental history is beginning to be seen as an important possible source of vulnerability; family history is also clearly important. Children with DSM-III-R Axis I diagnoses within the "disruptive behavior disorder" (DBD) category have been shown to have lower levels of CSF 5-HIAA than those within the "obsessive–compulsive disorder" group (Kruesi et al., 1990). The fact that a child with a DBD diagnosis does not show overt suicidal behavior prior to adolescence does not mean that such behavior will be lacking during adolescence. Some specific childhood behaviors, such as cruelty to animals (Kruesi, 1989), fire setting (Virkkunen, DeJong, Bartko, Goodwin, & Linnoila, 1989), and glucose craving (Kruesi, Linnoila, Rapoport, Brown, & Petersen, 1985; Kruesi et al., 1987), have been associated with aggressive/impulsive behaviors and low CSF 5-HIAA. Furthermore, the psychiatric status of mothers (Free et al., 1990), and possibly of fathers as well, has been shown to be a possible predictor of children's developmental course with regard to suicidality "scores." As noted in our discussion of the cases, above, Roy (1989) has shown in his comprehensive review that family history is critically important in assessing the probability of suicidal behavior in an individual.

The extent to which aggressive and suicidal behaviors may be attributed to family instability versus biological variables is important for both pathophysiological and therapeutic considerations. We (Brown, Goyer, Lamparski, Linnoila, & Goodwin, 1988) investigated 36 inpatient military men (mean age, 22.0 ± 4.4 years) from whom aggression ratings, suicidal history, CSF 5-HIAA, and histories of eight factors thought to be related to family instability were available. Results indicated that those whose mean rating of aggressive history was above a normal range (derived from a sample of age-matched military men without history of psychiatric difficulty) had a significantly higher frequency of suicide attempts, lower levels of CSF 5-HIAA, and higher family instability scores. Furthermore, those with a history of suicide attempts had significantly higher aggression ratings, lower levels of CSF 5-HIAA, and higher family instability scores. Finally, those with CSF 5-HIAA levels below the median had significantly higher aggression ratings and a higher frequency of suicide attempts, but did not show a significant difference in family instability scores. Thus, decreased CSF 5-HIAA is not necessarily associated with increased family instability, but is associated with an increased likelihood of aggressive and suicidal behaviors. Those individuals who are aggressive or suicidal usually do come from more unstable families. Low CSF 5-HIAA or family instability alone may not necessarily predispose an individual toward aggressive or suicidal behaviors, but if both are present, the individual is considerably more at risk of evincing those behaviors.

From the practical clinical point of view, there is no question of the importance of psychosocial and environmental factors in understanding, treating, and managing the patient. However, there is no convincing evidence that these factors help us to understand which individuals will manifest suicidality and which will not; no doubt, the majority of any group of individuals subjected to the same or a similar psychosocial or environmental stressor will *not* be suicidal. Ingestion of certain drugs (perhaps an "internal" environmental agent?) may constitute an exception.

FUTURE DIRECTIONS

An area that we believe to be particularly fruitful for future studies from a biological perspective is the study of children, in terms of understanding both a "trait" and its predictive value for adolescent and adult behavior. Closely related is the thorough study of families. An area that has been relatively understudied, neurobiologically more than clinically, has been that of the changes associated with old age. An individual's lifetime "data base," change, and rate of change are challenging areas to integrate with currently known data relating human biology and suicidal tendencies.

REFERENCES

Anders, T. F., Cann, H. M., Ciaranello, R. D., Barchas, J. D., & Berger, P. A. (1978). Further observations on the use of 5-hydroxytryptophan in a child with Lesch–Nyhan syndrome. *Neuropaediatrie, 9*, 157–166.

Asberg, M., Thoren, P., & Traskman, L. (1976). Serotonin depression—biochemical subgroup within the affective disorders? *Science, 191*, 478–480.

Asberg, M., Traskman, L., & Thoren, P. (1976). 5-HIAA in the cerebrospinal fluid: A biochemical suicide predictor? *Archives of General Psychiatry, 33*, 1193–1197.

Black, D. W., & Winokur, G. (1986). Prospective studies of suicide and mortality in psychiatric patients. *Annals of the New York Academy of Sciences, 487*, 106–113.

Blumenthal, S. J., & Kupfer, D. J. (Eds.). (1990). *Suicide over the life cycle: Risk factors, assessment, and treatment of suicidal patients*. Washington, DC: American Psychiatric Press.

Bowers, M. B., & Gerbode, F. A. (1968). Relationship of monoamine metabolites in human cerebrospinal fluid to age. *Nature, 219*, 1256–1257.

Brown, G. L., Ebert, M. E., Goyer, P. F., Jimerson, D. C., Klein, W. J., Bunney, W. E., Jr., & Goodwin, F. K. (1982). Aggression, suicide, and serotonin: Relationship of CSF amine metabolites. *American Journal of Psychiatry, 139*, 741–746.

Brown, G. L., Goodson, S. G., Rodriguez, P., Belmont, B., & Yanow, M. R. (1991). *Serotoneagic traits in offspring of control, unipolar and bipolar mothers: A developmental perspective*. Paper presented at the meeting of the American Academy of Child and Adolescent Psychiatry, San Francisco.

Brown, G. L., & Goodwin, F. K. (1984). Diagnostic, clinical, and personality characteristics of aggressive men with low 5HIAA. *Clinical Neuropharmacology, 7*, 756–757.

Brown, G. L., Goodwin, F. K., Ballenger, J. C., Goyer, P. F. & Major, L. F. (1979). Aggression in humans correlates with cerebrospinal fluid amine metabolites. *Psychiatry Research, 1*, 131–139.

Brown, G. L., Goyer, P. F., Lamparski, D., Linnoila, M., & Goodwin, F. K. (1988). *Family histories of aggressive impulsive individuals and CSF 5HIAA*. Paper presented at the annual meeting of the American Psychiatric Association, Montreal.

Brown, G. L., Kline, W. J., Goyer, P. F., Minichiello, M. D., Kruesi, M. J. P., & Goodwin, F. K. (1986). Relationship of childhood characteristics to cerebrospinal fluid 5-hydroxyindoleacetic acid in aggressive adults. In C. Shagass & R. C. Roemer (Eds.), *Biological psychiatry* (pp. 177–179). New York: Elsevier.

Brown, G. L., & Linnoila, M. I. (1990). CSF sertonin metabolite (5-HIAA) studies in depression, impulsivity, and violence. *Journal of Clinical Psychiatry, 5*(Suppl. 4), 31–41.

Brown, G. L., Linnoila, M. I., & Goodwin, F. K. (1990). Unpublished manuscript.

Brown, G. L., & Wilson, W. P. (1972). Parkinsonism and depression. *Southern Medical Journal, 65*, 540–545.

Brown, G. L., Wilson, W. P., & Green, R. L. (1973). Mental aspects of Parkinsonism and their management. In J. Siegfried (Ed.), *Parkinson's disease: Rigidity, akinesia, behavior. Selected communications on topic* (Vol. 2, pp. 265–278). Bern: Verlag Hans Huber.

Bryson, Y., Sakati, N., Nyhan, W. L., & Fish, C. H. (1971). Self-mutilative behavior in the Cornelia de Lange syndrome. *American Journal of Mental Deficiency, 76*(3), 319–324.

Bunney, W. E., Jr., Janowsky, D. S., Goodwin, F. K., Davis, J. M., Brodie, H. K. H., Murphy, D. L., & Chase, T. N. (1969). Effects of L-DOPA on depression. *Lancet, i*, 885–886.

Castells, S., Chakrabarti, C., Winsberg, B. G., Hurwic, M., Perel, J. M., & Nyhan, W. L. (1979). Affects of L-5hydroxytryptophan on monoamine and amino acids turnover in the Lesch–Nyhan syndrome. *Journal of Autism and Childhood Schizophrenia, 9,* 95–103.

Chadwick, D., Jenner, P., & Reynolds, E. H. (1975). Amines, anticonvulsants, and epilepsy. *Lancet, i,* 473–476.

Ciaranello, R. D., Anders, T. F., Barchas, J. D., Berger, P. A., & Cann, H. M. (1976). The use of 5-hydroxytryptophan in a child with Lesch–Nyhan syndrome. *Child Psychiatry and Human Development, 7,* 127–133.

Ciaranello, R. D., Lipsky, A., & Axelrod, J. (1974). Association between fighting behavior and catecholamine biosynthetic enzymes in two sublines of an inbred mouse strain. *Proceedings of the National Academy of Sciences USA, 71,* 3006–3008.

Coccaro, E. F., Siever, L. J., Klar, H. M., Maurer, G., Cochrane, K., Cooper, T. B., Mohs, R. C., & Davis, K. L. (1989). Serotonergic studies in patients with affective and personality disorders: Correlates with suicidal and impulsive aggressive behavior. *Archives of General Psychiatry, 46*(7), 587–599.

Cohen, D. J., Shaywitz, B. A., Caparulo, B. K., Young, J. G., & Bowers, M. B., Jr. (1978). Chronic, multiple tics of Gilles de la Tourette's disease. *Archives of General Psychiatry, 35,* 245–250.

Cohen, D. J., Shaywitz, B. A., Young, J. G., Carbonari, C. M., Nathanson, J. A., Liberman, D., Bowers, M. B., Jr., & Maas, J. W. (1979). Central biogenic amine metabolism in children with the syndrome of chronic multiple tics of Gilles de la Tourette. *Journal of the American Academy of Child Psychiatry, 18,* 320–341.

Cohen, S. I. (1980). Cushing's syndrome: A psychiatric study of 29 patients. *British Journal of Psychiatry, 136,* 120–124.

Dalton, K. (1961). Menstruation and crime. *British Medical Journal, iii,* 1752–1753.

Dalton, K. (1964). *The premenstrual syndrome.* Springfield, IL: Charles C Thomas.

Darwin, C. (1872). *The expression of the emotions in man and animals.* London: Murray.

Depue, R. A., & Spoont, M. R. (1986). Conceptualizing a serotonin trait: A behavioral dimension of constraint. *Annals of the New York Academy of Sciences, 487,* 47–62.

Eichelman, B. (1979). Role of biogenic amines in aggressive behavior. In M. Sandler (Ed.), *Psychopharmacology of aggression* (pp. 61–93). New York: Raven Press.

Eichelman, B., & Thoa, N. B. (1973). The aggressive monoamines. *Biological Psychiatry, 6,* 143–164.

Fichtner, C. G., Kuhlman, D. T., Gruenfeld, M. J., & Hughes, J. R. (1990). Decreased episodic violence and increased control of dissociation in a carbamazepine-treated case of multiple personality. *Biological Psychiatry, 27*(9), 1045–1052.

Flavin, D. K., Franklin, J. E., & Frances, R. J. (1990). Substance abuse and suicidal behavior. In S. J. Blumenthal & D. J. Kupfer (Eds.), *Suicide over the life cycle: Risk factors, assessment, and treatment of suicidal patients* (pp. 177–204). Washington, DC: American Psychiatric Press.

Foster, H. G., Hillbrand, M., & Chi, C. C. (1989). Efficacy of carbamazepine in assaultive patients with frontal lobe dysfunction. *Progress in Neuropsychopharmacology and Biological Psychiatry, 13*(6) 865–874.

Free, K., Brown, G. L., Rawlings, R., & Yarrow, M. R. (1990). *Suicidal thinking and behavior in the offsping of affectively disturbed mothers and control mothers.* Paper presented at the annual meeting of the American Academy of Child and Adolescent Psychiatry, Chicago.

Freud, S. (1957). Mourning and melancholia. In J. Strachey (Ed. and Trans.), *The standard edition of the complete psychological works of Sigmund Freud* (Vol. 14, pp. 237-260). London: Hogarth Press. (Original work published 1917)

Garbutt, J. C., & Loosen, P. T. (1984). A dramatic behavioral response to thyrotropin-releasing hormone following low-dose neuroleptics. *Psychoneuroendocrinology, 9*(3), 311-314.

Gardner, D. L., & Cowdry, R. W. (1986). Positive effects of carbamazepine on behavioral dyscontrol in borderline personality disorder. *American Journal of Psychiatry, 143*(4), 519-522.

Gottfries, C. G., Gottfries, I., Johansson, B., Olsson, R., Persson, T., Roos, B. E., & Sjostrom, R. (1971). Acid monoamine metabolites in human cerebrospinal fluid and their relations to age and sex. *Neuropharmacology, 10,* 665-672.

Hakola, H. P., & Laulumaa, A. (1982). Carbamazepine in treatment of violent schizophrenics. *Lancet, i,* 1358.

Higley, J. D., Suomi, S. J., & Linnoila, M. (1990a). Developmental influences on the serotonergic system and timidity in the nonhuman primate. In E. F. Coccaro & D. L. Murphy (Eds.), *Serotonin in major psychiatric disorders* (pp. 27-46). Washington, DC: American Psychiatric Press.

Higley, J. D., Suomi, S. J., & Linnoila, M. (1990b). Parallels in aggression and serotonin: Consideration of development, rearing, history, and sex differences. In H. M. van Praag, R. Plutchik, & A. Apter (Eds.), *Violence and suicidality* (pp. 245-256). New York: Brunner/Mazel.

Hohman, L. B. (1922). Post-encephalitic behavior disorders in children. *Johns Hopkins Hospital Bulletin, 380,* 372-375.

Johansson, B., & Roos, B. E. (1967). 5-hydroxyindoleacetic acid and homovanillic acid levels in cerebrospinal fluid of healthy volunteers and patients with Parkinson's syndrome. *Life Sciences, 6,* 1449-1454.

Jones, J. S., Stanley, B., Mann, J. J., Frances, A. J., Guido, J. R., Traskman-Bendz, L., Winchel, R., Brown, R. P., & Stanley, M. (1990). CSF 5-HIAA and HVA concentrations in elderly depressed patients who attempted suicide. *American Journal of Psychiatry, 147*(9), 1225-1227.

Jouvet, M. (1969). Biogenic amines and the states of sleep. *Science, 163,* 32-41.

Kay, A. D., Milstien, S., Kaufman, S., Creasey, H., Haxby, J. V., Cutler, N. R., & Rapoport, S. I. (1986). Cerebrospinal fluid biopterin is decreased in Alzheimer's disease. *Archives of Neurology, 43*(10), 996-999.

Kety, S. S. (1979). Disorders of the human brain. *Scientific American, 241,* 202-214.

Kruesi, M. J. P. (1989). Cruelty to animals and CSF 5-HIAA. *Psychiatry Research, 28,* 115-116.

Kruesi, M. J. P., Linnoila, M., Rapoport, J. L., Brown, G. L., & Petersen, R. (1985). Carbohydrate craving, conduct disorder and low 5-HIAA. *Psychiatry Research, 16,* 83-86.

Kruesi, M. J. P., Rapoport, J. L., Cummings, E. M., Berg, C. J., Ismond, D. R., Flament, M., Yarrow, M., & Zahn-Wexler, C. (1987). Effects of sugar and aspartame on aggression and activity in children. *American Journal of Psychiatry, 144*(11), 1487–1490.

Kruesi, M. J., Rapoport, J. L., Hamburger, S., Hibbs, E., Potter, W. Z., Lenane, M., & Brown, G. L. (1990). Cerebrospinal fluid monoamine metabolites, aggression, and impulsivity in disruptive behavior disorders in children and adolescents. *Archives of General Psychiatry, 47*(5), 419–426.

Laidlaw, J., & Richens, A. (1982). *A textbook of epilepsy* (2nd ed.). London: Churchill Livingstone.

Lamprecht, F., Eichelman, B., Thoa, N. B., Williams, R. B., & Kopin, I. J. (1972). Rat fighting behavior: Serum dopamine-β-hydroxylase and hypothalamic tyrosine hydroxylase. *Science, 177,* 1214–1215.

Lawlor, B. A. (1990). Serotonin and Alzheimer's disease. *Psychiatric Annals, 20*(10), 567–570.

Lawlor, B. A., Sunderland, T., Hill, J. L., Mellow, A. M., Molchan, S. E., Mueller, E. A., Jacobsen, F. M., & Murphy, D. L. (1989). Evidence for a decline with age in behavioral responsivity to the serotonin agonist, m-chlorophenylpiperazine, in healthy human subjects. *Psychiatry Research, 29*(1), 1–10.

Leventhal, B. L. (1984). The neuropharmacology of violent and aggressive behavior. In C. R. Keith (Ed.), *The aggressive adolescent: Clinical perspectives* (pp. 299–358). New York: Free Press.

Lewis, D. A., & Smith, R. E. (1983). Steroid-induced psychiatric syndromes: A report of 14 cases and a review of the literature. *Journal of Affective Disorders, 5,* 319–332.

Linnoila, M., Virkkunen, M., Roy, A., & Potter, W. Z. (1990). Monoamines, glucose metabolism and impulse control. In H. M. van Praag, R. Plutchik, & A. Apter (Eds.), *Violence and suicidality* (pp. 218–241). New York: Brunner/Mazel.

Linnoila, M., Virkkunen, M., Scheinin, M., Nuutila, A., Rimon, R., & Goodwin, F. K. (1983). Low cerebrospinal fluid 5-hydroxyindoleacetic acid concentration differentiates impulsively from nonimpulsive violent behavior. *Life Sciences, 33,* 2609–2614.

Lorenz, K. (1963). *On aggression.* New York: Harcourt, Brace & World.

Luchins, D. J. (1983). Carbamazepine for the violent psychiatric patient. *Lancet, i,* 766.

MacKenzie, T. B., & Popkin, M. K. (1990). Medical illness and suicide. In S. J. Blumenthal & D. J. Kupfer (Eds.), *Suicide over the life cycle: Risk factors, assessment, and treatment of suicidal patients* (pp. 205–232). Washington, DC: American Psychiatric Press.

MacLean, P. D. (1949). Psychosomatic disease and the "visceral brain": Recent developments bearing on the Papez theory of emotion. *Psychosomatic Medicine, 11,* 338–353.

MacLean, P. D. (1952). Some psychiatric implications of physiological studies on frontotemporal portion of limbic system (visceral brain). *Electroencephalogy and Clinical Neurophysiology, 4,* 407–418.

MacLean, P. D. (1954). The limbic system and its hippocampal formation: Studies in animals and their possible application to man. *Journal of Neurosurgery, 11,* 29–44.

Major, L. F., Brown, G. L., & Wilson, W. P. (1973). Carcinoid and psychiatric symptoms. *Southern Medical Journal, 66,* 787–790.

Matthews, W. S., & Barabas, G. (1981). Suicide and epilepsy: A review of the literature. *Psychosomatics, 22,* 515-524.

Mizuno, T., & Yugari, Y. (1975). Prophylactic effect of L-5-hydroxytryptophan on self-mutilation in the Lesch–Nyhan syndrome. *Neuropaediatrie, 6,* 13-23.

Neppe, V. M. (1982). Carbamazepine in the psychiatric patient. *Lancet, ii,* 334.

Papez, J. W. (1937). A proposed mechanism of emotion. *Archives of Neurology and Psychiatry, 38,* 725-743.

Papez, J. W. (1958). Visceral brain: Its component parts and their connections. *Journal of Nervous and Mental Disease, 126,* 40-56.

Pfeffer, C. R. (1985). Self-destructive behavior in children and adolescents. *Psychiatric Clinics of North America, 8,* 215-266.

Pokorny, A. D. (1964). Suicide rates in various psychiatric disorders. *Journal of Nervous and Mental Disease, 139,* 499-506.

Reimherr, F. W., Wender, P. H., Ebert, M. H., & Wood, D. R. (1984). Cerebrospinal fluid homovanillic acid and 5-hydroxyindoleacetic acid in adults with attention deficit disorder, residual type. *Psychiatry Research, 11,* 71-78.

Roy, A. (1989). Genetics and suicidal behavior. In L. Davidson & M. Linnoila (Eds.), *Report of the Secretary's Task Force on Youth Suicide: Vol. 2. Risk factors for youth suicide* (DHHS Publication No. 89-1622, pp. 247-262). Washington, DC: U.S. Government Printing Office.

Roy, A., & Linnoila, M. (1986). Alcoholism and suicide. *Suicide and Life-Threatening Behavior, 16,* 162-191.

Schulsinger, F., Kety, S. S., Rosenthal, D., & Wender, P. H. (1979). A family study of suicide. In M. Schou & E. Stromgen (Eds.), *Origins, prevention and treatment of affective disorders* (pp. 277-287). London: Academic Press.

Sheard, M. H. (1971). Effect of lithium on human aggression. *Nature, 230,* 113-114.

Sheard, M. H. (1975). Lithium in the treatment of aggression. *Journal of Nervous and Mental Disease, 100,* 108-117.

Sheard, M. H. (1988). Clinical pharmacology of aggressive behavior. *Clinical Neuropharmacology, 11*(6), 483-492.

Sheard, M. H., Marini, J. L., & Bridges, C. I. (1976). The effect of lithium on impulsive aggression behavior in man. *American Journal of Psychiatry, 133,* 1409-1413.

Singh, N. N., & Pulman, R. M. (1979). Self-injury in the de Lange syndrome. *Journal of Mental Deficiency Research, 23,* 79-84.

Sjordsma, A., Lovenberg, W., Engelman, K., Carpenter, W. T., Wyatt, R. J., & Gessa, G. L. (1970). Serotonin now: Clinical implications of inhibiting its synthesis with para-chlorophenylalanine (PCPA). *Annals of Internal Medicine, 73,* 607-629.

Soininen, H., MacDonald, E., Rekonen, M., & Riekkinen, P. J. (1981). Homovanillic acid and 5-hydroxyindoleacetic acid levels in cerebrospinal fluid of patients with senile dementia of Alzheimer type. *Acta Neurologica Scandinavica, 64*(3), 217-224.

Soubrie, P. (1986). Reconciling the role of central serotonin neurons in humans and animal behavior. *Behavioral and Brain Sciences, 9,* 319-364.

Sperry, W. M. (1959). The biochemical maturation of the brain. *Research Publications of the Association for Research in Nervous and Mental Disease, 39*(2), 47-57.

Spitzer, R. L., Endicott, J., & Robins, E. (1978). Research Diagnostic Criteria: Rationale and reliability. *Archives of General Psychiatry, 35*(6), 773–782.

Stanley, B., Traskman-Bendz, L., & Stanley, M. (1986). The Suicide Assessment Scale: A scale evaluating change in suicidal behavior. *Psychopharmacological Bulletin, 22*(1), 200–205.

Starkman, M. N., & Schteingart, D. E. (1981). Neuropsychiatric manifestations of patients with Cushing's syndrome. *Annals of Internal Medicine, 141*, 215–219.

Stoff, D. M., Pollock, L., Vitiello, B., Behar, D., & Bridger, W. H. (1987). Reduction of (3H)-imipramine binding sites in platelets of conduct-disordered children. *Neuropsychopharmacology, 1*(1), 55–62.

Sunderland, T., Tariot, P. N., & Newhouse, P. A. (1988). Differential responsivity of mood, behavior, and cognition to cholinergic agents in elderly neuropsychiatric populations. *Brain Research, 472*(4), 371–389.

Tunks, E. R., & Dermer, S. W. (1977). Carbamazepine in the dyscontrol syndrome associated with limbic system dysfunction. *Journal of Nervous and Mental Disease, 164*(1), 56–63.

Tyrer, P., & Seivewright, N. (1988). Pharmacological treatment of personality disorders. *Clinical Neuropharmacology, 11*(6), 493–499.

Valzelli, L. (1981). *Psychobiology of aggression and violence.* New York: Raven Press.

Virkkunen, M., DeJong, J., Bartko, J., Goodwin, F. K., & Linnoila, M. (1989). Relationship of psychobiological variables to recidivism in violent offenders and impulsive fire setters. *Archives of General Psychiatry, 46*(7), 600–603.

Walker, M., Moreau, D., & Weissman, M. M. (1990). Parents' awareness of children's suicide attempts. *American Journal of Psychiatry, 147*(10), 1364–1366.

Yakovlev, P. I. (1959). Morphological criteria of growth and maturation of the nervous system in man. *Research Publications of the Association for Research in Nervous and Mental Disease, 39*(1), 3–46.

Yakovlev, P. I., & Lecours, A. (1967). The myelogenetic cycles of regional maturation of the brain. In A. Minkowski (Ed.), *Regional development of the brain in early life* (pp. 3–70). Oxford: Blackwell.

Yassa, R., & Dupont, D. (1983). Carbamazepine in the treatment of aggressive behavior in schizophrenic patients: A case report. *Canadian Journal of Psychiatry, 28*(7), 566–568.

Yathma, L. N., & McHale, P. A. (1988). Carbamazepine in the treatment of aggression: A case report and a review of the literature. *Acta Psychiatrica Scandinavica, 78*(2), 188–190.

CHAPTER 30

Prediction of Self-Preservation Failures on the Basis of Quantitative Evolutionary Biology

Denys de Catanzaro, Ph.D.
McMaster University

"Self-preservation instincts" are commonly cited by laypeople to refer to the obvious tendencies of human beings and other organisms to perpetuate their own existence. Fear, pain, hunger, and thirst are among the clearest motivations fitting this notion. Scientific validation of this notion is now abundant in evidence from physiological and motivational psychology, which shows that numerous heritable, inborn, nonassociative processes subserve the seeking of nutrients and the avoidance of elements detrimental to the individual's existence (e.g. Carlson, 1981; Pinel, 1990). Such self-preservation is obviously supported by pressures of natural selection, since organisms must survive in order to reproduce (or for that matter, to exist at all). The existence of numerous genetic factors favoring self-preservation is undoubtable.

Self-preservation is so universal that it might be assumed to be an invariable orientation of behavior and physiology, with any deviation being ascribed to "pathology." I believe, however, that this conception is based upon a simplistic view of genetic expression. Typically, laypeople and social scientists think of genetically mediated traits as being fixed, present at birth, and unresponsive to environmental variation. More variable traits are generally ascribed to ontogeny. This conception is clearly inconsistent with modern biological evidence, which suggests that genetic expression is commonly modulated by the environment in which it occurs. For example, skin color varies in response to exposure to ultraviolet light (i.e., "tanning"), and levels of adrenal hormones vary dramatically in response to variations in psychological stress. Genetic expression also clearly varies in response to age, as is evident in hormonal and behavioral changes at puberty, and in alterations in hair color and many other features with maturity.

EVOLUTIONARY LIMITS TO SELF-PRESERVATION

An early concept of limitations to self-preservative genetic expression was developed by evolutionary biologists to explain degradation of diverse physiological traits during postreproductive aging. The evolutionary theory of "senescence" was advanced by Medawar (1952, 1957), clarified by Williams (1957), and modeled mathematically by Hamilton (1966). This theory considers that genetic expression can be "pleiotropic," varying across the spectrum of ages in the potential lifespan of individual members of a species. Such factors as predation, disease, various mishaps, and mechanical wear make it likely that progressively fewer individuals will survive with increasing age (see also Comfort, 1964). Accordingly, the probability that any particular gene in the species' gene pool will be expressed is an inverse function of the age of expression. Survival to reproductive maturity is clearly essential for the direct propagation of an individual's genes. But after this age there is a diminishing probability of gene expression, simply because of extrinsic factors determining the species' actuarial function.

Therefore, maximal selective relevance of any gene should be observed at about the age of sexual maturation. Probabilistically, this selective relevance should diminish progressively thereafter. Pleiotropic genes with self-preservative influences during juvenile development and early adulthood, but with more random effects later, may accumulate in the gene pool, simply because the probability of expression is greater in earlier life. This would explain the erosion of salubrious genetic expression seen with increased age. The probability that self-preserving genetically mediated attributes will be expressed thus relates to the remaining probability of reproduction at a particular age. Fisher (1950) introduced the concept of "reproductive value," which reflects the likelihood of reproduction beyond a certain age based on the population's mortality and fertility tables. Hamilton (1966) provided a refinement of Fisher's formula. Fisher, Williams, and Hamilton each briefly mentioned that parental care might add an additional dimension to reproductive value, but none of these theorists developed this idea in detail.

Subsequently, evolutionary theory has been enhanced by Hamilton's (1964) idea of "inclusive fitness." The direct biological fitness of an individual is defined in terms of the number of progeny he or she produces. Inclusive fitness accommodates the fact that an individual's kin share his or her genes by common descent, so that their reproduction serves his or her genetic interests. The summed effects of the individual on the reproduction of kin, weighted by the fractional coefficient of genetic relationship to the individual, can be considered, in addition to the individual's own progeny, to yield his or her inclusive fitness.

An integration of the theories of senescence, reproductive value, inclusive fitness, and social dominance has recently been developed and summarized in a relatively simple mathematical formulation (de Catanzaro, 1991a). This modifies the theory of senescence, while leading to a striking prediction that genetic expression can evolve to be conducive to outright self-destructiveness, conditional upon very restricted social circumstances. In highly social species, natural selection may actually support a spectrum of genetic expression, ranging from strong promotion and defence of survival to outright suicidal tendencies. Accordingly, dynamic evolutionary contingencies act on variance within and across individuals in age, sex, health, reproductive prospects, social dominance, and the quality of contact with kin. Essentially, a confluence of poor reproductive prospects and burdensomeness toward kin at any age may be sufficient for natural selection to support the individual's death.

Consider a hypothetical variable, ψ, which varies across individuals and over time; it represents what we might call the "residual capacity to promote inclusive fitness." In other words, ψ_i represents the ability of individual i, during his or her remaining natural lifetime, to perform any action that promotes the representation of his or her genes in subsequent generations. This can also be construed as the value of the individual's survival to the continued existence of his or her genes. Clearly, following inclusive-fitness theory, this is a function of the individual's remaining capacity to reproduce and the summated impacts of his or her survival upon the reproduction of kin, each weighted by their degree of genetic relatedness, such that

$$\Psi_i = \rho_i + \Sigma \, \delta\rho_k r_k$$

where ρ_i equals the expected reproduction of individual i in his or her remaining natural lifetime; $\delta\rho_k$ equals the increment or decrement in the expected reproduction of each kinship member k produced by the survival and behavior of i; and r_k equals the coefficient of genetic relatedness of each k to i, which is one-half for parent–child or sibling–sibling, one-quarter for grandparent–child, and so forth (Galton, 1889; Hamilton, 1964; 1971; Wright, 1922).

This formula is analogous to the inclusive-fitness formula of Hamilton (1964), but the concept of ρ, or residual reproductive potential, differs substantially from the concept of fitness. An individual's fitness refers to his or her total lifetime reproductive success, and typically is measured through a count of progeny a few generations hence. Residual reproductive potential, on the other hand, is prospective reproduction from a specific point in time, and is *not* inclusive of offspring already achieved. The mean value of ρ can be established empirically for any age cohort or defined subset of a population from actuarial statistics. This mean can be directly calculated through Fisher's (1950) "reproductive value" or Hamilton's (1966) modification, entitled, "expected reproduction beyond age a." The latter function, which is simpler, is represented by w_a, such that

$$w_a = \int_a^\infty \lambda^{-x} \, l_x \, f_x \, dx$$

where λ^{-x} = the Malthusian parameter, which adjusts the statistic for shifts in population size over time; l_x = the fraction of individuals of an age cohort living at age x; and f_x = the age-specific fertility rate. This quantity is integrated from the specific age being considered to the highest age at which any offspring are ever produced.

The term ρ is introduced, rather than simply employing w_a, because residual reproductive potential is dependent on other factors as well as age. The ρ value for particular individuals within each age cohort can differ substantially from the definable cohort mean. Let us consider social dominance: There is substantial variance in access to sexual partners in most species. Polygyny, whereby some males monopolize females while others are excluded, is common in mammals and occurs in various degrees in most human societies (Daly & Wilson, 1983; Symons, 1980). Although dominance hierarchies can shift over time, residual reproductive potential varies substantially, being lowest in physically weakest and/or socially most subordinate males. Even in the absence of social hierarchies, physical vitality is another obvious factor influencing residual reproductive prospects. Limited resources, such as food and shelter, are clearly also critical. For females, additional factors influencing residual reproductive probability include parity (insofar as it influences fertility) and dependency of extant offspring (since, e.g., lactation can influence fertility). ρ is clearly prospective and stochastic rather than absolute or definitive. There must be salient and reliable predictive features in the organism's experience for it to have evolutionary significance. Individuals must be able to perceive the predictive contingencies, and this perception must bear upon genetic expression.

For nonsocial species and in the absence of parental care, $\Psi_i = \rho_i$. However, any form of dependency of the residual reproductive potential of kin upon the behavior of i introduces the second element of the Ψ_i formula, or $\Sigma \, \delta\rho_k r_k$. This element encompasses the summated benefits and costs of the continued existence of i to the replication of his or her genes as they are represented in those of common descent. This quantifies the prospective impact that i, in his or her residual lifetime, may have upon the reproduction of each k, weighted by the coefficient of relationship between i and k. Like ρ_i, $\delta\rho_k$ includes only probable future reproductive impacts of the behavior of i; impacts achieved in the past are irrelevant by definition.

Clearly, the importance of this second element is greatest in species with complex social networks, such as our own. The evolutionary significance of ρ values of kin requires similar conditions to those pertinent to ρ_i, discussed above. The $\delta\rho_k$ values are probabilistic and require relatively reliable predictive cues to be meaningful. Furthermore, potential increments or decrements in the reproductive status of kin need to be evident to i and to have a bearing upon genetic expression in him or her. Estimation of $\Sigma \delta\rho_k r_k$ must again rest upon thorough empirical investigation of social ecology. In situations where we can operationalize ρ, quantification may be facilitated by a restatement of the Ψ formula, as presented previously (de Catanzaro, 1986), such that

$$\Psi_i = \rho_i + \Sigma\, b_k \rho_k r_k$$

where b_k is a coefficient of benefit or cost to the potential reproduction of k incurred by the survival of i, and ρ_k equals the residual reproductive potential of k.

The ρ_k values can be measured through methods described above for ρ_i. Values of b_k are estimable, if not calculable, for a number of common situations, and for most applications the limits are such that $-1 \le b \le 1$. Whenever there is total dependency of ρ_k upon i (e.g., when a nursing infant relies entirely upon its mother), $b_k = 1$. When the welfare of k is completely independent of the behavior of i, $b_k = 0$. At the other extreme, one can conceive of situations in which i is so burdensome that he or she fully precludes k's subsequent reproduction, such that $b_k = -1$. For intermediate degrees of dependency, b_k may have to be estimated on the basis of empirical evidence from previous comparable instances where the outcome is known.

Measurement of ρ can be such that each potential offspring is included until it is conceived; the value of each offspring is scaled as one-half of its reproductive value at any point subsequent to conception. In the absence of paternal care, conception is the end point of a male's input, typically precluding immediate subsequent conception by the same female. For the female, given the complete dependence of a fetus on its mother, the input to Ψ_i after conception grows over time as the probability of offspring mortality decreases. Thus, in effect, the result upon Ψ_i is the same whether ρ_i is defined with reference to the potential reproductive value of the offspring at conception or birth. Either Fisher's reproductive value or Hamilton's w_a is probably an excellent approximation of the ρ values of very young individuals, because differentiation in other factors affecting ρ probably increases with age. After conception, any parental care is quantified through $\Sigma \delta\rho_k r_k$.

The Ψ_i formula represents the value of continued survival of i to his or her genes' replication in future generations. In theory, Ψ_i should be an index of the strength and direction of pressures of natural selection bearing upon any self-preserving attribute. In nonsocial species, Ψ_i may vary on a spectrum from a maximal residual reproductive potential at the onset of reproductive maturity to 0, but is never negative. Here $\Psi_i = \rho_i$, and in the absence of social dominance age is the most probable determinant of ρ_i, so that Hamilton's w_a will closely approximate ρ_i. Under such circumstances, it can be assumed that self-preserving attributes will prevail at sexual maturity but that more random attributes will come into play thereafter.

Social dynamics make the situation much more complex. First, they allow the continued expression of self-preserving attributes where $\rho_i = 0$ (e.g., as in postmenopausal women), insofar as $\Sigma \delta \rho_k r_k > 0$. This factor permits indirect reproductive relevance of gene expression through kin solicitude. Given the common observation that individuals tend to confer benefits upon kin, it seems probable that positive values of $\delta \rho_k$ or of b_k prevail. Negative values can occur insofar as an individual consumes resources otherwise available to kin. However, a decrement in fitness of kin produced by consuming common resources may be compensated for by the indirect reproductive benefit that an individual provides them because he or she shares their genes.

Accordingly, negative Ψ_i values are possible in highly social species. These will occur wherever the total weighted anticipated effect of i upon the reproduction of kin becomes so negative that it outweighs ρ_i. The most straightforward examples come from situations where ρ_i approaches 0 (e.g., old age, infirmity, or low rank in a stable dominance hierarchy), while $\Sigma \delta \rho_k r_k$ is negative because of the consumption of resources otherwise available to kin. Theoretically, it is also possible that a negative Ψ_i value may be obtained despite a high ρ_i value, provided that i's existence is highly burdensome to a large number of kin. The implication of negative Ψ_i values is that natural selection may actually generate the expression of outright self-destructive traits. A negative Ψ_i value means that i's continued existence is a detriment to his or her own inclusive fitness. Self-destructive gene expression confined to such circumstances may actually confer a selective advantage, and hence a "death instinct" may evolve.

CORRESPONDENCE TO THE SOCIAL ECOLOGY OF SUICIDE

We must consider that modern human society and technology are rapidly evolving and deviate markedly from ancestral circumstances. Anthropologists inform us that hunting–gathering bands, consisting predominantly of extended kinship groups, prevailed over human evolution (see Flannery, 1972). Of course, the ancestral rather than the modern circumstances are more relevant to the shaping of human behavioral predispositions. The existence of numerous novel technologies for which there could not possibly be any evolutionary preparedness (e.g., guns, drugs, and cars) permits impulsive self-destructive acts that truly damage inclusive fitness. Furthermore, geographic mobility, occupational complexity, urbanization, and complexity of social networks are all novel in an evolutionary context. As previously argued (de Catanzaro, 1980, 1981), genetic expression may be random and maladaptive in novel environments, thus providing an alternative path to suicidal behavior. It is also quite conceivable, given human cognitive complexity, tendency to learn, and capacity for novel action, that some suicides derive merely from imitation or a logical decision to die (see also de Catanzaro, 1980, 1981; Hankoff, 1961; Phillips, 1974; Shneidman, 1957). My impression is that humans often contrive novel actions, and I doubt whether predispositions derived from our evolutionary past should ever be used to predict the finer details of modern human behavior.

Nevertheless, without any preconceptions about causal mechanisms, there is abundant evidence of a gross correspondence between the conditions specified by the Ψ formula and the actual documented circumstances of self-destructive behavior. The most unequivocal forms of such behavior are indeed found in species with complex social structure, prevailing where both ρ_i is low and the individual's existence bears negatively upon kin and society. Among humans, acts of suicide account for a substantial proportion of deaths in virtually all cultures in which careful surveys have been conducted (de Catanzaro, 1981; Dublin, 1963; Farberow, 1972; Rosen, 1971). Archival evidence on the social ecology of suicide has previously been reviewed from this perspective (see de Catanzaro, 1980, 1981). In brief summary, in diverse primitive and modern cultures, suicide is more common in males than females; it increases in frequency as a function of age; and it is most common in those without stable heterosexual relationships and dependent children (see also Durkheim, 1897/1951; Linden & Breed, 1976; Meer, 1976). Suicide is often associated with chronic infirmity, social isolation, social disgrace, perceptions of burdensomeness, and psychological states of hopelessness (see also Beck, Kovacs, & Weissman, 1975; Breed, 1972; Bohannan, 1960; Dublin, 1963; Maris, 1981).

Most importantly, there is now much evidence for neurochemical and genetic substrates of severe human dysphoria, and some similar evidence for suicide itself (see reviews by de Catanzaro, 1981; Lester, 1986; Motto, 1986; Stanley, Stanley, Traskman-Bendz, Mann, & Meyendorff, 1986; van Praag, 1986). Neurochemical systems, especially that involving serotonin, are responsive to the individual's experiences and covary with euphoria–dysphoria or happiness–depression. Evidence supporting this assertion comes from pharmacological manipulability of affective variation and measurement of neurochemical metabolites in association with such variation. The existence of dynamic physiological substrates of happiness and severe sadness agrees with the suggestion that conditions of genetic expression contribute to self-destructiveness.

It has also been known, from the work of Darwin right through to modern ethology and social psychology, that there are stereotyped facial and postural features associated with happiness, confidence, and dominance as opposed to sadness, despondency, and submission (see Panksepp, 1982;

Plutchik & Kellerman, 1980). Given commonalities among related mammals in these postures, and the cultural universality of behavior such as smiling and crying, it is highly doubtful that these are exclusively learned. I suggest that the Ψ formula may in fact account for a large part of the evolution of this whole aspect of human emotional dynamics.

Other self-destructive behavior, such as head banging, head hitting, self-scratching, and self-biting, is found in mentally deficient and psychotic people. Such behavior can be very persistent and is usually associated with profound physical and mental handicaps (de Catanzaro, 1978; van Velzen, 1975); this is consistent with negligible ρ_i values and burdensomeness toward kin. "Sudden-death" phenomena may also conform to the formula to some degree (see de Catanzaro, 1981; Hughes & Lynch, 1978; Richter, 1957). Moreover, it is a common medical observation that patients with marriages, families, and other social supports are less susceptible to illness and recover faster from comparable maladies than do those lacking such ties (Dimsdale et al., 1979; Kaplan, Cassel, & Gore, 1977). In fact, the pace of senescence in theory could covary with Ψ (de Catanzaro, 1991a). The Ψ formula can also be adapted to accommodate various phenomena that involve not a certainty of death, but a risk of it, with different inclusive-fitness effects dependent upon the outcome of the risk (de Catanzaro, 1984; 1991a).

PREDICTION OF SUICIDE

Scientific prediction of complex probabilistic human behavior is by nature a multivariate statistical task. To my knowledge, the best tools currently available for such a task are discriminant-function analysis and multiple regression (Edwards, 1979; Pedhazur, 1982; Tatsuoka, 1988). Discriminant-function analysis for a dichotomous outcome (e.g., "to be or not to be") is actually identical to multiple regression with a dichotomous criterion variable. For a multicategorical outcome, discriminant-function analysis is accomplished via canonical correlation. When the outcome to be predicted is continuous (e.g., a scale of degree of suicidal ideation or a scale of intent to die associated with a suicidal gesture), then multiple regression is appropriate.

In all of these cases, the ideal methodology is to obtain a large representative sample of the subject matter with measurement and quantification of a host of potential predictors, as well as an outcome or criterion variable. Multiple regression on such data will yield, through least-squares estimation, a regression line (or discriminant function), which provides a relative quantitative weighting of the predictors. The associated R^2 value is an index of the strength of prediction, whereas an F test on this R^2 value tests whether the prediction differs significantly from chance. The raw score regression line is expressed in the form $Y' = a + b_1X_1 + b_2X_2 + \ldots + b_kX_k$, where Y'

is the predicted criterion or outcome variable, a is an intercept constant, X_k is each raw predictor measure, and b_k is a weighting attached to each raw predictor score.

A significant regression allows one subsequently to measure a new sample simply on the predictors and compute a Y' value as an estimate of the unmeasured real outcome (Y). In theory, Y' should approximate Y in proportion to the value of R^2. In reality, there is usually somewhat greater error in prediction than R^2 would suggest—a phenomenon known as "shrinkage." Shrinkage is the result of some capitalization on chance involved in derivation of optimal regression lines, as well as of sampling error and inevitable differences in sampling and measurement procedures. Accordingly, authorities (e.g., Pedhazur, 1982) advocate cross-validation for major predictive uses of regression lines. Essentially, cross-validation involves full measurement of predictors and criterion for two or more samples, with reciprocal transplantation of regression lines and measurement of the discrepancy between predicted (Y') and actual (Y) outcome.

This methodology has exceptional potential for many medical phenomena, as well as for social phenomena such as suicide, insofar as prevention is possible and desirable. For suicide, where we actually have a wealth of information about social and psychological correlates, it should be possible to derive regression lines predicting suicide (and/or related behavior) on the basis of demographic factors, psychometric measures, and social interaction measures. If the general evolutionary–genetic hypothesis outlined above holds, measures related to perceived future reproductive prospects and family-benefiting behavior should correlate inversely with suicidal ideation. On the premise that human psychological nature evolved in ancestral societies that were predominantly extended kinship groups, questions related to perceived contribution to society should also correlate inversely with suicidal ideation. Friendship, health, and financial means can be viewed as resources facilitating both reproductive and productive activity, and thus may be predicted to correlate inversely with suicidal ideation. If the general hypothesis is false, all of such intercorrelations may instead be negligible, contrary, or inconsistent.

I have been conducting surveys of stratified samples of the general public as well as of various high-suicide-risk samples. These surveys reflect the theoretical model of motivation outlined above, asking Likert-form questions about the quality of relationships to members of the opposite sex, relationships to family members and society, and suicidal ideation. In an initial study of university undergraduates and the general public (de Catanzaro, 1984), a composite variable for suicidal ideation was predictable in highly significant multiple regressions. The major indication was that a sense of contribution to kin and society was of greater predictive value than heterosexual relations, which in turn predicted more than demographic factors.

Subsequently (de Catanzaro, 1991b), a refined questionnaire has been administered to a new large sample of the general public as well as to high-risk samples, including the elderly, psychiatric inpatients, the criminally insane, and male and female homosexuals. In every sample, between 67% and 84% percent of the variance in suicidal ideation was significantly explained in a multiple-regression model by information about relationships to members of the opposite sex, family members, and society at large. In all samples, the most reliable predictors of suicidal ideation (highest bivariate correlations and beta weights) were questions related to loneliness and a sense of contribution versus burdensomeness toward family members. Poor health and finances were especially important in the elderly. Younger males were more suicidal when they had had less sexual activity, whereas younger females were less suicidal when they had dependent children. Exclusively homosexual males, paradoxically, were more suicidal when their heterosexual relations had been poorer. A sample of males held in maximum security at Penetanguishine, Ontario, under Lieutenant Governor's warrants (a psychiatric population on indefinite sentences for potential or actual antisocial behavior), was highly suicidal, but remarkably similar to members of the general public in the influences of contribution to family and society. In this last survey, respondents were also asked to rate the perceived importance, in their understanding of the whole concept of suicide, of (1) their own emotions, (2) actions of relatives, (3) actions of friends/acquaintances, and (4) information from the news media and books. Consistently in all samples, respondents ranked their own emotions as the main source of information on suicide.

Later modifications of the questionnaire have been developed to look more intensively at familial interactions, reproductive relations, and career success as they predict suicidal ideation, with most samples consisting of students (Moyer & de Catanzaro, 1991). Homosexuality, failure of heterosexual relations, and academic/career failure are strong predictors within this population. However, none of these variables predicts suicidal ideation as well as does a quantification of the respondent's self-perceived value to all close family members, individually rated, weighted by the coefficient of relationship, and summated.

Although these empirical studies clearly indicate predictive value of Ψ-related measures, I believe that simple multiple regression is an inadequate model of the causal inputs of diverse variables to suicide. Multiple regression normally operates with linear interrelations of variables, and although curvilinear models are quite possible, they are cumbersome and tedious when there are many predictors. Moreover, the complex interactions of diverse predictors cannot adequately be incorporated into a simple multiple-regression model. For example, the interactions of age, sex, reproductive relations, and kin solicitude are very complex. Psychological welfare is surely dependent on such factors in conditional and idiosyncratic manners.

My colleagues and I are now developing more complex quantitative models, reflecting the Ψ formula more directly but allowing for conditional interactions of factors.

ANALYSES OF THE FIVE CASE HISTORIES

1. *Heather B.* This 13-year-old girl was undergoing the common turmoil of adolescence, exacerbated by the death of her father at age 7 and diminished parental guidance. She had not yet emotionally accommodated this death, and the brief, tumultuous remarriage of her mother must not have helped. She was currently alienated from school and many of her peers, with a few unconventional friends. Her arm-cutting behavior would appear to be parasuicidal, as suggested by the caption of her cartoon and her bitter note to her erstwhile friend Robin. Heather would surely have a positive ρ value, perhaps below average because of current maladjustment but nonetheless substantial. She might not be feeling sufficient appreciation from family, peers, and school authorities, which might elicit a perception (though not necessarily a reality) of burdensomeness. In theory, enhancement of this perception via more criticism and social alienation would increase her suicidal tendencies, outweighing ρ. With guidance and appreciation, she should not become truly suicidal, because she would have family and future reproductive interests to live for.

2. *Ralph F.* Dysphoria and suicidal ideation seemed more severe in this 16-year-old, who had also developed a suicide plan. There were physiological signs of self-preservation failure in his anorexia and weight loss. Ralph was socially isolated, and there had been much turmoil within his family. This included the recent suicide of his aunt, the accusations of sexual molestation by his sister and other female relatives against his grandfather, and conflict between his parents. Sour moods among family members might have been catching Ralph in the crossfire, giving him the perception of being unappreciated. This could have elicited an inaccurate sense of lack of worth to family. Reproductively, Ralph should have positive ρ, although his recent venereal diseases might have given him serious concern about being damaged (and thus a sense of having poor reproductive prospects). Also, we might ask whether or not his sexual activity was heterosexual, because he would not seem to have the qualities that would attract females at his age. His other physical ailments, juvenile rheumatoid arthritis and asthma, might suggest premature senescence as a consequence of social stress.

3. *John Z.* This 39-year-old man was a previously well-adjusted family man who suddenly lost his means of contributing to family and society. He once had a strong survival instinct, making him disobey his commanding officer in Vietnam to avoid death. He had a wife and three sons, and had

previously been confident, gregarious, and cheerful. At such a phase in life, he would probably not have appreciable ρ unless he had many resources, and his prime reason for living would be his role in raising his family. His job loss could have transformed his positive ψ value to a negative one. Finances made him lose his house, and his sense of worth to family was transformed to a sense of burdensomeness. Rejections in job applications would not have helped his sense of worth, and now his wife was expressing a desire to be relieved of him through his hospitalization. His 20-pound weight loss would appear to suggest physiological self-preservation failure.

4. *Faye C.* At 49, this woman had never had sexual relations, and at this age would have a ρ value of 0. She obviously also had no children, and there is no mention of other dependent relatives, so her potential for contribution to family is probably close to nil. Her major potential avenue for contribution to society at large was her master's degree in public health, but the case description in Chapter 12 indicates that she failed at this as her idealism turned to powerlessness. She seemed to be losing touch with reality, and mental illness was clearly developing. In summary, her Ψ value would be approaching 0, and early senescence would seem evident rather than outright suicide, as predicted under these circumstances.

5. *José G.* Like John Z, this man was a previously well-adjusted family man who suddenly lost his ability to contribute. His injury prevented him from working on the railroad, where he formerly had friends, appreciation, and a sense of worth. Although the financial consequences were not as severe as for José they were for John, José's age and developing physical ailments gave him a strong sense of burdensomeness and worthlessness. His physical degeneration would seem to have become worse following this psychological state, as emphysema and side effects of diabetes suddenly emerged. This man was dying, with senescence apparently accelerated and self-destructive emotions emerging as Ψ became increasingly negative.

In summary, information is incomplete for these cases, and we can thus only estimate Ψ and ρ values. Furthermore, it must be remembered that Ψ values are dynamic, changing with emerging social events. Also, Ψ is more relevant to natural selection on past events, whereas modern circumstances deviate substantially from circumstances prevailing in human evolution. Nevertheless, we can see a clear correspondence of each of these cases to diminishing Ψ. Heather's Ψ would probably be greatest among these cases; her behavior was parasuicidal rather than suicidal, and she could recover or degenerate further, depending on future social and family events. Ralph might be a good example of how the perception of self-worth is more important than the actual value to kin and society; his actual Ψ value could be somewhat greater than his emotions would suggest. John's Ψ value had recently plummeted to a clearly negative state, although he might still be rescued by re-employment. Faye's Ψ value would be close to 0 rather than negative, and she would seem to be experiencing mental senescence rather than outright self-destructiveness. José's Ψ value had recently become negative, and his rapid physical degeneration would suggest that recovery was unlikely.

One of the most important points to derive from this theoretical perspective, as from many other perspectives on suicide, is the importance of social dynamics in determining an individual's sense of worth. As illustrated by these cases, respect and appreciation from others should constitute the best defense against self-destructiveness. The nature of social regard (especially from family members), together with the potential for reproductive interactions with the opposite sex, may trigger emotions affecting both physiological and behavioral traits influencing survival.

REFERENCES

Beck, A. T., Kovacs, M., & Weissman, A. (1975). Hopelessness and suicidal behavior: An overview. *Journal of the American Medical Association, 234,* 1146-1149.

Bohannan, P. (Ed.). (1960). *African homicide and suicide.* Princeton, NJ: Princeton University Press.

Breed, W. (1972). Five components of a basic suicide system. *Life-Threatening Behavior, 2,* 3-18.

Carlson, N. R. (1981). *Physiology of behavior* (2nd ed.). Boston: Allyn & Bacon.

Comfort, A. (1964). *Ageing: The biology of senescence.* London: Routledge & Kegan Paul.

Daly, M., & Wilson, M. (1983). *Sex, evolution, and behavior* (2nd ed.). Boston: Willard Grant Press.

de Catanzaro, D. (1978). Self-injurious behavior: A biological analysis. *Motivation and Emotion, 2,* 45-65.

de Catanzaro, D. (1980). Human suicide: A biological perspective. *Behavioral and Brain Sciences, 3,* 265-290.

de Catanzaro, D. (1981). *Suicide and self-damaging behavior: A sociobiological perspective.* New York: Academic Press.

de Catanzaro, D. (1984). Suicidal ideation and the residual capacity to promote inclusive fitness: A survey. *Suicide and Life-Threatening Behavior, 14,* 75-87.

de Catanzaro, D. (1986). A mathematical model of evolutionary pressures regulating self-preservation and self-destruction. *Suicide and Life-Threatening Behavior, 16,* 166-181.

de Catanzaro, D. (1991a). Evolutionary limits to self-preservation. *Ethology and Sociobiology, 12,* 13-28.

de Catanzaro, D. (1991b). *Prediction of suicidal ideation by the residual capacity to promote inclusive fitness.* Manuscript submitted for publication.

Dimsdale, J. E., Eckenrode, J., Haggerty, R. J., Kaplan, B. H., Cohen, F., & Dornbush, S. (1979). The role of social supports in medical care. *Social Psychiatry, 14,* 175-180.

Dublin, L. (1963). *Suicide.* New York: Ronald Press.

Durkheim, E. (1951). *Suicide: A study in sociology* (J. A. Spaulding & G. Simpson, Trans.). Glencoe, IL: Free Press. (Original work published 1897)

Edwards, A. L. (1979). *Multiple regression and the analysis of variance and covariance.* San Francisco: W. H. Freeman.

Farberow, N. L. (1972). Cultural history of suicide. In J. Walderstrom, J. Larsson, & N. Ljungstet (Eds.), *Suicide and attempted suicide.* Stockholm: Nordiska Bokhandelns Forlag.

Fisher, R. A. (1950). *The genetical theory of national selection.* New York: Dover.

Flannery, K. V. (1972). The cultural evolution of civilizations. *Annual Review of Ecology and Systematics, 3,* 399-426.

Galton, F. (1889). *Natural inheritance.* New York: Macmillan.

Hamilton, W. D. (1964). The genetical evolution of social behavior. *Journal of Theoretical Biology, 7,* 1-16.

Hamilton, W. D. (1966). The moulding of senescence by natural selection. *Journal of Theoretical Biology, 12,* 12-45.

Hamilton, W. D. (1971). Selection of selfish and altruistic behavior in some extreme models. In J. F. Eisenberg & W. S. Dillon (Eds.), *Man and beast: Comparative social behavior.* Washington, DC: Smithsonian Institution.

Hankoff, L. D. (1961). An epidemic of attempted suicide. *Comprehensive Psychiatry, 2,* 294-298.

Hughes, C. W., & Lynch, J. J. (1978). A reconsideration of psychological precursors of sudden death in infrahuman animals. *American Psychologist, 33,* 419-429.

Kaplan, B. H., Cassel, J. C., & Gore, S. (1977). Social support and health. *Medical Care, 15*(Suppl.), 47-58.

Lester, D. (1986). Genetics, twin studies, and suicide. *Suicide and Life-Threatening Behavior, 16,* 274-285.

Linden, L. L., & Breed, W. (1976). The demographic epidemiology of suicide. In E. S. Shneidman (Ed.), *Suicidology: Contemporary developments.* New York: Grune & Stratton.

Maris, R. W. (1981). *Pathways to suicide: A survey of self-destructive behaviors.* Baltimore: Johns Hopkins University Press.

Medawar, P. B. (1952). *An unsolved problem in biology.* London: H. K. Lewis.

Medawar, P. B. (1957). *The uniqueness of the individual.* London: Methuen.

Meer, F. (1976). *Race and suicide in South Africa.* London: Routledge & Kegan Paul.

Motto, J. A. (1986). Clinical considerations of biological correlates of suicide. *Suicide and Life-Threatening Behavior, 16,* 83-102.

Moyer, A., & de Catanzaro, D. (1991). *Academic success, relations to the opposite sex, and relations to family as predictors of suicidal ideation among university students.* Manuscript in preparation.

Panksepp, J. (1982). Toward a general psychobiological theory of emotions. *Behavioral and Brain Sciences, 5,* 407-467.

Pedhazur, E. J. (1982). *Multiple regression in behavioral research,* (2nd ed.). New York: Holt, Rinehart & Winston.

Phillips, D. P. (1974). The influence of suggestion on suicide: Substantive and theoretical implications of the Werther effect. *American Sociological Review, 39,* 340-354.

Pinel, J. P. J. (1990). *Biopsychology,* Boston: Allyn & Bacon.

Plutchik, R., & Kellerman, H. (Eds.). (1980). *Emotion: Theory, research, and experience* (2 vols.). New York: Academic Press.

Richter, C. P. (1957). On the phenomenon of sudden death in man and animals. *Psychosomatic Medicine, 19,* 191–197.

Rosen, G. (1971). History in the study of suicide. *Psychological Medicine, 1,* 267–285.

Shneidman, E. S. (1957). The logic of suicide. In E. S. Shneidman & N. L. Farberow (Eds.), *Clues to suicide.* New York: McGraw-Hill.

Stanley, M., Stanley, B., Traskman-Bendz, L., Mann, J. J., & Meyendorff, E. (1986). Neurochemical findings in suicide completers and suicide attempters. *Suicide and Life-Threatening Behavior, 16,* 286–300.

Symons, D. (1980). Précis of "The evolution of human sexuality." *Behavioral and Brain Sciences, 3,* 171–214.

Tatsuoka, M. M. (1988). *Multivariate analysis* (2nd ed.). New York: Macmillan.

van Praag, H. M. (1986). Affective disorders and aggression disorders: Evidence for a common biological mechanism. *Suicide and Life-Threatening Behavior, 16,* 103–132.

van Velzen, W. Y. (1975). Autoplexy or self-destructive behavior in mental retardation. In D. A. A. Primrose (Ed.), *Proceedings of the Third Congress of the International Association for the Scientific Study of Mental Deficiency.* Warsaw: Polish Medical.

Williams, G. C. (1957). Pleiotropy, natural selection, and the evolution of senescence. *Evolution, 11,* 398–411.

Wright, S. (1922). Coefficients of interbreeding and relationship. *American Naturalist, 56,* 330–339.

PART VI

Synthesis and Conclusions

An Integrated Approach to Estimating Suicide Risk

Jerome A. Motto, M.D.

University of California at San Francisco, School of Medicine

Whatever differences clinicians may have about estimating suicide risk, there are at least some points on which they tend to agree—specifically, that the estimation of risk is important, complex, and difficult to quantify. The absence of a generally accepted instrument to accomplish the task attests to the elusiveness of a unitary solution to the problem. The most visible obstacle to such a solution is the very nature of human beings, in that every individual is unique. Thus, the objective and measurable observations that would accurately determine the level of suicide risk in one person may have very different significance for another, or no relevance at all for a third. That is, in a given case, the importance lies in the *meaning* of an observation and not in the observation itself.

It follows that if we have the opportunity to study our subjects thoroughly, and to establish a level of trust that assures candor and openness, we will be in an optimal position to assess risk in individual cases. That position is not always available to us in a busy emergency department, in a medical/surgical ward, on a crisis telephone line, or in the many other situations where we encounter suicidal persons. Yet the job has to be done, so we use shortcuts and simply acknowledge the many inherent limitations that this entails. Given an array of approaches to accomplish the task, our concern is this: How can a clinician take advantage of the many observations and recommendations that have been made?

BASIC ISSUES

Suicide occurs when a person's limit of tolerance of psychic pain is exceeded by the level of pain that is either experienced or anticipated with a degree of subjective certainty. Thus, the process of estimating the risk of suicide at a given time is essentially one of determining how close the actual or anticipated pain is to the person's tolerance threshold at that time. Both the threshold and the pain level are dynamic factors that are in constant flux. A constant level of pain that is well within a person's tolerance when he or she is assessed may generate a suicidal act when the threshold is reduced by fatigue, lack of sleep, or intoxication with drugs or alcohol. Similarly, for example, a constant pain tolerance may be gradually encroached upon by a progressive illness, or abruptly exceeded by unanticipated adverse events such as a painful interpersonal encounter or the loss of a job. These may be fantasized or real events; in either case, they are usually beyond the control of a clinician. The anticipated pain may be expected in the foreseeable future (e.g., a threatened divorce or censure), or may involve the indefinite future (e.g., early cancer or infection with AIDS).

If we accept psychic pain and the level of pain tolerance as basic elements of suicide, it would seem that the unstable relationship of these elements would justify eliminating the term "prediction" from our scientific terminology in addressing the problem of an individual's suicide risk. The phrase "estimation of risk" would more accurately reflect the reality of what we are learning from our research efforts and what we do in practice, regardless of the approach we use to assess the degree of risk.

METHODS

Approaches to suicide risk assessment may be considered in two general categories: "clinical" and "empirical." Clinical assessment in pure form is a time-honored interview method that elicits detailed information about a person's life experience, character structure, and adaptive needs; when effectively carried out, it enables the examiner to recognize the circumstances under which a suicidal act is likely to occur *in a given individual.* An empirical approach, at the other extreme, consists of inquiring about a number of items previously observed in persons who have committed suicide, with the implied assumption that these observations should identify the person being assessed as similarly at risk. The clinical approach is relatively time-consuming; assumes that the person being assessed is cognitively clear, articulate, and willing to cooperate; requires a setting conducive to calm reflection; and, for optimal results, calls for a well-trained and experienced professional. An empirical assessment, on the other hand, can be done relatively quickly, usually in a matter of minutes; may use data from various sources; is compatible with the hectic atmosphere of an emergency department or a crisis line; and does not require years of training and experience to carry out efficiently.

Considered in extreme form, these methods appear to contrast sharply. However, it is safe to say that very few persons with responsibility for estimating suicide risk use either of these approaches exclusively. That is, the dynamic therapist or consultant will elicit data that are included in the empirical approach—for example, feelings of utter hopelessness and despair, detailed suicide plans, a history of serious suicide attempts, termination behavior, or ready access to a lethal weapon. Similarly, an empiricist will give weight to the loss of significant persons or other meaningful elements in the individual's life, will recognize the potential role of suicide in the family history, will consider parallels with prior suicidal states, and will recognize the importance of substance abuse, extreme dependency, or other personality characteristics in the individual. In other words, though each clinician may identify more with one or the other approach, in practice there is a great deal of overlap in the data that contribute to the final judgment as to severity of suicide risk. It may simply be put in different terminology or phraseology. For example, one (dynamic) clinician may recognize the unbearable pain of intense dependency needs' being unmet in a rejection-sensitive individual with a history of emotional deprivation, whereas another (empirical) clinician recognizes that if a threatened divorce is carried out, the person is very likely to commit suicide.

The optimal approach, which is by far the most frequently used, is to utilize both methods of assessment to the extent that one can, mindful that what will work best is determined largely by the setting, the circumstances, the available time, the condition and cooperativeness of the person assessed, and—most importantly—one's own training, experience, and style. The usual pattern is to start with an abbreviated clinical inquiry along the lines of "What is happening in your life that is creating pain? What effect is it having on your thoughts, feelings, and behavior? And, finally, can you stand it?" This is generally followed by more empirically focused questions, such as whether suicide was attempted in the past or whether physical illness, drugs, or alcohol is involved. An empirical scale is used in many settings, especially psychiatric inpatient units and telephone crisis centers. When the brief clinical and empirical inquiries are combined with information available from third parties and with demographic observations of age, sex, and race, the clinician is ready to estimate the level of risk.

Given that different persons may require varied approaches, and that a given person may be approached differently in specific settings or by different clinicians, a number of modifying issues deserve consideration regardless of the approach used.

MODIFYING ISSUES

The Role of Intuition

When all the questions have been asked and answered, the final decision regarding degree of suicide risk is a subjective one. It may or may not agree with the score on a risk scale, with the content of the suicidal person's responses, or with others' impressions; it may not even be explainable in terms of clear inference or reasoning. It is simply the final summation of all the (sometimes conflicting or ambiguous) information that has been gathered and processed at a level not entirely conscious. This can be called an "intuitive" decision. Such a characterization often creates discomfort in clinicians who need a more objective criterion on which to base action. It has also been objected to by some who favor a dynamic approach, interpreting the term "intuitive" to mean judgment based on a purely instinctual sense rather than on a body of information (Maltsberger & Rosenberg, 1990, p. 6). The issue is broached here to emphasize the subjective nature of any risk assessment process, no matter how objective our methods appear to be. Whether clinically or empirically based, our information involves assumptions and interpretations that can lead us astray at every turn.

We also know that much information is gathered without the gatherer's fully realizing it, such as through a person's tone of voice, demeanor, or subtleties of speech and manner. As clinicians, we would do well to respect the impact of these nonverbal clues on our subjective judgment, even though we may be unable to explain why our impression has been influenced in a given direction. It is important to accept that when we have gathered all the information we can, this intuitive sense is our best guide to estimating suicide risk. If it contradicts more objective measures of risk, prudence would dictate reviewing the situation again, but if this does not reconcile the difference, the subjective judgment deserves precedence.

In one study examining the degree of concordance of an empirical suicide risk scale and subjective clinical impression, 57% of the cases were rated the same and 32% were one category apart (e.g., high vs. moderate, or moderate vs. low). Eleven percent were two categories apart (high vs. low), suggesting the proportion of cases that might need review. The mean time required for telephone crisis workers to administer the empirical scale was 5.4 minutes, with a range of 1–20 minutes (Motto, 1985).

The Role of Time

The identification of risk indicators by statistical means has generally considered a risk period (the time during which the indicator has been shown to be associated with suicide) of 2 years or more. This period has usually been dictated by statistical considerations combined with the low base rate for suicide, which is such that it requires at least 2 years to find enough suicides for systematic analysis. Clinical needs, however, focus on a much shorter risk period, as the clinician is most concerned about the chance of suicide occurring during the days or weeks following evaluation. This raises the question of how much relevance empirical studies or scales have for day-to-day work.

The first effort to narrow this gap was Exner and Wylie's (1977) retrospective study of 59 persons in the United States and Canada who committed suicide within 60 days after a Rorschach test had been administered. Eleven Rorschach variables were identified that could be interpreted as stress-related personality characteristics with implications for near-term suicide risk. A subsequent prospective study (Motto & Bostrom, 1990) yielded nine clinical items, of which the presence of four or more identified 38 suicides that occurred within 60 days of assessment, with a sensitivity of 79% and a specificity of 81%.

Fawcett (1988) used the term "early" suicide to mean within 1 year in a small but carefully studied sample of depressed suicides. He contrasted six "short-term" (less than 1 year) with five "long-term" (1–5 years) risk factors; only one item, "hopelessness," appeared on both lists. In a study of the relationship of this item to "ultimate" suicide, Beck, Brown, Berchick, Stewart, and Steer (1990) identifed a cutoff point at which hopelessness was associated with suicide, with a mean risk period of 3.5 years in psychiatric outpatients. An earlier study by these investigators used a 5- to 10-year follow-up period to find the risk of "eventual" suicide associated with feelings of hopelessness (Beck, Steer, Kovacs, & Garrison, 1985).

The clinical usefulness of any risk-correlated information is directly related to the immediacy of the danger, though longer-term risk potential is important to understanding the epidemiology of suicide. When a risk scale is derived by nonempirical means, it usually provides no clear guidelines as to the role of time (e.g., Friedman & Asnis, 1989). Although studies that specify period of risk can be useful, it is only by careful clinical probing that the trend of lethality over time can be determined. Acute situations require maximum near-term protection and support as the pain gradually diminishes, whereas chronic, intractable stress creates a progressive increase in risk over time. Still other circumstances are quite time-specific: "I'm not going to have my 30th birthday unless _____"; "It will be a year since my daughter's suicide on _____." Regardless of variations in assessment style, it is appropriate not only to estimate the immediate and near-term risk, but to formulate a trajectory of risk over a period of months and years, based on currently available information.

The Role of Strengths

One limitation of empirical methods is the tendency to underemphasize the role of strengths as a factor in estimating risk. Although this is recognized as a common-sense issue, suicide risk scales tend to focus on pathology or on the absence of strengths (e.g., no family, no funds, no job, etc.). Even a brief clinical interview will often reassure a clinician that in spite of numerous high-risk observations, an individual may have difficult-to-quantify characteristics that serve to protect him or her against suicide, and that may remain undetected by a risk scale. Such situations are conducive to the instances noted above in which an empirical instrument indicates high risk and the subjective impression of the examiner is that the risk is low.

The Role of Chronicity

A variant of the time dimension in risk assessment, as discussed above, is presented by those persons referred to as "chronically suicidal." This is a misnomer; the pattern is not one of a persistent suicidal state, but rather of repeated suicidal episodes interspersed with varying periods of normal functioning. The assessment problem, regardless of the method used, is that the person's pain tolerance is relatively low, resulting in repeated suicidal crises under the stresses of daily life. The crisis may last for only a few hours or days, after which the person appears completely free of pathology. Hence, the estimate of risk can vary from one extreme to the other in a very short time. Experience teaches us that the long-term risk is high in these circumstances, but most empirical measures would only indicate high risk if they were administered during a crisis. In chronic situations a brief clinical evaluation can give us the most accurate indication of risk, not only during the crisis period but in the intermediate and long term as well. The person is never far from a serious suicidal state even when symptom-free; thus any estimate of risk must be regarded as a very short-term indicator, and persistent monitoring is called for.

The Role of 5%: Statistical and Clinical Significance

The identification of "high-risk indicators," sometimes called "predictors of suicide" or (more realistically) "correlates of suicide," is one of the most consistent areas of empirical research in the field of suicide studies. Some correlates are explored as single indicators or as combinations of indicators (e.g., alcoholism combined with personal loss, hopelessness, or depressive illness). Others are included as one of a set of observations "significantly associated" with completed suicide. Still others are developed as scales with empirically derived weights, scores, and specific levels of implied risk. A common element in these statistical exercises is the use of a 5% level of confidence as the accepted standard for "significance."

It must be kept in mind that researchers tend not to discriminate between "statistical" significance and "clinical" significance. In the clinical world where risk assessment is carried out, any given "nonsignificant" statistical finding may prove to be of extreme importance in a given instance. The converse is also the case: A significant statistical finding (e.g. alcoholism), may have no clinical significance in a given case or may even operate to protect the person against suicide. The 5% convention can be especially misleading when a small sample or a very large sample is analyzed, even though there are statistical measures to correct for both.

The Role of Paradigm

One of the most obvious handicaps to reaching consensus in regard to empirical risk assessment is the diversity of suicidal behaviors examined. What are we trying to measure? There are instruments to evaluate depression, to differentiate suicide attempters and nonattempters, to predict "suicidal behavior," to assess the seriousness of intent after a suicide attempt has been made, to differentiate persons with suicidal ideas from those without them, and to quantify feelings of hopelessness. None of these gives us an estimate of the risk of completed suicide, though all are pertinent considerations. Until there is clarity as to what is being addressed, the role of such instruments in the estimation of suicide risk will remain ambiguous.

The Role of Therapist Differences

How a clinician goes about the task of risk assessment necessarily depends a great deal on his or her own professional and personal style. In the absence of any demonstrated superiority of a particular method, it is reasonable to postulate that the task will be done most efficiently and effectively when the clinician is operating in his or her spontaneous manner. Even if it could be shown in an investigative setting that a given test battery, an empirical scale, a clinical scale, a dynamic formulation, a brief clinical interview, or a combination of these provided the most accurate estimate of risk, a given clinician would do well to adopt such a procedure only to the extent that it is compatible with his or her natural style. This issue is akin to the question of identifying the best way to treat a suicidal person, which was clearly summarized by George Murphy (1972) as "The best you know how" (p. 359). The point has long been recognized in the behavioral world that the particular strengths and talents of the clinician are generally more important to a favorable outcome than the specific method used.

The Role of Individual Uniqueness

The fact that every person is different has been mentioned above as the most visible handicap to empirical methods; it dictates at least some degree of clinical inquiry to give individual meaning to the observations made. Yet an implied assumption is that empirical findings, or identified "risk indicators," have general applicability. Since, strictly speaking, they apply only to the population represented by the sample from which the risk factor was derived, Brown and Sheran (1972) suggested that the more homogeneous or "situation-specific" the sample analyzed, the more accurate the risk indicators should be when applied to individuals sharing the characteristics of that sample. This led to the examination of a wide variety of very specific populations, such as demographic, diagnostic, occupational, and personality categories. Though correlates of suicide have been identified for many such groupings, they have not yet been put in the form of a rating scale for use with the specific populations from which they were derived.

Another approach to individualizing an empirical risk factor, included in at least one scale (Motto, Heilbron, & Juster, 1985), has been to consider the person's special vulnerabilities in the light of the specific life circumstances involved. For example, a 32-year-old man had a persistent severe hand infection with the possibility of amputation. Though this event would not ordinarily appear on an empirical risk scale, the fact that he had prepared for 25 years for a career as a concert pianist increased the pain of this stress to a suicidal level. Similarly, a 30-year-old woman's impetuous act led her to anticipate rejection by her husband's parents. The fact that her deprived childhood had led her to substitute them for her own parents, with an intense dependent need for their approval, transformed a family stress into a suicidal crisis. It seems safe to assume that there are innumerable circumstances not ordinarily associated with suicide (and thus not generally considered "risk factors") that in certain vulnerable individuals may precipitate a suicide, and deserve to be adapted for inclusion in empirical scales.

Even among familiar risk factors in the empirical world, some can be found, paradoxically, to be associated with an outcome opposite to the expected one in some instances. For example, Farberow and MacKinnon (1974), in a rigorous study of suicide in Veterans Administration hospitals, identified "no alcohol abuse" and "no loss of physical health" as high-risk indicators. Litman (1974) found "no recent loss or separation" to be a high-risk item for callers to the Los Angeles Suicide Prevention Center. Lettieri's (1974) study of suicide in the same population revealed that "no divorce within 6 months" for males under 40; "no failure in performance of major role" and "no multiple divorces or rejections" for males 40 and over; and "no prior psychiatric hospitalizations" for females 40 and over were all "significantly" indicative of high risk for suicide. Such findings add to our already convincing evidence that we can make few assumptions about the implications of clinical data without considering the uniqueness of the persons from whom the data are obtained.

The Role of Prediction of Suicide versus Estimation of Risk

The idea and the expression "prediction of suicide" should have disappeared from our lexicon long ago. The first volume published on the prediction of suicide included a clear statement of this conviction: "A

crucial consideration sometimes underemphasized is that we can only predict the risk of suicide and not suicide as such" (Motto, 1974, p. 85). But
such a fantasy does not die easily. It has been pursued relentlessly, complete
with the precision of "false positives" and "false negatives," as though
suicide were a disease entity that is either present or absent. Diggory (1974)
captured the essence of the scientific fervor involved:

> If [prediction] is a realistic goal, no doubt we will approach it slowly, and
> before we reach it we will have used many procedures that will be better than
> those we now use but not as good as the one we seek. If one were to say that the
> prediction of suicide is no goal but a phantasm, a wraith, we have no present
> information with which to refute him. The belief that suicidal behaviors are
> predictable can be valid only as a belief in principle, . . . a special case of every
> scientist's article of faith that the universe contains regularities that can be
> discovered and understood by rational inquiry. (p. 59)

Diggory went on to attribute our lack of progress in suicide prediction to
our not having fully utilized multiple-regression analysis, pointing out that
"Our shortcomings arise . . . in our failing to come to grips with our data,
in not having thoroughly analyzed the data we do have, and in not contemplating the rich array of suicidal phenomena with a view to letting it guide
us to the theory we seek" (1974, p. 69). Such passion stirs our researchers'
blood, but does not alter the realization that suicide is a nonspecific symptom of a nonspecific human malaise, and that trying to create precision in
foreseeing its manifestations in individual cases is akin to clearing a path
through a swamp.

There only Yet optimism is the stock in trade of researchers and suicide prevention
workers alike. If we cannot predict suicide, what can we do? We can evaluate
our data by both subjective and objective measures to estimate how likely it
is that a person will commit suicide. We can thus predict the *risk* of suicide
rather than the suicide itself. This is in fact what is now done by clinicians
every day, though the process takes various forms. A carefully constructed
empirical risk scale can tell us that a person belongs to a population of
which a certain percentage will commit suicide within a specific time
period. A clinical interview, whether brief or lengthy, can give us an indication of whether the person's pain tolerance is so close to being exceeded that
he or she is likely to be included in that percentage. Adding pertinent data
from the person's family, the clinical laboratory, and the psychiatric record
will round out our picture, assuring us that we are not overlooking useful
information.

There only remains the summing up that gives us our final estimation
of risk. Though we may have been objective in our approach, there is no
avoiding subjectivity at this point, leaving us with what I have referred to
above as an intuitive judgment. It may be put in precise terms, such as "40%

risk," or in the commoner and less precise "low–moderate–high" terminology. If we consider a 40% likelihood of suicide as high risk, and a person assessed at this level does not commit suicide, does it imply (treatment considerations aside) that we have made an erroneous judgment, that the rating was a "false positive"? Similarly, if we consider a 2% likelihood of suicide as low risk, and the person does commit suicide, have we erred in the other direction with a "false negative"? A number of clinicians, including Murphy (1983) and Beck et al. (1990), have emphasized that recognizing the potential for suicide is not the same as predicting the event, even if the potential is seen to be high.

Uncomfortable as it is, we have no realistic choice but to deal in levels of risk that can vary from day to day or hour to hour, subject to the influence of numerous uncontrollable and unpredictable events. To try to predict more than the risk that is present at a given time, or that would be present under specific circumstances, is an unrealistic goal that can lead to frustration and discouragement. This tone has crept into the risk assessment literature to some extent in the form of questioning the value of efforts in this direction (MacKinnon & Farberow, 1976; Murphy, 1983; Pokorny, 1983 [see also Chapter 6, this volume]).

APPLICATIONS TO THE FIVE CASE HISTORIES
Heather B

Heather, the 13-year-old white schoolgirl, was apparently struggling with issues of low self-esteem, low self-confidence, unsatisfactory peer relations, loneliness, isolation, and emotional turmoil. She acted out many of her feelings in typically adolescent ways and criticized herself severely; she summed up her dilemma as being "mentally crazy," belonging in a mental hospital, needing to punish herself, and wanting to distance herself from her painful experience—even to the point of suicide. On the other side, Heather would appear to be intelligent, introspective, articulate, and communicative, and to retain a sense of humor and whimsy. Speaking through her cartoon figure, "Dimehead," she explained that cutting her arm was not a suicide attempt but a way of expressing her upset about a specific situation. She was aware of others' feelings and reassured them, "Doon worry bout her."

Demographically, Heather was in a low-risk group. We could entertain the diagnosis of depression, but the record does not clearly substantiate a mood, thought, or behavior disorder. Her ability to communicate with others seemed to be high; this has been found to be a low-risk factor in adolescents (Motto, 1984). No biological data are provided in the case description in Chapter 12. I find the psychological test data interesting but not helpful to me.

In summary, the dynamic background is limited to her father's premature death, but the clinical description suggests that whatever the conflicts involved, Heather was clearly asking for help. She demonstrated good premorbid adjustment. Empirical observations (e.g., suicidal ideas, fear of being "crazy," capacity for self-scrutiny, good communication skills) give a mixed picture. Her mother would seem to be a positive element as a stable, caring adult. My final (subjective, intuitive) judgment would be that Heather's risk of suicide over the ensuing 5 years would be low (0.5–1.5%) and would gradually decrease if professional assistance were to be obtained. If assistance were not obtained, my estimate of risk would indicate a gradual increase into the moderate range (2.5–5.0%), subject to influence by unforeseen intercurrent events.

Ralph F

Ralph is described in Chapter 12 as a 16-year-old white male with an impressive array of high-risk factors for suicide: depression; alcohol abuse since age 12; social isolation; a recent suicide in his household; a family history that included alcoholism, suicidal behavior, and instability; delinquency; chronic physical illness; and—most striking—feelings of hopelessness, existential despair, and obsession with suicidal ideas, including a specific plan. Any strengths would be expected to pale before such imposing pathology.

Yet we cannot ignore the fact that in spite of all this Ralph was able (with an average IQ and granting some recent "slippage") not only to keep at grade level, but to maintain a B+ average in high school and to develop some friends as well. Reference to "a strong histrionic quality" also raises a question of whether some of his statements might have been embellished or presented for dramatic effect. His attributing his suicidal thoughts to an effort to handle his anger toward his grandfather would tempt a dynamically oriented psychotherapist to see him as readily treatable.

My intuitive judgment would be that Ralph's risk of suicide would be high (5–10%) over the next 6 months, gradually diminishing with treatment to a moderate range (2.5–5.0%). Because of the characterological nature of Ralph's adjustment pattern, I would anticipate that he would remain at or near at least a moderate level of risk for a 5–7-year period, depending on the course of life events and interpersonal relationships.

John Z

John, the 39-year-old male, would appear to fit a pattern that has been referred to as "stable with forced change" (Motto, 1979). It focuses on the shattering effect that a major disruption can have on a person with a lifelong history of emotional and social stability. Unaccustomed to having little control over life events, yet feeling responsible for the care and security of his family, John was subject to depression and panic states so severe as to reach suicidal proportions. At the same time, his need to maintain an image of competence interfered with full compliance with a treatment program. His two reported suicidal episodes with a plastic bag and hanging would suggest that his control was tenuous, and by telling his wife about them, he seemed to be asking that someone else take over, in spite of his ambivalence about relinquishing control.

John exhibited four of the nine empirical high-risk factors most closely associated with completed suicide within 2 years in the stable-with-forced-change model: executive role, severe loss, recent change of occupation, and obsessive personality pattern. Though these do not consitute a rare set of circumstances, they take on some empirical weight when encountered in a person recognized to be at risk for suicide.

Finally, John's wife's observation of a 20-pound weight loss, decreased concentration, and obsession with trivia (an indication that John's usual psychological coping mechanisms were being strained to the limit), would seem to justify her concern that the treatment regimen was not sufficient. I would share her intuitive sense that the risk of suicide was very high (over 10%), and that involuntary hospitalization should be considered if John could not be persuaded to enter the hospital voluntarily.

Faye C

Faye, the 49-year-old unmarried woman, was seen in the emergency department primarily for a psychotic episode, during which she screamed, "You're not going to let me kill myself, are you?" This question can be interpreted in many ways, but my inclination would be to take it very literally as a request for reassurance by a person who was frightened by feeling out of control. My response would be, "No, we won't let you do that," and then I would proceed to arrange her admission to an inpatient unit for treatment of the psychosis. In the course of evaluating her emotional status upon her arrival on the ward, it would be necessary to explore the implications of her question about killing herself. If she were to be seen in another setting, the issue should be addressed without delay.

Faye's intense fear of hospitalization, memory of her earlier psychiatric hospital experience, delusion of being controlled by radio waves, and feelings of dyscontrol would be sufficient to identify her as being at risk for suicide, even in the absence of her verbal clue. The role of her temporal lobe epilepsy in this acute episode would also require evaluation, as would the possible role of involutional stresses. Although a lifelong characterological burden was imposed by her negative self-image and its related social constriction, Faye apparently functioned quite well in other settings. Completing a master's program in public health and idealistically challenging the mental health system would both suggest considerable strengths. When severely stressed at age 43, she sought appropriate help and continued this for a prolonged period. In spite of some tensions with her mother, she apparently derived much emotional sustenance from her father and maintained a stable relationship with both parents.

My judgment would be that Faye's suicide risk would be moderate (2.5–5.0% within 2 years) and would relate primarily to the psychosis. If this were resolved, the suicide risk might become very low (less than 1%). One empirical scale, the California Risk Estimator for Suicide (Motto et al., 1985), would similarly place her in the sixth decile of risk (moderate) in the acute state, and in the first decile of risk (very low) in the absence of persecutory ideas and suicidal impulses.

José G

José, the 64-year-old Hispanic male with a stable family (42 years), job (29 years), smoking (40 years), and alcohol ("long") history, had experienced a 6-month period of progressive physical disabilities. A nonhealing wrist injury prevented him from working, and complications of diabetic retinopathy and emphysema led to his being put on permanent disability. For several weeks he had experienced a pervasive dysphoria, including feelings of worthlessness, hopelessness, guilt, and being a burden, as well as thoughts of death. The loss of self-sufficiency and of earning power was clearly creating a great deal of psychic pain.

Though José demonstrated almost every depressive symptom known, we can only conclude from this that he was severely depressed. Estimating how suicidal he actually was would require information about his desire or intent to kill himself, rather than about his feeling that death would provide relief. We often see persons who wish fervently to die, but who insist with equal fervor that they themselves will never deliberately bring this about. José's Hispanic background would suggest lower risk; if he were close to the traditional church, this could reduce the risk even further. His increased drinking the past month would suggest lower near-term but higher long-term risk. In the short term, drinking might serve, as William Styron (1990) described in recounting his depression, "as a means to calm the anxiety and incipient dread that I had hidden away for so long somewhere in the dungeons of my spirit" (p. 40).

If José were experiencing actual suicidal thoughts or impulses, I would estimate his risk as at least moderate (2.5–5.0% in 2 years). If not, or if no further data were available, I would consider it low (1.0–2.5%), but would take the precaution of securing all firearms and asking the family to dispense his medications and observe him closely until it became possible to explore this issue in more detail.

SUMMARY

It is ironic that if we had a perfect predictive instrument, we would not be able to recognize it because it could never be validated by its critical outcome criterion. Though some exceptions could occur, we would be obliged to take all available measures to prevent a suicidal outcome in cases where suicide was predicted. After the crisis, we could have no way of knowing with certainty whether the person would have committed suicide or not. Even if we accepted the reality that people are not either 0% or 100% likely to commit suicide, and developed a perfect scale to estimate degree of risk, we would still be unable to validate it in individual cases. If it indicated "moderate" risk of 2.5–5.0%, for example, and no intervention were offered, we would have to observe 1 suicide in every 20–40 persons assessed at this level of risk to demonstrate its validity.

The key to assessment is obtaining information, primarily regarding the level of present or anticipated pain and the threshold of pain tolerance in the individual involved. Since different persons communicate in a variety of ways (verbal, nonverbal, symbolic, metaphoric, etc.), eclecticism in approach is essential. For some clinicians, communication will be facilitated most by one style; for others, a different method will be most effective. Thus, the "best" approach is the one that works best, given the unique characteristics of the persons involved and the conditions existing at the time. My own bias is that every assessment, whatever the approach, must include some form of direct inquiry regarding suicidal intent, and that the final decision in this regard must be a subjective and intuitive judgment. Contrary to possible assumptions in the legal world, accurate assessment does not necessarily mean safety. It can serve as a guide to the degree of risk that may be involved in a treatment program, but even low-risk management measures implemented without negligence or carelessness may have an adverse outcome.

There has been no mention here of biological markers of suicide, which are of much current interest but still in an investigational stage. Similarly, rational suicide has not been mentioned, though our aging population and the status of AIDS are making this issue progressively more important. The principles involved in assessment of risk are the same as with other forms of suicide, however. Finally, we can only presume that more precise assessment will operate to reduce suicidal deaths. The focus may have to shift to improved treatment and preventive programs to achieve that end, but we must remain aware that this is the ultimate goal of all our efforts.

REFERENCES

Beck, A. T., Brown, G., Berchick, R., Stewart, B., & Steer, R. (1990). Relationship between hopelessness and ultimate suicide: A replication with psychiatric outpatients. *American Journal of Psychiatry, 147,* 190–195.

Beck, A. T., Steer, R., Kovacs, M., & Garrison, B. (1985). Hopelessness and eventual suicide: A 10-year prospective study of patients hospitalized with suicidal ideation. *American Journal of Psychiatry, 142*, 559-563.

Brown, T., & Sheran, T. (1972). Suicide prediction: A review. *Suicide and Life-Threatening Behavior, 2*, 67-98.

Diggory, J. (1974). Predicting suicide: Will-o-the-wisp or reasonable challenge? In A. T. Beck, H. L. P. Resnik, & D. J. Lettieri (Eds.), *The prediction of suicide* (pp. 59-70). Bowie, MD: Charles Press.

Exner, J., & Wylie, J. (1977). Some Rorschach data concerning suicide. *Journal of Personality Assessment, 41*, 339-348.

Farberow, N., & MacKinnon, D. (1974). A suicide prediction schedule for neuropsychiatric hospital patients. *Journal of Nervous and Mental Disease, 158*, 408-419.

Fawcett, J. (1988). Predictors of early suicide: Identification and early prevention. *Journal of Clinical Psychiatry, 49*(10, Suppl.), 7-8.

Friedman, J., & Asnis, G. (1989). Assessment of suicidal behavior: A new instrument. *Psychiatric Annals, 19*, 382-387.

Lettieri, D. J. (1974). Suicidal death prediction scales. In A. T. Beck, H. L. P. Resnik, & D. J. Lettieri (Eds.), *The prediction of suicide* (pp. 163-192). Bowie, MD: Charles Press.

Litman, R. E. (1974). Models for predicting suicide risk. In C. Neuringer (Ed.), *Psychological assessment of suicidal risk* (pp. 177-185). Springfield, IL: Charles Thomas.

MacKinnon, D., & Farberow, N. (1976). An assessment of the utility of suicide prediction. *Suicide and Life-Threatening Behavior, 6*, 86-91.

Maltsberger, J. T., & Rosenberg, M. L. (1990). The interface between empirical suicide research and clinical practice. *Crisis, 11*, 3-10.

Motto, J. A. (1974). Refinement of variables in assessing suicide risk. In A. T. Beck, H. L. P. Resnik & D. J. Lettieri (Eds.), *The prediction of suicide* (pp. 85-93). Bowie, MD: Charles Press.

Motto, J. A. (1979). The psychopathology of suicide: A clinical model approach. *American Journal of Psychiatry, 136*, 516-520.

Motto, J. A. (1984). Suicide in male adolescents. In H. Sudak, A. Ford, & N. Rushforth (Eds.), *Suicide in the young* (pp. 227-243). Boston: John Wright.

Motto, J. A. (1985). Preliminary field-testing of a risk estimator for suicide. *Suicide and Life-Threatening Behavior, 15*, 139-150.

Motto, J. A., & Bostrom, A. (1990). Empirical indicators of near-term suicide risk. *Crisis, 11*, 52-59.

Motto, J. A., Heilbron, D., & Juster, R. (1985). Development of a clinical instrument to estimate suicide risk. *American Journal of Psychiatry, 142*, 680-686.

Murphy, G. (1972). Clinical identification of suicidal risk. *Archives of General Psychiatry, 27*, 356-359.

Murphy, G. (1983). On suicide prediction and prevention. *Archives of General Psychiatry, 40*, 343-344.

Pokorny, A. D. (1983). Prediction of suicide in psychiatric patients: Report of a prospective study. *Archives of General Psychiatry, 40*, 249-257.

Styron, W. (1990). *Darkness visible*. New York: Random House.

CHAPTER 32

Summary and Conclusions: What Have We Learned about Suicide Assessment and Prediction?

Ronald W. Maris, Ph.D.
University of South Carolina

Alan L. Berman, Ph.D.
Washington Psychological Center
The National Center for the Study of Suicide

John T. Maltsberger, M.D.
Harvard Medical School
McLean Hospital, Belmont, Massachusetts
Boston Psychoanalytic Society and Institute

It is a foolish if not an impossible endeavor to attempt to reduce the richness and diversity of the previous 31 chapters to a few consensual findings. In truth, this volume has presented many different perspectives on, professional approaches to, and arguments about assessing and predicting suicide. At this stage of our suicidological development it would probably be wise to preserve these differences. Also, we wish to avoid a mechanical chapter-by-chapter synopsis (although we do offer abstracts of each chapter in the Appendix). Instead, the focus here is on salient issues raised by the individual chapter authors. As we see them, they are as follows:

- What is being predicted or assessed?
- Comorbidity and multivariate interdisciplinary models
- Timing issues
- The problem of rare behaviors
- False positives and false negatives
- Instruments or tools of assessment and prediction
- Implications for treatment and suicide prevention

Of course, we also want to synthesize the comments about and to inform our readers of the outcomes of the five clinical cases described in detail in Chapter 12 and assessed by many of the individual chapter authors. Since this concluding chapter is primarily a summary, we resist adding many new citations.

WHAT IS BEING PREDICTED OR ASSESSED?

It might appear to a naive individual that the dependent (outcome) variable in our assessment/prediction equation is simple and homogeneous. Most obviously, in this book we have been attempting to predict the suicide outcome of our five individual cases. Fair enough, but doubts have been raised about whether one can *ever* predict individual suicide events. Motto (Chapter 31) and Litman (Chapter 21) argue that at best, we can predict suicide risk over periods of about a year. Trying to predict an individual suicide is a 0-1 (no suicide–suicide) or "zero-sum game," whereas predicting suicide risk is usually a 0-100% probability assessment over modestly long time frames. The problem with the current state of the art is that unacceptably high numbers of false positives and false negatives are produced when individual suicides are predicted, especially in short time frames. Of course, we could predict that suicide events would *never* occur, and we would be right almost all the time! On the other hand, it is probably too early to give up on predicting individual suicides—which, after all, is what most of us are ultimately interested in. Also, it is not clear that predicting suicide risk is really very different from predicting individual suicide events, when one considers the usual case of a fairly high probability of suicide risk in a fairly short time frame.

Predicting suicide risk for individuals is a variation on predicting suicide rates for groups, or assessing which suicide risk group an individual best fits in. In effect, when we predict an individual's probability of suicide in (say) a year, we are saying that the individual's biopsychosocial characteristics place him or her in a relative-risk group (usually a "high-suicide-risk group") for suicide of perhaps 1 out of 100 rather than 1 out of 10,000 (the uncontrolled normal population's suicide risk). This arena is the province of epidemiologists and sociologists (see Garrison, Chapter 23; Phillips, Lesyna, & Paight, Chapter 24; Wasserman, Chapter 25; Stack, Chapter 26). For example, constructing life tables for insurance companies to predict the life expectancies of various types of policy holders (including suicides), and basing public health policies and planning on expected suicide or death rates, might be two examples of predicting suicide rates for groups. When one predicts suicide rates for groups, one always runs the risk of committing the "ecological fallacy"—that is, of assuming that social characteristics (e.g., suicide rates) of groups or areas are applicable to particular individuals in those groups or areas.

In addition to predicting suicide or suicide risk for individuals and suicide rates for groups, a third outcome of interest is assessing suicide *types*, or predicting which such type an individual patient, client, inmate, or other individual may fit into (see Maltsberger, Chapter 2; Maris, Chapter 4; Stelmachers & Sherman, Chapter 13). This assessment/prediction procedure is akin to fitting a patient into a *Diagnostic and Statistical Manual of Mental Disorders*, third edition, revised (DSM-III-R; American Psychiatric Association, 1987) mental disorder category or code, in that once we know the suicide type in some detail, certain treatment, medications, interventions, and suicide prevention procedures are indicated. Moreover, various levels of suicide risk are associated with various types of suicide and self-destructive behaviors.

Fourth, we often predict or assess behaviors, attitudes, or conditions (e.g., depressive illness, panic disorders, gun ownership, etc.) that are *related* to suicide, rather than suicide itself. For example, in this book we have examined suicide-associated psychiatric factors (Tanney, Chapter 14), psychological factors (Eyman & Eyman, Chapter 9), social factors (Bonner, Chapter 19; Felner, Silverman, & Adan, Chapter 20), and biological or physical factors (Roy, Chapter 28; Brown, Linnoila, & Goodwin, Chapter 29; de Catanzaro, Chapter 30). Herein lies a danger: Most of us see suicide through our particular disciplinary lenses. This is a kind of "occupational psychosis" or blind spot), so to speak, since a way of seeing is also a way of not seeing. Like the three blind men who described an elephant by each feeling a trunk, leg, and tusk, we have to guard against being interested only in suicide outcomes related to our own discipline. As we note in the next section of this concluding chapter, this book has examined four basic types of self-destructive outcomes:

- Psychological (Chapters 3, 9, 10, 12, 27)
- Psychiatric (Chapters 2, 6, 14, 21, 31)
- Medical/biological (Chapters 15, 28, 29, 30)
- Sociological/epidemiological (Chapters 11, 23, 24, 25, 26)

Properly used, each discipline supplements every other. However, reduction of suicide to any one discipline's view is myopic and incomplete, since suicide is a complex, multidetermined outcome.

Let us not forget that our dependent variable, suicide, varies not only from individuals to groups and across types, but also along other dimensions. One basic outcome continuum is that extending from completed suicide to nonfatal attempted suicide, to parasuicide, to suicide ideation without self-destructive behavior, to no suicidal behaviors at all (see Leenaars, Chapter 16; Maris, Chapter 17). In short, what is being predicted or assessed is not one thing, but actually many multidimensional, intersecting, and interacting parameters. It is imperative to specify exactly and in sufficient detail what our self-destructive outcome is.

Finally, it is imperative that we not lose sight of our main purpose in making any assessment, namely to derive clinically relevant data. Embedded in the question of outcome is the issue of intent. The wish to die is but one of several motives in suicidal behavior. Often the function or objective of suicidal behavior, apart from the actual outcome, is life enhancing. The suicidal individual may wish to alter life circumstances, to replace feelings of helplessness with those of power, to deaden pain, to change behavior in others, and so on. These goals may be described as instrumental and interpersonal. Thus, when translating assessment into treatment, a functional assessment of the motives of self-destructive acts is useful.

Perhaps the most clinically relevant dimension of assessment is its temporality. Inherent in any assessment is the prediction of action potential. That is, if there is the possibility of suicidal behavior (assessed risk), what is the predicted probability of such thought translating into behavior? Typically this question has an implied scaling, as in from chronic to acute risk or from low to medium to high risk. Such considerations lead to treatment and management decisions as to the need for hospitalization, the level of suicide precautions required, and so forth (see below).

COMORBIDITY AND MULTIVARIATE INTERDISCIPLINARY MODELS

We have seen over the course of this book that the *independent* variables, as well as the outcome or dependent variables, in the assessment and prediction of suicide are complex and varied. When there is more than one predictor variable or DSM-III-R diagnostic category associated with a suicide outcome, it is customary to speak of "comorbidity." The question then naturally arises: How many predictors of suicide are there—5, 10, 100, 1,000?" In general, there should be as few predictors as possible (the principle of parsimony), and yet reasonably high sensitivity and specificity scores. If there are too many predictors of suicide, then measurement of interaction effects among the independent variables quickly becomes unwieldly (see Addy, Chapter 11). Given most multivariate regression (such as logistic regression) or log-linear statistical procedures, even four to six predictor variables in a suicide model can become cumbersome and complex to interpret.

Also, the more independent variables one has, the larger the total sample size must be to maintain statistical "power" (Schlesselman, 1982). Most suicide prediction scales have two or three dozen items. For example, Cull and Gill's (1982) Suicide Probability Scale has 36 items, and the Beck

Depression Inventory (Beck, Ward, Mendelson, Mock, & Erbaugh, 1961) has 26 items. On the other hand, Motto's Clinical Instrument to Estimate Suicide Risk (Motto, Heilbron, & Juster, 1985) is comprised of 101 items, and the Minnesota Multiphasic Personality Inventory (MMPI-2; Hathaway & McKinley, 1967) has 567 items. Usually the raw items on a suicide prediction scale can be reduced to a more manageable number of predictors by factor analysis or subscaling.

Other questions about suicide causal models are these: "Which predictor variables are salient?" (see Gould, Shaffer, Fisher, Kleinman, & Morishima, Chapter 7) and "How are the individual predictors weighted?" (Lettieri, 1974). We have attempted a crude answer to the first question in Table 1.1 (see Maris, Chapter 1). There we have specified fifteen common single predictors of suicide. Of course, depending on the type of suicide, the specific relevant predictors may vary. Even if the predictors of suicide are relatively constant, the relative importance (weight) of any given suicide predictor variable may vary with the type of suicide outcome or with the phase of the same "suicidal career" (Maris, 1981).

A general multivariate interdisciplinary causal model of suicide ought to include at least the following four overlapping domains (cf. Blumenthal & Kupfer, 1990, p. 693):

1. Psychiatry, including diagnosis (Dx)
2. Biology/family history (Hx)/genetics/neurochemistry
3. Psychology/personality
4. Sociology/economics/culture

The multifactorial etiology of suicide suggested by these four broad domains can perhaps best be visualized in Venn diagrams (see Figure 32.1). Ordinarily, suicide assessment and prediction involves consideration of factors from all four domains (e.g., set 1234). But single domains or other overlapping domains may also be salient determinants of particular cases of suicide, types, or situations. The domains also overlap. For example, psychiatry does not have exclusive rights to diagnosis—as clinical psychologists will be quick to point out—and substance abuse is part of both the biological and diagnostic domains.

Examples of suicide predictors in each domain considered in this volume include the following:

1. Psychiatry/diagnosis (Dx): major depressive episode, borderline personality disorder, chronic undifferentiated schizophrenia, panic disorder
2. Biology/family history (Hx) genetics/neurochemistry: low brain serotonin, suicide in the family, older age, male sex, white race, alcoholism and/or drug abuse, serious medical illness

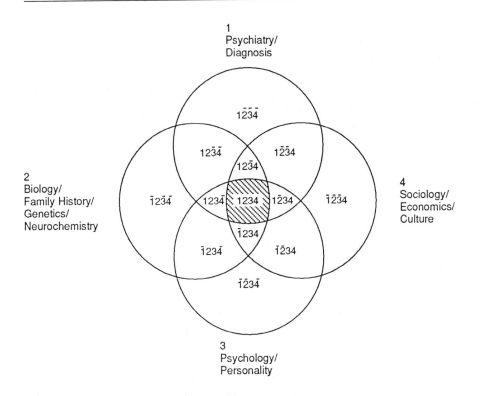

FIGURE 32.1. A multivariate interdisciplinary causal model for suicide. A bar over a number indicates that this number is *not* a factor in a particular section of the diagram.

  3. Psychology/personality: cognitive rigidity, hopelessness, unrealistically high self-expectations, psychic vulnerability
  4. Sociology/economics/culture: opportunity structures (e.g., gun availability), social isolation, high unemployment rates, stress, negative life events

It is important to realize that the interdisciplinary model of suicide depicted in Figure 32.1 and the importance of each sector vary over the human lifespan (Blumenthal & Kupfer, 1990; Leenaars, 1991). Suicidal careers need to be graphed with attention at least to the following lifespan continuum:

Suicidal Career

Background Early life Adolescence Young adulthood Midlife Young old Old old

One example of such a conceptualization of the multivariate determinants of suicide can be seen in Figure 32.2 (Maris, 1981). Given the multivariate interdisciplinary determination of suicide over the human lifespan, it may be useful to analyze suicide data using dynamic statistical procedures, such as path analysis (Maris, 1981), hazard analysis (Allison, 1984), and event history analysis (Wu & Tuma, 1990). Such causal models of suicide have been referred to as "kaleidoscopic" (Graves & Thomas, 1991) or "chameleonic."

TIMING ISSUES

Even when we can be reasonably sure an individual suicide will occur, we almost never know *when* the suicide will take place (Litman, 1990 and Chapter 21; Motto, Chapter 31; Maris, 1991). Will it be today or this weekend, if we do not hospitalize a client? Will it be some time this year, or some time in the next 5 years?

The focus of most suicide assessment and prediction is on the short run—usually hours, days, or weeks (Maltsberger, Chapter 2; Weishaar & Beck, Chapter 22). For example, Bonner (Chapter 19) points out that over 50% of jail suicides take place within the first 24 hours of incarceration. "Acute suicide lethality" is the probability of short-term suicide risk, whereas "chronic suicide lethality" is the probability of long-term suicide risk (Maris, 1981, pp. 10–11). Most suicide prediction actually focuses on estimating group suicide risk over years (the chronic lethality of "suicidal careers"; see Maris, Chapter 17), whereas clinicians need to know individual suicide probability over days (the acute lethality in suicidal crises). Thus, most suicide assessment is not very useful to clinicians.

We have also argued in this volume that the probability of suicide is often greater during times of stress (e.g., times when negative life events accumulate; Holmes & Rahe, 1967; Yufit & Bongar, Chapter 27; Bonner, Chapter 19), at points of transition (e.g., hospital discharge, a move within a hospital to another room or unit, or incarceration in jail; Litman, Chapter 21; Bonner, Chapter 19; and/or at times of change in general (e.g., improvement in vegetative symptoms before the elevation of a depressed mood, or a dramatic shift in marital status or in social support and living arrangements; Stack, Chapter 26; Maltsberger, Chapter 2).

Finally, Felner et al. (Chapter 20) remind us that we cannot reduce suicide rates simply by treating afflicted individuals (i.e., through secondary and tertiary prevention). Any major improvement in suicide rates will only come through primary prevention in whole populations, societies, and economies *before* individuals have entered into suicidal careers and environments.

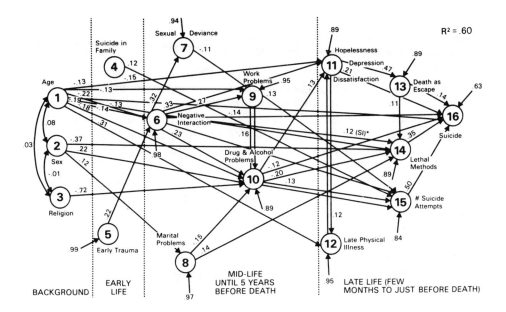

Note: Path 6–14 is from *social isolation* to lethal methods.

FIGURE 32.2. Direct-path coefficients for suicides versus natural deaths. From *Pathways to suicide: A Survey of Self-Destructive Behaviors* (p. 324) by R. W. Maris, 1981, Baltimore: Johns Hopkins University Press. Copyright 1981 by The Johns Hopkins University Press. Reprinted by permission.

THE PROBLEM OF RARE BEHAVIORS

One of the major challenges in attempting to predict suicide is that suicide is a rare occurrence, much like an earthquake (see Pokorny, Chapter 6; Garrison, Chapter 23; Addy, Chapter 11). Predicting individual suicides is like a single toss of a coin. We either get it right or wrong. A person has either died by suicide or is still alive. Thus, suicide prediction seems deceptively like a 50–50 probability game.

However, as we know, suicide in the general population occurs at a rate of only 1–3 per 10,000 per year (not 1 out of 2). The sheer probability is that if we predict "suicide," then we will be wrong almost all the time. In fact, predicting *any* death is difficult, because death itself is rare. Let us assume a crude mean life expectancy of 75 years, and multiply that number by 365 days per year. Such a fictitious person will have 27,375 possible lifetime days. But exactly which day will be his or her death day? It is very hard to say, since only one of those days will be correct. Nonetheless, each day of our lives does not have an equal probability of being our death day. The probability of death becomes greater as a person ages (the same is true for suicidal death), becomes ill or injured, becomes depressed, and so on.

Even individuals in "high-suicide-risk groups" have suicidal outcomes relatively rarely. That is, "high suicide risk" is really a misnomer, since the risk of suicide is not all that high. For example, it is well known that previous nonfatal suicide attempters have a lifetime probability of 15% of dying by suicide. But this is only about 1% in any given year. How much would anyone, even a gambler, be willing to wager on an outcome of 1–15 in 100? As psychiatrist Robert Litman puts it, only 1 or 2 people out of every 100 who enter "the suicide zone" (i.e., who are at acutely high risk for suicide) actually complete suicide (Litman, 1990).

FALSE POSITIVES AND FALSE NEGATIVES

As noted in Chapter 1, when we predict suicide there are four possible outcomes:

1. True positives ("sensitivity")*
2. True negatives ("specificity")
3. False positives
4. False negatives

The true positives plus the false negatives equal all of the suicides, whereas the false positives plus the true negatives equal all the nonsuicides. Ideally, we would like the true positives and the true negatives to approach 100% and the false positives and false negatives to approach 0%. Usually we settle for sensitivity and specificity scores in the 70–80% range—usually a little higher for sensitivity. As sensitivity scores go up, specificity scores tend to go down.

When Pokorny (Chapter 6) actually calculated scores for 4,800 psychiatric inpatients in Houston (67 of whom eventually committed suicide after 5 years), he got the following results:

1. True positives = 55%
2. True negatives = 74%
3. False positives = 30%
4. False negatives = 44%

---

*Sensitivity is actually $(TP/[TP + FN]) \times 100$ and specificity $= (TN/[FP + TN] \times 100$.

His true-positive and true-negative scores for suicides were higher than his false-positive and false-negative scores, but his sensitivity scores were not in the 70–80% range. In fact, Pokorny's suicide predictive value (the proportion of true suicides out of all positive predictions) was only 2.8% over the 5-year period.

Whether we are more concerned about false positives or false negatives generally turns on the relative *costs* of the two outcomes. Since suicide is a rare behavior, prediction usually results in a high number of false positives (Murphy, 1974; Pokorny, Chapter 6; Gould et al., Chapter 7). For example, Pokorny got 1,206 false positives out of 4,641 psychiatric inpatients when he attempted to predict their suicides on the basis of standard high-risk predictors such as those described in Table 1.1, Chapter 1 (about 26% false positives). Clearly, we cannot treat 25–30% of all psychiatric inpatients as if they were at high risk for suicide (e.g., put them in restraints, put them on one-to-one constant 24-hour monitoring, give them large doses of major tranquilizers, put them in seclusion, administer electroconvulsive therapy [ECT], etc.). However, except for economic considerations and the possible stigma arising from false labeling, in a sense false-positive suicides are more harmless than false negatives (in that they do not die).

False negatives include patients who are predicted not to commit suicide, but who in fact do commit suicide. In Pokorny's study, 28 of 63 eventual suicides (over a 5-year period; the samples varied somewhat, depending on exclusion criteria) were *not* predicted (44%). False negatives are especially troubling, since people thought to be relatively safe and at low risk for suicide have nevertheless killed themselves. False negatives include most malpractice cases and the jail and prison suicides. Although treating patients or inmates as if they were not at high risk for suicide is less costly in one sense, we must also consider the insurance, legal, and human costs of such unexpected deaths. False-negative suicides illustrate dramatically how much we have yet to learn about suicide assessment and prediction.

INSTRUMENTS FOR SUICIDE ASSESSMENT AND PREDICTION

Is there a single scale, instrument, or tool that alone gives us accurate suicide assessment and prediction? Unfortunately, there is no such instrument. It follows from our definition of "suicide" as a complex, multidetermined, multidisciplinary phenomenon that tools to indicate suicide will also be multiple and multifaceted and will vary over time. The types of tools or instruments for assessing and predicting suicide that have been reviewed in this volume include the following:

- Specific suicide scales (Rothberg & Geer-Williams, Chapter 10)
- General personality or psychiatric disorder scales (Eyman & Eyman, Chapter 9)
- Specific depression scales (Weishaar & Beck, Chapter 22; see also Marsella, Hirschfeld, & Katz, 1987)
- Biological markers of suicide (Roy, Chapter 28; Brown et al., Chapter 29)
- Psychological autopsy techniques (Clark & Horton-Deutsch, Chapter 8)
- Clinical judgment (Maltsberger, Chapter 2; Stelmachers & Sherman, Chapter 13; Litman, Chapter 21; Motto, Chapter 31)

We conclude that a combination or synthesis of *all* of these instruments is probably the best approach in assessing or predicting suicide. No one instrument or assessment procedure can substitute for any other.

Numerous suicide scales have been examined and applied to our five clinical cases (see especially Table 10.1, Chapter 10). Some of these scales are based on first-person responses (i.e., they are completed by the potential suicides themselves or by clinicians interviewing them). Others are third-person scales completed by examiners, often after a person has died. Among the suicide prediction scales considered in Chapter 10:

- Scale for Assessing Suicide Risk (SASR; Tuckman & Youngman, 1968)
- Los Angeles Suicide Prevention Center Scale (LASPC; Beck, Resnick, & Lettieri, 1974)
- Suicide Intent Scale (SIS; Beck et al., 1974)
- Suicide Death Prediction Scale (SDPS, long and short forms; Lettieri, 1974)
- Index of Potential Suicide (IPS; Zung, 1974)
- Suicide Probability Scale (SPrS; Cull & Gill, 1982)
- Clinical Instrument to Estimate Suicide Risk (CIESR, Motto, Heilbron, & Juster, 1985)
- Suicide Risk Scale (SuRS, Plutchik, van Praag, Conte, & Picard, 1989)

The SDPS (short form) and the CIESR did the best job of predicting outcomes in the five clinical cases (admittedly a small, biased sample). Interestingly, both of these scales are third-person instruments.

None of the general personality or psychiatric disorder instruments, do especially well by themselves in predicting suicide. However, they often provide useful supplementary information helpful in the mental disorder diagnosis and treatment of suicidal clients (see Eyman & Eyman, Chapter 9, for a full discussion). Psychological testing of potential suicides (and occasionally of completed suicides) often includes some of the following instruments:

- the MMPI (Graham, 1990; Hathaway & McKinley, 1943)
- the Thematic Apperception Test (TAT; Murray, 1943)
- the Rorschach (Rorschach, 1942/1981)
- the Schedule for Affective Disorders and Schizophrenia (SADS; Spitzer & Endicott, 1979)
- the Diagnostic Interview Schedule (DIS; Robins, Helzer, Croughan, & Ratcliff, 1981)
- DSM-III-R codes and/or the Structured Clinical Interview for DSM-III-R (SCID; Spitzer, Williams, Gibbon, & First, 1990)
- and many others

One can also test potential suicides specifically with depression and/or hopelessness scales, although the correlation of depression and hopelessness with suicide or suicide intent is far from perfect. Common instruments include the Beck Depression Inventory (BDI; Beck, Ward, Mendelson, Mock, & Erbaugh, 1961), the Hamilton Depression Rating Scale (Hamilton, 1960), and the Beck Hopelessness Scale (BHS; Beck, Weissman, Lester, & Trexler, 1974; Beck, Steer, Kovacs, & Garrison, 1985; Marsella et al., 1987). In one empirical test, hopelessness had a stronger positive association with suicide intent than did depression (Kovacs, Beck, & Weissman, 1975). This relationship is not true for all subgroups, such as black male teenagers.):

	Hopelessness (Beck Hopelessness Scale)	Depression (Beck Depression Inventory)	Wish to live
Depression	+.68	—	—
Wish to live	−.74	−.57	—
Suicide intent		+.57	−.76
(current)	+.68		

Of course, most depressed or hopeless individuals never commit suicide.

There are some biological markers of suicide (Roy, Chapter 28; Brown et al., Chapter 29; Mann & Stanley, 1988; Maris, 1986, & 1991). Perhaps the most widely recognized of these biological indicators are low levels of the serotonin metabolite hydroxyindoleacetic acid (5-HIAA) in cerebrospinal fluid. However, like most biological indicators, 5-HIAA is not predictive of suicidal behaviors alone. For example, it is related to other, nonsuicidal aggressive behaviors (van Praag, Plutchik, & Apter, 1990). Many of the biological correlates of suicide (such as the dexamethasone suppression test) are in fact indicators not of suicide per se, but of affective disorders or depressive illness. As we have seen, depressive illness and suicide have a complex, imperfect association.

After someone completes suicide, a valuable general procedure is the psychological autopsy (Clark & Horton-Deutsch, Chapter 8). The psychological autopsy consists of intensive retrospective interview(s) and data collection, designed to reconstruct the psychosocial features and circumstances surrounding the death of an individual (especially, the manner of nonnatural deaths). The psychological autopsy is not standardized and does not consist of any one questionnaire or form. It is particularly helpful in providing evidence of a deceased person's intent to commit suicide after the person is obviously unavailable for interview (Brent, Perper, Kolko, & Zelenak, 1988).

Finally, it has been argued in this book that suicide prediction and assessment tools always need to be tempered with clinical judgment (Motto, Chapter 31; Litman, Chapter 21; Maltsberger, Chapter 2). At the risk of lapsing into mysticism, what do we do if we simply do not trust or believe what suicide prediction instruments tell us? Motto (Chapter 31) recommends resolving conflicts of various instruments or of instruments and clinical judgment by trusting clinical judgment. After all, most scales and procedures are rigid, static, and mechanical. They are usually not flexible, or specific enough for many individual suicide prediction cases or circumstances. Of course, the problem here is that there are also bad clinicians with poor insight and inferior training. Thus, clinical judgment is not always the answer to our suicide prediction problems. Furthermore, we should follow science as far as it will take us.

Thus, we have now come full circle. Suicide assessment is properly a synthesis of scientific procedures and clinical insight. We should not forget, either, that instruments that help us assess or predict suicide need to be grounded in theory (see Shneidman, Chapter 3; Felner et al., Chapter 20; Yufit & Bongar, Chapter 27; de Catanzaro, Chapter 30; Maltsberger, Chapter 2). Without systematic theories of suicidal behaviors over the human life cycle, we literally would not know what to measure or how predictors of suicide might be interrelated.

CASE OUTCOMES

We now return to discuss the five case studies that have served as focal points for each chapter author to apply his or her expertise. We will attempt to summarize their commentaries within the framework of both the case material presented to chapter authors and the case outcomes not previously known to the authors.

Case 1: Heather B

Heather B's case is perhaps the richest among the five presented, since psychological test data are available to us. Extensive analyses have been provided by the Eymans (Chapter 9) and Leenaars (Chapter 16), who have focused in this volume on data available from psychological tests and personal documents, respectively. Several other chapter authors also discuss Heather's suicide risk, but from their more specific viewpoints. The resulting evaluations of Heather's suicide risk have the greatest variability among the five cases presented.

Stelmachers and Sherman (Chapter 13) conclude that Heather was more likely to be self-injurious than suicidal. They base this evaluation on the context within which Heather's ideation occurred (i.e., the absence both of a plan and of vegetative signs of depression). Rothberg and Geer-Williams (Chapter 10) rate Heather as having the lowest risk of the five cases presented. Tanney (Chapter 14) agrees, suggesting that the diagnosis he assigns to Heather of adjustment disorder (with mixed disturbances of emotions and conduct) is more likely to indicate nonfatal suicidal behavior than completed suicide. Clark and Horton-Deutsch (Chapter 8), on the other hand, express much greater concern about suicide; they make a diagnosis of comorbid affective and conduct disorders with an episode of major depression. Stack (Chapter 26), noting Heather's age cohort and the loss of her father (rather than a more acute familial loss, such as divorce), appears to agree with Tanney that her risk at the time of her presentation for treatment was low. However, he is concerned that her low family attachment/integration and her negative life experiences would predispose her to increased risk as she grew into her later teens. de Catanzaro (Chapter 30) similarly warns us that more criticism and social alienation might increase Heather's sense of burdensomeness, potentially outweighing her positive reproductive potential. He, however, is more optimistic that treatment ("guidance and appreciation") and positive family events would promote her future potential, including movement away from suicidality.

Weishaar and Beck (Chapter 22) note warning signs posed by Heather's behavior, cognitions, and affect, precipitated by the death of her father and the consequent familial instability. They presume a low score on the Beck Self-Concept Test and observe statements of hopelessness in her writings, in addition to her ideation and hints of self-injury; they conclude that more evaluation would be warranted. Similarly, Clark and Horton-Deutsch (Chapter 8) note that Heather's ideation, recent history of self-injury, marked anguish, anhedonia, and *severe* functional impairment in response to the comorbid diagnoses would warrant an evaluation of "high suicide risk," particularly in the context of her mother's minimizing the seriousness of her risk.

Yufit and Bongar (Chapter 27) also express greater concern for Heather's suicide potential, observing her "inability to maintain inner connections," self-condemnation, test themes of destruction, a desire for isolation, and few coping abilities. Leenaars (Chapter 16) sounds perhaps the loudest warning bell in applying his Thematic Guide for Suicide Prediction (TGSP) to Heather's test material. His analysis results in positive findings on 28 of 35 protocol sentences, 18 of 23 referring to specific highly predictive variables and 14 of 17 referring to a specific differentiating variable. He appropriately cautions us, however, that the TGSP has yet to be sufficiently tested to differentiate different groups of suicidal patients and behaviors; to establish norms, reliability, and validity; and so on.

Given their focus on psychological test data, Eyman and Eyman (Chapter 9) have the most complete slides to place under the microscope of psychological test analysis. Indeed, their evaluation is the richest in this volume. It is an excellent example of the value of psychological test material in the hands of competent interpreters, and highlights the value to the clinician of having as full and complete a picture as possible when approaching the task of risk evaluation. The absence of such a picture—in other words, the relatively limited amount of case material presented—is what restricts most of our chapter authors in making their evaluations of suicide risk.

The Eymans find sufficient projective evidence for two of the four variables they associate with suicide risk—a defensive stance toward aggression, and high self-expectations. Correspondingly, they do not find signs of dependent yearnings counteracted in Heather's behavior or a wish to escape intolerable pain through death. They describe Heather, quite appropriately, as struggling with unresolved mourning for her father, consequently sensitive and reactive to perceived rejection and abandonment, and parading her attitude toward death and self-injury as a communication of distress and a wish to retaliate. Although she was "at risk for some type of suicidal behavior," they further note a number of mitigating factors, such as her hopefulness and social relatedness, which reduced the seriousness of her risk at the time of evaluation.

These two points are worth iterating. All evaluations of risk are temporal, reflecting imminent (acute) versus long-term (chronic) possibilities or probabilities. We observe at a specific moment in time, but we make evaluations regarding these observations and the possibility of suicidal behavior at some future time. Second, given that no case ever presents itself in such a way as to permit an evaluation with absolute certitude, each and every case must be evaluated for both risk *and* protective factors. Thus, an evaluation of low risk now may turn into high risk when precipitated by unexpected and stressful events, given sufficient predisposing conditions and insufficient protective factors. As noted in Chapter 12 within the frame of several caveats mentioned, one value of the case method is that the authors' and the readers' evaluations of suicide risk can be juxtaposed to what we know actually happened in each case; this allows us either to validate our evaluations or to correct our misimpressions, as well as to rationalize or otherwise defend our false assumptions and conclusions.

What do we know of Heather's outcome? Having been referred by her mother, Heather entered outpatient psychotherapy jointly with her mother, ostensibly to work on increasing her compliance and decreasing her provocative behaviors at home. No less important as treatment goals were those of increasing her sense of appreciation, reinforcement, and belonging while allowing her an opportunity to explore, ventilate about, and correct the negative impact of her father's death on her family and herself. Heather was seen by her therapist as in mourning and depressed, feeling isolated and alienated; her thoughts were perceived as confused and self-deprecatory; her behavior was seen as both provocative and protective in commanding the attention of her remaining parent. Suicide risk may be modified by risk evaluation. When treatment is entered into, complied with, and competently given as a result of an evaluation, it may significantly alter a life course that is in danger of ending prematurely. At this writing, 4 years after she was evaluated and began treatment, Heather is a high school senior and reports no further self-injurious behavior.

Case 2: Ralph F

Ralph F exhibited a number of predisposing risk factors (Clark & Horton-Deutsch, Chapter 8). He had persistent suicide ideation and a plan; anhedonia, despair, and current homicidal rage; a recent inpatient hospitalization; a recent exposure to a completed suicide; and recent mood-congruent auditory hallucinations. In a context of parental marital conflict and consequent loss of support, and dual diagnoses of substance use and affective disorders, Ralph's risk is described in Chapter 8 as "extremely high." Tanney (Chapter 14) concurs, noting that the psychotic features and substance abuse "add to the risk already associated with major depressive disorder." Tanney, however, reminds us that Axis III diagnoses of physical disease further increase risk.

These themes are echoed by other authors, who appear to differ only in the degree of risk estimated in the short verus the long term. For example, Rothberg and Geer-Williams (Chapter 10) estimate Ralph's risk as high in the short term but moderate in the long term. Lester (Chapter 15) reverses these ratings, evidencing greater concern about long-term risk. In general, however, Ralph is viewed as at high risk. Weishaar and Beck (Chapter 22) provide a long list of clinical risk factors to document their view that Ralph had serious suicide potential. Yufit and Bongar (Chapter 27) point to Ralph's anxiety, guilt, and hopelessness as increasing vulnerability. de Catanzaro (Chapter 30) adds to this list of concerns that Ralph showed signs of self-preservation failure, social isolation (also noted by Stack, Chapter 26), and premature senesecence—factors leading to decreased reproductive potential, and thereby to increased suicide risk. Lastly, Litman (Chapter 21), who describes Ralph's risk as chronic and high, recommends a number of treatment strategies and objectives designed to ameliorate psychopathology (Alcoholics Anonymous and antidepressants), to reduce lethality (elimination of guns from the home), to change family dynamics (school placement), and to provide an increased understanding of Ralph's dynamics (psychological testing).

After appearing for follow-up outpatient psychotherapy 1 week after discharge from the hospital, Ralph then failed to keep his subsequent two scheduled appointments. Fifteen days after his discharge from the hospital, Ralph overdosed on his antidepressant medication, went into a 17-day coma, and finally died. His suicide note, addressed to his family, read as follows:

> Please forgive me. I'm sorry for the pain I've caused, and now it will end. I know this will hurt, but what would hurt more, this or seeing me in a straight-jacket in a padded room, staring into space or screaming? I don't want to put you all through that. I love you too much. I have one request, *be a family!*
>
> Heaven bound,
> Ralph

Case 3: John Z

The value of the case study method and the idiosyncratic approach to risk assessment is highlighted by Stelmachers and Sherman's (Chapter 13) comments on the case of John Z. They write that John was "arguably the most imminently suicidal" of the five cases presented, "but would receive the lowest rating" if only a rating scale approach were used. These authors note, in particular, the quality and severity of John's depression, in addition to the sequence and progression of events precipitating the request by his wife for a second opinion regarding his need for hospitalization. In contrast to Stelmachers and Sherman's observation about rating scales, the application of such scales by Rothberg and Geer-Williams (Chapter 10) leads them to make an evaluation of high risk, more so in the long term than the short term. They argue that the SAD PERSONS "suggests strongly considering hospitalization."

In agreement with Stelmachers and Sherman, the severity of John's depression is noted by Tanney (Chapter 14), who rates this patient's suicide risk as high, and by Clark and Horton-Deutsch (Chapter 8), who describe John as having a major depressive episode with panic attacks. In a context of two serious and recent suicide attempts and low compliance, Clark and Horton-Deutsch believe that John's suicide risk was extremely high, and state that they would recommend immediate hospitalization. McIntosh's (Chapter 18) singular focus on methods reminds us that John's self-reported first attempt by plastic bag, if his report could be verified, would be associated with a high risk for future suicide completion.

Noting John's depression and past attempts, Weishaar and Beck (Chapter 22) summarize relevant additional risk factors (immediate stressors, negative self-concept, family history of suicide attempts), particularly observing that suicide intent increases with repeated attempts. Stack (Chapter 26) also sees John's history as indicative of high suicide risk. Similarly, Yufit and Bongar (Chapter 27) describe John's increased self-absorption, loss of connectedness to job and work accomplishment, and decreased trust and hope as significant factors of risk. The combination of John's depression and panic with his nonresponsiveness to 5 months of outpatient treatment, his suicide ideation and attempts, and his noncompliance with recommendations of voluntary hospitalization prompts Litman (Chapter 21) to make the strongest statement regarding John's suicide risk and need for intervention. Litman notes that he would "move forcefully" toward hospitalization, placing John on observation, on antidepressant medication (and even ECT, if necessary), and in inpatient therapy, including job counseling. de Cantanzaro (Chapter 30) also sees re-employability as crucial to John's future decreased risk. He describes an acute loss of contribution to family and society, and the consequent transformation of felt worth into burdensomeness.

To borrow from Tanney's approach at summarization in Chapter 14, the "box score" on John's suicide risk is considerably less contradictory than that on Heather's. In fact, our authors are remarkably consistent in observing John to be high in suicide risk, both imminently and over the longer term if no significant therapeutic intervention were accomplished. Unfortunately, the clinician consulted by John's wife for the second opinion on her husband's need for hospitalization was apparently not so alarmed as to force immediate hospitalization. In spite of John's history of not complying with recommendations, this clinician trusted the patient's promise that he would voluntarily hospitalize himself the next day after taking care of "some odds and ends." On these grounds, John was allowed to go home in the care of his wife. John also promised his wife the next morning that he would be ready to go to the hospital that afternoon. He sent her to work for the morning and promptly retreated to his basement, where he hanged himself.

Case 4: Faye C

The case of Faye C appears to have been somewhat difficult for the chapter authors to view with consistency when making their ratings of risk. What is evident is that the case information provided is insufficiently precise for most to establish a clear picture. Thus, ratings exhibit a considerable range: "very high" (Rothberg & Geer-Williams, Chapter 10); "high" (Stack, Chapter 26); "moderate" (Clark & Horton-Deutsch, Chapter 8); "mild" and "chronic" (Litman, Chapter 21); and "low" to "high," depending upon the diagnosis (Tanney, Chapter 14.

Tanney suspects Faye was suffering from paranoid schizophrenia (Axis I) with temporal lobe epilepsy (Axis III). He further argues that the schizophrenia had had a subchronic course, had been well compensated for, and existed comorbidly with a long-standing depressive adaptation. Faye's temporal lobe epilepsy, according to Tanney, exacerbated Faye's suicide risk. Stelmachers and Sherman (Chapter 13) see Faye as "floridly psychotic" and anxious about the future. Although there is no mention of suicide ideation in the case description, Weishaar and Beck (Chapter 22) describe her as "vulnerable to ideation" because of her depression and psychosis. In this vein, Stelmachers and Sherman go on to suggest that suicide, to Faye, appeared as an escape from future torment.

The absence of current ideation and recent suicidal behavior, and the fact that her symptoms of psychosis were currently florid, serve to attenuate Clark and Horton-Deutsch's rating of Faye's risk, which would otherwise be of concern because of her level of anxiety, psychopathology (schizophrenic and delusional, depressed, and epileptic), insomnia, and poverty of interpersonal relationships. Stack focuses as well on Faye's low level of social integration (marital and familial). As a single, middle-aged woman, Faye was within a high-risk demographic group. Yufit and Bongar (Chapter 27), on the other hand, while observing her lack of connectedness to her therapist, suggest that Faye was overdependent on her family and had no developed sense of autonomy.

Rothberg and Geer-Williams (Chapter 10), estimating that Faye would have a "greater than 10% expectation of death within 2 years," strongly emphasize the need for hospitalization. Litman (Chapter 21) concurs, arguing that brief hospitalization would be called for, including the need for antipsychotic medication. He expresses concern that her risk for suicide would increase if she were left with a sense of helplessness and totally exposed to her fears and projections. Three sets of observations regarding risk have particular significance in light of the outcome of Faye's case. First are the comments by Litman and by Rothberg and Geer-Williams, which underscore the importance of treatment in the course of a suicidal patient's life (or death). Second is a comment by Clark and Horton-Deutsch, who refer to research (Drake, Gates, Whitaker, & Cotton, 1985) suggesting that the suicide risks of schizophrenics increases when their psychotic symptoms abate and depressive symptoms come to the fore. Third are the observations of several authors who express concern for Faye's social isolation.

Faye was evaluated at the emergency room and determined to be in need of inpatient hospitalization. She was admitted for psychiatric care, and had a predictable response to medication and various therapies designed to ameliorate her psychotic symptoms. As the end of her insurance coverage (30 days of inpatient care) approached, discussions were begun regarding discharge. Only retrospectively was it apparent that inadequate attention was given during this phase of her treatment to her fears about leaving the hospital for a world of relative isolation and to her underlying depression; perhaps these factors went unnoticed because she had responded ostensibly to antipsychotic medication and seemed much less floridly symptomatic. Two days before her planned discharge, Faye eloped from the hospital and threw herself from a city bridge to her death.

Case 5: José G

The case of José G reads like the typical worker's compensation case. His injury on the job led to subsequent depression, complicated by heavy alcohol use; his lack of improvement resulted in feelings of burdensomeness, worthlessness, and hopelessness; and his suicidality increased. But what of his potential to *act* in a self-destructive manner?

Stelmachers and Sherman (Chapter 13) appropriately remind us that stresses and stressors have to be understood in context. A myocardial infarction suffered by an elderly man with no means of support, both financial and interpersonal, will have a very different impact than would a myocardial infarction suffered by a man in his prime, with financial resources and a loving spouse capable of shouldering the various burdens of recovery. José was a self-sufficient, proud, autonomous character. Several of the chapter authors (Stack, Yufit & Bongar, de Catanzaro, Litman) have remarked that José's injury, disability, and consequent unemployment led to a forced retirement for a man who was more deeply committed to his work than perhaps to his marriage. Stelmachers and Sherman see José as a defeated man. Weishaar and Beck (Chapter 22) describe multiple losses (of job, health, and pleasure), in predicting high scores on scales of both depression and hopelessness. de Catanzaro (Chapter 30) frames these losses in terms of an "acute loss of ability to contribute." The result, as he sees it, was an increasing sense of worthlessness, "senescence," and depression.

As if this were not enough to cope with, José had multiple physical problems (diabetes mellitus, a diabetes-related visual disorder, and emphysema). Perhaps under normal circumstances he might have dealt with these in stride, but in José's situation these had to potentiate his sense of decline and hopelessness. And to complicate matters, he turned to alcohol, which only further potentiated his depression (see Lester, Chapter 15).

Tanney (Chapter 14) views José's presenting symptoms, outlined well by Clark and Horton-Deutsch (Chapter 8), as diagnostic of major depression and of a substance use disorder. There seems to be little to dispute in this characterization. Among male adolescents, the comorbid presentation of these two diagnoses is pathognomic of significant risk for suicide (Berman & Jobes, 1991). Perhaps among older males, the greater frequency of these diagnoses in the general population makes them less at risk for suicide, at least as determined by scaling techniques. Rothberg and Geer-Williams (Chapter 10), in their application of rating scales to José's case, indicate only a moderate to low risk for mortality by suicide. In contrast, several other authors (Tanney, Stack, Clark) rate José's suicide risk as high.

Litman (Chapter 21), who clearly is concerned, also sees a positive balance in José's history of resourcefulness and industry and in his supportive family. He posits a number of recommendations for his psychological and physical rehabilitation, none of which were either suggested or instituted in José's case. Instead, José felt (and ostensibly was) abandoned and betrayed by his employers and his doctors. Litman wonders whether anyone asked about the possibility of suicide, and in particular whether anyone asked about José's gun, a weapon of great lethality in the hands of a depressed drinker. No one did. José spent the last day of his life with his wife, visiting his son and family. It appears retrospectively that his son's announcement that he was leaving the next day to take a job with the railroad was what precipitated subsequent events. José soon wanted to return home, hours before he and his wife had originally planned. At his insistence they left and drove home in silence; once home, they parted—he to a six-pack of beer, she to some household chores. José drank close to two six-packs in approximately a 3-hour period and then put his gun to his head, ending his life with a single pull of the trigger.

In the end, what is most striking is how evident José's suicide potential should have been. As the typical adult suicide completer is described by Maris (Chapter 17), he is a male troubled by physical problems, isolated, struggling with some job-related situation, depressed and genuinely hopeless, using alcohol, and likely to use a gun; under this combination of circumstances, the first attempt has almost a 90% chance of being fatal.

IMPLICATIONS FOR TREATMENT
AND SUICIDE PREVENTION

Of course, the assessment and prediction of suicide should not be a sterile, self-contained game, unrelated to treatment and suicide prevention (cf.

Blumenthal & Kupfer, 1990, p. 710). Most of the time, suicide assessment and prediction are carried out in the service of suicide prevention. Even though a proper examination of suicide prevention issues would require yet another book, we would be derelict in our duty not to consider treatment at all.

The general assessment and treatment records of the potentially suicidal patient or client (most commonly an inpatient in a psychiatric hospital or psychiatric unit in a general hospital) usually involves the following components:

- Intake assessment and admission summary
- Nursing assessment
- Physical examination
- Social and family history
- Psychological testing
- Treatment plan and treatment team notes
- Doctor's orders
- Interdisciplinary progress notes
- Drug administration record
- Laboratory reports, neurological records, and so forth
- Sleep, eating, vital signs charts
- Other therapy notes (occupational, recreation, etc.)
- Discharge summary

Clearly, we cannot discuss all of these components here or in detail, but some of the items more specifically relevant to suicide assessment deserve elaboration.

The intake assessment and admission summary by the attending psychiatrist generally states the patient's chief complaint(s) or presenting problem; a provisional DSM-III-R (or, in the near future, DSM-IV) mental disorder diagnosis and code; current and prior psychotropic medications; prior hospitalizations; results of a mental status exam; an initial treatment plan; and first doctor's orders, including medications. Obviously, this initial encounter of physician, patient, staff, and hospital environment is critical. Even though it is provisional, the admitting diagnosis needs to be both accurate and thorough, since effective treatment depends upon correct diagnosis. If possible, a multiaxial diagnosis should be given, with any suspected comorbidity or alternative diagnoses to be ruled out being listed as well (although Tanney, Chapter 14, argues that Axis I-III codes/information are sufficient). It must be remembered that suicide is not a mental disorder itself, although suicidal behaviors are part of the criteria for diagnoses of major depressive episode (296.2X) and borderline personality disorder (301.83). The listing of prior and current medications often suggests that what has worked before should be tried again, at least initially.

If the presenting problem or chief complaint involves self-destructive ideation or behaviors or explicit suicide attempts, or if the admitting diagnosis includes one of the affective disorders, some schizophrenias, panic attacks, or some personality disorders (especially borderline or sociopathic), than a much more specific suicide assessment is warranted. Many hospitals routinely ask detailed questions about suicide ideation or behavior in either the physician intake assessment or the nursing intake assessment. Common questions concern prior suicide attempts; current suicidal ideas; and specific suicidal plans, including the anticipated method and when and under what circumstances the suicide attempt would take place. Of course, patients are not always truthful or clear-headed about their suicide intentions, and circumstances do change. Thus, a clinician cannot rely too heavily on answers to direct questions about a patient's suicidality, including suicide contracts a patient may make. But clinicians can rest assured that if one of their patients should commit suicide and they have *not* asked about suicide and written the response down in the medical records, they will wish they had. The intake evaluation, in which physician–patient rapport is established, is crucial. Many indirect indications of suicidality and assurances of the physician's willingness and ability to cope with the patient's suicidal ideation or behaviors turn on the doctor's being and being seen as concerned and capable.

If there is some indication of a suicide problem, a psychiatrist will want to assess the need for some sort of suicide precautions (see Litman, Chapter 21). Almost every hospital has a policy and procedural manual in which various types of actual or probable self-destructive behaviors are linked to two or three levels of precautions. Suicide watches vary from 24-hour, (i.e., "constant") within-arms'-reach, one-to-one supervision (for acute suicide probability, often based on a prior explicit suicide attempt) to 15-, 30-, or 60-minute logged observations (usually for patients who have suicidal ideas or behaviors, but are not thought to be imminently suicidal). Normally, the constant and 15-minute logged watches will take place on a locked ward or in a seclusion room (like an intensive care unit); that is, the suicide watch includes elopement precautions. Seclusion should be used judiciously (especially in jails; see Bonner, Chapter 19). Unless a patient or inmate is violent, aggressive, or agitated, the cause of suicide prevention is routinely better served by the would-be suicide's having a roommate or cellmate. In our forensic practice, there have been numerous cases in which patients or inmates completed suicide while their roommates or cellmates were away (e.g., on a home pass or having tests done).

In some very limited and controlled circumstances, physical restraints may need to be considered. Usually these conditions are specified in a clinic's policy and procedure manual. Restraints can include one- to five-point (the four limbs and the head) restrictions or drug/chemical restraints for highly agitated, psychotic, or aggressive patients. Restraints should be used only for short, specific time periods with 24-hour logged observation. We have had several patients even request to be put in restraints to keep from hurting themselves or others. However, Dr. Maltsberger is of the opinion that physical restraints should almost never be used with suicidal patients. Of course, sharp, dangerous, or protruding objects will also have to be removed from the person and place.

Unfortunately, it only takes 4 or 5 minutes of adequate pressure on the carotid arteries in a person's neck to produce death by oxygen deprivation to the brain. Thus, in our experience 15-minute suicide watches tend to allow a patient sufficient time to commit suicide, especially if the patient has a private bathroom with a lockable door. Almost any article of clothing and any protruding object can be utilized for self-asphyxiation. For example, a T-shirt sleeve over a door knob, with the neck of the shirt left on while the patient leans forward, will do the job (other actual forensic cases have included lowering an electric bed on one's throat; forcing three cellophane-wrapped dinner rolls down one's throat; and swallowing the leg of one's jogging pants, then immersing one's head in a toilet). Such hanging or asphyxiation deaths often occur during hospital or jail shift changes or during other kinds of changes (moving from one unit to another, going on leave or returning from a leave, coming off suicide precautions, experiencing a decrease in vegetative symptoms of depression [sleep, appetite, libido, etc.] before depressive mood lifts, etc.)

Medications for potentially suicidal clients need to be considered carefully. It is well known that many psychiatric patients attempt suicide by overdosing on the very drugs prescribed to treat their depressions, anxieties, psychoses, sleeplessness, or other symptoms. Psychiatrists need to be circumspect about giving patients large numbers of pills or refillable prescriptions. In a psychiatric hospital, a physician has to decide carefully when to medicate; how long to wait before starting drug treatment; of course, what drugs to use for which patients (here again, accurate diagnosis is critical); when to discontinue, reduce, increase, or change medications; what the potential interactions and side effects of medications are; and what dosages a particular patient should be on. In the discussion of drugs that follows we realize that simply listing different antidepressants and antipsychotics may be simplistic. However, this section is intended as a general overview, not an individualized psychoactive drug treatment plan. Psychopharmacologists are responsible for the complicated fine tuning of psychotropic medications for individual patients.

Since suicide rates are highest for individuals having one of the affective disorders, usually suicidal patients will be on one or more antidepressant drugs. These include heterocyclics, such as amitriptyline (Elavil), amoxapine (Asendin), doxepin (Sinequan), imipramine (Tofranil), and nortriptyline (Pamelor); less commonly the monoamine oxidase (MAO) inhibitors, such as isocarboxazid (Marplan), phenelzine (Nardil), and tranylcypromine

(Parnate); sometimes serotonin-specific agents, such as fluoxetine (Prozac), and trazadone (Desyrel); sometimes the benzodiazepine alprazolam (Xanax); and for manic–depressive illness, lithium carbonate (Eskalith, Lithobid, Lithane). If none of these antidepressant medications alleviate the patient's depression, or if the physician cannot wait for them to work (often over several weeks), ECT may be utilized (see Tanney, 1986).

Prozac is now the most widely prescribed antidepressant drug in the world (in 1990 Prozac had an 18.9% market share, followed by 7.9% for Pamelor and 3.3% for Desyrel; Cowley, Springen, Leonard, Robins, & Gordon, 1990). It is a powerful and unusual antidepressant, with few of the side effects of the heterocyclics or MAO inhibitors. However, it is not without controversy. Martin Teicher at Harvard had six of his depressed patients develop intense, violent suicidal preoccupations after 2–7 weeks of Prozac (Teicher, Glod, & Cole, 1990). It should be noted that five of Teicher's six patients had considered suicide *before* taking Prozac, and that only a very small percentage of patients on Prozac ever commit suicide. Prozac and Desyrel relieve depression by blocking postsynaptic reuptake of the neurotransmitter serotonin (Cooper, 1988).

Many would-be suicides are often highly agitated or manic, and sometimes they are delusional, hallucinatory, or otherwise psychotic. Thus, a psychiatrist also may need to consider an antipsychotic drug with an antidepressant drug. When extreme agitation or psychosis coexists with an affective disorder, the therapist has to assess whether or not to treat both simultaneously, and if not, which disorder to treat first. In general it is inappropriate to withhold antidepressant drugs from depressed patients who are psychotic. Sometimes a therapist can place an inpatient on suicide precautions in the controlled environment of a psychiatric hospital, and wait a few days before starting *any* psychiatric medication.

However, in most cases potential suicides who are psychotic or otherwise agitated will be started at hospital admission on a high-potency antipsychotic such as haloperidol (Haldol), usually at an initial dosage of 0.5 to 2 mg twice or three times a day. Doses can be much higher for extreme agitation—up to 100 mg (of Haldol) per day in otherwise healthy young people. Similar high-potency antipsychotics include thiothixene (Navane), trifluoperazine (Stelazine), and fluphenazine (Prolixin). Of course, one must attend to extrapyramidal side effects in administering high-potency antipsychotic drugs. These include involuntary posturing (dystonia); restlessness (akathisia); and muscular rigidity, tremors, and shuffling gait (parkinsonianism). Often such drugs as trihexyphenidyl (Artane) and benztropine (Cogentin) are prescribed to combat side effects of antipsychotics. When Haldol is used with some antidepressant drugs, anticholinergic effects (dry mouth, blurred vision, constipation) may be exacerbated.

Low-potency antipsychotics, such as chlorpromazine (Thorazine), thioridazine (Mellaril), and chlorprothixene (Taractan), are used for their sedative effects, but they can lower blood pressure dangerously. Finally, one may consider antipsychotic drugs of intermediate potency, such as perphenazine (Trilafon), loxapine (Loxitane), or the relatively new antipsychotic clozapine (Clozaril). Clozaril may work for treatment-resistant psychoses and does not cause tardive dyskinesia; however, it is expensive and can cause seizures and agranulcytosis (failure of the body to produce certain white blood cells that fight infection).

Finally, many suicidal patients will have been prescribed benzodiazepines, such as Xanax, diazepam (Valium), chlordiazepoxide (Librium), triazolam (Halcion), and flurazepam (Dalmane), for anxiety, insomnia, and/or panic disorder (although imipramine [Tofranil] is more common for panic disorders; see American Psychiatric Association, 1990). Since the benzodiazepines can cause depression, hostility, and paradoxical rage reactions, their use with potentially suicidal individuals needs to be monitored closely. Special suicide concerns have been voiced in connection with the benzodiazepine hypnotic Halcion, which has an ultrashort half-life (1.5 to 5.5 hours) and can produce severe withdrawal effects (Latimer, 1980; Lasagna, 1990). These can include angry outbursts, assaultiveness (even murder), anterograde amnesia, depression, suicidal ideation, delirium, and rebound insomnia. It must be remembered that benzodiazepines used in conjunction with alcohol or barbiturates can severely depress respiration.

Space permitting, we could profitably go into many other details relating suicide assessment to suicide prevention. Unfortunately, only a few broad, cryptic suggestions are possible. First, clinicians should do assessments and histories promptly, by the time specified in the hospital's policy and procedure manual. Nursing assessments of suicide potential are often more objective and thorough than physician assessments (complete with scales and standardized procedures). Second, treatment team meetings, decisions, and notes can protect and check the physician/psychiatrist. Treatment team meetings should be documented carefully, including who was in attendance. Third, clinicians should review the vital sign records and the sleep and eating charts for signs of changes in vegetative symptoms of depression. Improvements before depressive affect or mood lifts should be noted with caution, as they often indicate increased suicide vulnerability. Fourth, interdisciplinary progress notes are an extremely valuable record of a patient's detailed course in treatment. They should be complete, should make liberal use of verbatim patient quotes, and should utilize a "SOAP" categorization of comments (viz., "subjective, objective, assessment, and plan"). Fifth, clinicians should be especially attentive to suicide risk at times of changes (e.g., shift changes, mealtimes, coming and going from passes, movement from one level of security to another, holidays, etc.). Sixth, the physician/psychiatrist should write a thorough discharge summary in each case and do it promptly, especially if there was a completed suicide. In the case of a suicide, the activities and care of the patient in the last hours of his or her life (including any resuscitation procedures, etc.) should be described in exquisite detail. Who did what, when, and so on? Was there a postmortem or psychological autopsy? Were there any changes in policy, architecture, or the like as a result of the suicide? Finally, all clinicians should be sure to be familiar with their institution's policy and procedure manual.

It should be noted that the general assessment of the potentially suicidal patient or client on an outpatient basis should include attention to the same components listed above for inpatients, except for those aspects obviously specific to inpatient care (e.g., nursing assessment, occupational therapy notes, etc.). Unlike for hospital psychiatric units, outpatient practices rarely have policy and procedure manuals. However, given increasingly frequent malpractice suits, outpatient practitioners would be well advised to develop written policies regarding their procedures for assessing suicide risk, providing treatment, ensuring the patient's safety, and making referrals for hospitalization. In framing the presenting problems and developing an appropriate treatment plan, particular effort should be made to secure records of prior treatment(s) and evaluations of past treatment compliance. Few cases of outpatient suicide appear in malpractice case law; nevertheless, the practitioner should not be lulled into believing that there are but a few of these cases. The overwhelming majority of suits are settled, often at the last moment before trial, but they still leave a trail of painful experiences and considerable expense for the practitioner. Thus, the reasonably prudent outpatient practitioner needs to attend to issues of assessment, treatment planning, and implementation with the same rigor and documentation more often associated with inpatient institutional settings.

It should be obvious that suicide assessment is integral to suicide treatment and prevention. These interrelations are perhaps most evident when there is a complaint alleging malpractice. The alleged ability of the clinician to have foreseen a patient's suicide is the most fundamental issue in such a complaint. Questions regarding reasonable care and its implementation can only arise within the context of assessed risk. Thus, the typical claim will allege "failure to diagnose and safeguard," or "failure to recognize a patient's suicide tendencies and to take precautionary measures to protect the patient." Space does not permit us to provide detailed risk management strategies. However, the reader is referred to published guidelines (Berman and Cohen-Sandler, 1983; Bongar, 1991).

Finally, an important caveat: Any treatment of a suicidal patient that relies on impersonal means alone (e.g., the prescription of psychoactive medication, seclusion, restraint, checks, etc.) is second rate. Suicidal patients have been treated without medications (for instance, before they were available), and without electroconvulsive therapy, often with fairly good results. The heart of treatment is the relationship with the therapist. The suicidal patient is not receiving adequate care unless he or she is provided with a psychotherapeutic relationship that offers support, accessibility, investigation of the patient's current life impasse, and close monitoring of the patient's mood shifts.

CONCLUSION: A GENERAL MODEL
OF SUICIDAL BEHAVIOR

At the risk of oversimplifying or otherwise misrepresenting the complexities detailed in the preceding pages of this volume, we conclude with a general model of suicidal behavior. We believe that there is a need for theory to guide research; we should not settle for isolated "facts," empirical generalizations, or even hypotheses. Colleagues who have written similar treatises seem to be in agreement with the desirability of postulating general causal models of suicide (see, e.g., Blumenthal & Kupfer, 1990, p. 721, and van Praag et al., 1990, p. 60). Furthermore, any theory of suicide needs to encompass the lifespan, or what Maris calls the "suicidal career" (Maris, 1991a).

Figure 32.3 presents our general model of suicide. Among other characteristics, our model includes the following:

• The four major domains involved in suicide assessment and prediction (see Figure 32.1, above). The model suggests that the relative importance of the domains changes over the life cycle or suicidal career, and that they interact with one another.
• Blumenthal and Kupfer's (1990) concepts of "predisposing," "predictor" or "risk," "protective," and "trigger" or "precipitating" factors in suicide.
• Litman's (1990) notion of a "suicide zone." As noted earlier, for every 100 people who enter an acute suicidal crisis implied by the "suicide zone," only 1 or 2 ever commit suicide.
• Feedback loops. For example, those in the suicide zone who do not commit suicide can cycle back to increased vulnerabilities for eventual suicide or can acquire more protective factors. They can also exit by way of accidental, homicidal, or natural death. There are additional factors that presumably determine nonsuicidal outcomes.
• The salient predictors of suicide (such as those listed in Table 1.1 in Chapter 1, and described throughout the entire book), which are distributed across various stages of suicidal careers (there are many diverse suicidal careers). Some risk factors appear at more than one stage of the suicidal life cycle (e.g., depressive disorders).
• Motto's (Chapter 31) concept of a personal threshold of pain tolerance beyond which suicide is likely, even necessary.
• Stages of suicidal careers in relation to primary, secondary, and tertiary intervention and suicide prevention.

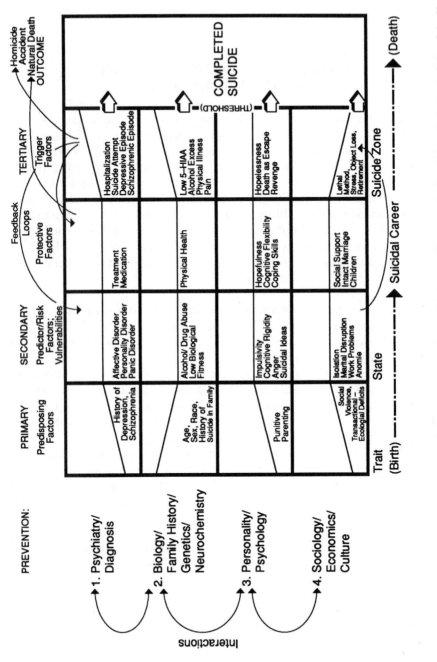

FIGURE 32.3. A general model of suicidal behaviors. Not all possible interactions are depicted here. Relative height of the line within each domain indicates approximate importance of those factors at the different stages of the suicidal career.

Without hoping to be able to anticipate all the questions raised by our model of suicide, we conclude with a few general comments. First, any suicidal outcome is a complex, multidomain, interactive effect of many biopsychosocial factors over fairly long times (usually 40–60 years). Second, most individuals who "fit" the model will not complete suicide. That is, our model is not sufficiently specified; it is a general model. Individual suicide prediction requires specification of suicidal types with their distinctive etiologies. Even then, prediction of individual suicides will have high rates of error. Third, most individuals in the "suicide zone" get treatment (medication, support, etc.), which protects them from a suicidal outcome; in other words, they tend to die natural deaths. Fourth, most completed suicides cycle through the suicide zone to protective factors and/or further risk factors and suicidal vulnerabilities many times before they complete suicide. Finally, triggering or precipitating factors of suicide may be a gradual, nondramatic accumulation of many interactive risk factors, not a dramatic, intense, single negative life event or stressor (here we disagree with Blumenthal & Kupfer's model).

We are now at the end of a long and ambitious scientific undertaking. Every monograph is an approach as much as an arrival. We have only been able to point to broad directions for suicide assessment and prediction. As usual, much remains to be done. Our hope is that at least some of our readers will be stimulated to carry on the work—to describe, with greater refinement and detail, the processes leading to suicide. Of course, we all have to die sooner or later, but not prematurely, in a manner that usually diminishes the ideal of the good life and devastates those who love us.

REFERENCES

Allison, P. D. (1984). *Event history analysis.* Beverly Hills, CA: Sage.

American Psychiatric Association. (1987). *Diagnostic and statistical manual of mental disorders* (3rd ed., rev.). Washington, DC: Author.

American Psychiatric Association. (1990). *Benzodiazepine dependence, toxicity, and abuse.* Washington, DC: Author.

Beck, A. T., Resnik, H. L. P., & Lettieri, D. J. (Eds.). (1974). *The prediction of suicide.* Bowie, MD: Charles Press.

Beck, A. T., Steer, R. A., Kovacs, M., & Garrison, B. (1985). Hopelessness and eventual suicide: A 10-year prospective study of patients hospitalized with suicidal ideation. *American Journal of Psychiatry, 142*(5), 559–563.

Beck, A. T., Ward, C. H., Mendelson, M., Mock, J., & Erbaugh, J. (1961). An inventory for measuring depression. *Archives of General Psychiatry, 142,* 559–563.

Beck, A. T., Weissman, A., Lester, D., & Trexler, L. (1974). The measurement of pessimism: The Hopelessness Scale. *Journal of Consulting and Clinical Psychology, 42,* 861–865.

Berman, A. L., & Cohen-Sandler, R. (1983). Suicide and malpractice: Expert testimony and the "standard of care." *Professional Psychology: Research and Practice, 14,* 6-19.

Berman, A. L., & Jobes, D. A. (1991). *Adolescent suicide: Assessment and intervention.* Washington, DC: American Psychological Association.

Blumenthal, S. J., & Kupfer, D. J. (Eds.). (1990). *Suicide over the life cycle: Risk factors, assessment, and treatment of suicidal patients.* Washington, DC: American Psychiatric Association.

Bongar, B. (1991). *The suicidal patient: Clinical and legal standards of care.* Washington, DC: American Psychological Association.

Brent, D. A., Perper, J. A., Kolko, D. J., & Zelenak, J. P. (1988). The psychological autopsy: Methodological considerations for the study of adolescent suicide. *Journal of the American Academy of Child and Adolescent Psychiatry, 27*(3), 362-366.

Cooper, G. L. (1988). The safety of fluoxetine: An update. *British Journal of Psychiatry, 153,* 77-86.

Cowley, G., Springen, K., Leonard, E. A., Robins, K., & Gordon, J. (1990, March 26). The promise of Prozac. *Newsweek,* pp. 39-41.

Cull, J. G., & Gill, W. S. (1982). *Suicide Probability Scale (SPS).* Los Angeles: Western Psychological Services.

Drake, R. E., Gates, C., Whitaker, A., & Cotton, P. G. (1985). Suicide among schizophrenics: A review. *Comprehensive Psychiatry, 26,* 90-100.

Garrison, C. Z., Lewinsohn, P. M., Marsteller, F., Laughinrichen, J., & Lann, I. (1991). The assessment of suicidal behavior in children. *Suicide and Life-Threatening Behavior, 21*(3), 217-230.

Graham, J. R. (1990). *Minnesota Multiphasic Personality Inventory-2.* New York: Oxford University Press.

Graves, P. L., & Thomas, C. B. (1991). Habits of nervous tension and suicide. *Suicide and Life-Threatening Behavior, 21,* 91-105.

Hamilton, M. (1960). A rating scale for depression. *Journal of Neurology, Neurosurgery and Psychiatry, 23,* 56-62.

Hathaway, S. R., & McKinley, J. C. (1967). *Minnesota Multiphasic Personality Inventory.* New York: Psychological Corporation. (Original work published 1943)

Holmes, T. H., & Rahe, R. H. (1967). The social readjustment rating scale. *Journal of Psychosomatic Research, 11,* 213-218.

Kovacs, M., Beck, A. T., & Weissman, A. (1975). Hopelessness: An indicator of suicide risk. *Suicide and Life-Threatening Behavior, 5,* 98-103.

Lasagna, L. (1980, April). The Halcion story: Trial by media. *Lancet,* 815-816.

Latimer, I. (1980, February–March). Trials and tribulations of triazolam. *Journal of Clinical Pharmacology,* 159-161.

Leenaars, A. A. (Ed.). (1991). *Life-span perspectives of suicide.* New York: Plenum Press.

Lettieri, D. J. (1974). Suicide death prediction scales. In A. T. Beck, H. L. P. Resnik, & D. J. Lettieri (Eds.), *The prediction of suicide* (pp. 163-192). Bowie, MD: Charles Press.

Litman, R. E. (1990). Suicides: What do they have in mind? In D. Jacobs & H. N.

Brown (Eds.), *Suicide: Understanding and responding* (pp. 143–156). Madison, CT: International Universities Press.

Mann, J. J., & Stanley, M. (1988). Suicide. In A. J. Frances & E. Hales (Eds.), *Review of psychiatry*, Vol. 7 (pp. 287–430). Washington, DC: American Psychiatric Press.

Maris, R. W. (1981). *Pathways to suicide: A survey of self-destructive behaviors.* Baltimore: Johns Hopkins University Press.

Maris, R. W. (Ed.). (1986). *Biology of suicide.* New York: Guilford Press.

Maris, R. W. (1991a). The developmental perspective of suicide. In A. A. Leenaars (Ed.), *Life span perspectives of suicide* (pp. 25–38). New York: Plenum Press.

Maris, R. W. (1991b). Suicide. In R. Dulbeco (Ed.), *Encyclopedia of human biology* (Vol. 7, pp. 327–335). San Diego: Academic Press.

Marsella, A. J., Hirschfeld, R. M. A., & Katz, M. M. (Eds.). (1987). *The measurement of depression.* New York: Guilford Press.

Motto, J., Heilbron, D., & Juster, R. (1985). Suicide risk assessment: Development of a clinical instrument. *American Journal of Psychiatry, 142,* 680–686.

Murphy, G. E. (1974). The clinical identification of suicidal risk. In A. T. Beck, H. L. P. Resnik, & D. J. Lettieri (Eds.), *The prediction of suicide* (pp. 109–118). Bowie, MD: Charles Press.

Murray, H. A. (1943). *Thematic Apperception Test.* Cambridge, MA: Harvard University Press.

Plutchik, R., van Praag, H. M., Conte, H. R., & Picard, S. (1989). Correlates of suicide and violence risk: 1. The Suicide Risk Measure. *Comprehensive Psychiatry, 30,* 296–302.

Robins, L. N., Helzer, J. E., Croughan, J., & Ratcliff, K. S. (1981). National Institute of Mental Health Diagnostic Interview Schedule: Its history, characteristics, and validity. *Archives of General Psychiatry, 38,* 381–389.

Rorschach, H. (1981). *Psychodiagnostics: A diagnostic test based on perception.* New York: Grune & Stratton. (Original work published 1942)

Schlesselman, J. J. (1982). *Case–control studies: Design, conduct, and analysis.* New York: Oxford University Press.

Spitzer, R. L., & Endicott, J. (1979). *Schedule for Affective Disorders and Schizophrenia—Lifetime version* (SADS-L). New York: New York Psychiatric Institute.

Spitzer, R. L., Williams, J. B. W., Gibbon, M., & First, M. B. (1990). *Structured Clinical Interview for DSM-III-R* (*SCID*). Washington, DC: American Psychiatric Press.

Tanney, B. L. (1986). Electroconvulsive therapy and suicide. In R. W. Maris (Ed.), *Biology of suicide* (pp. 116–140). New York: Guilford Press.

Teicher, M. H., Glod, C., & Cole, J. O. (1990). Emergence of intense suicidal preoccupation during fluoxetine treatment. *American Journal of Psychiatry, 147*(2), 207–210.

Tuckman, J., & Youngman, W. F. (1968). Assessment of suicidal risk in attempted suicides. In H. L. P. Resnik (Ed.), *Suicidal behaviors: Diagnosis and management* (pp. 190–197). Boston: Little, Brown.

van Praag, H. M., Plutchik, R., & Apter, A. (Eds.). (1990). *Violence and suicidality.* New York: Brunner/Mazel.

Wu, L. L., & Tuma, N. B. (1990). Local hazard models. In C. C. Clogg (Ed.), *Sociological methodology 1990* (Vol. 20, pp. 141–180). Ann Arbor, MI: Blackwell.

Zung, W. W. K. (1974). Index of Potential Suicide (IPS): A rating scale for suicide prevention. In A. T. Beck, H. L. P. Resnik, & D. J. Lettieri (Eds.), *The prediction of suicide* (pp. 221–249). Bowie, MD: Charles Press.

Chapter Synopses

Chapter 2. Maltsberger: *The Psychodynamic Formulation: An Aid in Assessing Suicide Risk*

Suicide prediction is difficult, since there are many types of suicide, but practically (clinically) there are not all that many. Suicide predictors usually concern groups, not individuals. Clinicians need to assess individual suicide potential over relatively short times. Suicide assessment includes a personal history, exterior factors, and mental status. Information bearing on suicide risk needs to be integrated via inductive clinical reasoning. A psychodynamic character strength formulation is needed.

Chapter 3. Shneidman: *A Conspectus of the Suicidal Scenario*

Shneidman considers three cases of attempted suicide: an immolator, a jumper, and a shooter. Commonalities of suicide include psychological pain, frustrated needs, self-denigration, mental constriction, isolation, hopelessness, and egression. These commonalities can be combined into a cubic model of three interacting variables: pain, perturbation, and press. The chapter concludes with a consideration of the 13 sectors of the suicidal "pie."

Chapter 4. Maris: *How Are Suicides Different?*

Since suicide is a complex dependent variable, we must specify the type of suicide to have any hope of accurate assessment or prediction. The suicide typologies of Durkheim, Freud, Baechler, and Shneidman are reviewed. Not only do completed suicides vary, but so do other self-destructive behaviors: nonfatal suicide attempts, indirect self-destructive behavior, suicide ideation, and other modes of death. Finally, a multiaxial classification of suicidal behavior and ideas is offered.

Chapter 5. Mayo: *What Is Being Predicted?: The Definition of "Suicide"*

To commit "suicide" is to end one's life intentionally. The definition of a suicide seems straightforward, but it is in fact complex. Some definitions are vague because the term being defined (*definiendum*) is vague; others are vague because the term is a matter of degree. "Intentionality" is vague in part because it is a matter of degree. Intentionality is an important component of suicide. The definition of suicide need not have a normative component. The proposed definition of suicide has four elements: fatality, reflexivity, activity–passivity, and intentionality.

Chapter 6. Pokorny: *Prediction of Suicide in Psychiatric Patients: Report of a Prospective Study*

This prospective research study attempted to identify persons who would subsequently commit or attempt suicide. The sample consisted of 4,800 patients who were consecutively admitted to the inpatient psychiatric service of a Veterans Administration hospital. They were examined and rated on a wide range of instruments and measures, including most of those previously reported as predictive of suicide. Many items were found to have positive and substantial correlations with subsequent suicides and/or suicide attempts. However, all attempts to identify specific subjects were unsuccessful, including use of individual items, factor scores, and a series of discriminant functions. Each trial missed many cases and identified far too many false-positive cases to be workable. Identification of particular persons who will commit suicide is currently not feasible, because of the low sensitivity and specificity of available identification procedures and the low base rate of this behavior.

Chapter 7. Gould, Shaffer, Fisher, Kleinman, and Morishima: *The Clinical Prediction of Adolescent Suicide*

Suicide is a major public health problem among adolescents. To predict suicide risk, it is necessary to focus on very specific factors in various high-risk groups. One strategy to identify suicide risk is using high-risk follow-up studies. Groups studied include prior suicide attempters, persons with mental illness, individuals with complicated birth histories, and individuals with certain biological markers. Another strategy is to use retrospective case study methods or "psychological autopsies." One such study is the New York psychological autopsy, which compared 120 consecutive suicides under age 20 with matched normal controls on affective disorders, substance abuse, antisocial behavior, prior suicide attempts, and a family history of suicide. Odds ratios and risk factors were calculated. For boys, the greatest risk was prior suicide attempts (250 per 100,000). For girls, affective disorder was the greatest risk factor (34 per 100,000). The high false-positive rate (low specificity) makes clinical prediction difficult. No multivariate analyses have been done yet.

Chapter 8. Clark and Horton-Deutsch: *Assessment in Absentia: The Value of the Psychological Autopsy Method for Studying Antecedents of Suicide and Predicting Future Suicides*

The psychological autopsy is a procedure for reconstructing an individual's life in order to clarify circumstances contributing to a (usually) non-natural death. Several community-based psychological autopsy studies are reviewed (e.g., Robins, 1981). Also reviewed are applications to suicides among youth and the elderly. One of the early uses of psychological autopsy was to help resolve equivocal deaths for the Los Angeles medical examiner. Without psychological autopsies, the official statistics are likely to be less accurate. There have also been psychological autopsies of psychiatric inpatients and jail suicides, although a suicide postmortem conference is in many ways different from a psychological autopsy. The psychological autopsy is also used to clarify various forensic issues. Various methodological issues are reviewed (e.g., standardized protocols, initial contacts, the time lapse since death, the ethics of interviews, etc.). The chapter concludes with recommendations of standards for psychological autopsies.

Chapter 9. Eyman and Eyman: *Personality Assessment in Suicide Prediction*

Four major approaches to personality assessment to the end of suicide prediction are: (1) the Rorschach (single indication and constellation), (2) the Thematic Apperception Test (TAT), (3) the Minnesota Multiphasic Personality Inventory (MMPI), and (4) a psychological test battery. The transparency and color-shading responses to the Rorschach have not proven clinically useful. However, some constellation approaches (e.g., Hertz, 1949, and Martin, 1960) are promising. None of the TAT or MMPI studies have been useful in suicide prediction, although the MMPI-2 (Hathaway et al., 1989) may be better. Most promising is a psychological test battery approach. For example, Smith and Eyman (1988) found four factors that discriminated male psychiatric patients who made serious suicide attempts: (1) overcontrol of aggressive ideation; (2) high self-expectations; (3) conflicted dependency yearnings; and (4) anxious, serious, ambivalent attitudes toward death. The case of Heather B (see Chapter 12) is analyzed using Smith and Eyman's variables. The authors conclude that she had incomplete mourning for her father, but not a serious wish to die.

Chapter 10. Rothberg and Geer-Williams: *A Comparison and Review of Suicide Prediction Scales*

After considering some issues in suicide risk prediction and summarizing previous reviews, the authors describe 19 suicide prediction scales, with special attention to cogency, reliability, validity, sensitivity, and specificity. For 6 of these scales, the subject is the respondent (either in person or through an interviewer), and for the other 13 another party is the respondent. A useful list of the strengths and weaknesses of the various suicide prediction scales is provided. Finally, 9 of the 13 second-party scales are applied to the five clinical cases discussed throughout this book. It may be worth noting that the most accurate predictions of the outcomes of our five cases by Motto, Heilbron, and Juster's (1985) Clinical Instrument to Estimate Suicide Risk and Lettieri's (1974) Suicidal Death Prediction Scale, short form. Since there is considerable variation in how the nine scales predict suicide risk for our five cases, it seems apparent that considerable work remains to be done on suicide risk prediction scales.

Chapter 11. Addy: *Statistical Concepts of Prediction*

In many situations, the ability to predict a particular response such as suicide is desirable. Statistical methodology enables the researcher to predict the probability that a response will occur, and this probability can then be interpreted by the clinician for a specific individual. Another approach to this prediction is to predict a continuous variable, such as a measure of suicide ideation. The methodology for both of these approaches is discussed. The general linear model is presented for the latter approach. Prediction of a specific response can be attempted by the logistic regression model, the probit model, discriminant analysis, or a log-linear model. All of these methods are probably better suited to identifying groups at higher risk for suicide than to identifying specific suicidal individuals.

Chapter 12. Berman: *Five Potential Suicide Cases*

Statistical profiles tend to describe average or modal suicidal types, and thus are of limited use in assessing or predicting the suicide of any given individual. Since only a unique individual commits suicide (or not), suicidology needs to focus on the case method. Accordingly, five detailed cases are presented for study. On the basis of the information presented about these cases, other chapter authors and readers are asked to assess each cases' suicide risks (in both the short and the long term), as well as to predict which, if any, of the cases actually attempted or completed suicide. The cases include (1) Heather B (a 13-year-old white female), (2) Ralph F (a 16-year-old white male), (3) John Z (a 39-year-old white married male), (4) Faye C (a 49-year-old unmarried white female), and (5) José G (a 64-year-old married Hispanic male). Although these five cases and the information provided are not comprehensive of all suicide types, they do cover age and sex variations reasonably well.

Chapter 13. Stelmachers and Sherman: *The Case Vignette Method of Suicide Assessment*

Since suicide prediction scales have limited clinical utility in assessing suicide risk for individuals, the case vignette method was developed. In one study there was considerable variation in assessing cases on a 7-point risk scale, although the strongest consensus occurred in assessing short-term high suicide risk. A second study tested whether or not anchoring case vignettes on a continuum from low to high suicide risk would increase rater agreement; it did. The factors in low- versus high-risk vignettes are presented and discussed. The crisis management procedure and proposed clinical disposition were also studied. In general, there was low reliability of selection of crisis management procedures and clinical dispositions. After reviewing the five common cases, the authors proposed that "chaos theory" be applied to suicide assessment. Although somewhat deterministic, chaos theory suggests that precise prediction of suicide risk cannot be achieved.

Chapter 14. Tanney: *Mental Disorders: Psychiatric Patients, and Suicide*

Mentally disordered persons are about five times more likely to engage in suicidal behaviors than the general population. Although the data are often inconclusive, and "box score" reporting of results is necessary, suicides are found to be most common among those with affective disorders and schizophrenia (with the rate of suicide generally higher for the former disorder). Completed suicide is more likely for those with psychotic disorders and unipolar affective disorders. Nonfatal suicide attempts are more common among those with personality disorders. The risk of suicide generally goes up when there is comorbidity or co-occurrence of mental disorders. Diagnoses of major depressive disorder and borderline personality disorder confound suicide risk assessment, since suicide is also one of the criteria for these diagnoses. Using mental status and psychiatric diagnoses, the author concludes that Heather had low suicide risk, that Ralph and John had high suicide risk, that José had high suicide risk (unless he had an organic syndrome), and that Faye's risk varied depending upon her principal diagnosis.

Chapter 15. Lester: *Alcoholism and Drug Abuse*

Substance abuse, especially alcoholism, is strongly related to both suicide and nonfatal suicide attempts. The relationship between nonalcoholic drug abuse and completed suicide is sparsely researched, and the existing research has produced equivocal results. One review of several studies found that about 18% of all alcoholics eventually commit suicide. Substance abuse in self-destructive populations is just one causal factor among many, and the interrelationships among the predictor variables at present are poorly understood. One good model for the kind of research that needs to be done is Motto (1980). To be useful, substance abuse predictive models for self-destructive need to be population-specific (e.g., young females, older males, etc.). Also, the relationship among alcoholism, drug abuse, and affective disorders in suicides needs to be teased out. Many of the biochemical predictors of suicide in alcoholics involve the serotonergic system. The author sees Ralph as being at high risk for suicide and José as possibly being at high risk, if he were to use alcohol and medications together. Much work remains to be done on the relationship of substance abuse to self-destruction.

Chapter 16. Leenaars: *Suicide Notes, Communication, and Ideation*

Suicide notes can be seen as "windows to the mind" or to the intent of suicidal individuals. Yet what was in a suicide's mind and what was communicated in a suicide note may be very different. Another problem is that only 12–15% of suicide completers leave notes. At least in some respects, the 85–88% of suicides who do not leave suicide notes may be very different from those who do leave notes. Although research is unclear on the differences between those who do and do not leave notes, at least age and sex differences may be suspected. The study of suicide notes needs to be systematic and scientific, not anecdotal. Theories need to be translated into protocol sentences that independent judges have determined to be characteristic of actual, genuine suicide notes versus simulated notes. One such empirical test is Leenaars's Thematic Guide for Suicide Prediction (TGSP; Leenaars, 1988d). The TGSP posits eight groups of statements regularly occurring in genuine suicide notes: unbearable psychological pain, interpersonal relations, rejection–aggression, inability to adjust, indirect expressions, identification–egression, ego, and cognitive constriction. The TGSP is applied in full to the case of Heather B and incompletely to the other four common cases. Suicide notes and other communications constitute an invaluable starting point for suicide prediction, but they are only one indicator of suicide.

Chapter 17. Maris: *The Relation of Nonfatal Suicide Attempts to Completed Suicide*

It is obvious that one must first make a suicide attempt in order to complete suicide. Prior nonfatal suicide attempts are powerful single predictors of eventual suicide. Nevertheless, only 10–15% of nonfatal suicide attempters go on to commit suicide. There are single nonfatal suicide attempts, multiple nonfatal attempts, multiple nonfatal attempts ending in completed suicide, and a single fatal suicide attempt (i.e., completion). Conventional wisdom suggests that multiple suicide attempts precede suicide completion, but in fact (especially for older males), a single fatal suicide attempt is the most common type of completion. The etiology of fatal suicide attempts is complex and multifaceted. Fatal suicide attempts are more common among older males who use guns, die instantly, and are socially isolated. Perceived causes of completed suicides are reviewed (with hopelessness, depression and anger being prominent). Immediate ("trigger") and long-term causes of suicide are not very different. Prior suicide attempters have an average completion rate of about 1% a year. Suicide is particularly likely in the first year or two after an initial nonfatal attempt. Suicide attempt data are applied to the five common cases, with the prediction order for suicide from high to low risk being as follows: José, Ralph, John, Faye, and Heather.

Chapter 18. McIntosh: *Methods of Suicide*

"Lethality" is the probability or likelihood (usually short-term) of suicidal death. Gunshot or firearm methods are the most lethal methods of suicide, although many other factors affect lethality (age, rescuability, isolation, availability of medical intervention, etc.). Typically, men choose firearms first and hanging a distant second as suicide methods. Women now choose firearms first too, but are nearly as likely to utilize poisons. Women also display a greater variety of methods of suicide than men do. Factors affecting method choice include gender socialization, availability, familiarities, certainty of outcome, ambivalent motivation, degree of disfigurement, culture, geographic region, age, race, and ethnicity. Self-poisoning and cutting are the most common nonfatal attempt methods. Asian-Americans are more likely than other ethnic groups to utilize hanging to complete suicide. Deaths by poisons have generally declined, in part because of better medical technology and in part because of the greater utilization of more lethal methods, such as guns. Carbon monoxide deaths are now less likely because of better gas emission controls on vehicles. Gun control legislation is today more necessary than ever to prevent suicide.

Chapter 19. Bonner: *Isolation, Seclusion, and Psychosocial Vulnerability as Risk Factors for Suicide Behind Bars*

Suicide is the leading cause of death behind bars. In jails and lockups, most suicides are white, young, and male. They tend to be unmarried and to be arrested on alcohol or drug charges. Their suicides tend to occur between 9 P.M. and 6 A.M., by hanging in the first 24 hours of incarceration, and in isolation. Prison suicides, on the other hand, tend to be older males, to include more blacks and Hispanics, and to be individuals serving longer sentences for major offenses. Their suicides tend to occur after about 5 years of incarceration and concurrently with institutional problems. Prison suicides also tend to have a history of psychiatric illness and prior suicidal behavior. The best explanatory model for jail and prison suicides in a biopsychosocial process model, which suggests which inmates will be vulnerable to incarceration stress. Suicide behind bars is the product of vulnerable individuals' experiencing chronic isolation, emotional pain, depression, stress, and hopelessness. Usually suicidal inmates should not be placed in isolation, and at a minimum, they should be screened for suicide potential before being secluded. Other suicide-preventing standards are also reviewed.

Chapter 20. Felner, Silverman and Adan: *Risk Assessment and Prevention of Youth Suicide in Educational Contexts*

Youth suicide epidemics cannot be reduced simply by treating afflicted individuals. There are several problems with traditional clinical youth suicide prevention strategies: Youths tend not to use them, resources are scarce, youths are already severely damaged, and the strategies are reactive. There are four orienting questions for school suicide prevention: (1) What do we mean by the concept of "prevention' when applied to youth suicide? (2) Whom does the program target? (3) What are the goals of suicide prevention programs? (4) What and where is the focus of intervention? (Felner & Felner, 1988). Primary prevention is preferred; the target is populations (not individuals); goals are either broad or specific conditions; and focus should be on changing processes that lead to suicide. The diathesis–stress model reminds us that early vulnerabilities are important. Transactional–ecological models suggests that we need to modify developmentally hazardous processes that affect whole populations. School-based suicide prevention efforts have five steps: to articulate vulnerabilities; to assess predisposing and precipitating processes; to reduce unwanted outcomes via prevention programs; to see how prevention programs reduce population vulnerabilities; and to see how youth suicide attempts and completions are reduced. Albee's (1982) modified probability model of psychopathology indicates that psychopathology develops when:

$$\frac{\text{Stress}}{\text{Social resources} \times \text{social competence} \times \text{resources}}$$

The area of suicide prevention needs naturalistic experiments to show that nothing happened that otherwise would have happened.

Chapter 21. Litman: *Predicting and Preventing Hospital and Clinic Suicides*

Proper diagnosis and treatment of psychiatric patients can alter the risk of suicide. Suicide risk assessment is not very useful to the clinician, because it focuses on long-term group risks, not on short-term individual risks. Assessment involves consideration of stress, support, vulnerability, and suicidality. The single most sensitive indicator of suicide potential is hopelessness. In emergency consultations, as in the case of José, it is very important to probe for suicidality. The decision to hospitalize can both decrease and increase suicide risk. Hospitalization has little impact on chronic suicide risk. Initial assessment (in the first 3 days) should include a provisional diagnosis, treatment plan, and doctor's orders. Assessment should involve a concerted effort by the patient's entire treatment team. Ralph's suicide risk is judged to be both high and chronic. It is important to assess whether inpatients should be on special suicide observations, and if so, on what level of observation. Often the presence of other people is the most powerful antisuicide measure. All clinics should be evaluated for suicide prevention security. The risk of suicide is increased at the time of discharge, and thus discharge should be planned carefully. The risk of suicide continues after discharge. Attention should be paid to chronically suicidal patients (especially alcoholics, the chronically depressed, schizophrenics, and borderline patients). A team treatment approach, monitoring transference, and complete record keeping all help in postdischarge suicide risk assessment.

Chapter 22. Weishaar and Beck: *Clinical and Cognitive Predictors of Suicide*

In order to predict suicide, we must assess suicide intent, medical lethality, and method of suicide. Relevant assessment scales include the Beck Depression Inventory, the Scale for Suicide Ideation, the Suicide Intent Scale, and the Beck Hopelessness Scale. Clinical and proximate risk factors (e.g., psychiatric disorder, history of suicide attempts, alcohol abuse, etc.) are more important in suicide prediction than are demographic characteristics. Hopelessness has been found to be more strongly related to suicide intent than depression is. Hopelessness is a potentially recurring state of negative expectancies. Negative expectations related to the development of a suicidal mindset include dysfunctional assumptions, dichotomous thinking, problem-solving deficits, and a view of suicide as a desirable solution to life problems. The five common cases are analyzed in terms of cognitive predictors. Cognitive characteristics that predispose an individual to suicide ideation and behavior tend to persist between suicidal episodes.

Chapter 23. Garrison: *Demographic Predictors of Suicide*

In 1987 suicide was the eighth leading cause of death, accounting for 1.5% of all deaths that year, or 30,796 individual suicides (a rate of 12.7 per 100,000). Probably suicides are undercounted at a rate of about 10%. Male suicide rates exceed those of females by a factor of 4 or 5, and white rates are about twice those of blacks. White males comprise about 72% of all U.S. suicides. Suicide rates for

Hispanics seem to be lower than those of whites. Suicide rates have increased over time and have consistently been higher among those over age 45. There was an especially large increase in suicide rates among white males aged 15–24 from 1957 to 1977. Age- and sex-specific rates need to be controlled for other important factors, such as marital status. High levels of unemployment have also been related to high suicide rates. Both men and women now use firearms as their suicide method of choice (in 57% of suicides). Generally, the higher the level of blood alcohol, the more likely one is to use firearms to suicide. The highest suicide rates tend to be found in the Mountain and Pacific regions of the United States. Even when considered together, demographic predictors provide little information about a particular individual's suicide potential; however, demographic profiles can identify groups at high suicide risk.

Chapter 24. Phillips, Lesyna, and Paight: *Suicide and the Media*

Publicized suicide stories tend to function as "natural advertisements" for suicide. Literature on imitation of publicized suicides is reviewed in two categories: nonfictional and fictional suicide stories. In the category of nonfictional stories, newspaper and television stories are reviewed. In reviewing stories on page 1 of the *New York Times,* Phillips found that suicides rose significantly just after these stories, probably because of imitation or suggestion. Stack and Wasserman expanded the early Phillips studies. European studies have produced equivocal results; Dutch studies suggest that imitation is more likely when suicide is explicitly conveyed in the headline. Looking at television, Bollen and Phillips found a similar modeling effect for suicide coverage. NBC and Nielsen rating studies found fewer effects, but failed to consider multiprogram stories and repetition of stories. Suggestion seemed to operate in a study of Viennese subway suicides. Fictional stories have included soap opera suicides, television movies dealing with suicide, and a German train suicide story; the studies of all of these have produced equivocal results. The general conclusions are that the more publicity, the greater the increase; that effects are geographic; that effects are largest for teens; and that fictional copying is weaker than nonfictional. Imitation is stronger if (1) the message is clear and focused, (2) the message is repeated, (3) it is on the front page, and (4) the copier can identify with the messenger. The chapter closes with recommendations for future research and data collection.

Chapter 25. Wasserman: *Economy, Work, Occupation, and Suicide*

Durkheim (1897/1951) related suicide to changes in "anomie" or social disruption, such as changes in the occupational division of labor or rapid market changes (e.g., the Great Depression in the United States in the 1930s). Most studies have related unemployment to increased suicide rates. Group suicide rate data are subject to the ecological fallacy when applied to individual suicides. Findings on occupational status and suicide are inconsistent. Generally, suicide rates and occupational status are related inversely, but with significant within-status variation. The association between occupational status and suicide needs to be controlled for other factors, such as psychiatric morbidity, exogenous social conditions, work-specific stress, the opportunity structure for suicides, occupationally related alcohol consumption, and demographic factors (e.g., cohort size; see Easterlin, 1980). Two empirical studies (in the province of Quebec and the state of Washington) related to work, economy, occupation, and suicide are reviewed.

Chapter 26. Stack: *Marriage, Family, Religion, and Suicide*

Traditionally (e.g., Durkheim), marriage and families have tended to protect individuals against suicide. Among white males, suicide rates tend to be highest for the widowed, followed by (in order) the divorced, single, and married. This pattern tends to be true for white women as well. Of course, other factors are relevant too, such as the opportunity structure (including the ready availability of guns). The part played by marital status in suicide is mediated through status integration theory. That is, less frequently occupied statuses and those with more role conflict tend to have higher suicide rates. As female labor force participation and divorce rates have increased, suicide rates for women and divorcees have declined. Classical religion and suicide studies (e.g., Durkheim) found that Catholics tended to have lower suicide rates than Protestants; however, more recent normative changes among Catholics have lessened, or even reversed, Catholic and Protestant suicide rate differences. Recent studies by Pescosolido and Georgianna (1989) have shifted the focus to network ties, and other religion studies have examined the degree of religiosity rather than simple religious membership. The five cases are reviewed, as are suggested directions for future research. Marriage, family life, and religiosity are overlapping, related factors in suicide.

Chapter 27. Yufit and Bongar: *Suicide, Stress, and Coping with Life Cycle Events*

The prior abilities to deal with life change, stressful events, and loss are major factors in assessing vulnerability to suicide. Paykel, Rich and Bonner, Linehan, and others agree that stressful life events frequently precede suicide attempts and suicidal ideation. Coping versus vulnerability models are examined. Various explanatory proposals or propositions predicting suicide are hypothesized. First, psychological equilibrium is a function of adequate coping skills, predominating over vulnerability to stress. Erikson's and Shneidman's developmental models are reviewed. Second, negative time equilibrium is a function of fear of the future plus nostalgia for the past. Suicidal individuals tend to lack a sense of connectedness or belonging. Also, having a perceived future assists coping with present stress. Third, positive time equilibrium is a function of planned future time orientation and acceptance and integration of past time events (including concepts of resiliency and buoyancy). Fourth, maintaining a vital balance is a function of resilient and buoyant coping abilities' predominating over vulnerability and loss of future time perspective. The vital balance in action is applied to the five common cases. A person learns through a series of successful coping behaviors over the life cycle.

Chapter 28. Roy: *Genetics, Biology, and Suicide in the Family*

Family history, genetics, and biology are part of the multidetermined act of suicide. Evidence for family history/genetic determinants of suicide comes from the following research: clinical studies, twin studies, the Iowa 500 study, a study of the Amish, and Copenhagen twin studies. From 5% to 15% of suicides have suicides among first-degree relatives. On average, 13% of twins are concordant for suicide; usually these are monozygotic twins. Of Amish suicides, 20–24% had a history of affective disorder among first-degree relatives, but there were also many families with much affective disorder and *no* suicides. Of 57 adoptees who committed suicide in Denmark, a statistically significant number had biological relatives who committed suicide, but almost none of the adoptee controls did. Biologically, suicide seems to be related to genetic traits resulting in impulsivity, violence, and antisocial personality traits—especially deficient central serotonin (5-HT) function through reduced presynaptic imipramine binding, reduced levels of 5-HT and 5-hydroxyindoleacetic acid (5-HIAA), and the unregulation of the postsynaptic 5-HT_2 receptors. Suicide prediction is very difficult, but *combinations* of prior suicide attempts and biological markers (e.g., low levels of 5-HIAA among discharged depressed patients) are helpful. In one study, about 20% of discharged patients with a prior suicide attempt and low 5-HIAA died by suicide within 1 year of discharge.

Chapter 29. Brown, Linnoila, and Goodwin: *Impulsivity, Aggression, and Associated Affects. Relationship to Self-Destructive Behavior and Suicide*

Suicidal behaviors, violence, and aggression have been found to be related to 5-HT levels in both humans and animals, but it is not clear whether this is a state or a trait. It is worth noting that cerebrospinal fluid (CSF) 5-HIAA decreases rapidly in early life, while suicide rates increase dramatically. The chapter reviews the five clinical cases with special attention to 5-HT levels, violence, impulsivity, and aggression. Axis II personality disorders that have aggression, impulsivity, and mood volatility as predominant features especially affect suicidal behaviors. Suicide is biological, as well as psychosocial. Several physical conditions increase suicide vulnerability, including parkinsonism; conditions associated with glucose metabolism (e.g., diabetes), corticosteroid metabolism

(Cushing's disease), or 5-HT metabolism (carcinoid syndrome or Lysch–Nyhan syndrome); and neurological disorders (e.g., epilepsy, Gilles de la Tourette syndrome). Some childhood diagnoses are related to lower levels of 5-HIAA and aggressive behaviors (e.g., disruptive behavior disorder). Studies of aggressive military men reveal higher frequency of suicide attempts, lower levels of 5-HIAA, and higher scores on family instability. Future biological research should study children, families, older age senescence.

Chapter 30. de Catanzaro: *Prediction of Self-Preservation Failures on the Basis of Quantitative Evolutionary Biology*

Self-preservation is so universal that it is often (wrongly) assumed to be an invariant orientation of behavior. Survival to reproductive maturity is essential for propagation of an individual's genes, but after this age there is a diminishing probability of gene expression. The "biological fitness" (Hamilton, 1964) of an individual is defined in terms of the number of progeny he or she produces. But genetic expression can evolve to be conducive to outright self-destructiveness. ψ_i represents the individual's residual capacity to promote inclusive fitness, such that $\psi_i = P_i + \Sigma \delta P_K r_K$, where P_i = expected reproduction of individual i, δP_k = the increment or decrement in expected reproduction of each kinship member k, and r_k = the coefficient of genetic relatedness. For nonsocial species, $\psi_i = P_i$. Negative ψ_i values are possible in highly social species. ψ_i is calculated for numerous different populations. Suicidal ideation tends to be explained by relations to the opposite sex, family, and society at large. Complex interactions of diverse predictors cannot be adequately incorporated into a simple multiple regression model. The ψ_i and p values for the five common cases are estimated and interpreted as to probable suicide outcomes.

Chapter 31. Motto: *An Integrated Approach to Estimating Suicide Risk*

Predicting suicide is made difficult by each individual's comparative uniqueness. Suicide results when an individual's threshold of pain tolerance is exceeded or is anticipated to be exceeded. Both the individual's pain level and tolerance threshold are in constant flux. Given this, we cannot "predict" individual suicides, but can only assess or estimate suicide risk probabilities—often over longer time frames than we would like. Suicide risk assessment can proceed clinically or empirically, although in practice these procedures overlap considerably. The final decision about estimating suicide risk is subjective or intuitive. Often suicide risk information is gathered without the therapist's even knowing it (e.g., through nonverbal clues). If there is conflict between objective and subjective criteria, the subjective criteria should decide the suicide risk. Risk assessment must usually be in the relative short run (e.g., this weekend, if the patient is not hospitalized, within 1 year, etc.). Strengths or protective risk factors also need to be assessed. Individuals can be chronically suicidal in the sense that their risk thresholds are easily broached. Statistical risk (e.g., $p = .05$) and clinical risk are often different. Often risk assessment paradigms are not for suicide, but actually for depression or the like. Therapists should assess suicide in their own "natural style." Various unique individual situations or factors often need to be given extra weight. We can only predict the risk of suicide, not suicide itself. Recognizing or predicting high suicide potential is not the same as predicting the *event* of suicide. Levels of suicide risk are in constant flux. The suicide risks of the five common cases are assessed. It would be nearly impossible to validate a perfect suicide prediction instrument, because we would be morally obliged to intervene in all predicted suicides. Accurate suicide risk assessment does not mean suicide prevention or safety. Of course, the ultimate goals of suicide risk assessment are better treatment and reduced suicide outcomes.

Index